Joe Weider's
ULTIMATE
BODYBUILDING

Joe Weider's ULTIMATE BODYBUILDING

The Master Blaster's Principles of Training and Nutrition

Joe Weider
with
Bill Reynolds

New York Chicago San Francisco Lisbon London Madrid Mexico City
Milan New Delhi San Juan Seoul Singapore Sydney Toronto

Library of Congress Cataloging-in-Publication Data

Weider, Joe.
      Joe Weider's ultimate bodybuilding.
          p.   cm.
      Includes bibliographical references.
      ISBN 0-8092-4715-1
      1. Bodybuilding.   I. Title.   II. Title: Ultimate bodybuilding.
    GV546.5.W445   1988   646.7'5   88-16229

28 29 30 31 32 33 34 35 36 37 38 39 40 41 42   CUS/CUS   0 9 8 7 6

ISBN-13: 978-0-8092-4715-8
ISBN-10:   0-8092-4715-1

Cover photograph by Michael Neveux

McGraw-Hill books are available at special quantity discounts to use as premiums and sales promotions, or for use in corporate training programs. For more information, please write to the Director of Special Sales, Professional Publishing, McGraw-Hill, Two Penn Plaza, New York, NY 10121-2298. Or contact your local bookstore.

All suggestions and recommendations in this book are made without warranty or guarantee, express or implied, and the author and publisher disclaim all liability in connection with the use of this information. The material presented herein is not a substitute for the advice of a personal health-care professional. Always consult a physician before taking or administering any drug, including steroids, or undertaking any exercise program.

This book is printed on acid-free paper.

Contents

Joe Weider's
ULTIMATE
BODYBUILDING

Preface
The Weider System—
Development of
My Training Philosophy

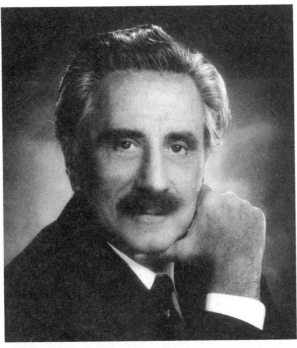

Joe Weider at 70 years of age displays the outward youth of a man 20 years younger, clear testimony for the benefits of a lifetime of systematic bodybuilding training. Joe has been personally training top bodybuilders, sports figures, and entertainment industry persons since 1936.

This massive and authoritative Master Blaster book is the greatest bodybuilding book ever written primarily because it is firmly based on the training principles of the Weider System of Bodybuilding, which has been followed by literally *every* bodybuilder in the modern history of the sport. I began developing my Weider System back in the 1930s and continue to refine and add new Weider Training Principles to it.

I am confident that I will continue to improve the Weider System right into the 21st century, because I am actually more motivated to serve the sport of bodybuilding right now than I ever have been. That's why you can rely on the information I present in this book to improve your physique.

I am often asked how I developed the Weider System of Bodybuilding. To understand *how* I developed the system, you must first understand *why* I developed it.

From the late 1880s, when bodybuilding arrived in America, through the late 1930s, it was a stiff and measured discipline. Bodybuilding took its cue from the organized, systematic Germans and the ultraconservative English when it entered America through the conformist Alan Calvert, the first man to sell adjustable barbells and dumbbells in North America. Eventually, bodybuilding landed with the reactionary York Barbell Company organization.

The distillate weight workout at that time consisted of three training sessions per week, no more and no less, each workout consisting of 9–12 basic exercises, and only one set of 8–10 reps was to be done of each exercise. Instructions were to increase one rep weekly until 12–15 were accomplished, at which time three to five pounds were added to the bar and the process repeated, starting with 8–10 reps for each set. This ironclad regimen occurred every Monday, Wednesday, and Friday. To deviate on only one day might have negated its blessing.

This inflexible training system *did* have its good points:

- Basic exercises worked all the muscles of the body.
- The progressive resistance principle was observed.
- Time for recuperation between workouts was allowed.
- It helped organize a bodybuilder's training habits.

Well and good, but what it didn't do was take into consideration those intrinsic qualities of individual strength, recuperative ability, body type, and genetic endowment. It froze a bodybuilder in a beginner's program. He remained a perpetual sophomore with no further curriculum. He became a victim of the adaptation response and the law of diminishing returns. His efforts eventually became less intense as progress appeared hopeless. Then the bodybuilder strayed, baffled by the realization that simple labor alone did not suffice or that it was not rewarded.

There were mavericks, however—guys like John C. Grimek, Barton Horvath, and some others—strength-oriented musclemen who went into weightlifting or powerlifting. The heavy weights generated a further muscle-building response that had eluded most of the fraternity of bodybuilders. It happened to be a step in the right direction, but no one seemed able to corral that runaway power and tame it in a way to build muscular detail.

Having been a competitive weightlifter myself, I pondered this classic problem. I had set some Canadian provincial lifting records and also had become a strong amateur wrestler. While still in my teens, I began to question the efficacy of the existing training methods. It was not unusual at that time to see a genetically gifted man do in two months of training what it took another man of lesser potential two years to do. With today's state of the art, that would never happen. Now in two years the average guy can almost become a superman.

I was a rebel when I was young, but I was also imbued with a deep sense of responsibility. When I was 11 years old, I had to leave primary school to help keep my family together financially during the Great Depression of the 1930s. Out of necessity I became intuitive and imaginative, so when I eventually landed in bodybuilding I instinctively peered around corners. I was incapable of accepting anything at face value. The only way I could accept it was to have it proven to me.

I began to examine the old training methods and realized that they didn't work. The system said to work out Monday, Wednesday, and Friday. But there were times when maybe I didn't feel like working out on a Monday, too beat

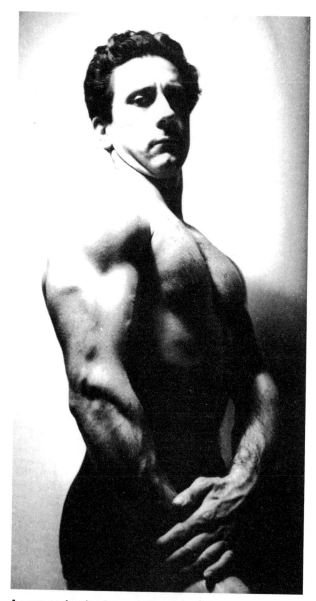

A very early physique photo of Joe Weider, from about 1940, at a time when the technology of the sport, which today includes tissue-building drug usage, scientific nutritional practices, and greatly advanced training systems, was in its infancy. Joe won many physique titles, then devoted himself to promoting the sport and modernizing its training, dietary, and mental approach practices.

energy-wise, but by Tuesday I was raring to go again. Since it was sacrilegious to work out on Tuesday, I helplessly let the day pass by.

Also, the existing system allowed a bodybuilder to increase his poundages no more than 5 pounds every month or so. If your progress was such that you could have added 10 pounds or more, you were again stymied. Before long I had had a stomach full of that. I then wrote an article called "Routines Are Made to Be Broken" in which I railed against the tyranny of tradition. Routines were made to serve, I said, not to be served.

During the 1940s, when the whole world went through upheaval and change, I had begun to develop a certain spirit of reconstruction. I had the opportunity to train and be with many of the emerging bodybuilding stars of that era. And when I couldn't actually train with a star, I corresponded with him faithfully.

I studied their methods and found that they were *instinctively* doing things in their workouts that they were unaware of, little cheats and turns that expedited the movement of weights. I remember an incident with Clarence Ross, a superstar of that period. I watched this great Mr. America do a set of barbell curls, 10 reps with 165 pounds, but I noticed he had to cheat them up a little. That was a heavy weight, of course. At the same time one of Ross's students, who was copying the star only with a lighter weight, got a scolding from his mentor for cheating up his curls.

Clancy Ross told him to do the curls strictly, with no cheating. I was thinking how entirely old-world that advice was. As Clancy returned to the bar for another set, I suggested he do the curls in the same way he told the student to do them, very strictly. With an awkward effort he could do only 4 strict reps, not the 10 reps he did with looser form. Only then did I make

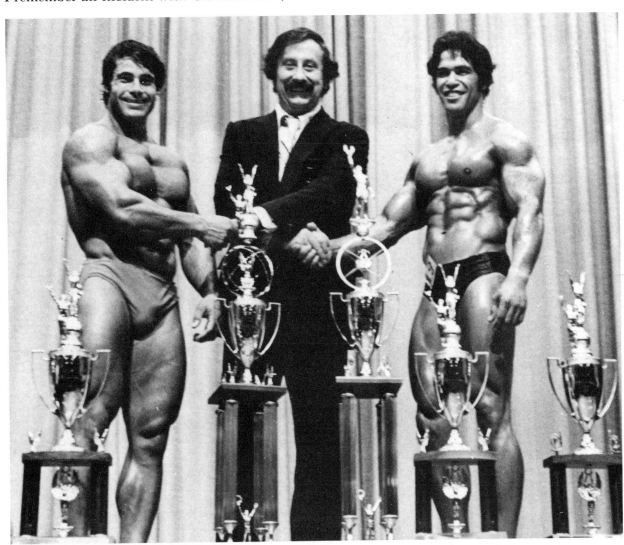

Joe and his brother, Ben Weider, founded the International Federation of Bodybuilders in 1947, and the organization has grown to include more than 130 affiliated nations, making it the fifth largest sports federation in existence. In this photo, Joe congratulates two of his early 1970s winners—Dr. Franco Columbu (left) and Ed Corney.

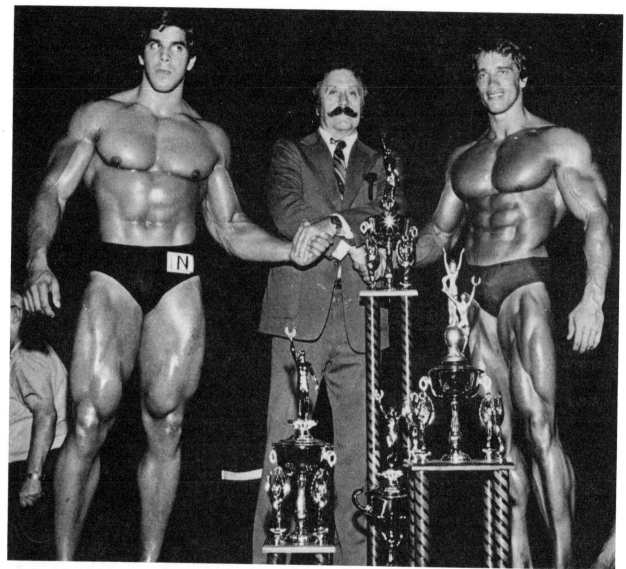

Two of Joe's greatest pupils have been Lou Ferrigno (left) and Arnold Schwarzenegger, both of whom turned to acting after retiring from bodybuilding competition. In this 1973 picture, Joe congratulates the pair, Arnold having just won his fourth consecutive Mr. Olympia title. (He currently holds the record of six consecutive wins and seven overall.) Ferrigno was only 21 at this show, but still gave the older and more mature Austrian Oak a run for his money.

Clancy aware that he was using cheating and forced reps in some of his movements, one of the big reasons for his well-documented body-building strength levels.

The same thing happened in weightlifting. Many top lifters had discovered that by clean-ing the weight to the shoulder and arching the torso forward they could heave-press a weight rapidly overhead by jerking the body erect without ever bending the knees. That trick, in fact, caused the elimination of the two-arm press from Olympic lifting competition follow-ing the 1976 Olympic Games in Montreal. But for a period of several years it was good enough

to fool and confuse the judges. The lifters also instinctively used a slight push-out as they did snatches, a movement contrary to the perfectly vertical pull required by the lifting rules.

Cheating and forced reps were techniques used by the lifters, yet everyone was advised to use strict style in workouts, according to tradi-tion. Unaware that they were so disorganized, the lifters truly believed in the rules—instinct never suffers the confusion of reason. Those weightlifters instinctively learned the best way to lift the most weight, legislated rules notwith-standing.

For a period of time, bodybuilding and

weightlifting were in a mess: no regimented method that worked was devised. Weightlifting articles used to be written stressing technique, how to get the weight up. Almost nothing was written on power assistance exercises, improving the total muscular structure, and building strength outside the required channels.

Fault did not lie entirely with the lifters and bodybuilders, however. Athletic coaches in general were blind and obstinate about weight training, thinking it would make their athletes muscle-bound. It wasn't until the Russian athletes who were trained with power assistance exercises began beating the pants off Americans that we finally woke up to the value of weight training in all sports.

Weight-trained East European boxers are still knocking the heads off our boxers, whose coaches to this day do not recognize the benefits of assistance power exercises to develop greater punching power. Old systems take a long time to die.

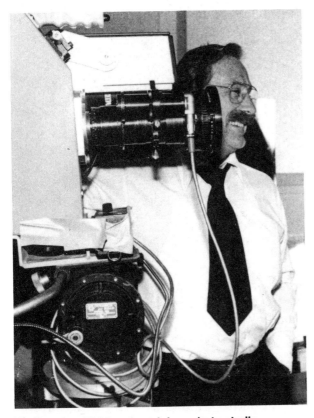

The real Joe Weider at work in a photo studio creating the sensational images which monthly grace his four magazines, *Flex, Shape, Muscle & Fitness,* and *Men's Fitness*. Despite long hours coaching the best bodybuilders in the sport, Weider always takes time to ensure that his publications have available the best possible photos to illustrate each article.

When I began publishing bodybuilding magazines nearly 40 years ago, I was adrift on a sea fraught with peril. I had set my course to follow the most direct route to that distant land of scientific training fact in the hope of returning with the evidence that would make weight training palatable. At landfalls along the way, the natives were not always friendly. Those bodybuilding champs eyed me with suspicion when I asked to examine their training methods and didn't overflow with enthusiasm when I suggested they test some new training idea. I fell under attack by some people in the business. After all, rebels are seldom invited to dinner by the entrenched powers.

Eventually I succeeded. The real point of my journey could not be misinterpreted. The evidence showed in every issue of *Muscle Builder* magazine. I pampered the sport. People offered to help me develop the Weider System. Some of these good bodybuilders were banned by the Amateur Athletic Union (AAU) for doing this, their careers ruined by bigots. Some lost deserved titles, while others were not permitted to enter AAU events. They were guilty of associating with me and of trying to increase the knowledge of the sport. Nevertheless, I finally was able to convince enough champions and near champions to cooperate with me to test my techniques.

I followed a three-step method in developing all of my techniques:

- By training with weights in all forms, I was able to develop an intuition that sensed exactly what worked for me. I also had the opportunity to train with the champs along with hundreds of other hard-training bodybuilders. I could see and feel the results. I saw the relationship between effort and recuperation. I felt that effort and recuperation were two distinct parts of bodybuilding training, yet conjoined physiologically.
- The character of the effort and the recuperative force at work needed a collective name. Forced reps and supersets were different methods, for example, varying in degree of intensity of effort and length of rest intervals between sets and even between individual repetitions.
- By giving each concept a name, I knew it would be easier to remember. Each name had

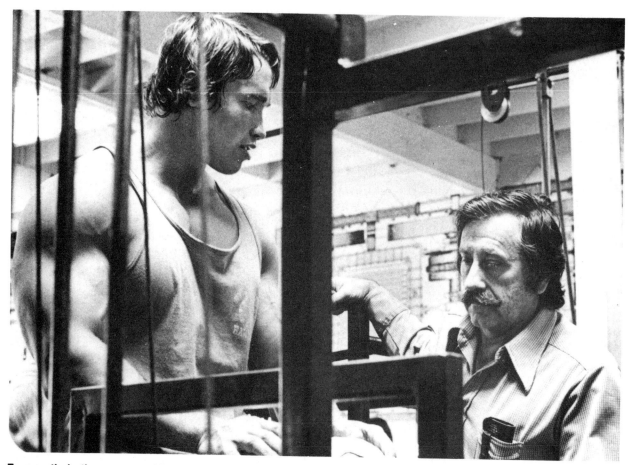

Frequently in the gym coaching the elite of the sport, Joe can be seen here dispensing his voluminous wisdom to Arnold Schwarzenegger when Arnold was widely considered to be the greatest bodybuilder of all time. It's no coincidence that Arnold was Weider trained.

to be a thumbnail sketch of the system. When you said "forced reps," you understood it meant going beyond the threshold of regular effort, beyond simple fatigue into the area of exhaustion. By naming them it was easier to unify them. That is what I called the "knot" that tied all the principles together, that enabled the Weider Instinctive Training Principle to be developed. In this way, a core sense and experiment were tied together to produce the instinctive way of training.

I once had a long list of the different principles that were developed. Some got absorbed along the way, combined with other concepts. The final outcome is the list of major principles as we know them today, such as supersets, trisets, giant sets, peak contraction, forced reps, overload system, retro-gravity system, split system, double-split system, cheating, staggered sets, and quality training.

All of these principles were created for one

reason: to gradually increase workout intensity in order to build greater power and large muscular mass faster. With the early methods, progress slowed considerably after the first 30 days. One of the first techniques I came up with to break free from that ancient tether was supersets. It practically eliminated the rest interval between sets, a mighty innovation, electronic compared to the spring-loaded timing procedures of old. Supersets pushed training along with new fuel for muscle growth.

But even supersets reached a point of diminishing returns, and in the search for another breakthrough I developed trisets and then giant sets. Thus the process continued, each new method taking us another step further on the road to intensity of training, a kind of carrot we had to keep chasing.

Some of the methods I developed applied to overall workouts, while others were developed to increase the intensity while working individual muscle groups. For instance, from regular straight sets of barbell curls we advanced to supersets, then to cheating, peak contraction, and forced reps, each succeeding method designed either to intensify or to isolate effort to build mass and shape respectively.

Each method was built on the previous one. When one had served its purpose and exhausted itself, I compounded it with a new one. The old one was not discarded. You don't give a beginner supersets. Nor do you give an intermediate bodybuilder the double-split system. The systems for the most part are used in logical order to maintain momentum, like the stages of a moon rocket.

Each method served a different purpose. Some were created to develop parts of a muscle through isolation, others for building muscle mass, and still others for taking advantage of the physiological recuperative power of muscle as it grows. Others may offer combined effects, such as both definition and mass.

Each Weider Training Principle has a life of its own in the sport. Each continues to grow, nourished by new input from great champions using it or through the ever-increasing outpourings of scientific research.

Intensity is the condition that prevails over all these principles to form the knot that binds them together for the common purpose—steady muscular growth. That is the keystone of the Weider System, eliminating stagnation and hastening progress.

The methods are geared like a car transmission that permits the beginner to start in low gear and shift up as he gains momentum. With a knowledge of the methods and the names given to them, he can pick what he thinks will work for him. Eventually, after several years, he should be able to function in the realm of instinctive training. That means he will still work with the different Weider methods that he learned as an intermediate bodybuilder, but

with greater sophistication. He will learn to intensify and pace. He will have a greater backlog with which to make comparisons. He will simply be a more fully loaded computer. But it will be his holistic intelligence that sets the programs for it—the instinct, so to speak.

I have found that the great superstars—Arnold Schwarzenegger, Franco Columbu, Frank Zane, Lou Ferrigno, Lee Haney, and many others—listen more carefully or search most avidly for any idea that may help them gain the slightest bit. They are humbled by years of training and by both the joys of winning and the disappointment of losing physique titles that give their lives force and meaning.

Now, well into the fourth generation of the Weider System, bodybuilders have been using the Weider Training Principles universally. Training has become highly refined and more penetrating due to the latest advances in sports medicine. Bodies are getting bigger and better faster. Third-place winners today would never have lost a contest 15 years ago. Times are changing.

So am I, in my attitudes toward training. I intend to keep all avenues open for the advancement of the sport. We all have *Muscle & Fitness* and *Flex* to work with. You can depend on anything worthwhile to appear on those pages, which I consider monthly updates of this book.

I want all of my student friends to realize that working out in the gym is only half of their training—recuperation is the other half. You have to build up recuperative power. It isn't something that comes overnight with eight hours of sleep. It is truly much more involved.

You must ultimately come to the realization that when you are not in the gym working out, when your body is recuperating, your workout is still going on. Successful training consists of two elements—the ultimate workout and total recuperation. And each of these factors is based on the Weider System of Bodybuilding.

PART I
ADVICE TO
NOVICE BODYBUILDERS

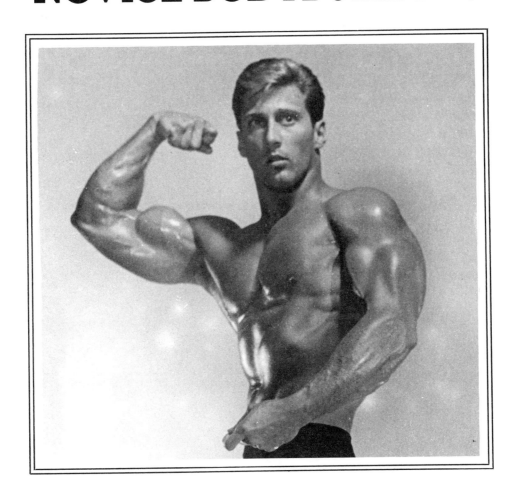

1
The Bodybuilding
Lifestyle

If there's a tougher sport to succeed at than bodybuilding, I haven't heard of it. A champion bodybuilder trains with mind-boggling intensity up to six or seven days per week, often twice per day when peaking for a competition. His workouts last from 1½ to 5 hours per day, and they are tremendously enervating. And a champion bodybuilder often must expend vast quantities of energy on his workouts when his energy reserves have already been depleted severely by a tight precontest diet. Very few sports demand this type of self-sacrifice and dedication.

To harden iron into steel, you have to heat it to hundreds of degrees, then plunge it into cold water. The heat and cold temper the metal. Making steel is analogous to bodybuilding, because every bodybuilder must undergo extremes of energy expenditure and strict diet, making his physique as hard as steel at contest time.

A bodybuilder willingly subjects himself to extremes of hard training and food deprivation, and in that process he hardens himself both physically and mentally. He gradually becomes what I consider to be an ideal man. The ancient Greeks felt the same way when they adopted the motto *Mens sana in corpore sano,* "a sound mind in a sound body."

Bodybuilding is such a difficult sport that it teaches its adherents lessons in persistence, mental drive, goal-setting, and many other qualities that apply to everyday life. These bodybuilding lessons will make you a success in business and any other aspect of your life. Champion bodybuilders are special individuals, men who succeed in every aspect of life.

Let me give you the best available example of a man who used the lessons he learned from

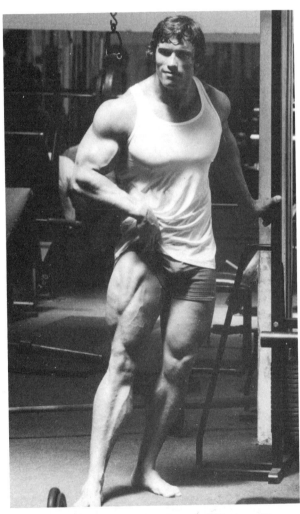

One of the greatest bodybuilders of all time—with superb development from top to bottom and side to side—Arnold Schwarzenegger, who moved from Austria to America specifically to become a great physique star. When Arnold first moved to California, he had very little leg development. The results of training with Joe Weider are evident in this photo.

bodybuilding in other aspects of his life. Arnold Schwarzenegger has won seven Mr. Olympia titles, making him the best bodybuilder of

3

all time. But two of Arnold's goals—in addition to becoming a superstar bodybuilder—when he came to America were to become a film star and to become a millionaire.

I have been amazed at the systematic manner in which Arnold has gone after each of these goals. He made many shrewd business moves—particularly real estate investments—and was a millionaire several times over before his 30th birthday. I'd stack up Arnold's business acumen against anyone's, including my own.

After he won his sixth Mr. Olympia title in 1975, Schwarzenegger systematically went about building a film career. He had been the main character in the great bodybuilding documentary, *Pumping Iron*, and Arnold set about capitalizing on his newfound fame. He hired a publicist and an agent and soon was on

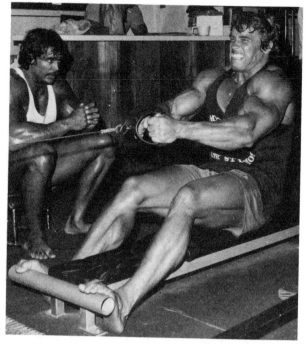

Schwarzenegger was noted as one of the hardest trainers at the original Gold's Gym on Pacific Avenue in Venice, California. Here he grinds out a set of seated pulley rows to add even more width to his barndoor-wide back. West Coast amateur sensation Denny Gable waits his turn at the pulley, hoping Arnold will complete enough reps for Denny to get his breath back prior to commencing his own set.

virtually every television talk show in the United States, Canada, and Europe.

While promoting himself into a media star, Arnold also promoted bodybuilding, the sport that made him a famous athlete. He was so obviously intelligent and articulate on all of the talk shows that members of the general public began liking the sport, and droves of them flocked to gyms around the world. Gradually, bodybuilding came out of the deep, dark closet it had been in prior to the middle 1970s.

Schwarzenegger made a series of shrewd moves with his acting career, finally hitting it big with *The Terminator*. He is now one of the hottest film stars in the world, an actor who now commands more than $3 million for each film he makes. He has a long, successful, and lucrative film career ahead of him, and many of the lessons he learned through 10 years of competitive bodybuilding helped him reach his present high position financially and artistically.

Bodybuilding is also health-building, because the regularity of training and mainte-

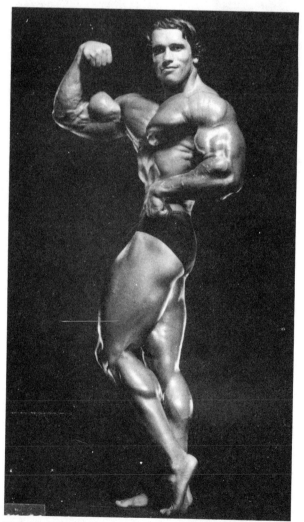

The awesome Arnold arms are clearly depicted in this photo taken in about 1975, the year he won his sixth consecutive Mr. Olympia title.

nance of a healthy diet increase health. Bodybuilding obviously improves your body dramatically. And the activity gives you excellent overall physical fitness.

A champion bodybuilder follows a strict training and dietary regimen day in and day out, year after year, in order to build an impressive enough physique to win national and international bodybuilding championships. But there is a certain purity in such self-discipline that actually builds upon itself, making training and diet even stricter.

It takes a very special breed of man to become a successful bodybuilder. Few are chosen to become champs in our sport. Even fewer men have the right genetic potential to succeed in the sport. Mike Mentzer (Mr. America, Mr. Universe) once stated that only one man in 100,000 has the genetic potential to become a superstar bodybuilder and that the vast majority of those men never set foot inside a weight room or public bodybuilding gym. I personally

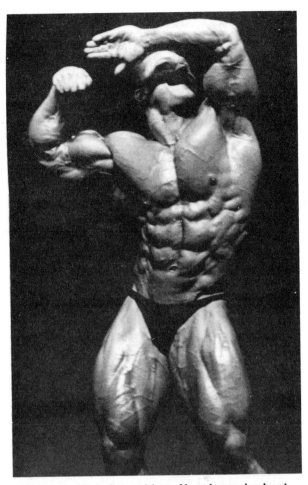

Current pro Rich Gaspari from New Jersey is about as close to a man of steel as humanly possible. Between 1986 and 1988, Rich placed second to Lee Haney three consecutive times in the Mr. Olympia show. But even placing second, he's become one of the most popular bodybuilders on the face of the earth.

feel that the picture is a lot brighter than Mike paints it, but a budding champion must have certain genetically predetermined traits in order to reach the top of the bodybuilding pyramid.

You will discover after only a few weeks of hard bodybuilding training whether or not you have sufficient interest in bodybuilding to keep you in the gym, training hard on a regular basis. Then it's just a matter of time before you reach competitive condition and embark on a bodybuilding career that might bring you to a national or world championship and perhaps even to a professional career.

I know what you want from the sport and have written this book in such detail that you probably won't need to own any other body-

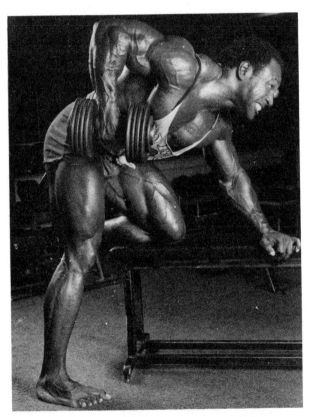

Current king of the hill is Atlanta, Georgia's Lee Haney, who has won five consecutive Mr. Olympia titles through 1988, and shows no sign of losing one any time in the next five years. At 5'11½" and 250 pounds in very hard shape, he's the biggest ever to win the title.

building books. All you'll need to do is purchase *Flex* and *Muscle & Fitness* magazines each month to learn about any new developments in bodybuilding technology, physiology, or biochemistry.

It's all up to you now. I'm sure you will succeed at building a championship physique over the next few years. It will be a long and fatiguing journey, but you won't make many bad turns en route, because in this book you hold a comprehensive road map in your hands. Read it, learn from it, and then get into the gym for some ferocious workouts.

Good luck!

2
The Basics of Bodybuilding

If you're new to bodybuilding and happen to overhear two seasoned bodybuilders discussing their workouts, you might conclude that they are speaking a foreign language. This is because the sport has developed a jargon consisting of many unique terms. So you can understand this terminology right from the first day in a gym, I will define and discuss the most common bodybuilding terms.

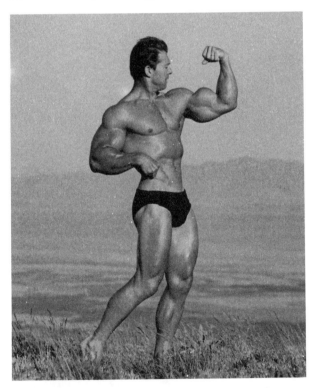

No one who would have seen a youthful Larry Scott, as he was growing up in Pocatello, Idaho, would have ever predicted he'd become a bodybuilding star. He had wide hips and narrow shoulders, and seemed to have an inability to put on muscle mass. And yet this genetic nobody won the first two Mr. Olympia titles contested in 1965 and 1966. This outstanding photo, taken at age 49, proves that bodybuilders only get better with age.

TERMINOLOGY AND DEFINITIONS

There are many other terms in somewhat less common usage in bodybuilding, and they will be defined in the Glossary in the back of this book. It might be a good idea after reading this chapter to turn to the Glossary and start soaking up these other terms. They might seem a little confusing at first, but after only two or three weeks of systematic training you will find that these terms have become second nature to you, and you'll be talking "bodybuildingese" with the best in the sport.

WHAT IS BODYBUILDING?

Weight training is an umbrella term for the general activity of training with resistance equipment. This equipment can be either *free weights* (barbells, dumbbells, and related equipment) or *exercise machines*, which provide the working muscles with a *resistance overload*. When a skeletal muscle is stressed with a resistance overload, it responds by increasing in *hypertrophy* (an improvement of strength, tone, and mass of the muscle group).

You can train with weights to accomplish the following varied objectives:

- Improve health and physical fitness.
- Increase strength and physical conditioning to improve sports performance.
- Reshape the body by building up or trimming down selected parts of the body.
- Rehabilitate a part of the body that has been weakened by an injury.
- Compete in *weightlifting* or *powerlifting* to compare strength levels against other lifters.
- Use heavy training, diet, and aerobics to create a physique for bodybuilding competition.

EQUIPMENT ORIENTATION

The basic piece of equipment for weight training and bodybuilding is a *barbell*. You will find the terminology for various components of a barbell illustrated below.

Exercise barbells are the simplest form, and they can be either *adjustable* (with the weights added or subtracted to change the *poundage,* or *weight,* on the bar) or *fixed* (with the weights either welded or bolted semipermanently in place). Home gym barbells are usually adjustable, while the barbells in a commercial gym are normally fixed, with a separate bar for each 5-pound weight increment from about 20 pounds to over 200 pounds.

A second type of barbell, called an *Olympic barbell,* is used for heavy bodybuilding exercises, as well as for use in weightlifting and powerlifting meets. The length and weight of this barbell are standardized internationally. An unloaded Olympic bar weighs either 20 kilograms (44½ pounds) or 45 pounds. The collars weigh either 2½ kilograms (5½ pounds) or 5 pounds.

Barbells are constructed around a steel *bar* about one inch thick and four to six feet long. Normally the bar with collars weighs about 5 pounds per foot. Its weight should be figured in when you are loading up the barbell for an exercise with a specific poundage. (A five-foot bar with two 10-pound plates on each side, for example, would weigh a total of 65 pounds.)

A tubular *sleeve* is often slipped over the bar to provide more freedom of bar movement in upper-body exercises. Crosshatched grooves called *knurlings* are normally cut into the sleeve to provide you with a more secure grip

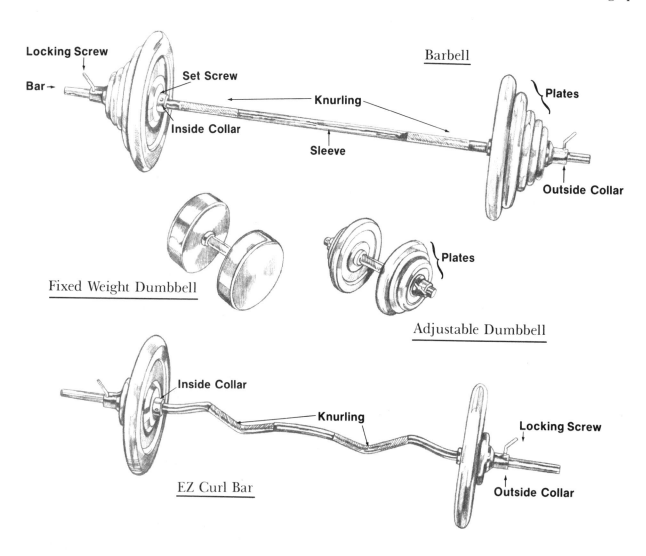

Fixed Weight Dumbbell

Adjustable Dumbbell

EZ Curl Bar

on the barbell when your hands are sweaty. If the barbell you are using does not have a sleeve, the knurlings are usually cut right into the bar itself.

Clamps called *collars* hold metal (or vinyl-covered concrete) discs called *plates* in place on the bar for an exercise. *Inside collars* are bolted to the bar with *set screws* to keep the plates from sliding inward toward your hands. *Outside collars* are fitted over the bar to hold the plates on the bar, keeping them from sliding off the ends during an exercise.

Dumbbells are merely shorter versions of a barbell intended for use in one hand or, most commonly, one in each hand. While barbells are used to work both the upper and lower body, dumbbells are usually intended for upper-body movements, particularly exercises for the arms, shoulders, and chest muscles. Dumbbell bars are usually 10–16 inches in length. You can count the dumbbell bar and collars as five pounds when loading up the correct poundage for each exercise.

TYPES OF EXERCISE

You have probably already heard of *aerobic exercise*, which is long-lasting, low-intensity movement done within the body's limited ability to provide oxygen to the working muscles at a rate at least as high as the exercise itself demands. In other words, aerobic exercise is something like bicycling or running during which you do not build up such an *oxygen debt* that you become breathless enough to be forced to terminate the activity.

The type of high-intensity exercise (such as weight training and sprinting) that builds up an appreciable oxygen debt is called *anaerobic exercise*. Aerobic exercise normally burns body fat to meet its energy needs, so it is often used by competitive bodybuilders to lower their body fat levels close to a major championship. In contrast, anaerobic exercise generally burns muscle sugar (glycogen) to meet its energy requirements.

While it is generally considered to be anaerobic exercise, a hard bodybuilding workout does provide significant aerobic fitness. And there is a type of weight training called *circuit training* that is specifically aerobic in nature.

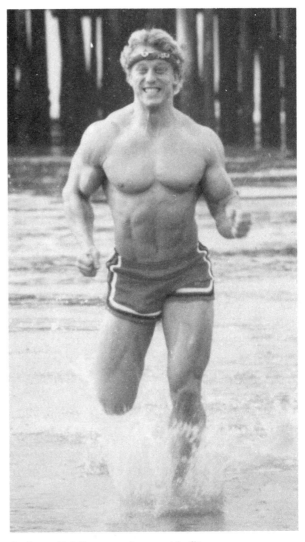

Andreas Cahling runs for aerobic fitness.

WORKING OUT

When you are doing a weight *exercise* such as a bench press, you are engaging in a *workout*, or *training session*. An exercise is also frequently called a *movement*.

Each complete full cycle of an exercise (such as bending your knees fully to sink down into a squatting position with a barbell across your shoulders, then straightening your legs to return to the starting point) is called a *repetition*, or *rep*. A group of repetitions (usually in the range of 5–15 for bodybuilding purposes) is called a *set*. Most of the time you will do multiple sets of each movement with *rest intervals* lasting one to two minutes between sets.

The full accumulation of exercises, sets, and reps performed during a workout is called a *routine*, *program*, or *training schedule*. More often than not, a routine refers to the written training schedule as it appears in a book, magazine article, or training diary.

There are two types of exercises used when working out in a gym. The first type of movement is called a *basic exercise*, and it works one or more large muscle groups in conjunction with other, smaller muscle groups. In contrast, an *isolation exercise* is a movement that stresses a single muscle complex (and often only a specific part of the body part) in relative isolation from the rest of the body.

When you perform several sets for a particular muscle group, your muscles become congested with blood, which is shunted into the area to remove carbon dioxide and other fatigue by-products and replace them with oxygen and glycogen. This pleasant, tight feeling in the muscle is called a *pump*, and for a couple of hours after a workout you will find that the pump makes a muscle group appear slightly larger than normal.

PHYSIQUE TERMS

Many years ago, a scientist named Sheldon began studying body types (often called *somatotypes*), and he eventually noticed that all men

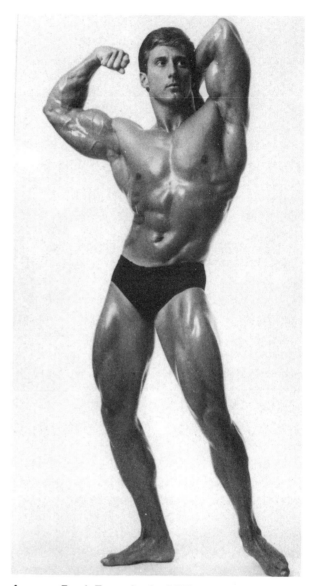

A young Frank Zane also had little genetic potential for greatness in bodybuilding. He had a small skeletal structure, an inability to add muscle mass to anything but his legs, and no ability to get cut up enough to win titles. This photo was taken in about 1965.

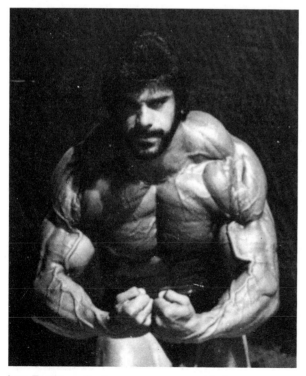

Lou Ferrigno displays awesome vascularity with this crouched most muscular pose.

and women can be placed in one of three basic body types or combinations of two basic types. Naturally slender and finely boned individuals are called *ectomorphs*. Naturally large-boned and frequently obese individuals are called *endomorphs*. And between these two extremes are naturally husky and muscular individuals called *mesomorphs*.

Generally speaking, the best bodybuilders are natural mesomorphs, usually with some shadings of ecto- or endomorphism. Still, one of the beauties of bodybuilding is that individuals who are predominantly ectomorphic or

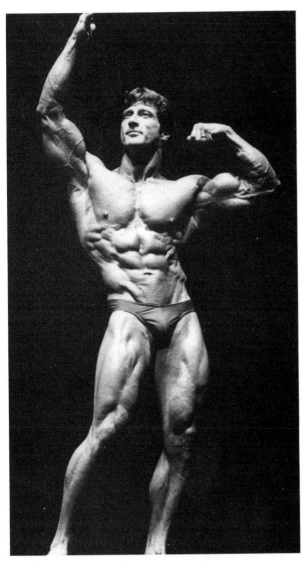

Zane proved everyone wrong by consistently hard, scientific training and diet. This outstanding photo was taken in 1979, when Zane won his third consecutive Mr. Olympia title, confounding the experts. What a difference 14 years can make!

endomorphic can still become very massive and muscular bodybuilders. So, you need not feel handicapped if you fall into one of these categories.

Ultimately, a great physique combines these qualities: muscle mass, body symmetry, muscular definition, and vascularity. *Muscle mass* is the actual size of the skeletal muscles, which has been developed through several years of dedicated overload training.

Body *symmetry* is the shape or general outline of the various body parts, as though seen in silhouette. A symmetrical physique has broad shoulders, a torso tapering down to a small waist-hip structure, and generally small joints surrounded by large muscle masses. Symmetry can be developed to a point, but most of it is a result of natural skeletal qualities and muscle insertions.

Muscular definition is the result of a low percentage of body fat, which is achieved through hard bodybuilding training, plenty of aerobics, and a low-calorie or low-carbohydrate diet. When you have plenty of hard muscle mass and a low degree of body fat, you have developed *muscle density*.

Vascularity is the prominence of veins and arteries over the muscles. The diameter of blood vessels actually increases with consistent heavy training. And the vascular system becomes prominent when your skin is thinned out through stringent precontest dieting.

ASSESSING YOUR POTENTIAL

Do you have the basic genetic potential necessary to become a great bodybuilder? You'll be able to find out whether you do by following the instructions in this section.

If you don't seem to have great genetics for the sport, however, you shouldn't mourn. Many of the very best bodybuilders over the years have had less than optimum genetic potential for the sport yet have succeeded in becoming Mr. America, Mr. Universe, and Mr. Olympia winners. Let me give you a few examples.

Larry Scott, who won the first two Mr. Olympia titles in 1965–66, has often been pointed to as a man who had inferior genetic potential for bodybuilding but overcame these insufficiencies to become one of the brightest stars in the history of bodybuilding. Scott was of only about average height, and his shoulder structure, when compared to the width of his waist-hip structure, was relatively narrow. And Larry was further handicapped by being a slow gainer, a bodybuilder who always had to scratch and claw his way upward.

Through dogged persistence, Larry Scott gradually improved his physique, capitalizing on his fast metabolism by always appearing terrifically muscular at each competition while he gradually improved his overall muscle mass and brought up weak points. Ultimately, Scott was able to muscle up to 210 rock-hard pounds at 5'8" in height. He won the Mr. California,

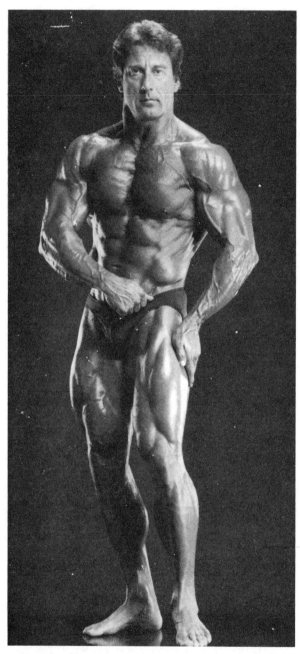

Still going strong at 49 years of age, Zane also proves that bodybuilders age like fine wine! This photo also provides an excellent example of *vascularity*.

ple of a bodybuilder with a small frame who ultimately succeeded in developing a widely admired physique. Frank's secrets were a superb depth of knowledge of training, diet, and psychological approach is to bodybuilding, plus the same type of dogged determination displayed by Larry Scott.

Through hard, consistent, scientific training and maintenance of a near-perfect nutritional program, Zane gradually built himself up. Ultimately, Frank never displayed the gargantuan muscle mass of a Lee Haney or Sergio Oliva, but his perfect symmetry, ideally balanced proportions, and incredibly detailed musculature allowed him to routinely defeat men 50 pounds heavier to take the Mr. America, Mr. Universe, and Mr. World titles before going on to four Mr. Olympia titles.

I've also seen many small-boned bodybuilders—most of them with better overall potential than Frank Zane—give up their training because they couldn't achieve the huge muscle mass of some of their competitors. But Frank never gave up, and he is famed as one of the top four or five bodybuilders of all time.

Danny Padilla is a short individual who has muscled up to the point where he won Mr. America, Mr. USA, and Mr. Universe titles, placing in the top five in the Olympia. Danny's only 5'2" tall, but he became a giant killer by developing one of the most massive and perfectly balanced physiques in history.

While a superbly developed big man does have a small advantage over shorter contestants, height really isn't a big issue in bodybuilding. The only things that really count are muscle mass, proportional balance, muscularity, symmetry, and posing ability. Danny kept these facts firmly in mind as he pumped iron year after year to build his great physique. He never let short stature get in his way.

I could point out hundreds more bodybuilders who have had less than ideal genetic potential and yet succeeded. The object lesson here is that *genetic potential is more of an enabling factor than a limiting factor*.

Superior genetic potential will allow you to develop a great physique more quickly, and at the upper reaches of the sport it is a bit of an advantage. But virtually all points of poor genetic potential can be overcome if you are persistent enough and both train and eat as

Mr. America, Mr. Universe, and Mr. Olympia titles and set a new standard of excellence for shoulder and arm development.

I've seen many young men with physical potential much greater than Larry Scott's grow frustrated when they don't seem to be making gains and drop out of the sport. Larry never did. He just kept pounding away, and he succeeded admirably.

Frank Zane, who won three Mr. Olympia titles in 1977, 1978, and 1979, is a perfect exam-

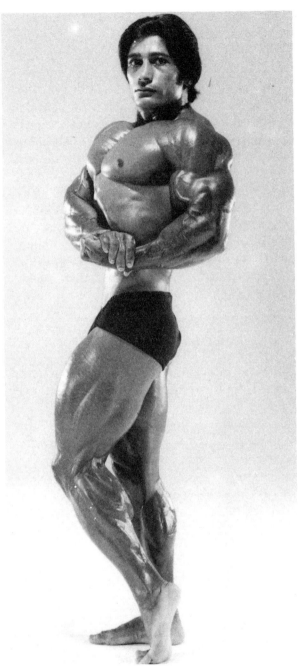

Bodybuilders come in all shapes and sizes from 6'5" Lou Ferrigno, down to 5'2" Danny Padilla, whose height was certainly no handicap to him. Danny won the Mr. America, Mr. USA, Mr. Universe, and Mr. World titles, plus placed in the top five at Mr. Olympia in 1981.

wider than your waist-hip structure. And it is advantageous to have small wrists, knees, and ankles since large muscles on either side of small joints create the illusion of tremendous body symmetry.

It is advantageous to have a basal metabolic rate that allows you to maintain a relatively low body fat percentage. However, you *can* overcome a sluggish metabolism through stringent

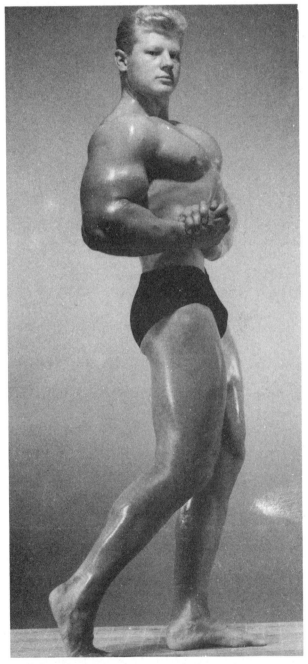

Dave Draper was once a real fatty, but was able to reduce his body weight to normal levels—even to contest bodybuilding levels—through hard, consistent training and solid diet.

scientifically as possible. A small minority of bodybuilders may, indeed, not have the genetic potential to become superstars, but everyone has potential enough to develop a superb physique.

The first point of genetic potential involves your skeletal structure. When you are in an untrained state, your shoulders should be a bit

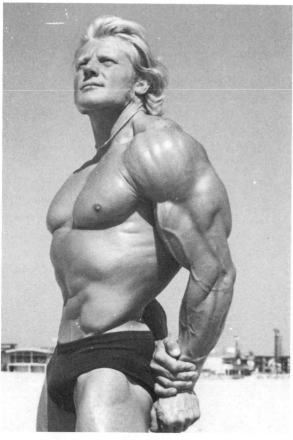

Here's proof that Dave knew what he was doing in his training and diet. He won the Mr. America, Mr. World, and Mr. Universe titles before turning to a film career. He currently coaches upcoming athletes in Capitola, California.

dieting. A good example of this is Dave Draper, who was a fairly pudgy young man. Through strict dieting, Dave was able to lean out his physique and won the Mr. America, Mr. World, and Mr. Universe titles during a long and distinguished career.

I personally believe that it is also an advantage to be able to build muscle mass relatively quickly. Many bodybuilders, such as Scott and Zane, are slow gainers, but it's better to be able to increase muscle mass quickly enough to keep your level of enthusiasm for training relatively high.

While it is not a genetically determined trait, intelligence is also a point of potential for bodybuilders of the future. The sport is rapidly becoming more scientific, and future great bodybuilders must have enough intelligence to be able to read texts on anatomy, kinesiology, physiology, biochemistry, psychology, and other diverse scientific disciplines.

Self-discipline, an acquired trait, can be improved gradually through consistent training. But it's advantageous to come into the sport with good self-discipline and consistent work habits. These qualities are developed in general sports participation, which is probably the main reason so many athletes from other sports are nearly immediate successes as bodybuilders.

After a year or so of steady training, you will be able to assess the final genetically determined trait of a top bodybuilder. It's an advantage to have long muscle bellies—a quality dictated by your unique muscle insertions—but you won't be able to tell whether or not you have such advantageous muscle conformation until after you have achieved at least a moderate amount of muscle mass.

PHYSICAL EXAM

Bodybuilding is probably the most intense and demanding form of exercise you have ever taken up. It places tremendous stress on the heart, vascular system, and lungs, stress that might be harmful if you have hidden cardiac disease or any of many other health problems that can be detected by a routine physical examination prior to taking up a program of heavy bodybuilding training.

It should come as no surprise that I strongly recommend having a physical examination before starting in the sport of bodybuilding involvement. An exam is doubly important if you are over the age of 35 and/or have been sedentary for more than a year. I also strongly suggest that you have your physician include a stress test electrocardiogram with your examination. Men and women over 40 years of age *must* take an ECG.

I certainly don't wish to give you the idea that bodybuilding isn't safe, because properly performed workouts are perfectly safe. But if you have an existing heart problem that has thus far been undetected, it is within the realm of possibility that a heavy workout could be the last one you ever take.

If your physician detects some problem that might be aggravated by heavy barbell and dumbbell training, you probably will still be able to train lightly and then gradually increase the intensity of your workouts. Just be sure that you follow your physician's recommendations to the letter. He or she can see you in person; I can't.

WHERE TO WORK OUT

With the tremendous surge of popularity for weight training and bodybuilding, a majority of individuals taking up the sport do their first workouts in a commercial gym or health spa. But this wasn't true in the past, when there were far fewer gyms with superior equipment. A large majority of current and past superstar bodybuilders began working out at home in a basement, garage, or bedroom, moving on to commercial gyms only after winning a few titles. Often the top people would move to Los Angeles in order to train at the great gyms that have always been a part of the southern California lifestyle.

I still think that it is a good practice to start bodybuilding in a home gym, particularly if you are not initially in good physical condition and feel that you might be intimidated by the muscular types found in commercial gyms. You will have perfect privacy in a home gym and can work out at any time of the day or night since you are not limited by the set hours gyms are open.

If you can spend a few bucks setting up a home gym, you will also save on gym dues, which must be paid on a regular basis at a commercial bodybuilding gym. For $300-$500 you can equip a home gym sufficiently to put in some Olympian workouts, and your outlay is a one-time expense.

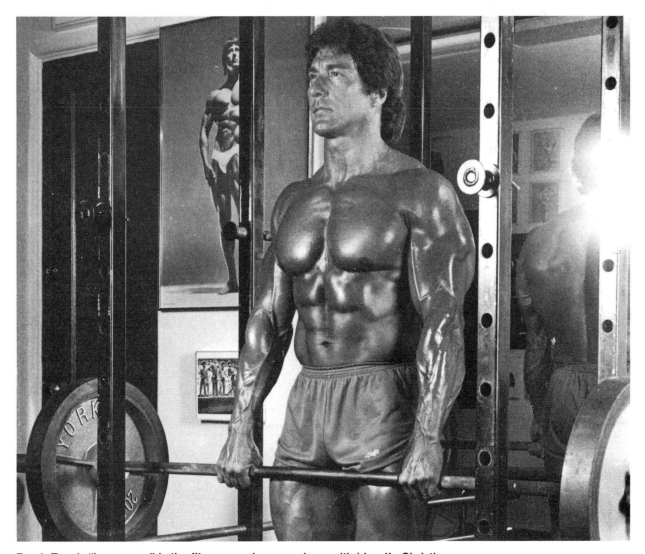

Frank Zane's "home gym" is the fitness spa he runs along with his wife Christine.

After a year or two of steady, progressively heavier training, you might find you need a wider variety of equipment in order to juice up your workouts. In this case you will probably want to join a larger commercial gym like Gold's Gym, World Gym, or Powerhouse Gym. Dues for these facilities range from $200 to $300 per year, but the top men normally are allowed to work out free since they are a good advertising vehicle for most gym owners.

At the best commercial gyms you will find all of the equipment you'll ever need in order to become a champion. Many of them have fixed dumbbells in 5-pound jumps up to over 150 pounds, for example, and very few men are strong enough to do any type of exercise with that much weight in each hand.

You will also find a great deal of camaraderie in the best gyms. At some health spas, bodybuilders are treated almost like freaks, while you'll be among your own kind at a gym like Gold's or World in Venice, California.

Occasionally you will find a school or YMCA that has a well-equipped bodybuilding gym. In this case, if you are either enrolled in school or have a YMCA membership card, you can work out very heavily in the gym for a much lower cost than at a commercial gym.

Should you have access to several good gyms in your area, I suggest taking one or two workouts at each one during peak attendance hours (usually 3:00 to 7:00 P.M.) in order to determine which one has the best equipment and atmosphere before deciding on the gym you want to join. You might even decide to join more than one gym, like a lot of the bigger guys in L.A. I know plenty of top champs who train their upper bodies at Gold's and their legs at World Gym.

WORKOUT FREQUENCY

Each time you place heavy stress on a muscle group in your bodybuilding workouts, you must rest that body part for 48–96 hours before blasting it in a succeeding training session. This rest period allows the muscle to fully recover and then increase in mass, tone, and strength between workouts. (I will tell you more about this recovery cycle a bit later in this chapter.)

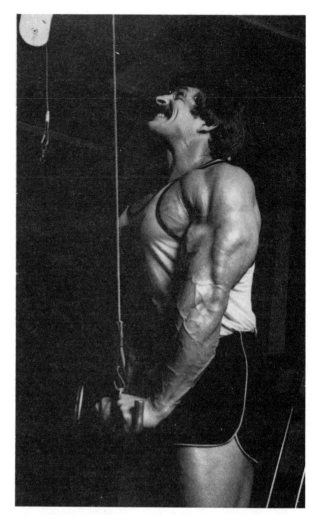

Mike Mentzer performs a set of Pulley Pushdowns with a huge weight.

Because you must rest for two or three days between workouts for each body part in order for your muscles to grow properly, beginning-level bodybuilders *must* train on three nonconsecutive days per week. Most commonly, this means training on Mondays, Wednesdays, and Fridays each week, resting on Tuesdays, Thursdays, and weekends. However, you can work out on any other three nonconsecutive days per week, such as Sunday, Tuesday, and Thursday. I just prefer to recommend Mondays, Wednesdays, and Fridays so you can keep the weekends free.

Later, when you become more experienced and your workouts begin to take more than one hour per day to complete, you will probably wish to switch to a split routine, in which you train only part of your body on each workout day. By doing half of your body parts on one day and the other half on the next, you will work out four to six times per week but still essentially allow 48–72 hours between training sessions for each muscle group.

WHEN TO TRAIN

A majority of top bodybuilders seem to train either in the morning (between 8:00 A.M. and noon) or in the afternoon (between 3:00 and 6:00 P.M.). But you can find top men and women working out at literally every hour of the day and night. Let me introduce you to a few examples.

Tom Platz (Mr. Universe) is one of the most consistent morning trainers, getting into Gold's or the World Gym about 9:00 A.M. each workout day. Lee Haney prefers to do the first half of his double-split routine at about the same time in the morning, then comes back for part two at about 3:30 or 4:00 P.M. And at the time Gold's Gym owner Pete Grymkowski was winning the IFBB Mr. World title, he liked to train between midnight and 6:00 A.M. daily.

There is some scientific evidence that the average person is at a physical and mental peak at about 3:00 in the afternoon. And there is other evidence that your body tends to peak out physically and mentally for that time of the day at which you tend to train regularly.

My thought on the correct time of day to train is that you *should* work out consistently at about the same hour in order for your body to marshal all of its forces for a great training session. And you should pick that time of day when you can consistently work out without any interruptions. Other than that, let the chips fall where they may.

LENGTH OF REST INTERVAL

The object of a rest interval between sets is to allow your body to partially recover its energy reserves for the succeeding set. Under normal circumstances you should rest for 60–120 seconds between sets, longer when working large body parts such as thighs, back, and chest, and shorter between other muscle groups' sets.

With experience you will learn that you should go to the next set at the point when your breathing returns to normal. But in the first

few months of steady bodybuilding training, I would suggest actually timing yourself with a sweep second hand on a clock or watch.

Regardless of what length the rest interval you choose, do not make the mistake of resting for more than three or four minutes between sets, even when you are in power training. Resting too long will cause your body to cool off too much, and you might be more susceptible to injury. Keep moving along, and you'll remain warmed up, thereby avoiding progress-stalling injuries.

WHAT TO WEAR

You should always wear the appropriate clothing for the climate in which you are working out. In sunny southern climes you can probably just train in shorts and perhaps a tank top or T-shirt. But as you go north or approach winter you should bundle up more and more, until at a maximum you might wear three or four layers of T-shirts, leg tights, and warm-up suits.

It's always best to wear several thin layers of clothing rather than only one thick one. Multiple thin layers are actually warmer than one thick layer of clothing, and you can take off thin layers as you get warmed up.

One item of clothing you should always wear is shoes. They both protect your feet from compression injuries and add to body stability when you are doing exercises in a standing position. I always recommend a good pair of running shoes for use in bodybuilding workouts. They have excellent built-in arch supports, as well as treads that help your feet stick to a toe board when you are working calves. Running shoes range in price from about $30 to more than $100.

BREATHING PATTERNS

The only hard and fast rule about breathing during a set is: *do not hold your breath*. If you hold your breath while exerting under a heavy load, the flow of blood to and from your brain can be inhibited. This is called the *Valsalva effect* or *Valsalva maneuver*, and it can cause you to faint for a few seconds.

I don't think I need to tell you how disastrous it could be if you passed out with a heavy bar-

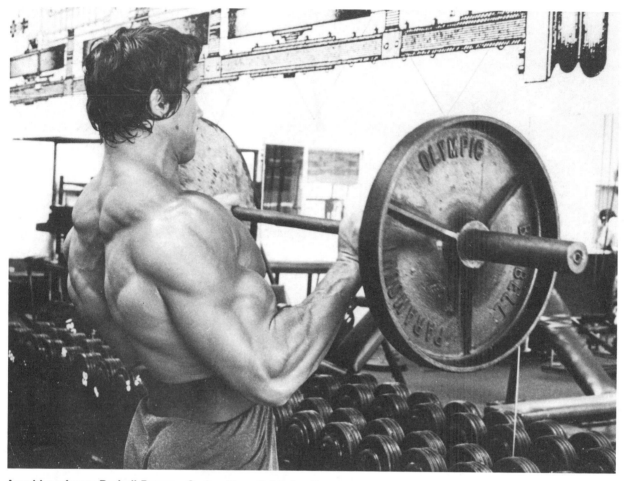

Arnold performs Barbell Reverse Curls with a slight cheating movement with his back.

bell partway up in a bench press. When you're lying on your back in a very vulnerable position, the bar can crash down across your face or, more crucially, across your exposed throat. There are several recorded instances of bodybuilders—some of them very experienced men—who have been killed when bench pressing alone, simply because they held their breath while exerting against the weight.

You won't get hurt only on bench presses when you pass out, however. I know of one case in which a young bodybuilder held his breath while doing overhead barbell presses, incurring nearly $5,000 worth of facial damage when he fell nose first against a dumbbell rack, the bar crashing against the back of his head in this position.

So, you don't want to hold your breath when you exert. But is it best to inhale as you exert against the weight or to inhale as you return from the top position of an exercise back to the starting point? Most of the best bodybuilders prefer to inhale as they lower the weight and exhale as they raise it. So if you feel you need a rule for when to breathe on each repetition, use this one: bar up, inhale; bar down, exhale.

You'll undoubtedly find that breathing becomes automatic after only a couple of workouts. You will need to think about it only for the first week or so of your bodybuilding training. After that you will be able to do it automatically, without thinking about the mechanics of breathing in and out.

PROPER EXERCISE FORM

Biomechanics is the study or application of adopting correct body positions in exercise. In weight training and bodybuilding, biomechanics is maintenance of the correct form in each exercise, which guarantees two things: (1) Your working muscles will receive full stress from the exercise in question; (2) Your body positions are such that your joints and muscles are in the strongest possible position, thereby minimizing the chance of a training injury.

What is correct form? In essence, it is moving your limbs or trunk over the widest possible range of motion in each exercise while moving only those parts of the body specified by the movement description. Short-range movements are less effective than full-range movements, and any cheating through extraneous body motion reduces the value of the exercise and leaves your body more open to injury.

Let me give you an example of correct and incorrect exercise form, using the popular biceps movement, barbell curls. In this exercise, you take an undergrip on a moderately weighted barbell with your hands set about shoulder width apart. Setting your feet about the same distance apart, you stand erect with your arms straight down at your sides and the barbell resting across your upper thighs.

From this starting position, a proper barbell curl is performed by bending only the elbows and moving only the forearms to carry the barbell forward and upward in a semicircular arc to a finish position beneath your chin. To finish the movement, you simply return the barbell back along the same arc to the starting point.

Correct biomechanics in barbell curls demand that the upper arms remain motionless, more specifically pressed against the sides of the rib cage throughout the movement. The torso is held bolt upright and is kept motionless throughout both the upward (positive) and downward (negative) cycles of each movement.

Some of the biomechanical mistakes when performing barbell curls revolve around allowing the upper arms to move during each repetition. Usually the elbows travel outward away from the torso, thereby shortening the range over which your biceps must contract. You might also cheat by bending your torso backward toward the top of the positive arc, thereby shortening the distance over which your biceps must contract.

There is a movement called *cheating curls* that is a bastardization of barbell curls in a standing position. With cheating curls you bend forward at the waist at the start of each repetition, then whip your torso backward to sling the weight upward. Then the movement is finished by bending even farther backward and pulling with the biceps and trapezius muscles to bring the weight up to shoulder level. Most of the benefit for the upper arm muscles occurs when the weight is lowered slowly while the biceps resist the downward momentum of the bar in relatively strict biomechanical position.

I feel that it is essential to use very strict biomechanics when you are a beginner, because such cheating to make an exercise easier to perform robs the working muscles of some of the stress they should be receiving. As you become more advanced, you will be able to use the Weider Cheating Training Principle to advantage to make each set harder—rather than easier—on the working muscles. But until then, you should be very careful to use strict form in all of your movements.

THE RECOVERY CYCLE

There is one physiological constant in bodybuilding: in order for a muscle to increase in hypertrophy (grow in mass and strength), the muscle must first fully recover from a previous workout. Without complete recovery between training sessions, you won't make any gains from your workouts.

Scientific experiments have shown that it takes between 48 and 96 hours for complete recovery to occur and hypertrophy to take place. And this period of time must be one of complete rest from resistance exercise for the muscle in question.

My own experiments have convinced me that young and less experienced bodybuilders can get by very well on 48 hours of rest, intermediates make their best gains on about 72 hours of rest between workouts, and the most advanced bodybuilders grow most quickly when they take the full 96 hours of rest between workouts.

All of this means that beginning bodybuilders can make good gains from their workouts if they train on nonconsecutive days—e.g., Mondays, Wednesdays, and Fridays. Intermediates tend to make good gains training four days per week, but only twice for each body part, on what is called a *split routine*. And most of the best men and women in the sport follow a four-day training cycle—three workout days followed by one day of rest, training their bodies in thirds on each training day—in which each major muscle group is worked every fourth day.

In order to assist the normal recovery process, you should maintain good routines of rest, diet, and stress control. Get a solid eight or nine hours of restful sleep each night, plus perhaps a 30-minute nap during the middle of the day. And avoid such energy leaks as pickup basketball games.

Basic rules of proper bodybuilding nutrition are outlined in Chapter 6, as well as in much greater detail later in this book. In particular, you should avoid junk-food meals when attempting to foster optimum between-workouts recovery ability.

Stress is one of the biggest and least understood enemies of proper postworkout recovery. The best way to avoid stress is to have a relaxing hobby other than bodybuilding training that you can get into whenever you begin to feel stress levels building up. A couple of hours of fly tying or painting watercolors is almost as good as a week in the Caribbean when you are feeling stressed.

TRAINING DIARIES

If you are serious about becoming a superstar bodybuilder, it is essential that you keep a faithful and detailed training diary throughout your bodybuilding training. "By keeping a training journal, you will increase your awareness of what you are doing in your bodybuilding workouts," says three-time Mr. Olympia *Frank Zane.*

Seven-time Mr. Olympia *Arnold Schwarzenegger* further stresses the value of maintaining a comprehensive training log: "Write everything down. Unless you take accurate notes about your training and record the results you receive from it, you will have difficulty in determining which training techniques work best on your unique body."

Ultimately, you will be successful as a bodybuilder only as a function of how quickly and thoroughly you learn precisely which training and nutritional practices work best for you.

Your search will be filled with cul de sacs, but you can limit these dead-end experiments by keeping a detailed training diary.

As you update your training log, it's vitally important to refer back to your recorded notes from time to time. I don't think it would be excessive to review these notes weekly, and certainly you should review all of them each month. This will give you a clear indication of which training routines, exercises, and techniques—to say nothing of which nutritional variables—are working best for you.

Referring to your older records can also be quite inspirational, because they allow you to graphically note your progression in training poundages and intensity levels. From day to day or week to week you probably won't be able to see much progress. But over a period of several months you will be able to see that you have made significant strides. It's not uncommon for an experienced bodybuilder to gain 50–60 pounds on selected basic movements (e.g., squats, benches) over a one-year period. And when you see results this great, your enthusiasm for each workout will be greatly increased.

At the most basic level you should record the date of each workout, the exercises performed, the weights used in each movement, and the sets and reps performed. You can do this in any type of notebook, particularly in the inexpensive bound ledger books available at office supply stores. Or you can use the convenient *Muscle & Fitness Training Diary* (Contemporary Books, 1982) that I put together for use by serious bodybuilders.

When recording your workouts, you should use a type of bodybuilding shorthand that looks like this:

1. Bench Press: 135×12; 165×10; 185×8; 205×6
2. Dumbbell Incline Presses: $60 \times 9 \times 8 \times 8$
3. Flat-Bench Flyes: $40 \times 8 \times 8 \times 8$

In the foregoing example, you might have done 12 reps with 135, 10 reps with 165, 8 reps with 185, and 6 reps with 205 pounds in the bench press. This was followed by three sets of dumbbell incline presses using a steady weight of 60 pounds in each hand for successive sets of 9, 8, and 8 reps. The chest routine was concluded with three sets of 8 reps each of flat-bench flyes using 40-pound dumbbells in each

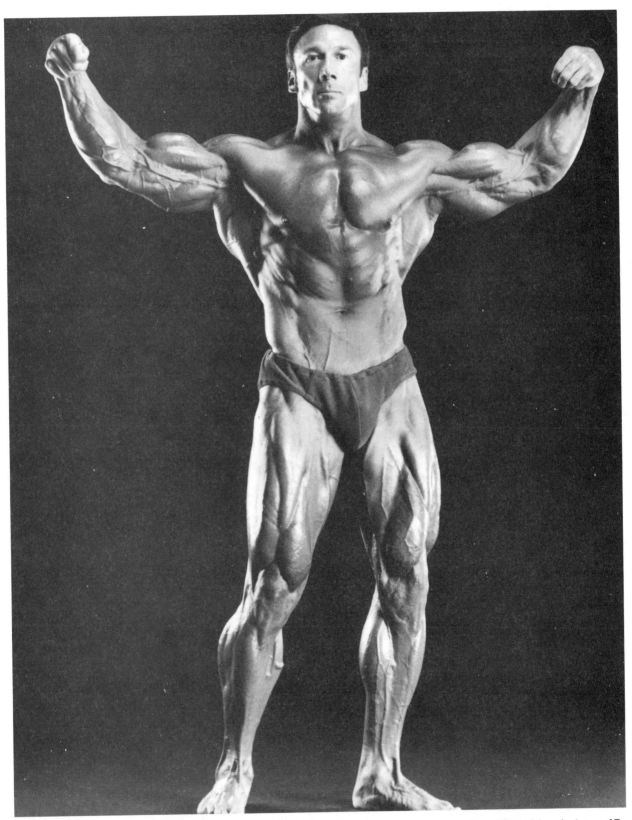

Bodybuilders come in all ages, too. Boyer Coe first competed successfully on the national level at age 17, eventually winning Teenage Mr. America, Mr. America, Mr. World (many times), Mr. Universe (many times), and many IFBB pro Grand Prix titles. At age 42, he's in the best shape of his life.

hand. I think you will agree that this is a pretty simple system.

If you feel like further simplifying your notes, you can use abbreviations for different exercises. Here are some samples:

- DB Flyes = Dumbbell Flyes
- BB Presses = Barbell Presses
- F Chins = Front Chins
- PB Necks = Presses Behind Neck

I'm sure you'll be able to come up with many more of these abbreviations. As long as you know what they mean when you review your notes, anything is fair game.

Many other variables can also be recorded in your training diary. One of these is your daily food and food supplement intake. If you decide to record your nutritional program, you should be careful to note the time of day each nutrient was consumed, plus the amount of each food you eat. This will allow you to later determine how many calories or grams of protein at what times of the day led to a particular change in the appearance of your physique.

I'm also a big believer in recording your morning pulse rate, your pulse rate when still in bed just after you awaken. An abrupt increase in morning pulse rate is a sure indication that you are overtraining and should cut back on your workouts a bit. If you happen to have equipment to take your blood pressure, morning blood pressure spikes are also a sure indication that you are entering an overtrained state.

"Write down how you felt before and after your training session," advises *Frank Zane*. "Note anything unusual that occurs in your body, such as injuries or exceptional strength or weakness in any movement."

Here are some other factors that you might wish to record in your training log: sleep patterns that might have an influence on training energy levels, your daily mood shifts, emotional drains, unique stressors, the length of time it takes to complete a workout, the type and amount of aerobic exercise you are engaged in, and any other factor that might conceivably have an effect on your bodybuilding progress.

As a concluding tip, *Boyer Coe* (IFBB Pro World Grand Prix Champion) suggests, "Try placing a star after each exercise in which you will increase your training poundage at your next workout. I find that this is an excellent way to increase my own workout enthusiasm levels. Whenever I can glance at my training diary and see that I've starred two or more movements, I *know* I've been making great progress. And that in turn fuels my workout enthusiasm to keep training hard and make even more gains in muscle mass and quality!"

3
How Muscles Grow Larger and Stronger

When a muscle grows larger and stronger in response to having a resistance overload placed on it, we say that it has increased in hypertrophy. To understand muscle hypertrophy, you must first understand the structure and function of muscle contraction.

SURFACE ANATOMY

The structure of the skeletal muscles is called *anatomy*. In the figures on pages 24–25, you will find the major muscles of a bodybuilder's physique identified according to how visible they are when an athlete has achieved a low percentage of body fat.

Each skeletal muscle has a point of origin and point of insertion. According to how a muscle originates and inserts, it moves certain parts of the body in set patterns. For example, the biceps muscle complex originates from the upper surface of the humerus, or upper arm bone. And it inserts via a thick tendon to the bones of the forearm. With these unique points of origin and insertion, the biceps muscle contracts primarily to flex the forearm toward the upper arm. It also contracts secondarily to supinate the forearm bones, which means to turn the hand so the palm is facing forward when your arm is down at your side. No other type of arm articulation is permitted by the structure and function of your biceps muscles.

The function of each major skeletal muscle group is called its *kinesiology*. You will find a comprehensive chart of the kinesiology of your major muscle groups in the chart on page 26.

MUSCLE CONTRACTION

Skeletal muscles are made up of thousands of muscle fibers, and each fiber consists of many

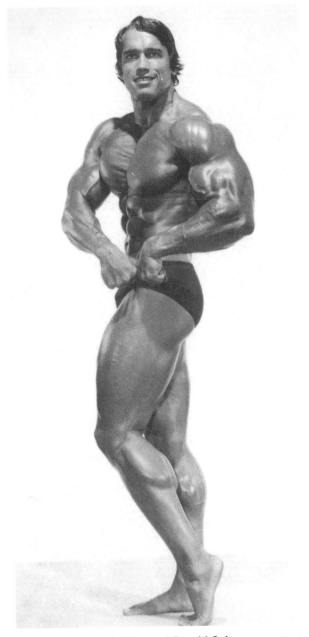

Surface anatomy to the max! Arnold Schwarzenegger illustrates how to bring out every major muscle group and minor striation in a concentrated side-chest pose.

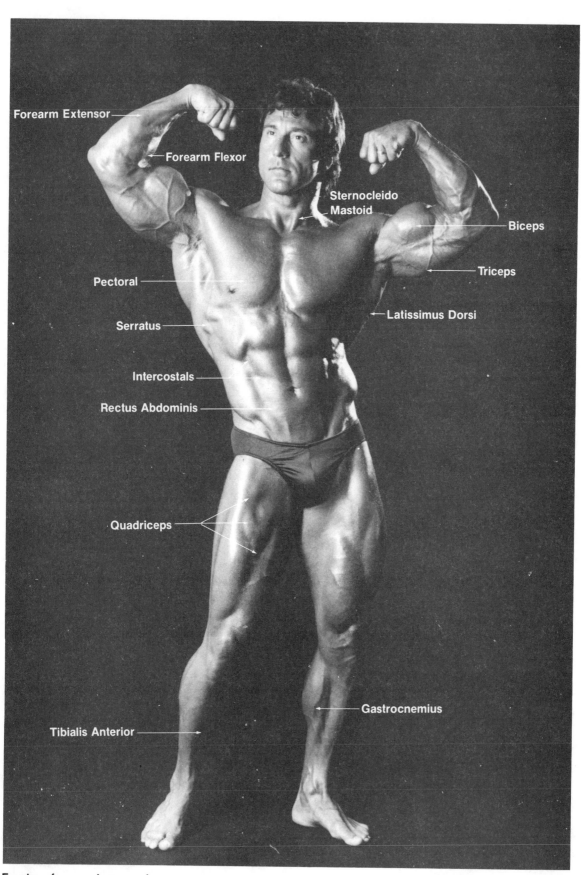

Front surface anatomy as demonstrated by Frank Zane.

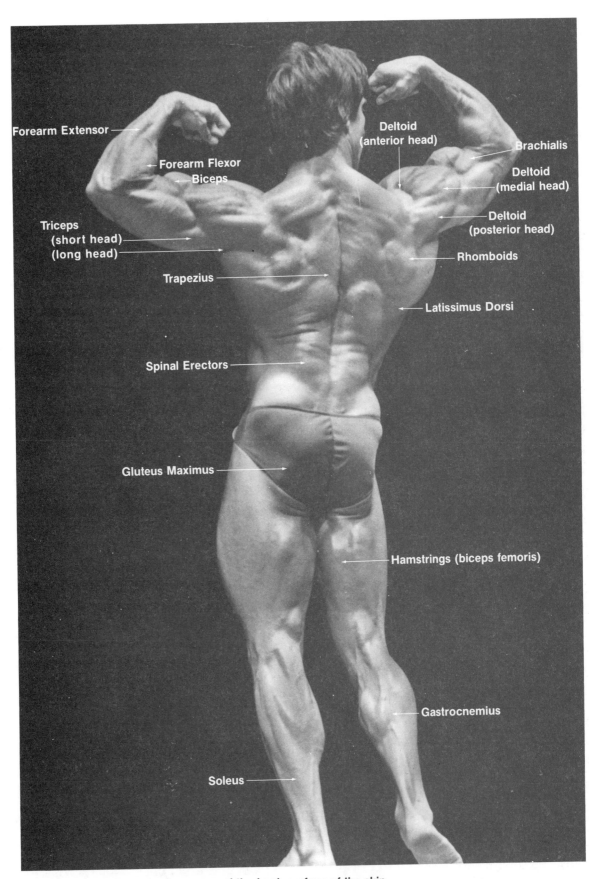

Forearm Extensor

Forearm Flexor
Biceps

Triceps
(short head)
(long head)

Trapezius

Spinal Erectors

Gluteus Maximus

Deltoid
(anterior head)

Brachialis

Deltoid
(medial head)

Deltoid
(posterior head)

Rhomboids

Latissimus Dorsi

Hamstrings (biceps femoris)

Gastrocnemius

Soleus

Zane displays various muscle groups of the back surface of the skin.

KINESIOLOGY OF MAJOR MUSCLE GROUPS

Muscle Group	Function
Neck muscles	Flex neck in every direction; rotate head
Trapezius	Pulls shoulders upward and backward
Latissimus dorsi	Pulls upper arms' bones downward and backward; helps to arch upper back
Erector spinae	Straightens spine from a position with torso flexed completely forward; helps to arch lower and middle back
Deltoids	Help to raise upper arm bone out to the side; help to raise upper arm bone forward; help to raise upper arm bone toward the rear
Pectorals	Help to move upper arm bones forward and across each other in front of the body
Biceps	Flexes arm; supinates hand
Brachialis	Flexes arm with hand in pronate position (facing the floor when forearm is parallel to the floor)
Triceps	Straightens arm from a fully flexed position; helps to raise upper arm bone to the rear
Forearm muscles	Flex wrist in different directions; impart rotational force to hand
Rectus abdominis	Helps to flex torso forward at the waist; helps to force shoulders toward hips when torso is arched slightly forward
External obliques	Help to flex torso from side to side at the waist; help to twist torso in relation to hips
Intercostals	Help to flex torso forward at waist; help to bend torso to each side; help to twist torso in relation to hips
Quadriceps	Help to straighten leg from a fully bent position
Buttocks	Help to extend upper leg bone in relation to spine
Hip flexors	Help to flex upper leg bone in relation to hip
Biceps femoris	Helps to flex leg completely at the knee
Soleus	Helps to extend foot when leg is bent at more than a 30-degree angle
Gastrocnemius	Helps to extend foot when leg is straight at the knee
Tibialis anterior	Helps to flex foot in relation to shin bone

muscle cells strung end to end. When a muscle fiber contracts—shortens in length—it follows a principle called "all or nothing." This means that each individual muscle cell either contracts completely or does not contract at all. And it is crucial to understand that using maximum weights ensures that a maximum number of individual muscle cells is contracted.

This brings us to the most fundamental of all training principles, the Weider Overload Training Principle. The overload principle says that a muscle responds by growing in hypertrophy after it is stressed with a load greater than it is used to handling. And by progres-

sively increasing resistance overload on the muscle, you can continue to cause it to grow in mass and strength.

To induce a skeletal muscle to continue to grow in mass and strength, you must use a procedure called *resistance progression*. In progression of resistance you are required to gradually increase the number of repetitions done in an exercise from a "lower guide number" to the "upper guide number." When the upper guide number is reached, 5–10 pounds are added to the bar, reps are reduced to the lower guide number, and the process is repeated.

Assuming that you are required to do one set of 8–12 repetitions of a bench press movement, you will find an example of four weeks of progression for the movement in the figure below. In this example, "50 × 8" means to do 8 repetitions with 50 pounds.

EXAMPLE OF SIMPLE PROGRESSION

Week	Mon	Wed	Fri
One	50 × 8	50 × 9	50 × 10
Two	50 × 11	50 × 12	55 × 8
Three	55 × 9	55 × 10	55 × 10
Four	55 × 11	55 × 12	60 × 8

In most cases you will work your progression procedure on multiple sets of each movement. In this case you must ultimately reach the upper guide number for reps on each set before increasing the weight and dropping the reps back to the lower guide number. In the chart below you will find a model for four weeks of progression on three sets of 8-12 repetitions in barbell bent rows.

Lee Haney (three-time Mr. Olympia) says, "The key to building massive, powerful muscles is to doggedly increase the training weights you use. But it is only good to increase training poundages if you do so in perfect form. Cheating to increase training poundages is a dead end. There is a direct correlation between the amount of weight you use with perfect biomechanics in an exercise and the mass of the muscles that move that weight. Keep this firmly in mind throughout your bodybuilding involvement, and you will ultimately develop a massive and powerful physique that will win many titles for you!"

EXAMPLE OF COMPLEX PROGRESSION

Week	Mon	Wed	Fri
One	60 × 8	60 × 9	60 × 10
	60 × 8	60 × 8	60 × 9
	60 × 8	60 × 8	60 × 8
Two	60 × 11	60 × 12	60 × 12
	60 × 9	60 × 11	60 × 12
	60 × 9	60 × 9	60 × 11
Three	60 × 12	65 × 8	65 × 9
	60 × 12	65 × 8	65 × 8
	60 × 12	65 × 8	65 × 8
Four	65 × 10	65 × 11	65 × 12
	65 × 9	65 × 10	65 × 10
	65 × 8	65 × 9	65 × 9

4
Bodybuilding Safety and Warm-Up Procedures

As long as you follow several well-recognized safety rules, bodybuilding will be a very safe physical activity for you. But the editors of my two muscle magazines, *Muscle & Fitness* and *Flex*, receive reports of serious injuries in the sport each week. Consider these recent examples:

- A Florida bodybuilder squatting without collars on the ends of his Olympic bar seriously wrenches his lower back when one end of the bar dips, the weights on that end slide off, and the heavy end of the bar then whips violently downward.
- A California bodybuilder tears his left pectoral muscle completely loose when he uses too heavy a weight in the bench press without sufficient warm-up.
- A Pennsylvania bodybuilder suffers a deep cut on his cheek when he trips over a dumbbell lying on the floor as he walks to the gym water fountain for a drink.
- A New York bodybuilder suffers a permanent lower-back injury when he loses his balance doing a set of military presses while bending backward, a classic example of poor exercise form.

I have received documented reports of two recent deaths. In both cases relatively experienced bodybuilders were killed when performing limit bench presses alone in basement or garage home gyms without spotters. Apparently each man fainted as a result of holding his breath during a heavy effort, and the bar crashed down across his neck.

If it is possible either to seriously injure yourself or to end up dead, you should master all of the safety rules that will protect you in the gym. There are 12 commonly accepted safety procedures.

Rule 1. Always warm up thoroughly before you begin to work out with heavy weights. A warm-up will prepare your muscles and joints for heavy exercise that could injure you if you did a set cold. A thorough warm-up will also improve your coordination as you train, preventing you from unwittingly assuming poor exercise form as you do each set. The vast majority of bodybuilding injuries are related directly to nonexistent or incomplete warm-ups.

Rule 2. Avoid training in an overcrowded gym. Once you are thoroughly warmed up, you must remain warm by wearing appropriate clothing (enough to retain body heat if the gym is too cool) and resting no more than two or three minutes between sets. To avoid excessive rest intervals between sets you should train in a gym only when you have timely access to equipment. When too many people are working out with you, you will probably be forced to stand in line for a piece of equipment, which will allow your body to cool off. Then you will be susceptible to injury.

Rule 3. Always use proper exercise form. The second most common cause of injury is use of improper biomechanics (exercise form). Be sure that you precisely interpret the written and photographic descriptions of each exercise presented in this book. Correct biomechanics are the only kind I will teach you, so be sure you learn to do the exercises correctly and then always seek to perform them perfectly. If you feel that you might not be doing the movements correctly, be sure to ask an experienced bodybuilder to monitor your workout form.

Rule 4. Always train with competent supervision. The best way to avoid adopting incorrect

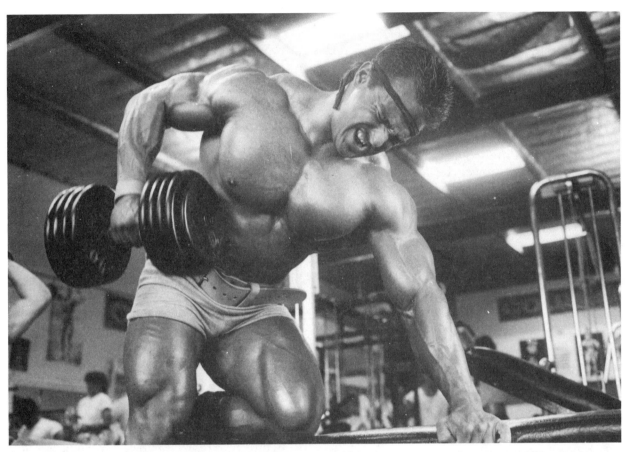

Young Shane DiMora, who won the National Middleweight Championship at the tender age of 19, has paid his dues with plenty of sets of heavy One-Arm Dumbbell Bent Rows. Shane's back is particularly well developed and has taken him far in the sport in a very short time.

biomechanics in your exercises is to train in a gym with an instructor available at all times. There are also many other mistakes you might make in your workouts, all of which can be caught and corrected by a good gym instructor. In the absence of an instructor, try to find an experienced bodybuilder who is willing to keep an eye on you.

Rule 5. Obtain as much bodybuilding knowledge as you can assimilate. The more you know about your sport, the less your chance of inadvertently doing something that can cause you harm. Read every issue of *Flex* and *Muscle & Fitness* from cover to cover and purchase and read as many bodybuilding books as you can afford. You'll no doubt read about some bodybuilding topics over and over, but in the long run such repetition will make the sport much safer for you.

Rule 6. Never work out alone. Most serious injuries happen when you are working out alone, usually in your home gym. The presence of spotters when you are lifting maximum weights is essential (see rule 7), so at a minimum you should grab a family member to keep you company and give you safety spots from time to time.

Rule 7. Always use spotters when lifting maximum weights. Spotters should be standing by to rescue you whenever you fail with a heavy weight in a basic movement. This is particularly crucial when you are doing bench presses and squats. It is best to have one spotter at each end of the bar when you do these movements with maximum poundages, but you can use one-person spots on each movement. When you are doing benches, the spotter should stand at the head end of the bench with his hands in the middle of the bar; when you get stuck, he can merely pull up on the weight to help you place the barbell back on the bench rack. With squats he can stand directly behind you and deadlift the weight off your shoulders if you get stuck in the bottom position.

Rule 8. Use catch racks when doing squats and bench presses. If you don't have catch racks on which to rest the barbell, it is difficult to do squats or benches with maximum weights. It's much easier to have a spotter help you lift the weight from the rack than it is for one or two spotters to help you get the barbell into position for either movement. Many gyms also have pressing benches and squat racks with safety pins in the low position of the movement. With these safety pins you can put the weight on them to rest if you are unable to complete a full repetition.

Rule 9. Always use collars on the ends of your barbells. This is probably the one safety rule most abused in large bodybuilding gyms. Because the weights on an Olympia bar must be changed frequently, bodybuilders tend to leave the collars off the bar. But this is inviting trouble if you happen to extend your arms unevenly or otherwise allow one end of the barbell to dip below the other end as you are doing an exercise. When one end is lower, the weights can easily slide off, causing a vicious whipping action of the bar. This can, in turn, injure your lower back, knee, ankle, shoulder, elbow, or wrist.

Rule 10. Never hold your breath when you are doing a heavy repetition. Holding your breath can cause a Valsalva effect, or an impedance of blood flow to and from the brain. This can, in turn, cause you to black out briefly. Do I need to paint you a picture of what might happen then if you have a heavy barbell pressed halfway out in a bench press repetition? And if you happen to pass out while in a standing position, you can fall and hit your head on the floor or a piece of equipment.

Rule 11. Use a weightlifting belt when doing heavy movements. A weightlifting belt supports your lower back and abdomen, thereby preventing injuries to the middle of your body. It is particularly necessary to use a weightlifting belt when doing squats, heavy overhead pressing movements, or any type of deadlift or rowing motion.

Rule 12. Always maintain good gym housekeeping. Many injuries occur when someone fails to see a loose weight lying on the gym floor and either trips over it or stumbles over it when he loses balance while doing a heavy set of some standing movement. All barbells and dumbbells should be replaced in proper racks or storage areas when you have finished your set with them. Loose plates and other pieces of equipment should also be placed in proper storage areas when not in use.

If you carefully follow the 12 safety rules presented in this chapter, you will have many years of injury-free training ahead of you. You will even be able to avoid microtraumas of your joints, which eventually lead to joint pain in many bodybuilders. And when you are totally pain-free, you will always have hard, productive workouts, which in the end will help you develop the body you want.

WARMING UP FOR A BODYBUILDING WORKOUT

Bodybuilding training with weights is a much more intense physical activity than anything you've ever done before. Since you will be lifting very heavy weights at times in your bodybuilding workouts, there is increased potential for injury. Therefore, it is essential that you warm up thoroughly prior to every heavy training session. Indeed, you should consider a proper warm-up to be an integral part of every bodybuilding workout.

The primary function of a preworkout warm-up is to prevent training injuries that might happen if you attempt to hoist heavy weights while cold. A warm-up decreases the resistance of tissues in the muscles and joints by lubricating them where they fit together. This in turn increases the effective range of motion of each body joint.

A thorough preworkout warm-up also prevents injury by increasing blood circulation through the muscles and connective tissues and augments the supply of oxygen available to the working muscles during a heavy training session. All of this means you can actually lift much heavier weights in your workouts once

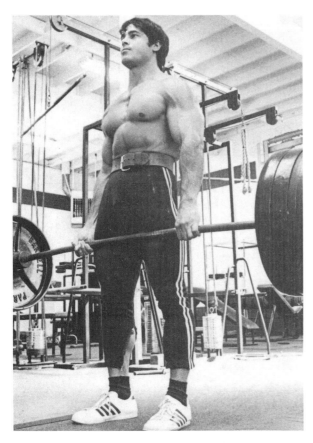

Dr. Franco Columbo, two-time Mr. Olympia winner, owed much of his sensational back development to his power as a deadlifter. He's done 10 reps with 720 pounds at a body weight of only about 190 pounds.

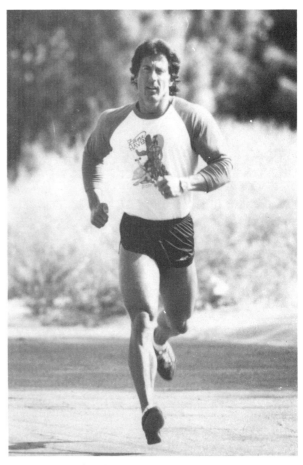

Running is not a method for warming up unless preceded by appropriate stretching exercises.

you're fully warmed up than is possible with a cold skeletal muscle system.

The final way in which a warm-up prevents injury is by improving neuromuscular coordination. This means it is much easier to move a heavy weight through the correct arc to prevent injuries once it is warmed up optimally. By far, the majority of muscle and joint injuries while training with weights occur when a bodybuilder attempts to lift a heavy barbell with incorrect biomechanics while the body either is insufficiently warmed up or has been allowed to cool off during a workout.

There is also a psychological benefit attendant to a proper warm-up. When you warm up correctly, you prepare yourself psychologically to lift maximum weights in your bodybuilding workout. If you have assuaged any fear of injury when training heavily, it is much easier to lift maximum weights.

WARM-UP PROCEDURES

You should combine work with light weights and three types of nonresistance work in your warm-up. The best nonweight warm-up exercises include aerobic exercise movements, stretching exercises, and free-hand calisthenics.

Recent research has demonstrated that it is possible to injure muscles and connective tissues by stretching cold muscles and joints. Therefore, each warm-up should commence with light aerobics, usually jogging in place or skipping rope, starting with slow, short movements and then gradually accelerating the leg movements and increasing range of arm/leg articulation.

After 3–5 minutes of gradually more intense aerobics, you should be breathing a little more heavily. Follow up on the aerobics with a combination of stretching and free-hand exercise to form the core of your nonresistance warm-up. The exercises I suggest using are illustrated and described in this chapter.

Only after a 10- to 15-minute nonweight warm-up should you turn to the weights to finish up your complete warm-up. Each time you start training a body part, you should do your first one or two basic exercises for at least one light, high-rep set as part of your warm-up.

Let's say you are about to do a full chest workout. You should begin it with bench presses, starting with about 40% of your maximum effort for 15-20 repetitions. Successive warm-up sets should include about 15 reps with 60%, 12 reps with 70%, and 10 reps with 75% to conclude the resistance part of your warm-up. This weight work will completely prepare your chest, shoulder, and arm muscles for a heavy chest workout. It also completely warms up the shoulder, elbow, and wrist joints for the heavy work to follow.

You will frequently be tempted to cut your warm-up short or completely avoid doing it when you get to the gym late and have only a limited amount of time for your heavy training session. Never miss doing your warm-up, however, because doing so will leave you open to training injuries. If nothing else, going heavy without thoroughly warming up will cause microtraumas to your joints, which will eventually result in the chronic sore joints that plague some bodybuilders late in their careers.

YOUR WARM-UP EXERCISES

The following exercises will help you warm up your muscles and joints before a heavy weight workout. Perform them in the sequence listed, resting minimally between movements. Hold stretching exercises for 60–120 seconds in the stretched position and do 20–30 repetitions of each of the calisthenics movements. Should you not feel completely warmed up after going through the series of exercises one time, don't hesitate to do another circuit of movements.

At the end of a proper warm-up you should feel ready to take on the world. Your breathing should be accelerated, and you should have broken into a sweat. You will be both physically and psychologically prepared to use maximum poundages in all of your bodybuilding movements.

Jumping Jacks

Start with your feet together and your arms down at your sides. Bend your knees a few degrees and suddenly straighten them to leap about 6–8 inches off the floor. As you leap from the floor, you should simultaneously spread your legs to go about shoulder width and raise your arms directly out to the sides and upward until your hands touch directly above your head as your feet again contact the floor. Bend your knees to absorb the shock of landing, then jump off the floor again and return to the starting position, again bending your knees to absorb the shock of landing. Continue rhythmically for 25-30 repetitions. This is a good full-body warm-up.

Alternate Toe Touches

Stand erect with your feet spread about six inches wider than your shoulders. Keep your legs straight throughout the movement. Extend your arms directly out to the sides, parallel to the floor, and keep them straight throughout the movement. Bend forward and twist your torso toward the left to touch your right hand to your left foot. Return to the starting point and repeat the movement to the opposite side. Continue the movement rhythmically until you have performed 20–25 repetitions to each side. This is a good warm-up for the back, buttock, and hamstring muscles.

Free-Hand Squats

Stand with your feet set about shoulder width apart, your toes angled slightly outward. Place your hands on your hips and hold your arms akimbo. Keep your torso in as vertical a position as possible while slowly sinking into a full squatting position. Slowly return to the starting point. (Alternatively, you can start with your arms straight down at your sides and raise them forward up to shoulder level as you sink into each squat repetition, returning them to your sides as you extend your legs and stand erect to finish the movement.) Do 20–25 repetitions of the exercise. This is a good warm-up for the quadriceps, hamstring, and buttock muscles.

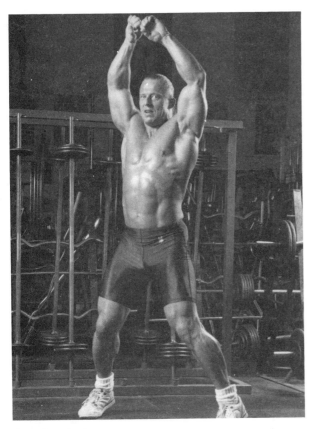

Jumping Jacks
Model: Andreas Cahling

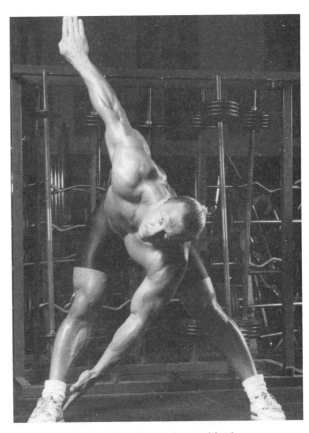

Alternate Toe Touches (opposite position)

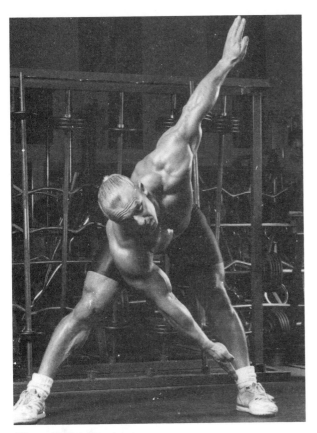

Alternate Toe Touches

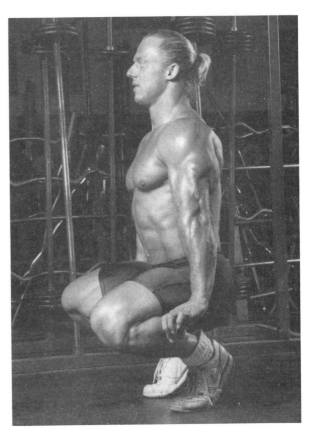

Free-Hand Squats

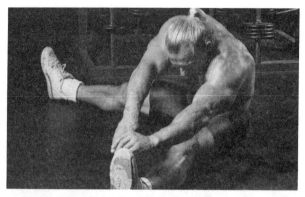

Seated V Stretches (variation reaching toward one leg at a time)

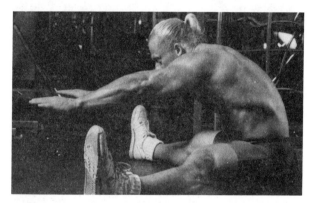

Seated V Stretches (variation stretching directly forward)

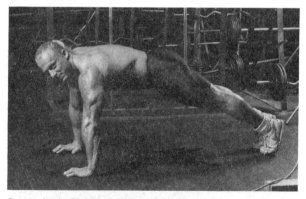

Swan Arch Stretches (initial position)

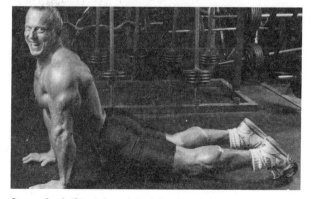

Swan Arch Stretches (stretched position)

Seated V Stretches

Sit on the gym floor and spread your legs so they are at a 90-degree angle to each other as you sit on the floor. Hold your legs straight throughout the movement. Keeping your spine as flat as possible, slowly bend forward until you begin to feel a slightly painful stretching sensation in your hamstrings. Ideally, you will bend forward until you actually rest your torso on the floor between your legs, but this degree of body articulation demands terrific leg, hip, and back flexibility. Once you feel the stretching sensation, back off slightly until it stops, then hold the stretched position for one to two minutes. Be careful not to hold the painfully stretched position since this not only can cause tiny tears in the muscles and connective tissue but also does *not* increase flexibility. This stretching exercise helps to warm up and stretch the hamstrings, groin, spinal erectors, other back muscles, and the buttocks.

Swan Arch Torso Stretches

Assume the starting position for push-ups, in which your weight is supported on your toes and hands with your arms held straight, your hands set about shoulder width apart and fingers pointing forward, and your torso straight as illustrated. Keeping your arms and legs straight, slowly lower your hips toward the floor until you feel the slightly painful stretching sensation in the muscles on the front of your torso, particularly the frontal abdominals. Back off a degree from this painful position and hold the stretching posture for one to two minutes. This stretching exercise warms up and stretches the frontal torso muscles and hip flexor muscles.

Towel Dislocation

Set your feet a comfortable distance apart and stand erect with your hands grasping the ends of a towel. Keep your arms straight throughout the movement and maintain tension on the towel so it is straight throughout the movement. Standing erect, slowly raise your hands forward and upward in a semicircular arc. As the towel passes over your head, continue the movement backward and downward in a continuation of

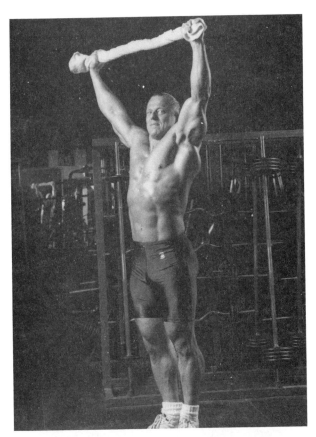

Towel Dislocation (for shoulder mobility—start)

the same circular arc, "dislocating" your shoulders so you can complete the movement, rotating your hands downward until the towel touches your back. Reverse the movement to return to the starting point. Repeat the movement for 5–10 full repetitions. This is a good warm-up exercise for all of the muscles surrounding your shoulder girdle, including the pectorals, deltoids, trapezius muscles, latissimus dorsi muscles, and biceps.

Push-Ups

Assume the starting position as illustrated. Both your feet and your hands should be set about shoulder width apart, with your fingers pointing forward. Your torso and legs should be held straight throughout the movement so they maintain one long, straight line as you perform the exercise. Your arms should be straight at the start of the movement. Allowing your elbows to travel toward the rear, slowly bend them and lower your chest until it lightly touches the floor. Immediately extend your arms to return to the starting position. Repeat the movement for as many repetitions as are comfortably possible. This is a good warm-up exercise for the pectorals, deltoids, triceps, and those upper back muscles that impart rotational force to your shoulder blades.

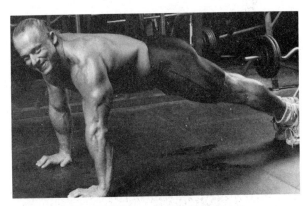

Push-Ups (start/finish)

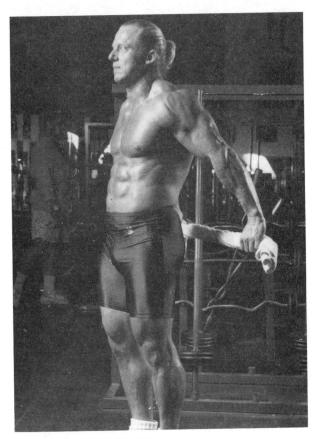

Towel Dislocation (finish)

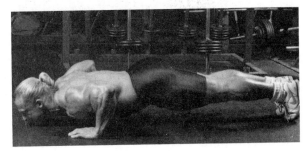

Push-Ups (midpoint)

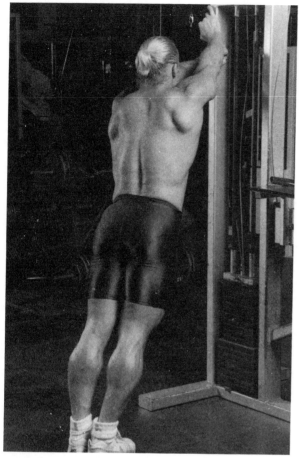

Calf Stretch (to stretch calves, progressively move feet farther from the wall while keeping legs held straight)

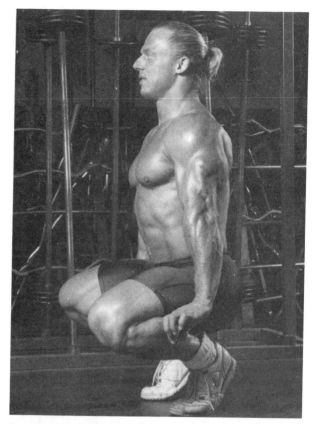

Squat Jump (start)

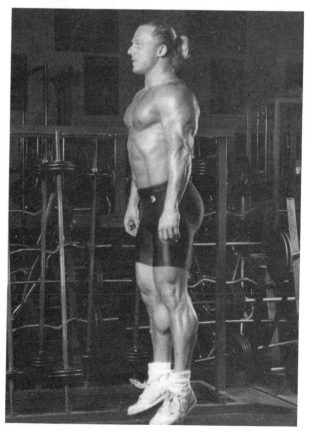

Squat Jump (midair)

Calf Stretches

Stand facing the gym wall, your feet about shoulder width apart about 2½ feet away from the wall. Lean forward and place your hands on the wall at about shoulder level. Your hands should be about shoulder width apart, with fingers pointing toward the ceiling. Keeping your arms, legs, and torso straight, lean forward. If you can comfortably press your heels flat on the floor in this position, walk a few more inches away from the wall and repeat the procedure. When you can just place your heels on the floor without feeling a painful stretching sensation in your calf muscles, hold this position for one or two minutes. You can also stretch your calves in a similar position one leg at a time, bending the nonstretching leg a bit to help you lean into the movement. This is the premier exercise for stretching and warming up the calf muscles.

Squat Jumps

Set your feet about shoulder width apart, your toes angled slightly outward. Your arms should be straight down at your sides at the start of the movement. Simultaneously bend your legs about 45 degrees and raise your arms forward until they are parallel to the gym floor. When you reach the bottom position of the movement, explosively snap your arms back down to your sides and forcefully straighten your legs to leap a few inches off the floor. Return to the starting position, bending your knees to absorb the shock of landing, and immediately continue the movement by bending your knees until they are again at about a 45-degree angle. Rhythmically continue the movement until you have completed 25–30 repetitions. This is an excellent full-body warm-up but is particularly good for warming up the calves, thighs, hamstrings, buttocks, lower back, and deltoids.

Thigh Stretches

Stand next to an incline bench or vertical upright. Grasp this solid object with your left hand to balance yourself as you do the stretching exercise. Reach to the rear and downward to grasp your right toe with your right hand, your leg fully bent. Pull upward on the toe until you feel a slight stretching sensation in the quadriceps muscles at the front of your thigh. Hold this stretched position for 1–2 min-

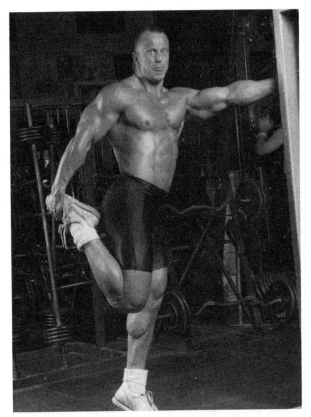

Thigh Stretch (do an equal amount of stretching for each leg; for a more intense stretch, pull up on foot)

utes. Repeat the exercise for the same length of time stretching the quads of your left leg, balancing yourself by grasping the object with your right hand. This is a good exercise for stretching and warming up the quadriceps muscles at the front of your thighs.

5
Beginning
Exercises and Routines

You will find 25 basic bodybuilding exercises fully described and precisely illustrated in this chapter. It is vitally important to learn these movements perfectly because they will form the basis of all of your workouts for the rest of your years in the sport. You will be using many of these exact movements, plus even more variations on the basic exercises. Learning how to do them incorrectly can be dangerous enough to cause you injury in a workout. And if you fail to do the movements with perfect form, you won't get as much out of the exercises as you should.

All of the many exercise descriptions in this book are described with correct biomechanics. And using the descriptions and exercise photos, you can learn each movement perfectly on your own, without additional coaching. Still, you will benefit from having an experienced bodybuilder check out your form if one of these men or women is available to you.

The first step in learning an exercise is to read the exercise description through two or three times while carefully analyzing the illustrations. Then you should do the movements without anything heavier than a broomstick in your hands, preferably in front of a mirror in which you can actually *see* yourself doing the exercise. This should give you a good feel for how you will articulate your arms and/or legs in the exercise.

Once you have the coordination of the movement down, you should begin to use a very light weight for the exercise. Gradually work the poundage upward until it is high enough to require at least a small degree of exertion to accomplish 8–10 repetitions. Within a couple of weeks you should be able to do the movement automatically, without thinking about how you have to move your body on each repetition.

ABDOMINAL EXERCISES
Sit-Ups

Emphasis—This is the most basic of front abdominal movements. It stresses the rectus abdominis muscle wall, particularly the upper half of the muscle group. When performed twisting, sit-ups also place intense emphasis on the intercostal muscles. Still, sit-ups are not the best isolation movement for the rectus abdomi-

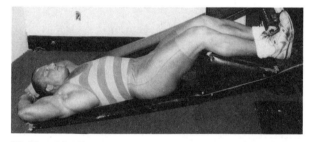

Sit-Ups (start)

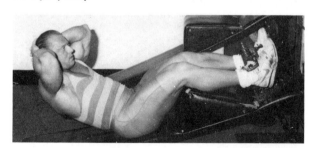

Sit-Ups (about halfway up)

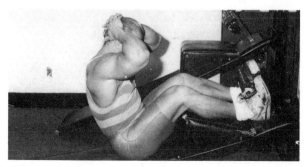

Sit-Ups (finish)

nis since the hip flexor muscles also contract powerfully to help you sit erect. The best isolation movement for the frontal abs is crunches.

Starting Position—Lie on your back on the floor or a flat abdominal board. Hook your feet under a heavy piece of furniture or the roller pads/loop of webbing at the end of the abdominal board. Alternatively, you can have a training partner hold your ankles to restrain your feet during your set. Place your hands behind your head and keep them there throughout the movement. You should also bend your legs about 30 degrees and hold them bent like this throughout your set.

Movement Performance—Use abdominal strength to slowly curl your torso upward, lifting first your head, then your shoulders, upper back, and lower back, until you are sitting erect. Reverse the process to slowly return to the starting point. Repeat the movement.

Common Mistakes—Never do sit-ups straight-legged, because doing so places an unnecessary strain on your lower back. You should also avoid sitting upward with a jerk.

Training Tips—Intensity can be added to the movement by holding a barbell plate behind your head and/or by incrementally raising the foot end of the abdominal board. You can also do twisting sit-ups, alternately twisting to one side and the other, touching each elbow in turn to the opposite knee.

Leg Raises

Emphasis—Leg raises also stress the rectus abdominis, particularly the lower half of the frontal abdominal wall. Significant stress is also borne by the hip flexors.

Starting Position—Lie on your back on the floor or an abdominal board, your head toward the end where your feet were for sets of sit-ups. Grasp a heavy piece of furniture or the abdominal board restraint to keep your torso motionless as you do your set. You should also bend your legs 20–30 degrees and keep them bent throughout your set in order to keep harmful strain off your lower back.

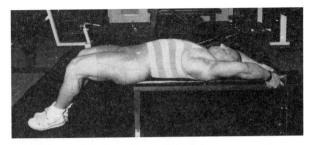

Leg Raises (bench variation, which allows a longer range of motion—start)

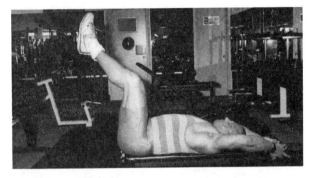

Leg Raises (finish)

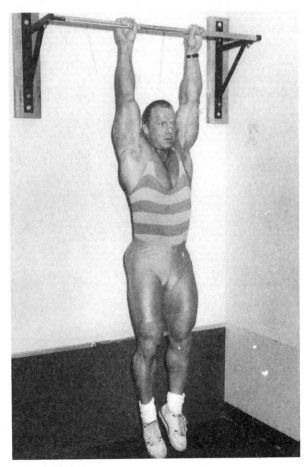

Hanging Leg Raises (variation on normal Leg Raises—start)

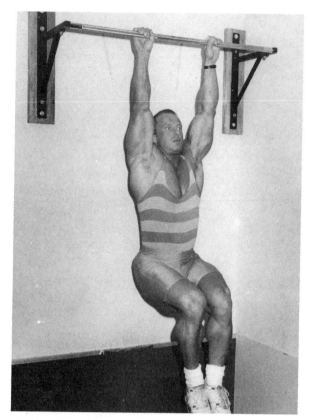

Hanging Leg Raises (about at midpoint)

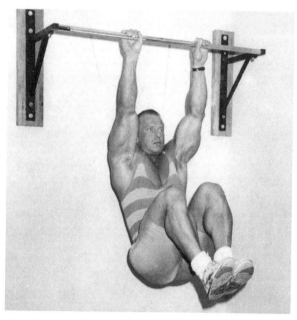

Hanging Leg Raises (finish)

Movement Performance—Use anterior abdominal strength to slowly raise your legs from the floor or abdominal board, moving your feet upward and to the rear in a semicircular arc until your feet are directly above your hips. Slowly return to the starting point and repeat the movement.

Common Mistakes—Don't bounce your feet from the floor/board and avoid holding your legs straight as you perform your leg raises.

Training Tips—You can increase intensity on your abs by either wearing iron boots, holding a light dumbbell between your feet, or incrementally raising the head end of the abdominal board.

THIGH EXERCISES

Leg Press

Emphasis—This fundamental exercise powerfully stresses the quadriceps, buttocks, and hamstrings. It places such intense stress on the cardiorespiratory system that it is also good for burning body fat and hardening your physique for a competition.

Starting Position (Universal Gym)—Sit on the machine seat and place your feet on the lower set of pedals (if there are two sets). Grasp the handles at the sides of the seat and keep your torso erect. Slowly straighten your legs.

Starting Position (Vertical Machine)—Lie on your back with your shoulders at the lower end of the angled pad and your hips directly beneath the sliding platform of the machine. Place your feet on the platform with your heels about 12 inches apart and your toes angled slightly outward. Slowly straighten your legs and rotate the stop bars of the machine to release the sliding platform. (Be sure to relock the stop bars at the end of your set before exiting the machine.)

Starting Position (Angled Machine)—Sit in the machine with your back against the angled pad and your hips in the corner of the bench made by that back pad and the seat pad. Bend your legs and place your feet on the sliding platform, your heels about 12 inches apart and your toes angled slightly outward. Slowly straighten your legs and rotate the stop bars of the machine to release the sliding platform. (Be sure to relock the stop bars at the end of your set before exiting the machine.)

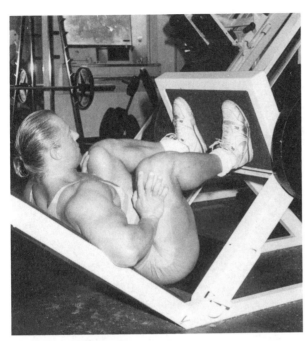

Leg Presses (45-degree angled machine—start)

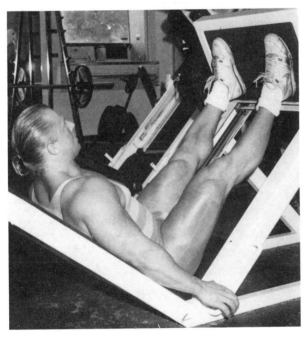

Leg Presses (finish)

Starting Position (Nautilus)—Sit in the machine and rest your back against the pad. Place your feet on the pedals. Slowly straighten your legs.

Movement Performance—Use thigh and buttock strength to resist the weight of the machine as you bend your legs fully. Without bouncing in this low point of the movement, slowly straighten your legs. Repeat the exercise.

Common Mistakes—Be careful not to hold your breath as you perform this movement; doing so will raise your blood pressure to dangerous levels. Never allow your shoulders to hunch forward in the middle of the movement, or you will place your spine in a very vulnerable position.

Training Tips—On both Nautilus and Universal Gym machines you can adjust the seat forward and backward. The closer it is to the pedals at the start of the movement, the longer the range of motion as you perform the exercise. On all variations of leg presses you should allow your knees to travel outward past the sides of your chest in the low position of the movement. Allowing your knees to press against your chest can cause you to black out in the middle of a set.

Squats

Emphasis—This is definitely the best lower-body exercise and probably the best single bodybuilding movement. It places very direct stress on the quadriceps, buttocks, lower back, and hamstrings. Such intense stress is placed on your entire cardiorespiratory system that squats actually improve your metabolism, making it anabolic.

Starting Position—Place a barbell on a squat rack and load it up for a heavy set of squats. Bend your legs and dip under the bar, positioning it across your shoulders. You should grasp the ends of the bar out near the plates to steady it in position for your set. Straighten your legs to lift the weight from the rack and step back one or two paces. Position your feet about shoulder width apart, your toes angled slightly outward. Tense your back muscles to keep your torso rigid as you do the movement. You should also focus your eyes on a spot at head level in order to keep your head up as you perform each repetition.

Movement Performance—Keeping your torso as erect as possible, slowly bend your legs, allowing your knees to travel outward over your toes. Slowly squat down until you are in a full squatting position. Without bouncing at the bottom of the movement, slowly stand erect. Repeat the movement.

Common Mistakes—One of the most common errors is to allow your torso to incline forward, which shifts major stress from your quads to buttocks and places your lower back in a vulnerable position. Bouncing in the bottom position of the movement can seriously injure your knees.

Training Tips—You can also do partial squats, one-quarter, one-half, or three-quarters of the way down. You can do bench squats in which you straddle a flat exercise bench and squat down until your buttocks lightly contact the bench. And you can do parallel squats in which you sink downward until your thighs are parallel to the floor. In all squat variations you can elevate your heels by placing them on a 2 × 4-inch board as you do the exercise; this improves balance a bit for some bodybuilders. You can also wear a lifting belt cinched tightly around your waist to reinforce your midsection and prevent abdominal and/or lower back injuries. If the bar cuts into your neck or upper back, pad it by rolling a towel around the bar.

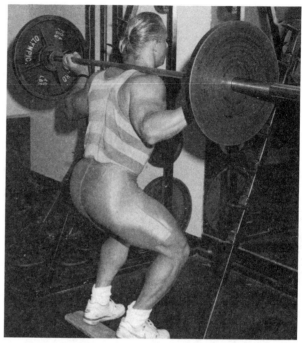

Squat (partway up or down)

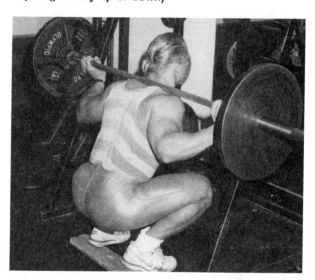

Squat (bottom position)

Leg Extensions

Emphasis—This excellent movement virtually isolates stress entirely on the quadriceps muscles at the front of your thighs.

Starting Position—This movement can be performed on a wide variety of machines, but the starting position and exercise performance are identical, regardless of the machine used. Sit in the machine with the backs of your knees against the edge of the machine pad nearest the lever arm. Hook your insteps under the lower

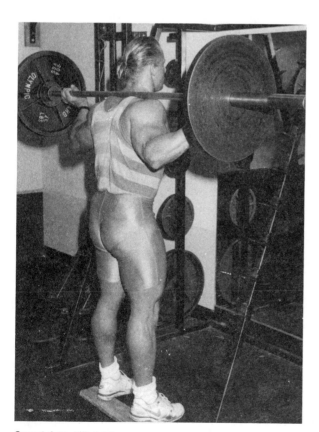

Squat (start/finish)

set of roller pads (if there are two sets). Incline your back against the back board if there is one on the machine. Grasp either the sides of the padded seat or the handles provided to steady your torso as you do the movement.

Movement Performance—Slowly straighten your legs. Hold the top, peak-contracted position of the movement for a slow count of two, then slowly lower back to the starting point. Repeat the exercise.

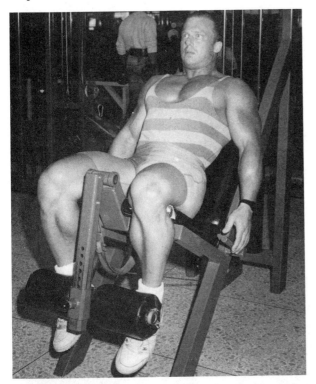

Leg Extensions (start)

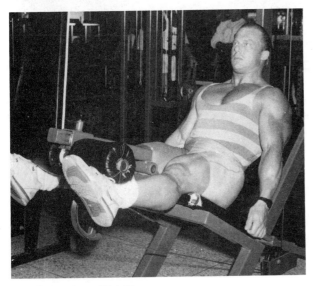

Leg Extensions (finish)

Common Mistakes—You won't get as much out of the movement if you fail to completely straighten your legs on each repetition. Do the movement relatively slowly in order to prevent momentum from robbing your working quadriceps muscles of some of the stress they should be working against.

Training Tips—You can also do this movement with one leg at a time. Doing exercises for your legs or arms with one limb at a time allows you to place much more intense mental focus on the muscles involved, which allows significantly more development of the working muscles.

Leg Curls

Emphasis—Leg curls are the best isolation movement for the biceps femoris (hamstrings) muscles at the back of your thighs.

Starting Position—This movement can be performed on a variety of exercise machines, but the starting position and exercise performance are identical for each machine. Lie facedown on the padded surface of the machine with your knees near the edge of the pad toward the lever arm. Hook the backs of your heels under the upper set of roller pads (if there are two sets). Straighten your legs fully. Grasp either the sides of the padded bench or the handles provided to keep your torso restrained as you do your set.

Movement Performance—Use biceps femoris strength to flex your legs and move your feet in a semicircular arc upward and forward until your legs are bent as completely as possible. Hold this top, peak-contracted position for a slow count of two, then slowly lower your legs back to the starting point. Repeat the movement.

Common Mistakes—If you allow your hips to rise off the bench surface, you will shorten the range of motion of this exercise, so keep your hips pressed against the pad at all times. You should also avoid partial movements when you do leg curls.

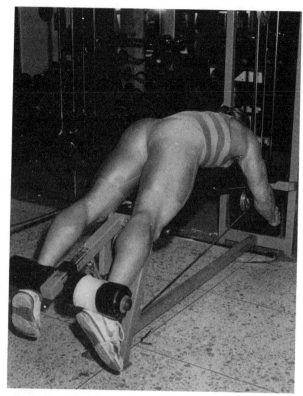

Leg Curls (start)

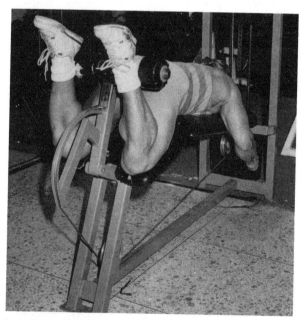

Leg Curls (finish)

Training Tips—You can also do leg curls with one leg at a time, which intensifies the contraction in your working muscles. As you read further in this book you will discover that there is also a standing variation of leg curls in which you use one leg at a time to do the movement.

BACK EXERCISES
Deadlifts

Emphasis—This is the most fundamental back exercise. It powerfully stresses the buttocks, spinal erectors, upper back muscles, quadriceps, and forearm flexor muscles. Significant secondary stress is placed on the latissimus dorsi and posterior deltoid muscles.

Starting Position—Load up a heavy barbell that is lying on the gym floor. Step up to the bar and place your feet about shoulder width apart, your toes pointing relatively straight ahead. Bend your legs and flatten your back, keeping your arms straight as well, so your hips are above your knees and your shoulders are above the level of your hips. Roll the bar toward your body so it touches your shins. Take a shoulder-width grip on the barbell handle. This is the fundamental pulling position you should adopt whenever you are lifting a weight from the floor, so study it closely in the photo to be sure you have it right.

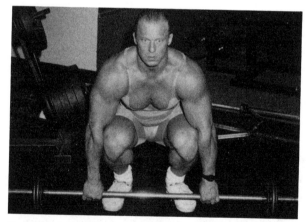

Deadlift (start—note position with butt low and back flat at the beginning of the lift)

Movement Performance—Keeping your arms straight throughout the movement, slowly lift the barbell from the floor to a position across your upper thighs by first straightening your legs, then following through by also straightening your torso in relation to your upper legs. Pull your shoulders back in the finish position of the exercise. Reverse this procedure to slowly return the barbell to the floor. Repeat the movement.

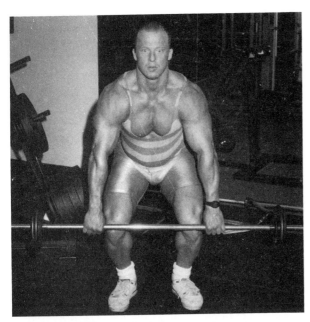

Deadlift (part way up or down)

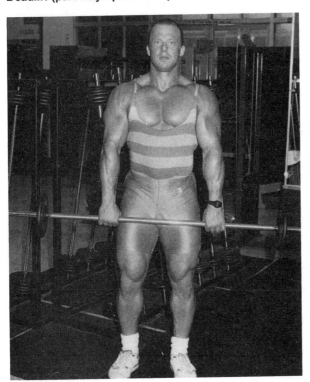

Deadlift (finish)

Common Mistakes—You will place your lower back in a vulnerable position if you allow your hips to come up so quickly that your shoulders pitch forward. Never attempt to jerk the bar from the floor or bounce the weight off the floor.

Training Tips—If you have difficulty grasping the bar with maximum poundages, you can

either reverse your grip (turn one hand so your palm is forward while the palm of your other hand faces the rear) or reinforce your grip with straps. You can also do top deadlifts in which you pull the bar from a rack set so the weight is a bit above knee level at the start of the movement. This is a favorite exercise of Frank Zane.

Barbell Bent Rows

Emphasis—This is an excellent movement for stressing virtually all of the back muscles. Particular stress is placed on the latissimus dorsi muscles, anterior deltoids, biceps, and forearm flexors. Strong secondary stress is on the trapezius muscles, spinal erectors, and teres major muscles. Most top bodybuilders do various types of barbell, dumbbell, and cable rows to build thickness in the lats.

Starting Position—Place a barbell on the floor of the gym, set your feet about shoulder width apart, angle your toes slightly outward, and take a shoulder-width overgrip on the bar (with your palms facing the rear). Straighten your arms and bend your legs slightly. Flatten your back and raise your shoulders so your torso is parallel to the floor and the barbell is held at straight arms' length directly beneath your shoulders.

Movement Performance—Moving only your arms, slowly bend your arms and pull the barbell upward and slightly backward until the barbell handle lightly touches your lower rib cage. Hold this peak-contracted position for a moment, then slowly lower back to the starting position. Repeat the movement.

Common Mistakes—Avoid raising your shoulders during the movement, because this imparts momentum to the bar, which decreases the resistance your upper back muscles should be feeling. Don't do bent rows with your legs straight, because doing so will place harmful stress on your lower back.

Training Tips—When you use an Olympic barbell, the diameter of the plates is so great that you cannot keep the barbell free of the gym floor in the bottom position of the movement. If this is the case, you should do the

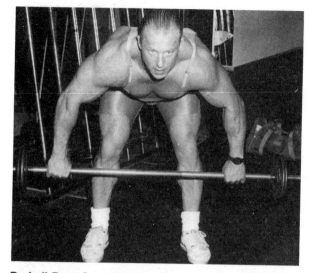

Barbell Bent-Over Row (just above starting point)

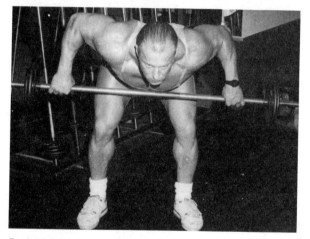

Barbell Bent-Over Row (finish)

exercise while standing on either a flat exercise bench or a thick block of wood. You should also experiment with a variety of grip widths, from one as wide as the length of the barbell handle will permit to one as narrow as having your hands touching each other in the middle of the barbell handle.

Lat Machine Pulldowns

Emphasis—This is also an excellent movement for the latissimus dorsi muscles. It is particularly good for building width in the lats. Strong stress is also placed on the posterior deltoids, biceps, brachialis, and forearm flexor muscles.

Starting Position—Take an overgrip on the lat machine handle with your hands set three to five inches wider than your shoulders on each

side. If there is a leg restraint bar on your machine, straighten your arms and then sit down on the seat with your knees beneath the bar. If there is no restraint, bend your legs and then either kneel or sit directly beneath the pulley.

Movement Performance—Keeping your elbows back, slowly bend your arms and pull the lat bar directly downward to touch your upper chest in front of your neck. Hold this position for a moment, then slowly return to the starting point. Repeat the movement.

Common Mistakes—Don't pump your body upward and downward in order to impart excess momentum to the bar. Be sure you do no incomplete movements; the bar must always touch low on your chest.

Training Tips—The movement just described is called *front pulldowns*. You can also do pulldowns behind the neck, in which you pull the bar downward to touch your upper traps in back of your neck. You can also experiment

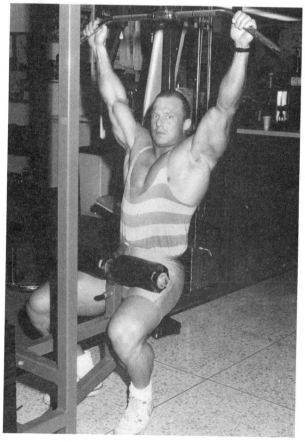

Lat Machine Pulldowns (start)

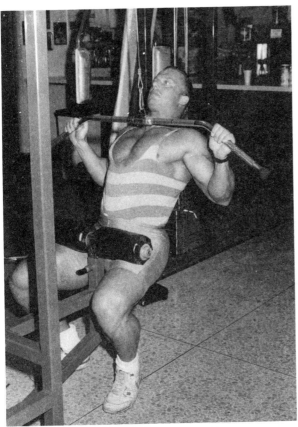

Lat Machine Pulldowns (finish—variation in which bar is pulled to chest; bar can also be pulled down behind the head to touch the upper trapezius muscles)

with various grip widths, from one as wide as the length of the bar permits inward to one in which your hands are touching. You can also use an undergrip on the bar, which places your biceps in a more powerful pulling position. There are also several types of handles that permit a grip in which your hands are parallel to each other. There are both medium and narrow gripping handles for this type of pulldown, which can also be done to the front or back of your neck. Finally, you can get much more out of your pulldowns if you are sure to keep your back arched throughout the movement, particularly toward the finish position. You won't be able to fully contract your lats unless your back is arched like this.

Shoulder Shrugs

Emphasis—Doing shoulder shrugs while holding a barbell or two dumbbells in your hands isolates stress on your trapezius and forearm flexor muscles. Some secondary stress is borne by the upper chest muscles and deltoids.

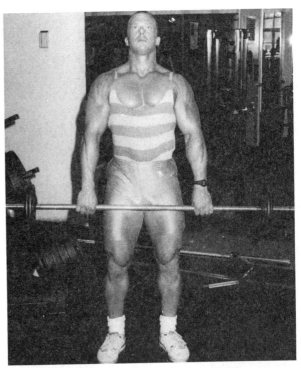

Barbell Shoulder Shrug (start—for finish, see next series of photos of dumbbell version of movement)

Starting Position—Take a shoulder-width overgrip on a moderately heavy barbell, assume the correct pulling position described for deadlifts, and stand erect with your arms held straight and the barbell resting across your upper thighs. Allow the weight to pull your shoulders forward and downward.

Movement Performance—Use trapezius strength to shrug your shoulders upward and backward as far as possible. Hold this position for a moment, then lower back to the starting point. Repeat the movement for the suggested number of repetitions.

Common Mistakes—Avoid bending your arms as you do barbell shrugs; they should act only as cables attaching the barbell to your shoulders. And don't allow your body to sway forward and backward or your knees to jerk as you do the movement.

Training Tips—A similar movement can be performed at the bench press station of a Universal Gym while you stand between the handles. If you are relatively short, however, you won't be able to bear the weight correctly, and you should stand on a thick block of wood when doing your shrugs.

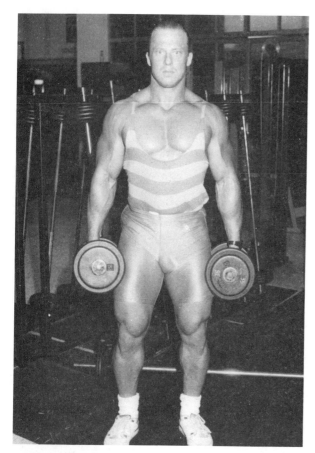

Dumbbell Shrug (start)

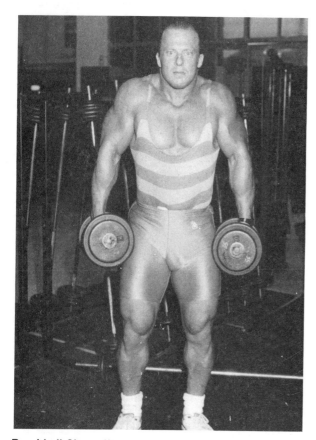

Dumbbell Shrug (finish)

CHEST EXERCISES
Bench Presses

Emphasis—This is an excellent basic movement that places intense stress on the pectorals (particularly the lower and outer sections of the muscle group), anterior and medial deltoids, and triceps. Secondary stress is also placed on the muscles that impart rotational stress to the scapulae. Bench presses are such a great exercise that they are often called "upper body squats." Indeed, you could get a very good workout by doing only bench presses, squats, and barbell bent rows. These movements place direct stress on virtually every skeletal muscle.

Starting Position—Load up a barbell resting on the rack attached to the end of a pressing bench. Lie on your back on the bench with your shoulders 3–5 inches away from the bench uprights. Place your feet flat on the floor on each side of the bench to balance yourself on the bench during your set. Take an overgrip on the barbell with your hands set 3–4 inches wider than your shoulders on each side. Straighten your arms to lift the barbell from the rack and bring the weight to a position at straight arms' length directly above your shoulder joints.

Movement Performance—Being sure that your upper arm bones travel directly out to the sides, slowly lower the barbell downward and a bit toward your feet until it lightly touches the middle of your chest. Without bouncing the barbell off your chest, slowly press it back to the starting point. Repeat.

Common Mistakes—Bouncing the bar and arching your back are both cheating and make your muscles lose part of the stress they should be receiving.

Training Tips—You can change your grip from one as wide as the length of the bar permits to one in which your hands are touching in the middle of the bar. Narrow-grip bench presses place more stress on the triceps and less on the pectorals. Medium-grip benches tend to stress the inner pectorals more than the outer pecs, which are stressed most intensely with wide-grip bench presses. Regardless of the grip, you should avoid holding your breath as you do the movement. Holding your breath can

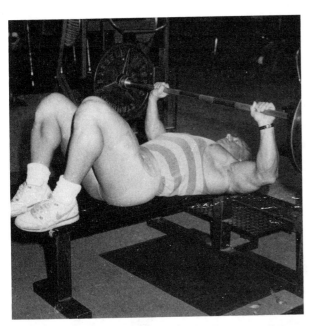

Bench Press (start/finish)

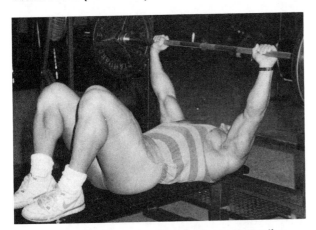

Bench Press (partway up or down in movement)

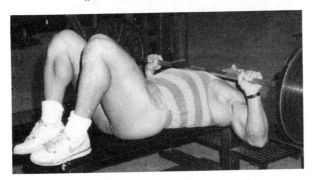

Bench Press (bottom position of movement)

cause the Valsalva effect, which causes you to black out. If you are training alone and black out, you could be seriously injured when benching. Always use a spotter when doing bench presses. The spotter can stand at the head end of the bench and pull up with his or her hands to assist you in bringing the weight back up to straight arms' length.

Incline Barbell Presses

Emphasis—Pressing a barbell on an incline bench stresses the same muscles as bench presses, but with much more stress placed on the upper pectorals. Any kind of inclined movement—with a barbell, two dumbbells, or a machine—will help to fill out the upper chest muscles and create a complete tie-in with your anterior deltoids.

Starting Position—Sit on the incline bench, straddling the seat (if the bench has such a seat), and lie back. Take an overgrip on the barbell with your hands set 3–5 inches wider than your shoulders on each side. Straighten your arms to lift the barbell from the rack, bringing it to a position at straight arms' length directly above your shoulders.

Movement Performance—Keeping your elbows back, slowly bend your arms and lower the barbell directly downward to touch a point on your chest at the base of your neck. Without bouncing the bar off your chest, slowly straighten your arms to return the bar to the starting point. Repeat the movement.

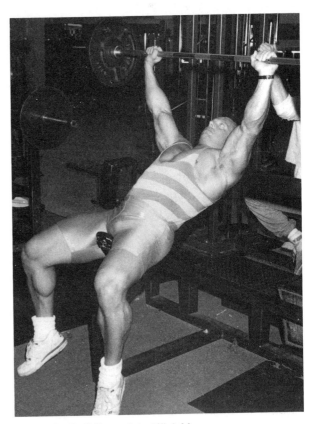

Incline Barbell Press (start/finish)

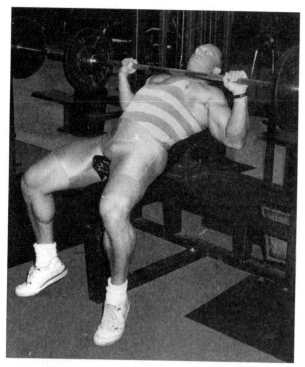

Incline Barbell Press (bottom point of movement)

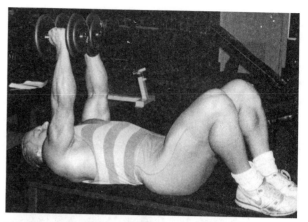

Lying Dumbbell Flyes (start)

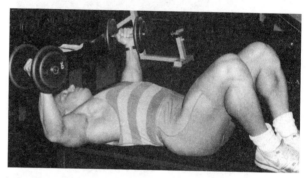

Lying Dumbbell Flyes (partway downward or upward)

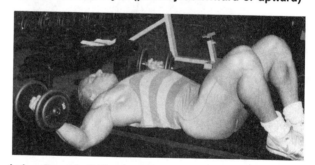

Lying Dumbbell Flyes (bottom position)

Common Mistakes—Allowing your elbows to travel forward as you lower the weight removes resistance from your pectorals and deltoids. Arching your back to cheat up the weight also robs your chest muscles of some of the resistance they should be receiving.

Training Tips—You can place more resistance on your pecs with a 30-degree bench than with the 45-degree version. By occasionally changing the width of your grip you can stress your pectorals from different angles and ultimately develop more complete chest musculature. A similar movement can be performed on a Smith machine.

Dumbbell Flyes

Emphasis—Doing flyes with dumbbells isolates the triceps from the movement and places direct stress on your pectorals, particularly on the lower and outer sections of the muscle group. Significant secondary stress is placed on the anterior and medial heads of the deltoids, with only a minor amount of stress on your triceps. Flyes performed on an incline bench place much more of the stress on your upper pecs, while decline flyes stress the lower sections more intensely.

Starting Position—Grasp two moderately weighted dumbbells and lie back on a flat exercise bench, your feet flat on the floor on each side of the bench to balance your body as you do the movement. Extend your arms straight up from your shoulders, your palms facing inward and the weights touching each other directly above your chest. Bend your arms about 30 degrees and maintain this rounded-arms position throughout the set.

Movement Performance—Slowly lower the dumbbells directly out to the sides in semicircular arcs to as low a position as is comfortably possible. Slowly return them back along the same arcs to the starting position. Repeat the movement.

Common Mistakes—Holding your arms straight when doing dumbbell flyes will place harmful stress on the ligaments of your inner elbows. If you allow the dumbbells to travel a bit forward of the recommended position, you will reduce the amount of stress placed on the working pectoral muscles.

Training Tips—You can do dumbbell flyes on both incline and decline benches set at a variety of angles.

SHOULDER EXERCISES

Standing Barbell Presses

Emphasis—This is one of the most basic deltoid exercises, one that very strongly stresses the anterior heads of the muscle group and more moderately stresses the medial delts. Strong secondary stress is placed on the triceps muscles, and a bit less stress is placed on the upper pectorals and the upper back muscles that impart rotational force to the scapulae.

Starting Position—Place a moderately heavy barbell on the gym floor at your feet. Set your feet a comfortable distance apart and bend over to take an overgrip on the bar, your hands set 3-4 inches wider than your shoulders on each side. Flatten your back and dip your hips to assume the correct starting position for pulling a barbell from the floor.

Movement Performance—Begin to pull the bar quickly off the floor by straightening your legs, then your back, and finally pulling with your arms to clean the bar to your chest. Fix the bar at your shoulders by whipping your elbows under the bar. This movement is called a *power clean*. Move your elbows under the weight. Slowly straighten your arms to push the barbell directly upward past your face to straight arms' length above your shoulders. Slowly lower it back to your shoulders and repeat the movement.

Common Mistakes—Avoid bending your torso backward, as this both removes stress from the muscles that should be benefiting from the movement and places harmful stress on the vertebrae of your lower back. Avoid kicking your knees to cheat up the weight.

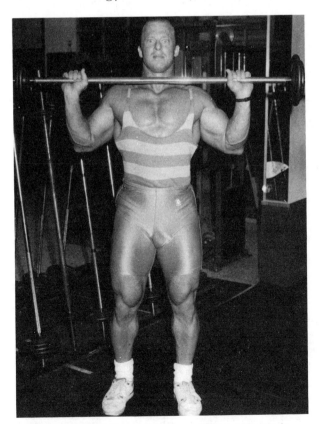

Standing Barbell Press (start—variation with bar in front of neck at beginning of movement)

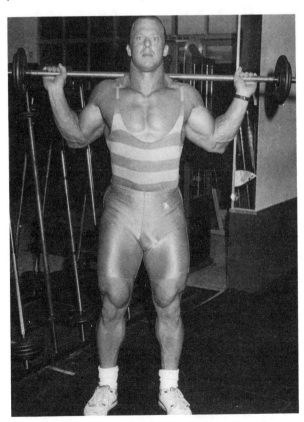

Standing Barbell Press (start—variation with bar in back of neck at beginning of movement)

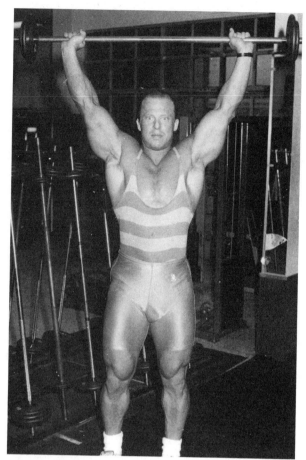

Standing Barbell Press (finish—for both from press and press behind neck)

Movement Performance—Keeping your legs and torso motionless, slowly pull the barbell directly upward 1-2 inches in front of your boddy until your hands touch the underside of your chin. Your elbows should be above the level of your hands throughout the movement, particularly in the top position of the movement. Slowly reverse the movement and lower the barbell back along the same arc to the starting point. Repeat the movement for the required number of repetitions.

Common Mistakes—Dropping the weight from the top position rather than lowering it slowly and under full control will rob your working muscles of about 50% of the stress they should receive. Swinging your torso forward and backward to cheat the weight up also robs the working muscles of some of the stress they should be receiving.

Training Tips—A wider grip on the bar (about shoulder width) transfers stress from the trapezius muscles and to the deltoids. A similar movement can be performed by holding a straight bar handle attached to the end of a cable running through a floor pulley.

Training Tips—You can practice using a variety of grip widths on the barbell handle. A similar movement can be performed on a Smith machine. You can do seated barbell presses while sitting at the end of a flat exercise bench.

Barbell Upright Rows

Emphasis—Upright rows performed with a barbell place direct stress on the anterior-medial deltoids and trapezius muscles. Secondary stress is placed on the posterior deltoids, teres major, biceps, brachialis, and forearm flexor muscles.

Starting Position—Take an overgrip in the middle of a barbell handle with 4-6 inches of space between your hands. Set your feet a comfortable distance apart and stand erect with your arms straight down at your sides and the barbell resting across your upper thighs.

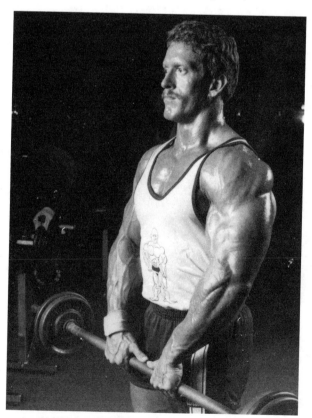

Barbell Upright Rows (start)
Model: Bob Jodkiewicz

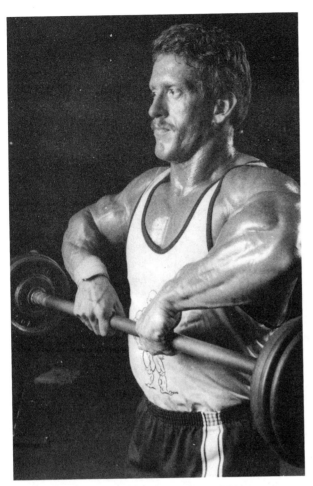

Barbell Upright Rows (approaching finish)

Dumbbell Side Laterals

Emphasis—This is an excellent exercise for isolating the medial and anterior heads of the deltoids. There is also minor force imparted by the trapezius and other upper back muscles that rotate the scapulae.

Starting Position—Grasp two light dumbbells, set your feet a comfortable distance apart, and stand erect. Press the dumbells together 4–6 inches in front of your hips, your palms facing each other. Incline your torso slightly forward and maintain this position throughout your set. Bend your arms about 15-20 degrees and keep them rounded like this throughout your set.

Movement Performance—Keeping your palms facing the floor, use deltoid strength to move the dumbbells out to the sides and slightly in front of your body in semicircular arcs until

your hands are above the level of your shoulders. Hold this peak-contracted position for a moment, then slowly lower the dumbbells back along the same arcs to the starting point. Repeat the movement.

Common Mistakes—Avoid swinging the dumbbells quickly upward to the finish position, since this cheating motion robs some of the working muscles of the stress they should be receiving. Raising the dumbbells with your palms facing forward at any angle shifts too much of the stress to your anterior deltoids. That is counterproductive, since you are attempting to isolate your medial deltoids when you do dumbbell side laterals.

Training Tips—In order to fully isolate your medial delts, tilt the front of your hand downward in the top position of the movement. This will be something like the movement you should make when pouring milk out of a bottle. You can also do dumbbell side laterals with one arm at a time, grasping a sturdy upright with your free hand to brace your body in position for the exercise and therefore make the movement stricter.

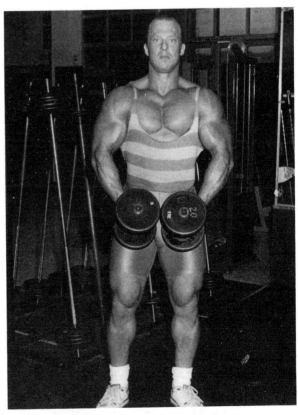

Standing Dumbbell Side Laterals (start)

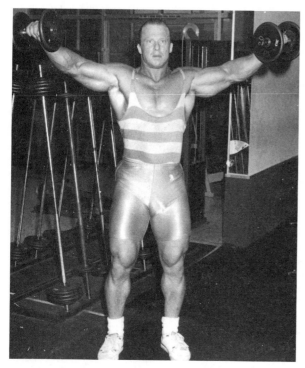

Standing Dumbbell Side Laterals (finish)

ARM EXERCISES

Standing Barbell Curls

Emphasis—This is the most basic of biceps movements. It places primary stress on the biceps muscles and secondary stress on the brachialis and forearm flexor muscles.

Starting Position—Place a moderately heavy barbell on the gym floor at your feet. Bend over and take a shoulder-width undergrip on the bar (palms facing away from your body). Stand erect with your arms straight down at your sides and the barbell resting across your upper thighs. Your feet should be set a comfortable distance apart, and you should avoid swaying your torso forward and/or backward to help you move the weight upward. Press your upper arms against the sides of your torso and keep them in this position throughout the set.

Movement Performance—Use biceps strength to curl the weight upward in a semicircular arc to a position just beneath your chin. Hold this position for a moment, powerfully contracting your biceps, then lower back to the starting point. Repeat the movement for the desired number of repetitions.

Common Mistakes—Torso movement during the exercise is cheating, and it robs the biceps of some of the stress they should receive. Allowing your elbows to move out to the sides away from your torso also is cheating.

Training Tips—If you have difficulty avoiding torso swing, you can alleviate the problem by

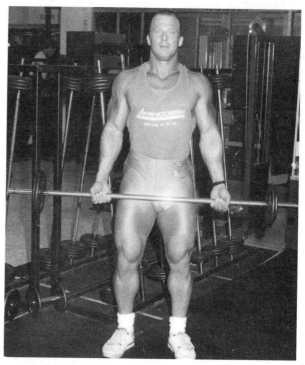

Standing Barbell Curls (start)

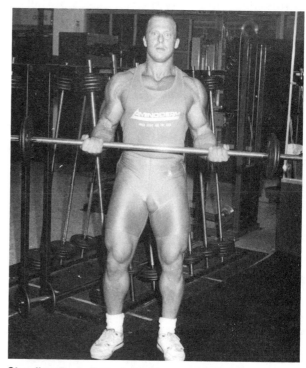

Standing Barbell Curls (halfway up or down)

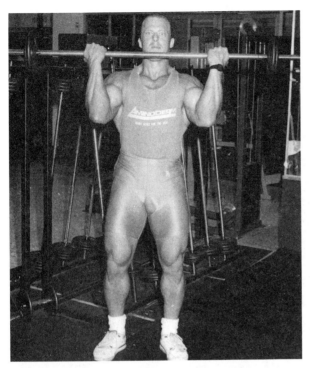

Standing Barbell Curls (finish of movement)

wearing one of my Weider Arm Blaster units. This inexpensive piece of equipment effectively restricts any movement of the upper arms and torso as you do all types of barbell curls and dumbbell curls, either standing or seated at the end of a flat exercise bench. Alternatively, you can avoid torso swing by doing barbell curls with your back pressed against the gym wall or the upright member of any exercise machine. Regardless of how you do the movement, you should experiment with different grip widths. Arnold Schwarzenegger did most of his barbell curls with a relatively wide grip, his hands set 6–8 inches wider than his shoulders on each side, and his biceps were terrific. Ricky Wayne (Mr. World and Pro. Mr. America), on the other hand, favored a narrower grip, his hands only 4–6 inches apart in the middle of the bar, and his biceps were also extremely impressive. Try using a wide variety of grip widths to determine which one works best for you.

Standing Dumbbell Curls

Emphasis—Like barbell curls, this dumbbell movement places very intense stress on the biceps and lesser stress on the brachialis and forearm flexor muscles. But you will be able to supinate your hands using dumbbells, which gives you a better biceps contraction than barbell curls. The function of your biceps is to flex your arm *and* supinate your hand.

Starting Position—Grasp two moderately weighted dumbbells, set your feet about shoulder width apart, and stand erect with your arms hanging straight down at your sides, your palms facing inward toward your legs. Press your upper arms against the sides of your torso and keep them in this position throughout the set.

Movement Performance—Use biceps strength to simultaneously curl the dumbbells forward and upward in a semicircular arc to the shoulders. As the dumbbells reach the halfway point, rotate your wrists so your palms are facing upward during the second half of the movement. This wrist twist is called *supination*. Slowly lower the dumbbells back along the same arcs to the starting point and repeat the movement. As the dumbbells reach the halfway point back to the finish position, rotate your wrists again so your palms are facing inward toward each other for the second half of the

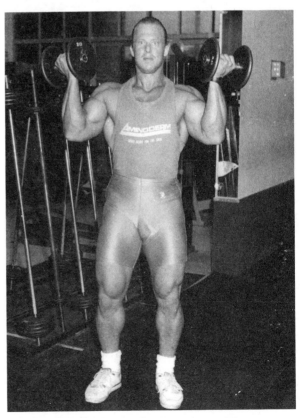

Standing Dumbbell Curls (finish—only position illustrated)

lowering movement. This wrist twist in the opposite direction from supination is called *pronation*.

Common Mistakes—Using torso sway to swing the dumbbells up to the finish position is cheating and should be avoided. Curling the weights upward with your palms facing each other throughout both the raising and lowering stages places less stress on your biceps and more on the brachialis muscles. But if you want to work brachial muscles, you should concentrate on this movement, which is called *hammer curls*.

Training Tips—To make this movement somewhat stricter you can sit at the end of a flat exercise bench with your feet set flat on the floor to balance your body in position. As with barbell curls, you can do dumbbell curls either using a Weider Arm Blaster or with your back pressed against the gym wall. You also can

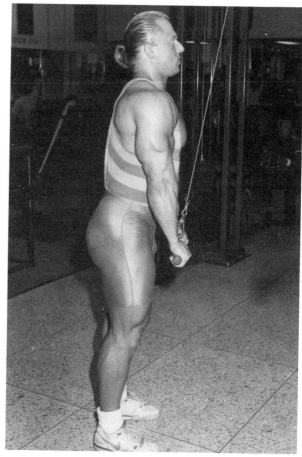

Pulley Pushdown (finish)

alternate arms with one hand going up while the other goes down. With all variations of dumbbell curls you can experiment with raising the weights a little out to the sides rather than directly forward on each repetition.

Pulley Pushdowns

Emphasis—Pushdowns allow you to isolate stress almost totally on your triceps muscles, particularly the medial and outer heads of this three-headed muscle complex.

Starting Position—Take a narrow overgrip on a bar handle attached to the end of an overhead pulley. Set your feet a comfortable distance apart and pull your elbows downward so you can keep them pressed against the sides of your torso throughout the set. Lean slightly forward at the waist. Your arms should be fully bent at the start of the movement, and your hands should be beneath your chin.

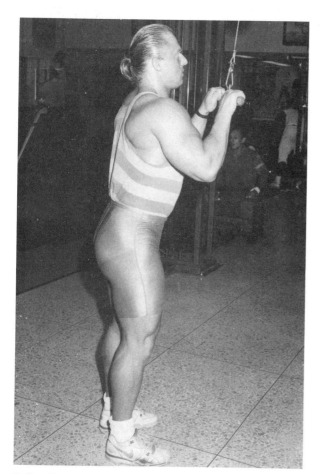

Pulley Pushdown (start)

Movement Performance—Use triceps strength to slowly move the pulley handle forward and downward in a semicircular arc until your hands touch your upper thighs. Slowly return the handle along the same arc to the starting point. Repeat.

Common Mistakes—The most common mistake when doing pushdowns is to allow your elbows to travel outward to the sides away from your body. This cheating motion will allow you to use more weight, which could be impressive, but it removes stress from your triceps. You should also avoid bobbing your shoulders forward and downward to help cheat the pulley handle to the finish position of the movement.

Training Tips—There is an excellent short bar handle used specifically for triceps training; the bar is bent in the middle and angled downward on each side. You will find this handle both comfortable and effective when compared to a standard straight bar handle. You can also use a rope handle consisting of two ropes that you grasp with your palms facing inward toward each other. The final handle with which you can experiment is a loop handle with which you do one-armed pulley pushdowns.

Lying Barbell Triceps Extensions

Emphasis—This is another good movement for isolating your triceps muscles from the rest of your body. Lying triceps extensions stress primarily the medial and long inner heads of the triceps.

Starting Position—Take a narrow overgrip in the middle of a moderately weighted barbell with your index fingers about 4-6 inches apart. Lie back on a flat exercise bench with your torso and head on the padded surface of the bench and your feet on the floor on each side of the bench to balance your body on the bench as you do the movement. Extend your arms directly upward from your shoulders. Keep your upper arms motionless throughout the set.

Movement Performance—Moving only your forearms, slowly lower the barbell to the rear and downward in a semicircular arc until it

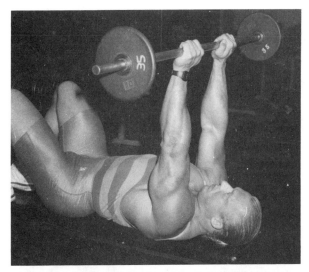

Lying Barbell Triceps Extensions (start/finish)

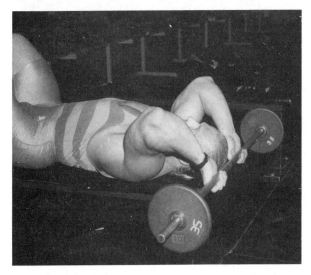

Lying Barbell Triceps Extensions (bottom position)

lightly touches your forehead. Use triceps strength to return the weight slowly back along the same arc to the starting point. Repeat the movement for the suggested number of repetitions.

Common Mistakes—Avoid allowing your elbows to move out to the sides, since this cheating movement takes stress off your triceps. Never bounce the weight off your head.

Training Tips—This movement can also be done on a decline bench (decline triceps extensions) or on an incline bench (incline triceps extensions). On all variations of triceps extensions with a barbell you can occasionally vary your grip to change the angle of stress on your triceps.

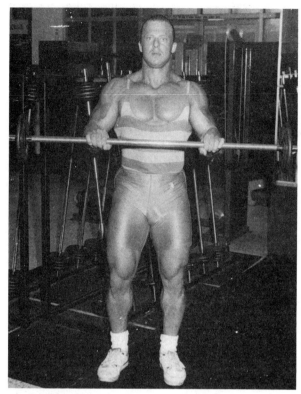

Standing Barbell Reverse Curls (midpoint)

Barbell Reverse Curls

Emphasis—Reverse curls are a direct movement for your brachialis and forearm supinator muscles. Strong secondary stress is placed on the biceps.

Starting Position—Set your feet a comfortable distance apart and bend forward to take a shoulder-width overgrip on a moderately heavy barbell. Stand erect with your arms running straight down at your sides and the barbell resting across your upper thighs. Press your upper arms against the sides of your torso and keep them oriented like this throughout the set.

Movement Performance—Use brachialis, biceps, and forearm strength to curl the barbell slowly forward and upward in a semicircular arc from your thighs to a position beneath your chin. Slowly lower the weight back to the starting point and repeat the movement.

Common Mistakes—Avoid using torso swing to cheat the weight up and avoid letting your elbows move out to the sides as you do the movement.

Training Tips—You can use a Weider Arm Blaster or press your back against the gym wall to avoid cheating. You should also experiment with changing your grip. It will be very difficult to use a grip wider than shoulder width, but you can move your hands inward even to the point where they are touching each other in the middle of the bar.

Barbell Wrist Curls/Reverse Wrist Curls

Emphasis—Performed with your palms facing upward, wrist curls isolate stress on the powerful forearm flexor muscles. Performed with your palms facing downward, reverse wrist curls isolate stress on the somewhat weaker forearm extensor muscles.

Starting Position—For wrist curls, take a shoulder-width undergrip on a moderately weighted barbell. Sit at the end of a flat exercise bench with your feet set about shoulder width apart. Run your forearms down your thighs so your wrists and hands are off the end of your knees. Allow the weight to pull your hands downward. (For reverse wrist curls, the instructions for starting position and movement per-

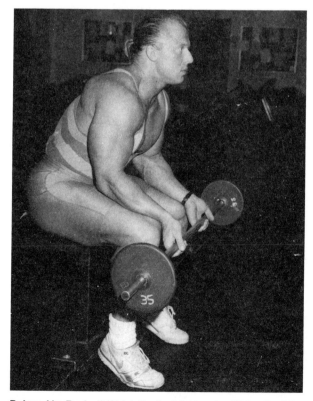

Palms-Up Barbell Wrist Curls (start—aka Wrist Curls)

formance will be the same, except your palms will face down toward the floor rather than upward.)

Movement Performance—Use forearm flexor (or extensor) strength to curl the barbell upward in a semicircular arc to as high a position as possible. Slowly lower back to the starting position and repeat the movement.

Common Mistakes—Allowing the weight to pull your hands so far downward that your fists open and the weight is rolling down your fingers is a waste of time and energy.

Training Tips—You might find that you get a better forearm flexor contraction if you place your thumbs under the bar rather than around it. You can also experiment with different-width grips, as well as with your forearms resting across the surface of a flat exercise bench rather than down your thighs. You will probably find that for reverse wrist curls you can use only 50% of the weight you use for wrist curls, since the flexor muscles are significantly stronger.

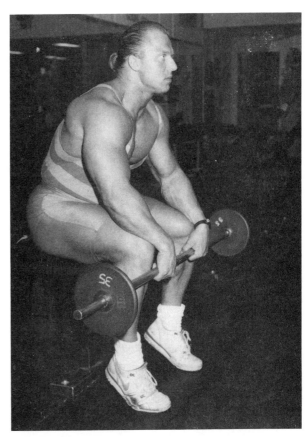

Palms-Down Barbell Wrist Curls (start—Reverse Wrist Curls)

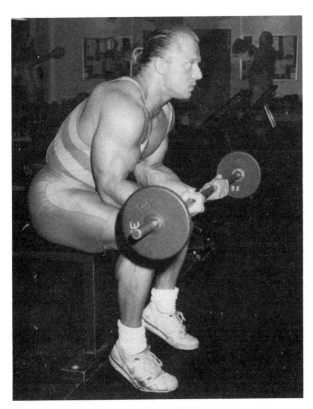

Palms-Up Barbell Wrist Curls (finish)

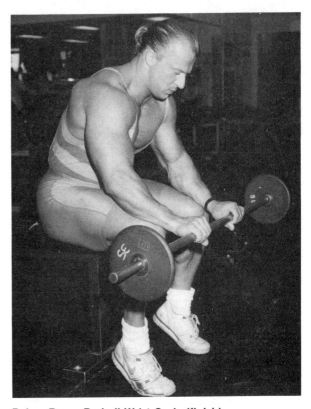

Palms-Down Barbell Wrist Curls (finish)

CALF EXERCISES

Standing Calf Raises

Emphasis—Performed on a standing calf machine, standing calf raises directly stress the gastrocnemius muscles of your calves in relative isolation from the rest of your body.

Starting Position—Bend your legs and place your shoulders beneath the padded yoke of the machine. Step up on the block of wood with your toes and balls of your feet on the block. Straighten your legs to bear the weight of the machine and allow your heels to sink as far below the level of your toes as possible. Your feet should be 12–14 inches apart with your toes pointing straight ahead at the start of the exercise.

Movement Performance—Use calf muscle strength to slowly rise as high as possible on your toes. Hold this peak-contracted position for a moment, then lower your heels back to the starting position. Repeat.

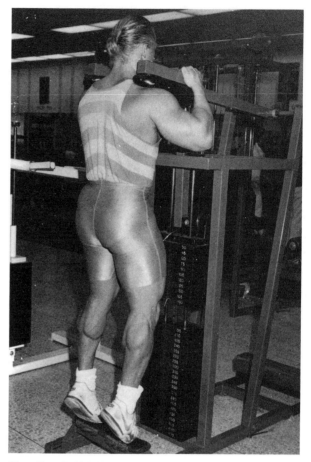

Standing Calf Raises (finish)

Common Mistakes—Don't use so much weight that you are unable to do a complete movement on every repetition. Avoid cheating by kicking upward with your knees.

Training Tips—Try a somewhat wider foot stance from time to time. You should also vary the angle of your feet as you go from one set to the next. In addition to pointing your feet straight ahead, you can angle your toes inward or outward at approximate 45-degree angles.

Seated Calf Raises

Emphasis—This movement has become popular only within the last 10–12 years. It directly stresses the broad, flat soleus muscles beneath the gastrocs. The soleus muscles can be contracted completely only when your legs are bent at a 90-degree angle as in this movement. Secondary stress is placed on the gastrocnemius muscles.

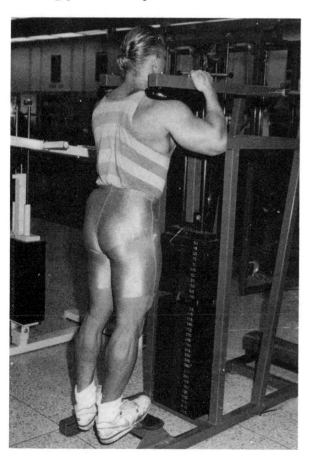

Standing Calf Raises (start)

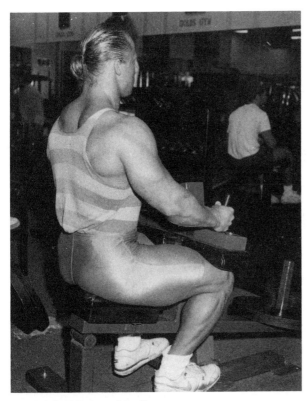

Seated Calf Raises (start)

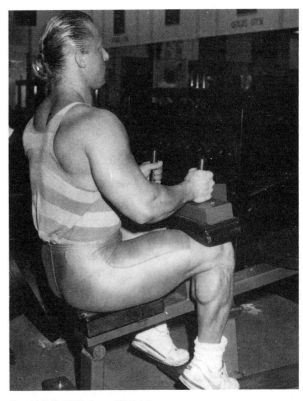

Seated Calf Raises (finish)

Starting Position—Sit on the padded surface of the machine and adjust the height of the two knee pads by pulling the pin out of the column and then replacing it after adjusting the pad height. Place your toes and the balls of your feet on the toe plate, your feet about shoulder width apart and toes pointing directly forward. Slide your knees beneath the pads and extend your feet to raise the pads enough to push the stop bar forward to release the weight. (Be sure you relock the stop bar before exiting the machine at the end of your set.) Allow the weight of the machine to push your heels as far below the level of your toes as possible.

Movement Performance—Use calf muscle strength to rise as high as possible on your toes. Hold this peak-contracted position for a moment, ment, return to the starting point, and repeat the movement for the appropriate number of reps.

Common Mistakes—A shorter-than-full range of motion will rob your calves of much of the stress they should receive. Bouncing the weight will eventually lead to sore ankles and Achilles tendons.

Training Tips—Try using the two additional toe angles explained in the exercise description for standing calf raises. If a seated calf machine isn't available, you can do this movement with a barbell by padding the handle and resting the weight across your knees while seated at the end of a flat exercise bench with your toes and the balls of your feet on a calf block. With very heavy weights you can have a training partner lift the weight up for you once you're in position to use it.

BEGINNING ROUTINES

I assume that many readers have no experience training with weights. Therefore, I will provide several training programs that will gradually improve muscle mass, tone, strength, and recovery ability between workouts. If you do have some barbell and dumbbell experience, you may be able to launch into these sequential routines at the intermediate level or higher. And you will ultimately be able to formulate your own routines using the suggestions presented later in this book.

You can follow each of these training schedules for four to six weeks before advancing to the next level. As you become an advanced bodybuilder, you will probably use a different routine every training day, tailoring your workout to your daily energy reserves and specific physical requirements. But if you're a beginning or intermediate bodybuilder, you must be more regimented in your approach to bodybuilding training, because following a set routine will teach you to train hard and consistently.

BREAKING INTO BODYBUILDING

If you make the mistake of just jumping into a full bodybuilding workout—particularly if you've never trained with weights before—you will experience severe muscle soreness the day following a workout. Therefore, you must slowly break into your first training program, gradually increasing workout intensity.

Experienced bodybuilders know they should start each new training program with one or two sets fewer of each exercise, then gradually add sets until they are up to the complete routine. They also tend to use lighter-than-normal training poundages in order to avoid or at least minimize soreness, then gradually work up to more normal weights in each movement.

Newcomers to the bodybuilding lifestyle should also break slowly into the first program presented in this chapter. A gradual break-in can last as few as two weeks if you are in good physical condition from participating in other sports or as many as four weeks if you have been particularly sedentary. But it *is* necessary in order to avoid muscle soreness and/or mid-workout nausea.

If you have never lifted weights, your first workout should involve only one set of each listed exercise, using the relatively light weights suggested for the movements in the first routine. In fact, you should *not* increase your training poundages until after you are doing the full number of sets listed for each exercise in the program.

With each succeeding workout you can add a total of three or four new sets, being sure to do two sets of every exercise for which three sets are listed, until you reach the highest number of sets listed for each exercise. You can add only one or two sets if your fitness level is initially

low or as many as four or five sets if you are particularly fit. But break into the full program slowly in order to avoid stiff and sore muscles.

MUSCLE SORENESS

Even when you follow the suggested break-in procedure, you could experience mild to moderate muscle soreness. The best remedy for muscle soreness is one or two long, hot baths each day. But you should go ahead and do your next scheduled workout even if you do feel stiff and sore. A good workout will actually help to alleviate muscle soreness.

Most cases of muscle soreness are caused by overly intense workouts, but soreness can also be caused by overstretching when warming up. Never push a stretch so far that your muscles are screaming. Doing so will cause small tears in muscles and connective tissue, which are both painful and destructive over the long haul.

STARTING POUNDAGES

Based on my 50 years of experience training top bodybuilders and film stars, I have a good feel for how much weight a beginner should use in his or her first few workouts. But this poundage varies according to body weight. It should go without saying that lighter individuals cannot handle as much weight as larger people. Also, a man will always be able to hoist heavier weights than a woman of the same body weight.

In the first training program I have suggested starting poundages in terms of a percentage of body weight, with differing poundages for men and women. Simply multiply the percentage for each movement by your body weight in pounds. And round that figure upward or downward to the nearest multiple of five pounds.

The suggested starting poundages should feel a little light to you, but don't increase the weights until after you are doing the full training schedule. If, on the other hand, the suggested poundage for any exercise feels heavy or prevents you from doing the required number of repetitions, you should reduce it by 5-10 pounds.

I have suggested starting poundages for only the first routine, because after six weeks of steady training you will know far more about your physical capabilities than I do. I simply can't climb into your body and immediately tell how quickly your strength levels are improving, so you should judge your own starting weights for each new program past the first routine.

THE ROUTINES

The three routines presented in this section can be used for the first 16-20 weeks of your training, not counting a break-in period of 2-4 weeks. And be sure to warm up thoroughly, using the warm-up schedule outlined in Chapter 4 prior to each weight-training session.

While each routine has stated workout days of Monday, Wednesday, and Friday, any other three nonconsecutive days each week can be used. Just be sure to program at least one full rest day between training days. So, you can just as easily train on Tuesdays, Thursdays, and Saturdays if these workout days fit more easily into your weekly schedule.

In the following routines, be sure to do all of the listed sets for each exercise before proceeding to the next movement. Rest intervals between sets should be held down to 60-90 seconds.

WORKOUT NUMBER ONE

(WEEKS 1-6)

Exercise	Sets	Reps	% Men	% Women
Sit-Ups	2	20-30	0	0
Squats	3	8-12	30	20
Leg Curls	2	8-12	40	30
Barbell Bent Rows	3	8-12	25	15
Bench Presses	3	6-10	25	15
Upright Rows	2	8-12	20	10
Barbell Curls	2	8-12	20	10
Pulley Pushdowns	2	8-12	15	7½
Wrist Curls	2	10-15	20	10
Standing Calf Raises	3	10-15	35	25

WORKOUT NUMBER TWO

(WEEKS 7-12)

Exercise	Sets	Reps
Leg Raises	3	20-30
Leg Presses	4	10-15
Leg Extensions	2	10-15
Leg Curls	3	8-12
Deadlifts	2	6-10
Lat Pulldowns	4	8-12
Shrugs	2	10-15
Standing Presses	3	6-10
Side Laterals	2	8-12
Dumbbell Curls	3	8-12
Lying Triceps Extensions	3	8-12
Wrist Curls	2	10-15
Reverse Wrist Curls	2	10-15
Seated Calf Raises	4	10-15

WORKOUT NUMBER THREE

(WEEKS 13-18)

Exercise	Sets	Reps
Sit-Ups	2	20-30
Leg Raises	2	20-30
Squats	4	10-15
Leg Curls	3	8-12
Leg Extensions	2	10-15
Deadlifts	3	6-10
Barbell Rows	3	8-12
Lat Pulldowns	2	8-12
Upright Rows	3	8-12
Standing Presses	3	6-10
Side Laterals	2	8-12
Barbell Curls	3	8-12
Lying Triceps Extensions	3	8-12
Reverse Curls	2	8-12
Wrist Curls	3	10-15
Standing Calf Raises	5	15-20

6
Other
Bodybuilding Basics
for Mind and Body

Your mind is by far the strongest organ in your body. Like the rudder of a giant oil tanker, it guides your body wherever you wish it to go. But your mind will help you become a bodybuilder only if you give it the right kind of data to work with.

I personally like to think of the mind as an organic computer that can be programmed—much like an electronic computer—to accomplish specific tasks. In this chapter I will instruct you on how to program your mind to make it easier to reach your bodybuilding goals, regardless of how lofty they might be.

DESIRE AND COMMITMENT

A winning mental approach to bodybuilding begins with a strong desire to succeed, which naturally leads to a powerful commitment to maintain the type of lifestyle necessary to become a great bodybuilder. So, let's begin our discussion of the mental aspect of bodybuilding with a short dissertation about desire and commitment.

It's pretty difficult to develop desire. Generally speaking, you either have it or you don't. But desire does grow from a great love of the sport, and you can definitely increase your love of the sport by constantly reading the available books and magazines concerned with bodybuilding, going to bodybuilding competitions, attempting to talk to all of the stars of the sport with whom you come into contact, and contemplating the positive aspects of bodybuilding.

What level of desire to succeed must you have in order to make a commitment to competitive bodybuilding? You have to have a strong enough desire for success that you simply can't stay out of the gym. You end up eating, sleep-

ing, and doing bodybuilding. You desire to become a successful bodybuilder so fiercely that you actually become one with the sport.

Making a commitment to become a successful competitor is very serious business indeed. Don't make it until you clearly understand what a competitive bodybuilder's lifestyle entails. When you are totally dedicated to the sport, you have to give up a lot of things that are important to the average person. You simply won't succeed unless you make all of the sacrifices required of all serious bodybuilders.

A champion bodybuilder lives the sport 24 hours a day, during both off-season and pre-contest preparatory cycles. You must maintain a regimented diet, even during the off-season, because unrestricted eating will make you so fat that you won't be able to get ripped up for a competition. And prior to a show you will be forced to monitor virtually every calorie that goes into your mouth.

The training is difficult both mentally and physically. You have to be in the gym five or six times a week, bombing away at peak intensity for 1½–2 hours per session. And during a pre-contest cycle you will often be forced to train twice a day and even three times a day if aerobic training is part of your peaking strategy. You can never dog it in a workout, because the hammer has to be down at all times. Without 100% intensity on every set, you will never achieve the mass, proportional balance, and muscular definition that constitute a superior physique.

Once you do make a commitment to the bodybuilding lifestyle, it will be effective only if you keep that commitment sacred. You must consider your commitment etched in steel, or you won't succeed. But when your intense desire

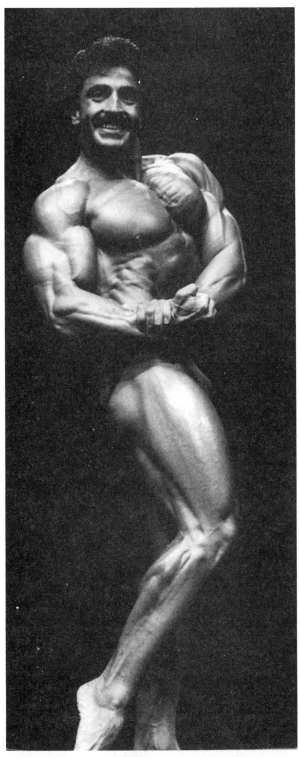

Samir Bannout, the Lebanese who convincingly won the 1983 Mr. Olympia show (over fellow Middle Easterner, Egyptian Mohamed Makkawy), is well aware that diet and nutrition are a 50/50 battle during the off-season, but that diet rises in importance to as much as 90 percent over the final couple of weeks. Still, proper mental approach is the glue which holds everything together. With a bad mental attitude, all of the hard training and tight diet in the world wouldn't build an ounce of new muscle mass.

to succeed has resulted in an ironclad commitment to the sport of bodybuilding, you have adopted the correct mental posture to benefit from the tips included in the balance of this chapter.

POSITIVE MENTAL FOCUS

One of the most important mental keys to bodybuilding success is positive thinking. Gearing your mind to think consistently positive thoughts—totally banishing negativity from your mental life—will make your training and nutritional programs at least 50% more effective than normal at building a sensationally muscular physique. Let me give you an example of how positive and negative thinking can affect your bodybuilding efforts.

Let's say that you grew up with a very protective mother who constantly cautioned you against participating in activities that might injure you. Instead of wishing that you might see something interesting along the way as you reaped the exercise benefits of an afternoon bicycle ride, she'd point out the pitfalls of such a trip. "Don't fall off your bike and get hurt," she'd caution. "Watch out that you don't get hit by a truck!"

Given this type of negative childhood—many years of it—it's logical to assume that you would grow up tending to think negatively. As a result, you would be careful to avoid situations in which the risk of injury is elevated. Confronted with the institutionalized violence of a football game, you would opt for tennis or golf.

The only sure way to achieve a massive physique is to train consistently with heavy—often near maximum—weights in all of your basic exercises. For massive thighs you need to squat heavy, for thick pecs you need to bench heavy, and for a thickly muscled back you need to row with heavy poundages. There's simply no way you can use light weights and achieve the type of muscle mass it takes to win the big national and international bodybuilding shows.

There is a small risk of injury whenever you use maximum poundages in your workouts, however. For example, you *could* get a heavy barbell slightly out of the groove on a maxed-out set of heavy bench presses, straining a rotator cuff muscle and leaving your shoulder in

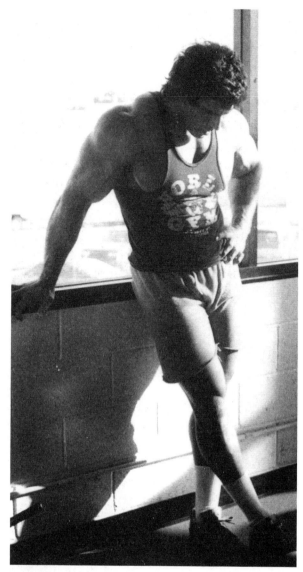

Prior to becoming a noted film actor, particularly as television's "The Incredible Hulk," Lou Ferrigno won a host of physique titles: Teenage Mr. America, Mr. Eastern America, Mr. America, Mr. International, and twice Mr. IFBB Universe. Only Mr. Olympia eluded him, and he'd probably have won that title had his film career not intervened. Here Lou concentrates deeply between heavy sets of bench presses to further expand his already potroast-sized pectorals. Preset psyching is something every successful bodybuilding champ undergoes to one degree or another.

strong pain for several weeks. And if you failed to have a spotter handy for that particular set, you might even totally lose control of the bar and end up having it smash two or three facial bones.

Realistically speaking, there is only an infinitesimally small chance of injury on heavy sets as long as you are fully warmed up and use correct biomechanics on every repetition you do with those maxed-out weights. But if you've been brought up fearing injury, how much chance is there that you'll go for those heavy sets on each basic exercise in order to develop awesome muscle mass? I think you'll agree that there's very little chance that you'll bomb your muscles with the big weights. And as a result, you'll never achieve a contest-winning physique.

The lesson here is that by thinking positively—e.g., that you *won't* be injured when you max out on a set—you'll hurdle past training obstacles that stall the physical progress of normal men and women. How can you condition yourself to think positively at all times?

It's really rather simple. First you must become aware of the fact that you have negative thoughts that must be eliminated from your mind. What are your most common negative thoughts? Start to make a list of them in an effort to identify which negative thoughts most often force themselves into your mind.

Take the biggest negative thought and start to work on it. Every time it enters your mind, boot it out. Say to yourself, "I won't think about that one again." When you say it, *mean* it.

Just through this simple process—repeated several times on each thought as you turn to it—you can eliminate negative thoughts and get on with making big gains from your bodybuilding efforts. It'll take a while to begin thinking consistently positive thoughts, but once you do you'll have taken a very big step toward a Mr. Universe physique.

GOAL-SETTING

It's difficult to take the direct route to any bodybuilding objective without using a road map. Unless you have your map handy, you will make many false starts and go up many dead end alleys en route to winning your Mr. Universe competition. And the road map that will put you on the superhighway to bodybuilding success is the proper application of goal-setting techniques.

Goal-setting should be somewhat like a

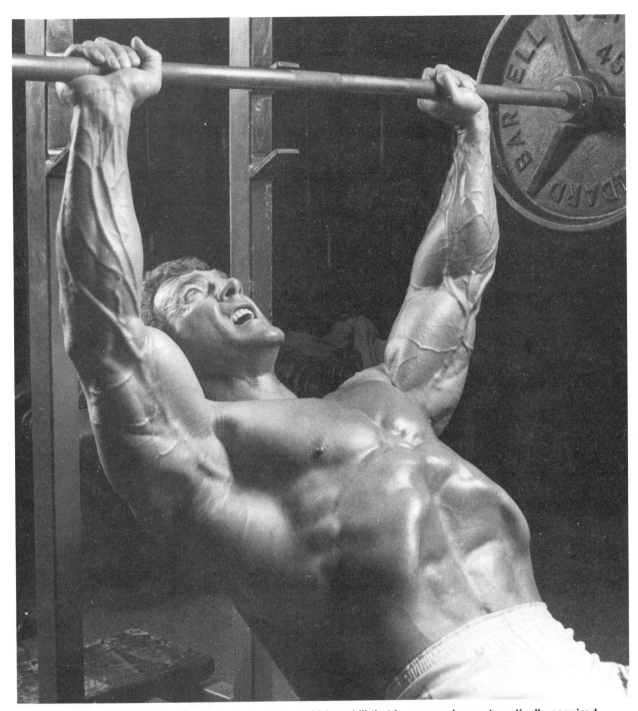

Concentration within a set is also vitally important, and it's a skill that is more or less automatically acquired within a few months by consciously working to concentrate on the active muscle(s) during every set. Here, massive Scott Wilson shows us intraset mental intensity. Scott works as a manager and personal trainer at the Gold's Gym in San Jose, California.

backpacking trip along the John Muir Trail in the Sierra Nevada. The 200-mile trip (your ultimate goal) consists of innumerable individual paces (short-range goals), which add up to a day's journey (a long-range goal). And all of the one-day stages ultimately add up to the entire trip of 200 miles. Step by step, you reach the ultimate goal, at times almost without noticing how steadily you are making progress. For a fuller discussion of this concept, read Chapter 30, "The Inner Game of Bodybuilding."

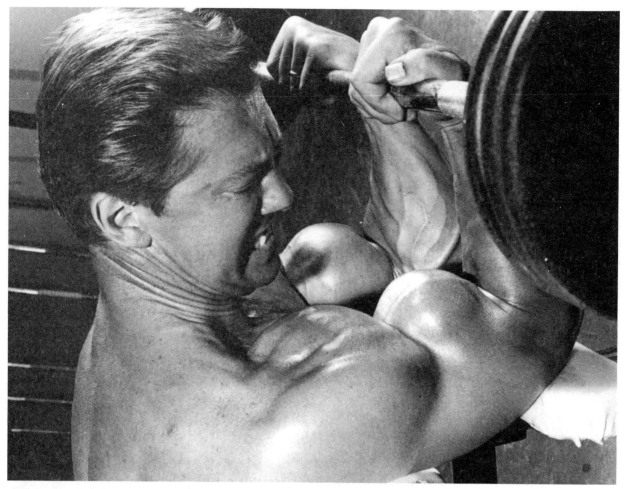

Larry "the legend" Scott shows equally intense intraset mental concentration during a hard set of Barbell Spider Curls. With his upper arms supported against a padded bar to totally immobilize and isolate them from the movement, he enhances his biceps' peaks.

TOTAL CONCENTRATION

There is an enormous difference between a set performed with total concentration and one done while your mind wanders. The former works your muscles to the limit, thereby engendering maximum growth, while the latter does little or nothing to develop additional mass and detail in the muscles the exercise works.

The first step to mastering mental concentration during a workout is to learn precisely which muscle—or which part of a muscle group—is being affected by each exercise. I've given you this information very precisely in the exercise descriptions in every workout chapter of this book, so you can visually identify the exact area of your body being worked by each of your exercises by referring to the illustrations of surface anatomy in the last chapter.

Once you know which muscles should be bearing the weight in an exercise, attempt to concentrate your mental focus on each of those muscles. Feel them powerfully contracting and extending under the load you place on them with a barbell, a dumbbell, or an exercise machine. Feel the burning sensation of accumulating fatigue by-products in the working muscles toward the end of your set.

At first you will find it impossible to keep your mental focus on the working muscle(s) throughout your set. Within a couple of reps your mind will probably skip off to something else. When this happens, merely force it back to the working muscles. Over a period of weeks and months you will find that your mind will wander less and less, a sure indication that your concentration is improving.

Don't worry about how fast you develop total

concentration on your working muscles in each set, because this will happen relatively slowly. As you know, a watched pot never seems to boil. Just be sure that you diligently keep forcing your mind back to the muscles whenever your concentration wavers, and in time you will have great workout concentration.

Ultimately, you will develop the totally focused mental concentration of a champion. When you are deeply into a set, you won't notice anything else in the gym. You won't even notice the weight in your hand. You will be conscious only of the working muscles. I think that a Boeing 747 could crash into the opposite side of the gym and a top bodybuilder probably wouldn't notice it. This is the level of concentration you should be aiming for within a heavy set. This is total concentration.

BASIC BODYBUILDING NUTRITION

Most champion bodybuilders believe that nutrition is at least as important as training when it comes to building a championship physique. Let's listen to the advice of *Rich Gaspari* (National and World Light-Heavyweight Champion, winner of many IFBB Pro Championships, and runner-up in the Mr. Olympia contest): "To my way of thinking, bodybuilding is 50% training and 50% nutrition during an off-season preparatory cycle. Then as a competition approaches, the value of bodybuilding nutrition increases dramatically, until it is 75%-80% responsible for how I appear onstage at an Olympia."

A substantial portion of this encyclopedic tome has been devoted to an exhaustive discussion of bodybuilding nutrition. But I feel that it's necessary to give you some beginning-level nutritional advice so you can immediately begin eating correctly to complement your training efforts. And once you have mastered the information in this brief chapter, you can turn to Part VI and begin an in-depth study of bodybuilding nutrition.

BASIC DIETARY RULES

There's an axiom in bodybuilding nutrition that says, "You are what you eat." This means that your body mirrors your diet—when you follow a well-disciplined diet, you will have sharp muscularity to go with your exceptional degree of muscle mass; and when you consume nothing but junk foods, you will lose muscle tone and grow flabby in appearance.

In order to make the fastest possible progress in bodybuilding, follow these fundamental rules for proper nutrition:

Always eat for your body's benefit rather than for taste. When compared to some of the revved-up junk foods found in every supermarket, the food you should eat for bodybuilding purposes will seem rather bland. But if you want to win some of the big titles someday, you will learn to make this bland food taste good to you.

Include as much variety in your diet as possible. The more different foods you consume each day, the better will be the balance of protein, fat, carbohydrate, vitamins, and minerals in your diet. Unfortunately, most people eat the same 10-12 foods day in and day out, seldom allowing themselves to deviate from a restricted diet; many bodybuilders actually eat as few as 5-6 different foods day in and day out, often eating precisely the same daily meals for years at a time. Give yourself the taste treat of new and exotic foods every day, and your health and physique will also profit.

Consume smaller meals at frequent intervals during the day. Small meals are much more efficiently digested than the large meals in which many bodybuilders indulge. When you are attempting to gain muscle mass, you can eat as many as five to six times a day, and when you are trying to lose body fat, you can still eat four to five times a day as long as you keep the meals low in calories. It's particularly important that you have at least a little high-quality protein in each small meal, since your body can digest and assimilate only about 20-25 grams of protein each time you eat.

Include plenty of high-quality animal-source protein in your diet. Animal protein from meat, fish, poultry, eggs, and milk products has all of the essential amino acids necessary for utilization of the protein in your body to build new muscle tissue. In contrast, vegetable-source proteins do not have all of these essential amino acids and can be assimilated in your body only when consumed along with some animal-source protein.

Curtail the amount of animal fat in your diet. The saturated animal fats in red meat, egg yolks, and full-fat milk products have a deleterious effect on your heath. And fat is more than twice as rich a source of calories as either protein or carbohydrate. You should, however, consume at least a little vegetable fat each day, since it helps you to metabolize the small amounts of animal fat in your daily diet.

Eat food as fresh and lightly cooked as possible. The longer food is stored, the more nutrients it loses. Even frozen foods have less nutrient value than their fresh counterparts. Cooking also destroys nutrients, with more nutrients lost as cooking time or temperature increases.

Load up on the natural carbohydrates found in fruits, vegetables, grains, nuts, and tubers. Your body will use the natural sugars in these foods to give you maximum workout energy levels. And the vitamins, minerals, and enzymes contained in these foods contribute greatly to general health, as well as to bodybuilding results.

Drink at least 8–10 glasses of pure water daily. Water is your body's natural solvent and detoxification agent. Replace it frequently in your body by drinking either natural spring water or distilled water.

Take at least one multipack of vitamins, minerals, trace elements, and digestive enzymes a day. You can even take two multipacks a day, but be sure that you take them with meals for optimum assimilation. Taking supplementary vitamins and minerals is good insurance against nutritional deficiencies that can retard your progress.

Avoid junk-food calories. Junk food includes any foods that are fried or contain refined sugar and/or white flour. These junk foods provide only calories and no vitamins, minerals, or enzymes to speak of. They are definitely deleterious to the bodybuilding lifestyle.

Don't drink your calories. You can drink 1,000 calories worth of orange juice almost without noticing it but would find it very difficult to eat 1,000 calories worth of whole oranges. It's always difficult to control caloric consumption when you are consuming large numbers of fluid calories.

Don't miss meals. There's no way you can pack on plenty of quality muscle mass when you fail to eat the food necessary to fuel your workouts, provide for body recovery between workouts, and build your muscles. If you have to miss a meal at any time, take a protein drink in its place.

Don't add extra salt to any of your food. Your normal diet is too high in sodium content as it is without aggravating the situation by eating even more table salt with your meals. Sodium retains unnecessary water in your system.

Avoid alcohol. I know this is going to be a difficult one for some of you readers who like a postworkout brewski or six. But alcohol is a very concentrated source of calories that your body just doesn't require for optimum function. I've never known a champion bodybuilder who abused alcohol and got away with it.

Given the foregoing rules for proper bodybuilding nutrition, here is a sample one-day bodybuilding menu:

- *Meal 1* (8:00 A.M.)—poached eggs on whole-grain toast, half a cantaloupe, one or two glasses of nonfat milk, multipack.
- *Meal 2* (11:00 A.M.)—yogurt. raw nuts, one piece of fruit, 5–10 free-form amino acid capsules.
- *Meal 3* (2:00 P.M.)—broiled fish, dry baked potato, green vegetable (steamed), one or two glasses of nonfat milk.
- *Meal 4* (5:00 P.M.)—tuna salad, scoop of low-fat cottage cheese, one piece of fruit, 5–10 free-form amino acid capsules.
- *Meal 5* (8:00 P.M.)—skinned and broiled chicken breast, brown rice, one green and/or

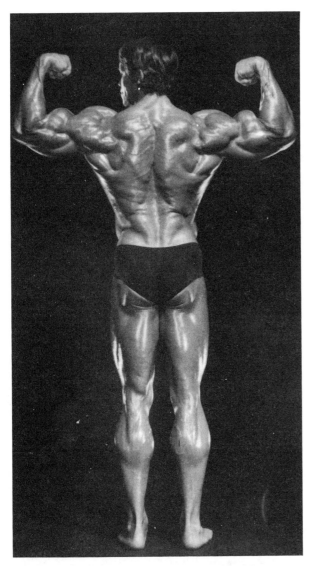

The end result of the proper mental approach to bodybuilding is obvious in this classic Arnold Schwarzenegger back double-biceps shot. From top to bottom, you won't find a weak muscle group. Arnold has a well-deserved reputation as one of the supreme Zen masters of bodybuilding.

one yellow vegetable or a large salad, iced tea, multipack.
- *Meal 6* (11:00 P.M.)—protein shake

Of course, the foregoing menu can be adjusted to fit your personal tastes of food. And the caloric total can be adjusted upward or downward according to your nutritional needs.

MUSCLE CONFUSION

I always advise beginning and intermediate bodybuilders to change training programs each 4-6 weeks. The reason for this is that most men tend to grow bored with a set routine, and boredom erects a wall against continued progress. Still, there are many exceptions to the rule about changing training schedules each 4-6 weeks.

Many bodybuilders prefer to stick with the same routine for long periods of time. *Arnold Schwarzenegger* is typical of this type of bodybuilder: "I personally believe you should stick to any routine which is productive, at least until you reach the point where you are no longer making good gains on it. With constant experimentation as a beginner, intermediate, or low-advanced bodybuilder you will eventually learn which exercises, routines, and training techniques work best for your unique body. Once you discover what works well for you, why abandon it in favor of a routine which may be relatively worthless to you? I believe you shouldn't. I personally stuck to some body part routines for 5-6 years at a time."

Larry Scott, himself a two-time Mr. Olympia victor, feels the same way Arnold does about changing to new routines at set intervals: "Certain routines simply work well for a bodybuilder while others don't work very well. It took me several years of systematic experimentation to come up with some of my body part training programs, and I prefer to stick with a good routine once I find it. I've personally used the same biceps program—with only minor variations—for more than 15 years."

At the opposite end of a continuum are the many bodybuilders who constantly vary their routines from one workout to the next, seldom if ever repeating a particular routine. The great *Lou Ferrigno* is typical of the type of bodybuilder who follows the Weider Muscle Confusion Training Principle: "Once I reached the advanced level of bodybuilding and started entering competitions, I discovered that I quickly became bored with a set training program. So, I began to use the Weider Muscle Confusion Principle, changing to a new and more challenging routine every time I came into the gym to bomb a particular body part.

"There are many ways you can change to a new program, while perhaps sticking to the same pattern of training for each muscle group. I personally prefer to do at least one—and sometimes up to three—basic exercise for each body part, using maximum poundages, then one to three additional isolation movements for the same muscle group. In this manner, I can maintain, perhaps even increase, muscle mass while at the same time refining the development of each muscle complex.

"When I come into the gym, I might first substitute variations of particular exercises into my routine for a body part. If I had done incline barbell presses on a 45-degree angle in my previous chest workout, I might do dumbbell inclines at the same angle, machine inclines at a variety of angles, or barbell inclines at a variety of angles. And when using a barbell or Smith machine, I can even vary the width of my grip in order to stress my pectoral muscles from even more diverse angles.

"Additionally, I can train heavy, medium, or relatively light; I can vary the order of exercises; change the tempo of a workout; switch off to a different training principle; do less or more sets or reps; superset, triset, or giant set the body part; or move the weights very quickly or slowly. The number of variations on each routine is almost infinite. I daresay that I probably have never performed the same routine for any body part, ever.

"A very real advantage of avoiding a set routine is that this allows you to train instinctively in the gym, matching your workout to your energy levels, ability to concentrate, and your innate feel for what your body needs at that moment. This is what the legendary Dave Draper used to call 'freewheeling it.' And I failed to make really good gains from my training efforts until I learned to train instinctively like this.

"As you gradually develop a flawless instinct for your body's physical requirements, you can begin to freewheel it in the gym yourself. But don't make the common mistake of allowing instinctive training to make you lazy. You always have to push yourself to go all out, regardless of the routine or intensity techniques you are using for each body part. That's the only sure way to become a winner."

Using the Weider Muscle Confusion Training Principle will allow you to avoid mental boredom. It also prevents your body from adapting to a set routine, thus failing to make the gains you should be making from your workouts. When you stick to a set order of exercises, number of sets, reps, and weight, your body can adapt to the routine so completely that you are essentially no longer overloading the muscles. As a result, you will fail to keep pushing yourself to new gains.

As with every principle, exercise, or routine I present in this book, you should give Muscle Confusion a trial in your own workouts, using your training instinct to determine whether it works well for you. I think it will, but you have to make that decision for yourself. If Muscle Confusion does work well, you can use the words "shake it up baby" to characterize all of your future training programs. Simply by shaking up your routine from one workout to the next, you can make continuous, high-gear gains in muscle mass and quality. Who could ask for more?

PART II
ADVICE TO
INTERMEDIATE
BODYBUILDERS

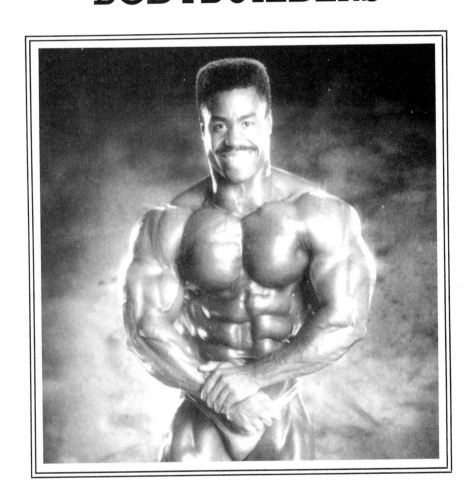

7
Instinctive Training and Overtraining

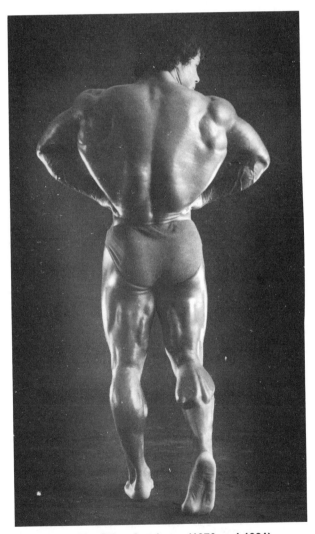

A two-time Mr. Olympia winner (1976 and 1981), Franco Columbu was one of the most powerful bodybuilders of all time, having set world records in power lifts on several occasions. Once a shepherd boy in Sardinia, Franco became a successful Doctor of Chiropractic and businessman. He has one of the most inspiring success stories in the history of the sport. Franco's back lat spread mandatory pose was so sensationally broad that his fans dubbed it "The Cobra Head pose."

Talk to the top 100 bodybuilding champions in the world, and every one of them will tell you that the Weider Instinctive Training Principle is the most important principle to all bodybuilders. Indeed, the Instinctive Principle is so important to bodybuilders that I often refer to it as the master principle. The Weider Instinctive Training Principle governs the effective use of every other Weider Principle.

Dr. Franco Columbu (winner of two Mr. Olympia titles) discusses the value of mastering the Weider Instinctive Training Principle: "One of the most fundamental secrets of successful bodybuilding is getting to know your body, how it reacts to various training and nutritional practices. And the only way to determine what works best for your body and physiological system is through trial and error.

"You will make hundreds of training and nutritional experiments in your body lab over the years. And unless you have finely honed your instinctive training ability, it will take many weeks, even months, to evaluate each experiment. Since each training and nutrition variable should be tested individually, it could take you 20–30 years to determine precisely how your body reacts to each new external stimulus if you did not take the time to master the Weider Instinctive Training Principle.

"When you have developed instinctive training ability, it will take you only a few short days or weeks to evaluate each training or nutritional variable. This in turn shortens the length of time you will require to learn your body's requirements to as few as 1–1½ years, thereby leaving you with plenty of time in which to actually build up your body. So, it definitely pays to master the Weider Instinctive Training Principle."

WHAT IS INSTINCTIVE TRAINING?

When I was originally researching the Weider Instinctive Training Principle back in the 1950s, I noticed that selected champions of that era—men like Clancy Ross, Marvin Eder, and Jack Dellinger—could tell more quickly than most other bodybuilders whether a new technique or dietary rule would be of value in their overall training philosophies. Such a champion seemed to have an instinctive "feel" for what would or would not work for him.

I knew I'd have a terrific new addition to my Weider system of bodybuilding if I could first learn how these hyperinstinctive champions became so intuitive, and then codify such a new principle so all bodybuilders could understand it and apply it to their own training and dietary efforts. So, I interviewed all of the champions who had developed such great instinct for proper training and diet.

Gradually, I began to recognize a common thread, which ran through every champion's mastery of instinctive training ability. Each of the champions had drawn a parallel between the subtle signals the body was giving him and the rate at which he was making progress as a result of his training and dietary practices. With experience, each champ had learned that signals such as a good muscle pump or next-day muscle soreness would affirm that a muscle group had been trained optimally and would be increasing in mass and strength quite rapidly.

Today we refer to these subtle signals our bodies give us as *biofeedback*. And by systematically searching for biofeedback signals and attempting to interpret them, we can over a period of time learn to listen to our bodies. And the body is almost never wrong in telling us its day-to-day requirements for exercise and nutrition.

Complete mastery of biofeedback signals is complete mastery of the Weider Instinctive Training Principle. And mastering the Instinctive Principle will allow you to unerringly modify your training and nutritional philosophies so they approach the ideal formula for improving your physique at the fastest possible rate.

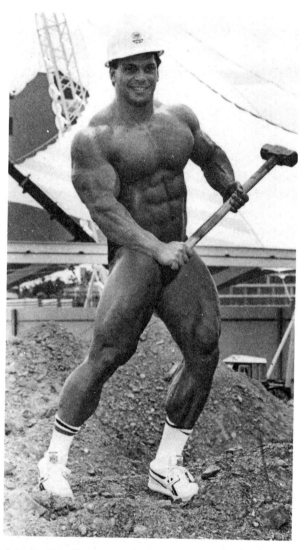

A body literally under construction. Many times an IFBB Pro Grand Prix Champion, Rich Gaspari was clowning around at a construction site, but the parallels between putting up a highrise and building a championship physique are very similar. First must come a comprehensive plan, then plenty of quality materials (workouts, good food, a solid mental approach). And after several years of hard work— much longer than it takes to put up most buildings— you end up with a physique comparable to that of Richard Gaspari.

HOW TO RECOGNIZE BIOFEEDBACK DATA

What should you be looking for when you begin to master the Weider Instinctive Training Principle? The easiest positive signal that a particular training variable is working is muscle pump, the pleasantly tight feeling in your muscles that lasts for several hours after you have finished a workout.

It's essential that you experiment with only one training or dietary variable at a time. Play with different combinations of movements for a particular body part and see which scheme of exercises gives you the best pump. Later you can try various numbers of sets for each movement, different rep ranges, and various combinations in workout tempo.

With time you will work out precisely which combination of exercises, routines, and training principles give you the best pump. But never stop experimenting, even if you feel you have come up with a perfect workout combination. You will constantly read or hear about new training and dietary techniques, and you should continue to experiment in an effort to further refine your overall bodybuilding philosophy. Becoming so complacent that you give up the quest for new knowledge spells certain death for your bodybuilding career.

Other biofeedback signals you must learn to recognize are listed below, along with suggestions for the interpretation of each signal.

- *Greater-than-normal muscle soreness.* The change of routines or training techniques has stimulated the muscles either more intensely or from a difficult angle than before, which means the changes which you made had positive value.
- *Residual fatigue and/or loss of enthusiasm for workouts.* You are doing too many total sets each workout, which means you are beginning to overtrain. And when you are overtrained, you will cease to make good progress from your workouts.
- *The sensation of your muscles contracting powerfully against the weights in each exercise.* Your mental concentration is at an optimum level, which will result in fast muscle growth. Conversely, the lack of this contractile sensation can indicate that you are not concentrating as completely as you must in order to make optimum gains in muscle mass and quality.
- *A noticeable increase in the amount of weight you can use with strict form in a particular bodybuilding exercise.* Since there is a direct, linear relationship between strength levels and muscle mass, your muscles are growing larger and stronger as a result of your efforts in the gym.

- *Increases in the measurements of various body girths.* As long as you are not concurrently gaining excessive body fat, your muscle mass is increasing.
- *Appearance in the mirror.* The way you appear in the mirror, as well as in progress photos taken at regular intervals, gives you a very clear picture of whether your appearance is improving, and appearance improvement is undoubtedly the end result of serious

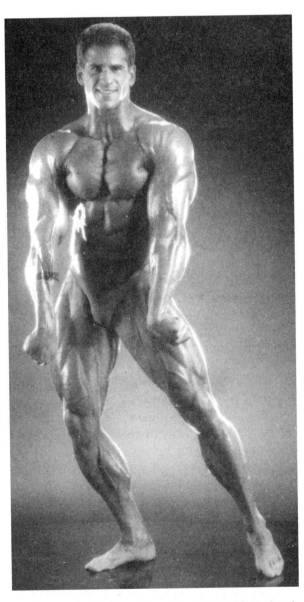

One of twins, Tom Terwilliger (the 1986 NPC National Light-Heavyweight Champion) has a brother who is also well-developed, although the pair has yet to approach the collective competitive success of the Mentzer brothers. Tom is a gym owner in Long Island, New York, and regularly competes in IFBB professional shows.

bodybuilding. If you are growing fatter, for example, you know you should begin cutting back on your calories.

- *Relative energy levels.* As long as you are energetic during your workouts, and for the rest of the day, you are eating and sleeping optimally. But if you are tired a lot of the time, you need to improve your diet and/or sleep-rest patterns.

- *Fluctuations in mood.* If you are moody too often, it can slow your progress, so you should take steps to reduce stress and situations that can cause emotional depression.

Generally speaking, it takes much less time to evaluate nutritional variables. Slight changes in dietary practices will result in dramatic changes in energy, muscle pump, amount of body water retention, or degree of body fat. And these slight dietary adjustments can be as subtle as taking in 100 extra milligrams of vitamin C, or as gross as eating half of the normal number of calories to which you are accustomed.

After a year or two of detecting and monitoring your body's biofeedback signals, you will develop such an intuitive instinct for how your muscles should feel when being optimally trained that you will be able to tell after only a few sets whether a new training or nutritional variable should be included in your training philosophy. And when you reach this level of intuition, you have perfect command of your instinctive training ability.

"When I look back at my first 2-3 years of serious bodybuilding," notes *Tom Terwilliger* (National Light-Heavyweight Champion), "I made twice as much progress the second year than the first. Usually progress comes slower each successive year. But in my case, I needed a year of experimentation in the gym and in the kitchen in order to master the Weider Instinctive Training Principle and use it to determine which routines, exercises, sets, reps, training principles, and foods worked best for me.

"When I learned how to train and eat correctly, I began making comparatively sensational progress in light of my first year of steady training. Of course, I have never made really fast progress, at least not as fast as some top bodybuilders I know, but the rate of progress was fast enough to keep me interested in my

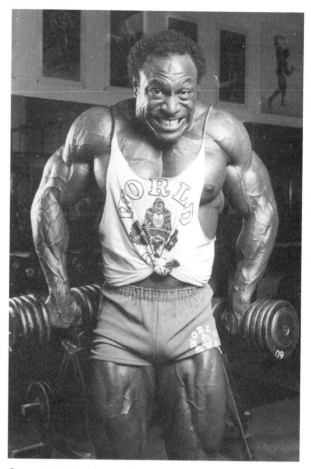

Superstar Lee Haney demonstrates his unique version of dumbbell shrugs with the weights held behind his hips and his arms held slightly bent. Set after set, Lee adds a brick here, a window sash there, and soon he also has a physique comparable to Rich Gaspari, whom he has defeated on many occasions, including three straight Mr. Olympia shows between 1986 and 1988.

workouts. I owe the Instinctive Training Principle for a large portion of my success as an amateur and professional bodybuilder!"

OVERTRAINING

"The single most common mistake made by almost all bodybuilders—from beginners to the most advanced men—is to overtrain," reveals *Lee Haney*, five times Mr. Olympia. "Anyone who allows himself to become overtrained will make little or no progress from his efforts in the gym. And in extreme cases of overtraining, it is actually possible to *lose* muscle mass!

"Young bodybuilders are usually surprised when they read my training programs. In spite of my huge muscles, I do what seems to them very few total sets for each body part, usually as few as 12–15 for the large muscle groups. But training on low sets like this is the very reason I have been able to develop huge muscles—it keeps me from overtraining while stimulating my muscles to keep increasing in hypertrophy at a very fast rate. I firmly believe a bodybuilder has to consciously *under*train to continue making great gains from his workouts."

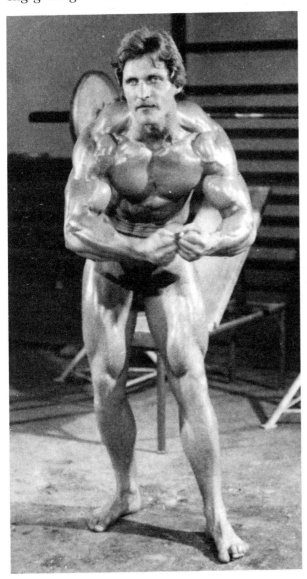

Born and raised in East Germany, Peter Hensel was forced to bring his family west in order to further his bodybuilding aspirations. Within one year of West German food and training, Hensel had won the IFBB Heavyweight World Championship, and has since gone on to become a successful pro bodybuilder. This very early photo should be compared with some of Peter's more recent pictures to show how much he's improved since coming west.

Overtraining occurs when you do too many long, exhausting workouts and push your system past the point where your body can fully recover between training sessions. As you continue to push your body past its limited ability to recuperate between workouts, it will give you one or more biofeedback signals that it will soon become overtrained. Unfortunately, many bodybuilders fail to correctly read these signals, inexorably pushing their bodies into a full-blown overtrained state in which they are unable to make gains in muscle mass, no matter how hard they continue to push heavy iron.

Following are the 10 most common signals that you are becoming overtrained:

- Lack of enthusiasm for workouts
- Low energy levels (chronic fatigue)
- Irritability
- Persistently sore muscles and/or joints
- Deterioration of motor coordination
- Insomnia
- Loss of appetite
- Deterioration of ability to concentrate
- Elevated morning pulse rate
- Elevated morning blood pressure

If you notice two or more of these symptoms, chances are good that you are entering an overtrained condition. A bit later in this chapter, I will tell you what steps you must take to prevent overtraining and continue to make good gains from your heavy gym sessions. But for now, I will tell you how to avoid overtraining.

The best tool you have for avoiding overtraining is the Weider Instinctive Training Principle. If you could talk to all of the Weider-trained bodybuilding superstars, they would tell you the same thing *Peter Hensel* (World Heavyweight Champion) tells men who attend his training seminars: "You must *always* listen to your body. If you develop instinctive training ability and learn to listen to what your body tells you about its requirements, you will know exactly how to train, eat, and approach the mental aspect of high-level bodybuilding. When your body is becoming overtrained, it will tell you that you need to take a layoff and get more rest, allowing it to fully recuperate. Only then can you start back with your heavy bodybuilding workouts, knowing you will be making good gains from them."

Signals of Overtraining

The biggest red flag signaling an overtraining problem is lack of enthusiasm for your workouts. When it comes time to leave for the gym and you decide you'd rather wrestle King Kong than pump iron, you should immediately know you are becoming overtrained. And when you feel this way for three or four days in a row, you are definitely overtrained.

Lack of enthusiasm for workouts goes hand in hand with low energy levels, which in turn is a function of insomnia. Irritability, loss of appetite, and persistently sore muscles and/or joints are also easily recognized signals that you are overtraining. But you'll always need to be alert for such signals, or you'll completely

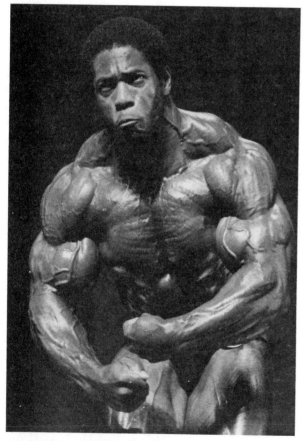

Brutally massive and muscular is the only way to describe the competitively conditioned physique of Britain's Bertil Fox, who has won several Mr. World and Mr. Universe titles before turning to IFBB competition. His best IFBB placing to date was fifth at the hotly contested Munich, West Germany show in 1983, a competition won by Samir Bannout. Fox is every bit as strong as he looks, capable of reps with more than 500 pounds in the bench press with very little warm-up.

ignore them. And you'll need to be especially alert for signs of deteriorating motor coordination and diminished ability to concentrate during a set.

When you begin to push a barbell upward on benches or inclines and it gets out of the groove occasionally, your motor coordination is going south. The same can be said of many other exercises, but you will most easily recognize signs of poor motor coordination in the really heavy basic movements like benches, squats, and overhead presses.

Mental concentration can deteriorate to the point where you find your mind is focused on your grocery list rather than on the biceps, which are straining against the weight in barbell preacher curls. All serious bodybuilders have developed pinpoint concentration during every set, and a deterioration of this ability should tell you that you are becoming overtrained.

One of the most scientific methods of determining when you are becoming overtrained is monitoring your morning pulse rate and blood pressure. Exercise scientists working with endurance athletes discovered that a spike in pulse and/or blood pressure is a signal that an athlete is overtrained. Both of these signals can be used by bodybuilders to indicate when they are pushing too hard with the long workouts.

Blood pressure readings are a little complicated, but you should record in your training diary your pulse rate upon awakening each morning. While still lying in bed, you can use a watch or clock with a sweep second hand to take your pulse. If it goes up more than 3-5 beats per minute, you know absolutely that you are becoming overtrained.

If you do want to take your blood pressure every day, an inexpensive pressure cuff can be purchased in most drug stores. They range in price from about $100-$130, and come with instructions for foolproof use. Any spike in morning (resting) blood pressure also indicates that you are becoming overtrained. And combined with pulse-rate readings, blood pressure lets you know scientifically when you are becoming overtrained. These two methods are the best available for detecting this condition.

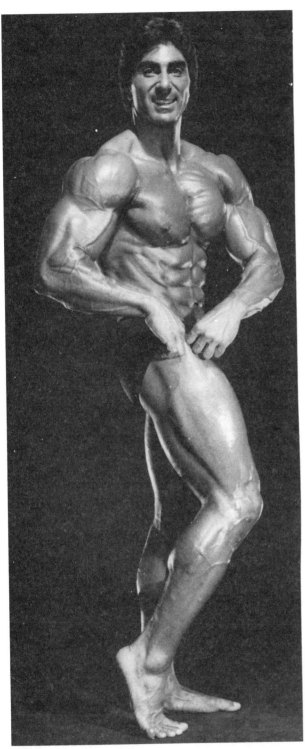

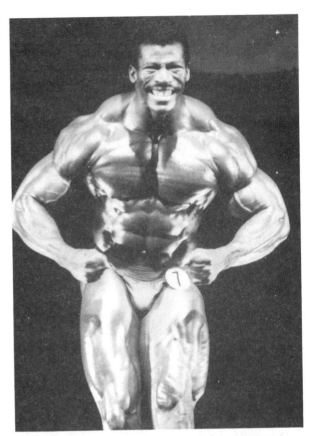

Detroit's most muscular cop is massive Ron Love, who has won his weight class at the NPC Nationals and also taken an IFBB Pro World Championship. Shot in the line of duty, Ron eventually ended up in the station gym for a little rehab and liked what he saw. It's legend that he bench pressed 335 pounds (at 200 pounds body weight) the first time he touched a weight. He's now capable of benching 600 pounds, although doing so would leave him more open to injury than if he consistently trained with weights about 80% to 90% of that maximum.

Why You Overtrain

Ron Love (National Heavyweight Champion) tells us we should think of our checking account when trying to understand why a bodybuilder overtrains: "It's easier for most young bodybuilders to understand how various energy flows can cause overtraining if they think about their checking accounts. In your checking account, you are constantly writing checks and depositing money to cover your checks when they come back to the bank for payment.

"As long as you don't write checks for greater amounts of money than you have deposited, everything will be copacetic. But if you write checks totalling more money than you actually have in your account, the account will become

Owner of a gym equipment and sunbed concern, Dennis Tinerino of Northridge, California, is one of the most titled bodybuilders of all time. Among his awards are Teenage Mr. America, Mr. North America (won while still a teen), Mr. USA, Mr. America, Junior Mr. America, Natural Mr. America (a drug-tested event, the first of its kind in bodybuilding history), Amateur Mr. Universe, and Pro Mr. Universe. Despite heavy business pressures, Denny still trains both hard and regularly.

overdrawn and the bank will take an immediate interest in you.

"In the same way you have a flow of money into and out of your checking account, you have a flow of energy into and out of your body. And you must keep your energy flows either balanced or have more energy coming in than going out, or you will go 'energy broke,' or become overtrained.

"The most obvious way in which you expend energy each day is in your bodybuilding work-

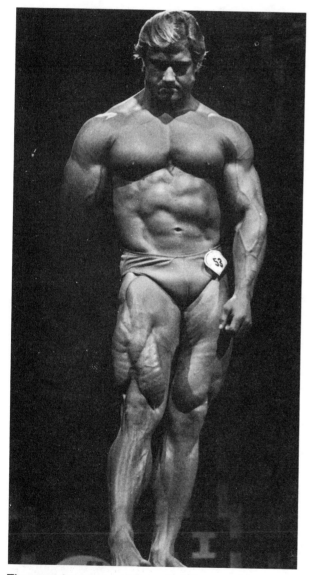

The most famous quadriceps isolation in the business, as demonstrated by Mr. Universe Tom Platz, now a successful businessman and aspiring actor. Never in the history of the sport has such leg mass been combined with such a wealth of cross striations within each quadriceps muscle.

outs. But you can also expend energy through aerobic exercise, by burning off nervous energy, and by failing to follow good nutritional rules or neglecting to get sufficient rest and sleep each day.

"On the other side of the coin, you deposit energy by eating correctly and getting enough sleep and rest. Primarily, you should avoid junk foods while consuming at least one gram of protein per pound of bodyweight. But you should also consume plenty of complex carbohydrate foods and adequate food supplements per day."

Sleep and rest requirements vary from one individual to another. An average amount of sleep per day is 8 hours, but I have known top bodybuilders who sleep as little as 5-6 hours and others who require 10 or more hours of sleep per day. Certainly, bodybuilders peaking for an upcoming show tend to get less sleep than the average, due to precompetitive tension.

I recommend enough sleep each night to keep you from nodding off during the day, whatever that amount might be. If you require a rule for sleep and rest, I can best give it to you in three parts:

- Sleep 8-9 hours per night.
- Take one short nap (20-30 minutes) each afternoon.
- Include brief (3-5 minutes) rest breaks every 2-3 hours, in which you put your feet up and attempt to relax completely.

Again, sleep and rest requirements are individual, and they can even vary from one day to the next as a function of length and intensity of training sessions, stress levels, travel across several time zones, diet, and many other variables. It may take you several months to determine how much sleep and rest you require.

By now you have probably concluded that overtraining can be caused by several variables. Primarily, it is caused by excessively long training sessions, but not by short, high-intensity workouts. And it can be exacerbated by faulty diet, excessive stress, and insufficient sleep and rest. Any combination of these variables can cause you to slip into an overtrained state in which you will cease to gain muscle mass and strength.

For elite bodybuilders, there is a very thin line between doing the maximum amount of high-intensity training necessary to induce optimum muscle hypertrophy, and doing too much training and lapsing into an overtrained state. But by using the Weider Instinctive Training Principle to advantage, you will be able to consistently push yourself close to that line without slipping over it, allowing yourself to make consistently great gains from your workouts.

WHEN YOU HAVE OVERTRAINED

When you are in an overtrained state, your body is deeply fatigued. So the first step you should take when overtrained is to take a layoff from your bodybuilding workouts. Stay totally out of the gym for at least 1–2 weeks in order to allow your body to rest and fully recover its normal energy reserves.

The champs have different thoughts about

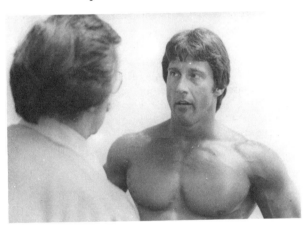

Always one to increase his knowledge of the sport, and hence his instinct for what works best for him, is Frank Zane. Here Frank talks with Joe Weider.

layoffs. Three-time Mr. Olympia *Frank Zane* says, "I always take a one-month training layoff after each Olympia, before getting back into the gym to gradually build up my training intensity from a relatively low base level. This layoff allows my body to recover from the super-hard training it takes to reach Olympian physical condition. It also allows minor injuries to heal completely. Such injuries are an inevitable consequence of the highly intense training any bodybuilder needs to go through to reach peak shape."

In contrast, *John Terilli* (Australasian Champion and a leading pro bodybuilder) believes, "It is necessary for me to take a one-week layoff from the gym every 2–3 months. Such a regularly scheduled layoff keeps me from overtraining, allows minor nagging injuries time to heal, and gets me back into the gym with newfound enthusiasm for my workouts."

A few other bodybuilders simply take a day off here and there when they feel that they are not recovering fully between workouts. *Gary Strydom* (NPC National Champion) is typical of these men: "I can always tell when I have accumulated too much residual fatigue and

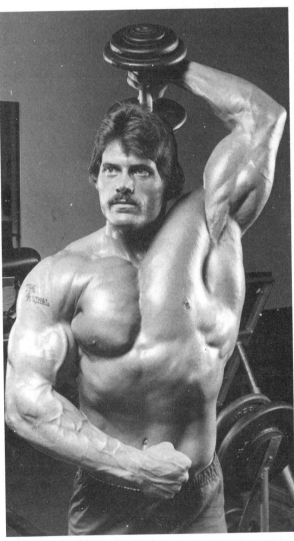

Another aspiring actor, Rod Koontz was an overall Mr. USA winner in the middle 1970s, and still competes professionally on occasion. He and his lovely wife, Yvonne, have a young son, who already shows much promise to follow in Daddy's footsteps.

need an extra day off. So if I'm following a three-on and one-off system, it might become one-on, one-off, two-on, one-off. That extra day of rest really does the trick, keeping me from becoming overtrained."

The best rule for determining the length of a layoff once you have overtrained is to stay out of the gym until you have built up so much enthusiasm for your upcoming workouts that you literally find it difficult to stay away from the iron. Again, this is your body's way of telling you that it has completely recovered from the overtrained state and is ready to start making new gains. This could occur after as few as 3–4 days or as many as 3–4 weeks.

Don't fret about losing a little muscle mass and tone while on a layoff, because you will regain it very quickly when you are back in the gym. And you will make far better overall gains from your workouts when you are not overtrained than when you are, so a layoff is always a good investment when you are going all-out to gain body mass for your next competition.

After your layoff, you should start back with a routine consisting of 20%–30% less total sets, but including such Weider high-intensity training techniques as forced reps, descending sets, and retro-gravity (negative) reps.

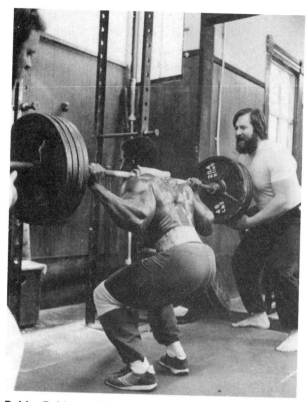

Robby Robinson (Mr. America, Mr. World, Mr. Universe, and a victor at many IFBB professional competitions) got his leg development the hard way— he *worked* for it. Even this is a relatively light weight for Bob—something in the neighborhood of 400 pounds. Note his use of safety spotters at each end of the bar to lift the weight off should he unexpectedly incur an injury in mid rep.

PREVENTING OVERTRAINING

The most obvious solution to overtraining is to prevent it from ever occurring in the first place. And the easiest way to prevent overtraining is to consistently *under*train. By this I mean you should always do a few less total sets for each muscle group than you think you should be doing. But each set that you do perform should be of very high intensity.

The simple factor most responsible for muscle hypertrophy is training intensity. Low-intensity training builds small muscles, very much like running marathon distances builds skinny little legs. And high-intensity training builds big muscles, the type of muscular development necessary to win major bodybuilding titles.

"When you train with high intensity," reveals *Mike Mentzer* (Mr. America, Mr. Uni-

verse), "it is impossible to do many sets. So doing 20 sets for a muscle group requires each set to be of relatively low intensity. The only way a bodybuilder can do 20 sets per body part is to pace himself each set, conserving strength and energy to expend on the last few sets."

Six-day split routines are excellent for high-level bodybuilders who are in a precontest body-refining cycle, but it is very difficult to gain any muscle mass on such a training program. Most of the champions find it beneficial to slightly overtrain when peaking for a competition, but know they should be systematically undertraining when attempting to increase muscle mass. Therefore, I strongly recommend training less frequently during an off-season building cycle.

Bodybuilders with less than 1½–2 years of steady training behind them will undoubtedly

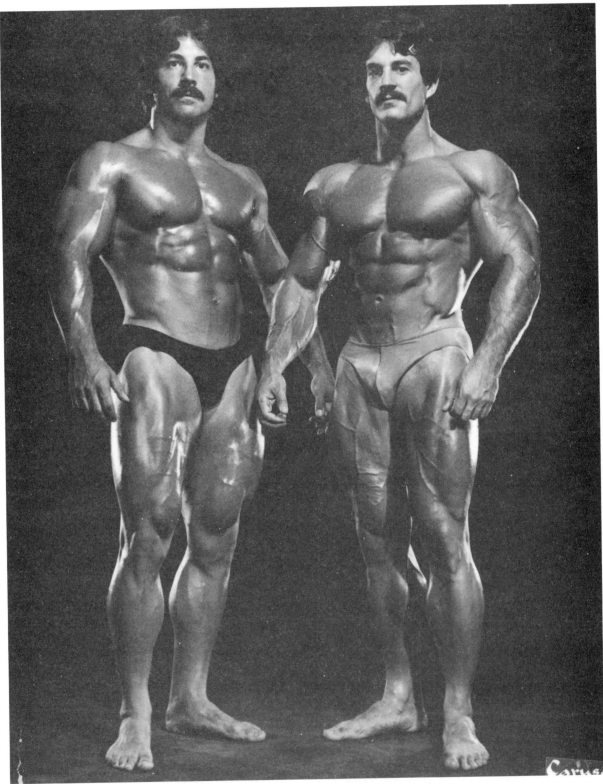

The Genetics Brothers—Ray (left) and Mike Mentzer are the only brothers to have both won Mr. America titles. Mike took his in 1979. This particular photo was taken about two years before Ray reached his peak of muscular development, which was very near his brother's pictured development.

make their best gains while following a four-day split routine in which each major muscle group is trained twice a week. Virtually all other bodybuilders will make excellent progress following a program in which they divide their body parts routines into three equal installments on three consecutive days, followed by one day of rest before the cycle is repeated.

By systematically training with relatively short, high-intensity workouts and using the Weider Instinctive Training Principle to determine when you are beginning to overtrain, you will find it relatively easy to avoid becoming overtrained. And this in turn will allow you to continue making fast progress from your bodybuilding training, diet, and mental approach.

8
Weider
Specialization
Methods

One inevitable fact in serious bodybuilding is that no two body parts will respond to hard weight work at the same speed. Inevitably, some muscle groups forge ahead, gaining mass by leaps and bounds as a result of seemingly low-intensity effort in the gym. And just as inevitably, other body parts will lag behind in spite of seemingly Herculean efforts.

One of the most fundamental qualities of a contest-winning physique is an equal development of every muscle group, with none visibly under- or over-developed. All of the greats of the sport—Lee Haney, Richie Gaspari, Mike Christian, Lee Labrada, Ron Love, and many others—have almost ideally balanced proportions. And if you wish to win some of the bigger titles, you must embark on a specialized training program, which will help you to balance out your own physical proportions.

MUSCLE PRIORITY TRAINING

At the time of writing this book, ultramassive *Lee Haney* is the greatest of the greats, having won five consecutive Mr. Olympia titles, so I will let this superbly developed athlete explain the Weider Muscle Priority Training Principle the way he uses it:

"I entered my first Mr. Olympia show in 1983 at Munich, West Germany, following a very successful '82 campaign in which I won the Heavyweight and Overall NPC National Championships, plus the IFBB World Heavyweight Championship, all premier amateur events. At Munich, I placed third behind the winner, Samir Bannout, and Mohamed Makkawy. When I checked with the judges after the competition, the rap on me was that I had weak upper arm development compared to the rest of

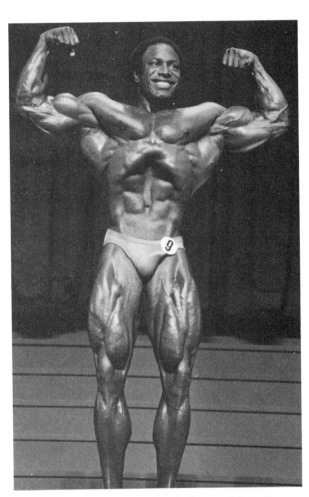

Early in his career, when this photo was taken, the now-legendary five-time Mr. Olympia Lee Haney was roundly criticized for having deficient arm and calf development. One of the most intelligent men in the sport, Haney analyzed his problems and worked systematically to correct them. For proof of his success in both respects, just glance at his photo in "The Mr. Olympia Bodybuilding Hall of Fame" in Chapter 26.

my body, which I readily conceded after viewing photos of that Olympia. So, I embarked on a heavy program of arm specialization using

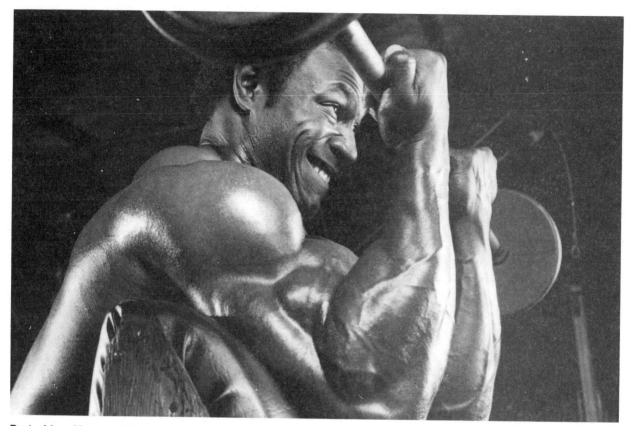

Part of Lee Haney's all-out attack on his arms consists of plenty of sets of barbell preacher curls . . .

the Weider Muscle Priority Training Principle.

"Cut to the 1984 Mr. Olympia extravaganza at Madison Square Garden in New York City. I had improved every muscle group, particularly my arms, so much and had achieved such superior muscle density and detail that I easily won my first Mr. Olympia title. To say the least, I was ecstatic with the victory, my third pro title, but by far the most important up to that point.

"I thought I had made considerable added improvement to my physique for the 1985 Olympia in Brussels, Belgium. I had particularly improved my delts, abdominals, and calves, plus streamlined my hip girdle. History records a second Lee Haney Mr. Olympia victory at Brussels, but it was definitely not by the overwhelming margin I enjoyed the previous year. I felt happy to have survived the challenge of the oldest and youngest men in the show, ageless Albert Beckles, second place, and 21-year-old Rich Gaspari, my old training partner, third.

"The problem I identified after the '85 Olympia was deficient thigh mass and muscularity. So, I immediately embarked upon a specialized program of muscle priority leg training. The program succeeded admirably, and my thighs *were* vastly improved—as was the rest of my physique to a lesser degree—for the 1986 Olympia at Columbus, Ohio. I easily overwhelmed Gaspari, who placed second, and upstart Mike Christian, third, recording a perfect score sheet: First-place votes from every judge in every round, including the posedown.

"I'm sure you wonder how I have consistently worked such minor miracles on my physique over the years. To understand how I do it, you must first understand how the Weider Muscle Priority Training Principle works, since muscle priority training forms the foundation of my TotaLee Awesome specialization programs.

"To bring a lagging muscle group up to the level of the rest of your physique, you must train it with absolute maximum intensity. The object is not to do a long and involved workout consisting of 25–30 total sets. Rather, you have to bomb the lagging body part with totally brutal intensity for a quick 10–12 total sets.

"It isn't easy to muster up this type of energy. You certainly cannot expend such a huge must also program your stronger muscle group(s) later in your training schedule while proportionately cutting back on both the amount and intensity of work you give them. Cutting back on intensity and duration of training for stronger areas serves two functions:

- It allows you to "bank" energy for expenditure on weaker areas.
- It allows the strong body parts to regress a bit in development, so it is even easier to balance your physical proportions.

"You should never worry about allowing a dominant muscle group to slide a little in development, because it will come up very quickly with 8–10 weeks of specialized training once the weaker areas have been improved. This was exactly the case I faced when bringing up my arms, because I proportionately decreased training intensity for my more strongly developed chest and shoulder muscles. I didn't resume hard training on pecs and delts until nine weeks before the Olympia, and by the time I stepped onstage to compete in '84, both body parts were even better than before, plus in perfect harmony with my biceps and triceps development.

"In some cases when a large muscle group needs improvement, muscle priority dictates that you train it by itself in a session during which you work no other body parts. When I wanted to bring up my legs, this is exactly how I priority trained them. I did only legs on two workout days out of every eight, divided up the rest of my body parts into two equal groups and did each one twice on four additional days, and finally I rested for two days.

"It worked great for me!"

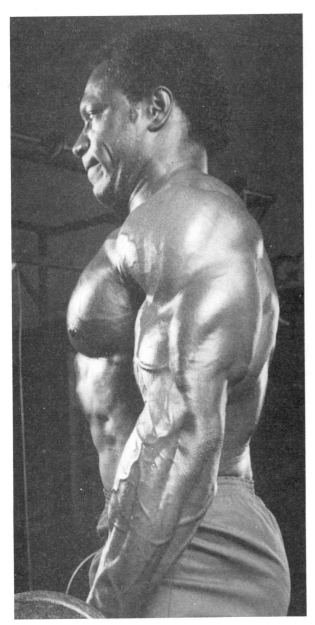

... **standing barbell curls** ...

SPECIALIZATION TRAINING

After years of practical, in-the-gym experimentation—abetted by what exercise physiologists working on Weider Research Clinic studies have discovered—I concluded that it is best to train a lagging body part every fourth day. This means you will follow the popular three-on, one-off split routine. Following are examples of how you would use this type of split routine to specialize on various body parts:

amount of energy toward the end of a workout when your fuel tanks are edging toward empty. It just stands to reason that such a high-intensity workout must take place at the beginning of a training session when you have a maximum amount of physical and mental energy for expenditure in intense, specialized training to improve a weak area. And that is the essence of the Weider Muscle Priority Principle, the way I have applied it to my own workouts: Work a weak body part first in a training session when you have optimum energy reserves.

"As you schedule a weak body part first in your routine and bomb it unmercifully, you

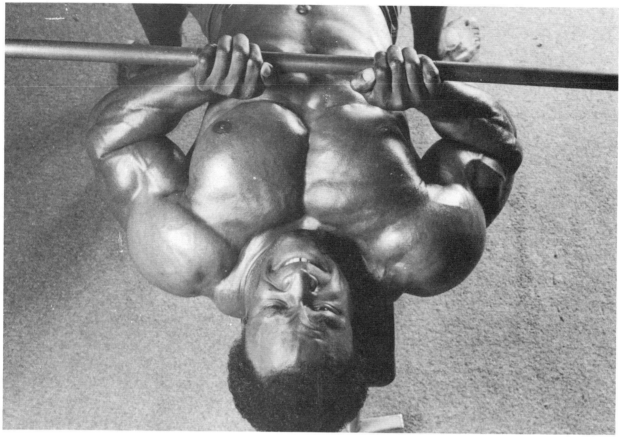

. . . close-grip bench presses . . .

CHEST SPECIALIZATION

Day 1	Day 2	Day 3	Day 4
Chest	Back	Thighs	Rest
Biceps	Shoulders	Triceps	
Abdominals	Calves	Forearms	

SHOULDER SPECIALIZATION

Day 1	Day 2	Day 3	Day 4
Shoulders	Back	Thighs	Rest
Biceps	Chest	Triceps	
Abdominals	Calves	Forearms	

BACK SPECIALIZATION

Day 1	Day 2	Day 3	Day 4
Back	Chest	Thighs	Rest
Triceps	Shoulders	Biceps	
Abdominals	Calves	Forearms	

ARM SPECIALIZATION

Day 1	Day 2	Day 3	Day 4
Upper Arms	Chest	Thighs	Rest
Forearms	Back	Shoulders	Rest
Abdominals	Calves		

LEG SPECIALIZATION

Day 1	Day 2	Day 3	Day 4
Quadriceps	Chest	Shoulders	Rest
Hamstrings	Back	Upper Arms	
Abdominals	Calves	Forearms	

Note: This last program is exactly the type Lee Haney talked about for leg specialization.

I'm sure you can see a pattern developing in these routines. The weak area is not only bombed first on a certain training day, but that certain training day also follows a full rest day, allowing you maximum energy to expend on bombing it. Almost all of the top stars in the sport (men and women alike) work weaker body parts in this manner.

Should you require specialized training on calves and/or abdominals, these body parts should also be scheduled first on a particular workout day. Both muscle groups should be bombed with short, highly intense workouts featuring a wide variety of exercises aimed at

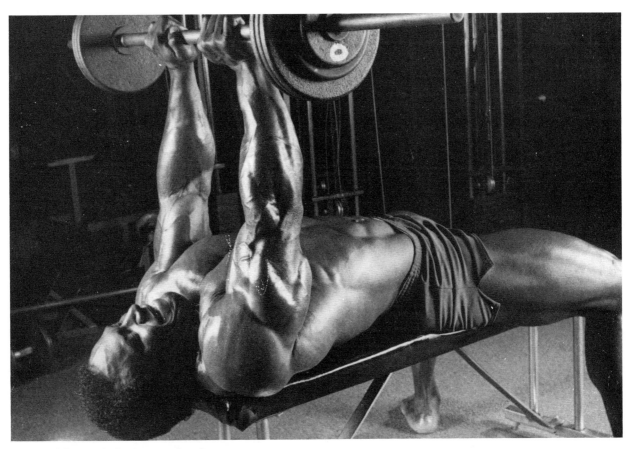

. . . and lying barbell triceps extensions.

every facet of the muscle complex on which you are specializing.

It should be obvious that you will be able to specialize effectively on only one muscle group at a time, but feel free after 2–3 months of specializing on one to shift off to another lagging area. I have seen countless top bodybuilders attempt to specialize on two or more weak areas, and they have always failed to reach their goals of improving several weak areas at once. You should always stick to one specialized body part at a time. Even though this might seem like a slower approach, it is by far the fastest over the long haul.

WHEN TO SPECIALIZE

The time to begin specializing on a weak body part is the moment you first notice it is lagging behind other muscle groups. This could occur after as few as 6–8 months, so you should be constantly alert for muscle groups which develop either very easily or only with great diffi-

culty, then take appropriate measures to harmonize your physical proportions.

If you train in a home gym rather than a big commercial muscle emporium, you will be forced to use your own judgment on which body part will need special attention. Traditionally, this has taken place in front of a mirror. But a mirror does have its limitations, because many bodybuilders see only what they want to see when in front of a mirror. Flabby abs can appear flat and as ridged as an old-fashioned washboard, or weakly developed legs can look like the pillars of Hercules. I'm sure you get the picture.

When making your own physical evaluation, I strongly urge you to have a friend take photographs of you in standard physique poses. And as mentioned in Part I, you can tape some of these photos into your training diary as a means of determining long-range progress in improving your physique. Any type of print can be used, from a simple color Polaroid print 3 × 4-inches in size up to a professionally pho-

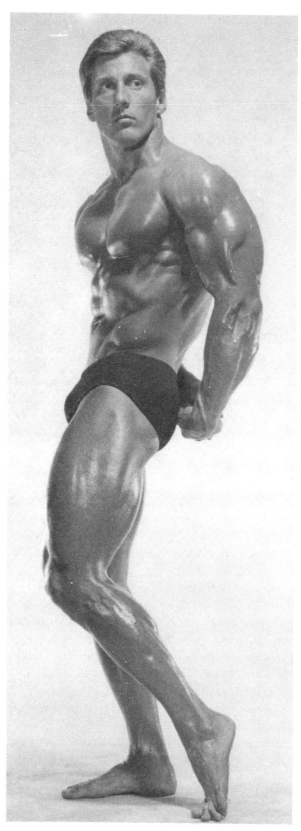

Early in his own competitive career (this photo was taken about 1965), Frank Zane was unable to develop true contest muscularity and failed to win many competitions he would have otherwise won if he'd been more muscular.

tographed and produced 8 × 10-inch black-and-white or color print.

I firmly believe you can best evaluate your physique only with photographs, because outstandingly strong or weak body parts are glaringly easy to spot. They almost hit you in the face in comparison to attempting to identify such muscle groups when looking at yourself in a mirror. But either way, be honest with yourself, if not downright critical of your physique.

Should you train in a large public gym, you will be able to find an experienced bodybuilder, the gym owner, or even an experienced physique judge who will give you a fair critique of your development. But you should always shy away from training buddies, since people close to you will often be even more blind to your weak and strong points than you might be yourself.

Once you are in competition, I strongly suggest that you approach judges after each show to discover which weak point(s) you should improve before your next show. Just be sure you talk to each judge with a humble desire to improve yourself. Never argue with any judge when he tells you what you need to improve. I've actually seen bodybuilders heatedly arguing with judges about whether their legs look like those of a seagull at the beach! It's much better to be polite.

TRAINING INTENSITY LEVEL

Bodybuilders specializing on a lagging body part should be cognizant of the following 11 rules for optimum training:

- Do fewer total sets than you normally would. I suggest reducing total sets for a weak muscle group by about 30%. So if you have been doing 10 total sets for a lagging set of biceps, cut back to 7 sets.
- Train fast. Even with the heaviest poundages, you should rest no longer than 90 seconds between sets when working large muscle groups, 60 seconds on smaller body parts.
- Attack each lagging muscle group from a maximum number of angles. A routine consisting of five sets each on two exercises is not as productive as one consisting of two sets each of five different bodybuilding movements.

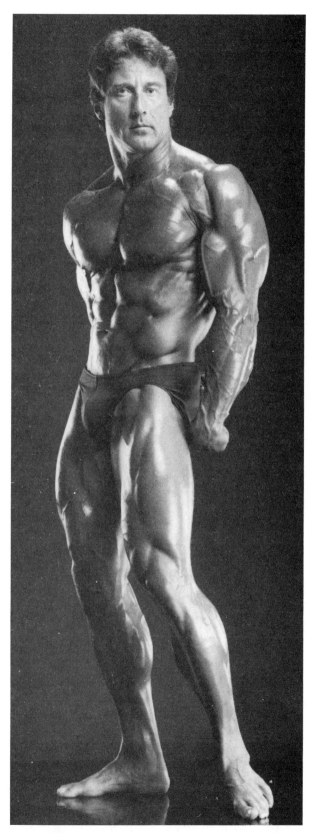

Even in this casual photograph—taken, incidentally, when Frank was 48—shows the type of deep muscle density that can be developed via total dedication to the sport and its training, diet, and mental approach.

- Psych up before every training session, and stay highly motivated throughout your training session. Maintain total mental concentration on working muscles. And spend at least 15 quiet minutes per day visualizing the weak part the way you wish it to one day appear.
- Choose at least one heavy basic exercise for the muscle group upon which you are specializing, and do at least 2–3 isolation movements for each body part in your specialization program.
- Use the Weider Pre-Exhaustion Training Principle (discussed in detail further on in this chapter) when bombing lagging torso muscle groups, such as pecs, delts, lats, and traps.
- Use maximum poundages on each exercise following a thorough warm-up, but do not use so much weight that you are forced to sacrifice optimum exercise form.
- Always maintain perfect biomechanics on every set of every exercise in your specialization routine. After all, you are attempting to stress the lagging body part as intensely as possible, something you simply can't do when using sloppy exercise form.
- Train at least to the point of failure on each post-warm-up set. And on many sets, you can extend yourself to continue pushing well past the normal failure point by using forced reps. (Forced reps are discussed in detail later in this chapter.)
- Make friends with pain. When going all-out to improve a lagging muscle group, you will be constantly crashing past the pain barrier. Rather than fearing this point and therefore holding back a little on intensity, accept it as a sure indication that you are training hard enough to induce muscle hypertrophy.
- Maintain a positive mental attitude. You *will* improve, won't you? So get into the gym and get to it!

HIGH-INTENSITY TRAINING TECHNIQUES

You can think of your bodybuilding involvement as a long, steady upward progression of training intensity. In effect, you are climbing an endless ladder, each successive rung a step upward in intensity. It is now time to teach you how to use several high-intensity Weider Training Principles in your bodybuilding workouts.

For your first 1–1½ years of steady training, you will increase training intensity in two ways:

- By gradually increasing the total number of sets you perform for each body part.
- By gradually increasing the amount of weight you use for every exercise in your routine.

But you already know from reading Chapter 7 that there is an upper limit to the total number of sets you can perform for each muscle group without consequently overtraining and ceasing to make continued progress from your workouts training naturally. Thus, you will probably make the best gains performing no more than 10–12 total sets for a large and complex body part and 6–8 for smaller muscle groups.

Once you have reached the upper threshold of total sets for each body part, you must elevate training intensity by using several Weider Training Principles used in high-intensity bodybuilding training. The Weider Principles I will discuss in this section are Supersets, Cheating, Forced Reps, Burns, Descending Sets, and Retro-Gravity (Negative) Reps.

SUPERSETS

Advanced bodybuilders often increase training intensity by decreasing rest intervals between sets. This is particularly true during a precontest peaking cycle, but the method is also used relatively frequently via the Weider Supersets Training Principle during an off-season mass-building phase.

Supersets are compounds of two exercises performed with little or no rest between the movements, and with each superset followed by a normal rest interval of 60–90 seconds duration before a succeeding superset is initiated. If you normally rest 90 seconds between sets, for the sake of illustration, and you can switch from one supersetted exercise to the other in only five seconds, you decrease the average length of rest interval to only 47½ seconds. Compared to a 90-second average rest interval, one of 47½ seconds can cause a dramatic increase in training intensity.

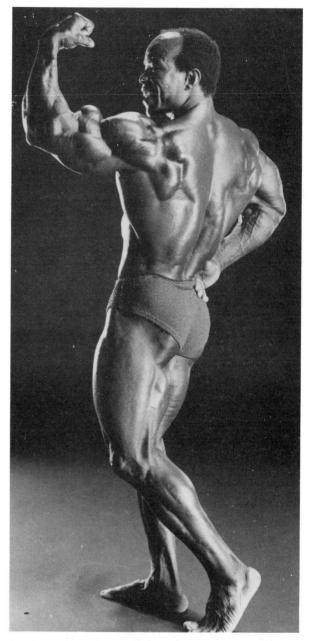

Age has little bearing on competitive success. Albert Beckles is 57 in this photo and has won nearly 10 IFBB Pro Grand Prix titles. In fact, he didn't win his first IFBB pro show until he was 50. Note in particular the depth of Albert's spinal erector muscles and the cross-striations on his hamstrings.

"Since supersets constitute a big jump up in training intensity," cautions *Albert Beckles* (IFBB World Pro Grand Prix Champion), "you should first experiment with them. There are two types of supersets—those done for antagonistic, or opposing muscle groups, such as biceps–triceps or quadriceps–hamstrings; and those which compound two movements for a single, relatively large muscle group. Of these two types of supersets, the least intense form compounds two exercises for antagonistic muscle complexes.

"As a result of all these factors, I always tell bodybuilders new to the Weider Supersets Training Principle to experiment with supersets compounding movements for the biceps and triceps, or forearm flexors and forearm extensors. Only after you grow more experienced with supersets for smaller antagonistic body parts should you gradually progress to supersets for larger antagonistic muscle groups

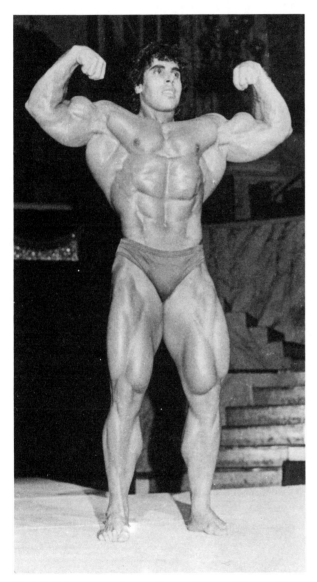

Bodybuilders come from all over the world in making top competitive reputations for themselves. Ed Kawak came from war-torn Beirut, and won a host of international titles in France prior to turning to competition in the IFBB system. Ed lives and owns a gym on the French Riviera. It's a dirty job, but someone has to do it!

such as quadriceps–hamstrings and chest–back."

Here are examples of supersets for antagonistic muscle groups, two each for the muscle groupings just mentioned:

- Biceps + Triceps = Barbell Curls + Pulley Pushdowns
- Biceps + Triceps = Dumbbell Curls + Lying Dumbbell Triceps Extensions
- Forearm Flexors + Forearm Extensors = Barbell Wrist Curls + Barbell Reverse Wrist Curls
- Forearm Flexors + Forearm Extensors = Barbell Reverse Curls + Dumbbell Reverse Wrist Curls
- Quadriceps + Hamstrings = Leg Extensions + Leg Curls
- Quadriceps + Hamstrings = Hack Squats + Stiff-Legged Deadlifts
- Chest + Back = Bench Presses + Chins Behind Neck
- Chest + Back = Parallel Bar Dips + Front Lat Pulldowns

As a footnote, the chest–back combination of bench presses and chins has long been a favorite torso superset of the legendary three-time Mr. Olympia Sergio Oliva.

Eduardo Kawak, the great Lebanese bodybuilder who has won three Mr. World and four Mr. Universe titles, now runs a California-style bodybuilding gym in Nice, France. He explains everything you'll ever need to know about doing supersets for a single muscle group: "For many bodybuilders, there will come a time when training intensity is most appropriately augmented by supersetting two movements for a single body part.

"I believe that you should first do single body part supersets for larger and more complex muscle groups, such as chest, back, or thighs. I recall that I first did such supersets for my pectorals, compounding bench presses with flat-bench dumbbell flyes, then later incline barbell presses with incline dumbbell flyes, and parallel bar dips with cable crossovers. These all are good combinations for blasting your pecs to the limit.

"My favorite back supersets are chins compounded with seated pulley rows, upright rows with barbell shrugs, and lat pulldowns with machine pullovers. For quadriceps I like to superset leg presses with leg extensions, or hack squats with sissy squats. For hamstrings I like to superset seated leg curls with lying leg curls, or stiff-legged deadlifts with lying leg curls. And for shoulders, I like to superset standing presses with dumbbell side laterals, or barbell upright rows with dumbbell bent laterals in a standing position.

"As a word of caution, you are only doing supersets when you rest a maximum of 8–10 seconds between compounded exercises. I often see even champion bodybuilders doing what I call 'alternate sets' in which they move back and forth between two movements while resting 60–90 seconds between the movements.

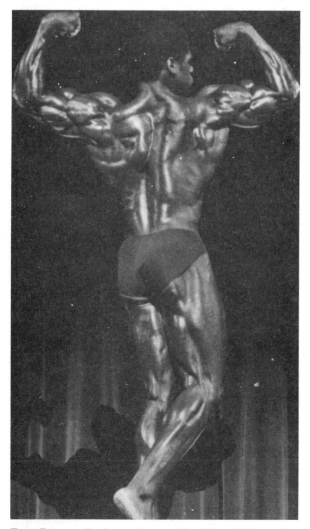

Tony Pearson had won three national-level titles prior to turning 21 and is still going strong more than 10 years later in IFBB professional events. Pearson was Mr. America at 20, while Casey Viator shaded him by a full year, winning the title at a record 19 years of age.

These alternated exercises are fine for adding variety to a body part routine, but do not increase training intensity in the same manner as do supersets."

Pre-Exhaustion Supersets

There is a specialized case in which you will use a form of one body part supersets called "pre-exhaustion supersets." This occurs in torso muscle groups—less frequently when working quadriceps with squats—when you fail to bomb a torso muscle group to the limit with a basic exercise because the smaller and weaker arm muscles, which assist in that movement, fatigue completely and fail to continue moving the weight long before the corresponding torso muscle complex can be completely fatigued and bombed to the max.

Tony Pearson (a Professional Grand Prix winner, plus a five-time winner of the IFBB World Mixed Pairs Championship) explains why and how to use the Weider Pre-Exhaustion Training Principle: "When I do bench presses for my pecs, I am also working my anterior deltoids, triceps, and those upper-back muscles which rotate the scapulae. But I am unable to push my pecs to the limit with bench presses— nor with inclines, declines, or parallel bar dips—because my triceps give out long before I have forced my pectorals to contract to the limit. And this is where pre-exhaustion comes into play.

"For example, when using pre-exhaustion for my pectorals, I superset an isolation movement like flat-bench dumbbell flyes with my bench presses. If I rest a maximum of five seconds between the set of flyes and the set of benches, my pectorals will be weakened, or pre-exhausted, to the point where my triceps *are* briefly stronger than my pecs and anterior delts. Under such a condition, I can push my pecs and anterior delts to the max on basic chest movements.

"Resting longer than five seconds between such exercises can be disastrous, because the pectorals will recover very quickly if allowed to rest too long after the isolation exercise before you start the bench press part of the superset. Physiologists tell us that a muscle group can recover about 40% of its energy after only 10–12

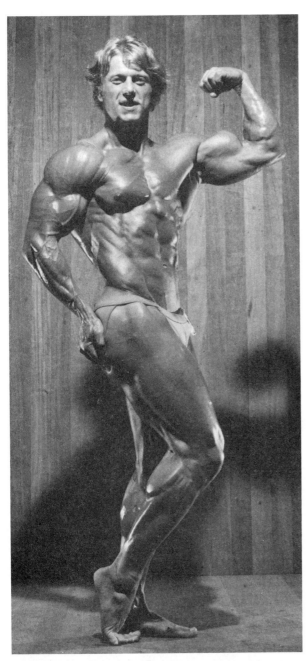

Scandinavian athlete Andreas Cahling moved from Sweden to southern California to make his reputation in the sport. He eventually won the IFBB Pro. Mr. International title, and turned himself into a bodybuilding entrepreneur, selling posing suits throughout the world.

- Lower Pectorals = Decline Flyes + Decline Presses
- Deltoids = Dumbbell Side Laterals + Standing Barbell Presses
- Deltoids = Cable Upright Rows + Seated Dumbbell Presses
- Trapezius = Barbell Shrugs + Barbell Upright Rows
- Latissimus Dorsi = Bent-Arm Pullovers + Lat Pulldowns
- Latissimus Dorsi = Nautilus Pullovers + Chins Behind Neck

"I'd suggest starting out doing only 2-3 of these pre-exhaustion supersets," Pearson cautioned. "The Pre-Ex Principle is a highly intense form of training, and it can cause your muscles to become painfully sore if you overuse the technique. It's best to start with a relatively low degree of intensity doing only a couple of pre-ex supersets, then gradually increase training intensity by adding to the total number of pre-ex supersets performed for a selected muscle group."

As *Casey Viator* (history's youngest Mr. America winner at age 19) notes, "You can also use pre-exhaustion on your quadriceps as well as on torso muscles. Many bodybuilders fail to push their quads to the limit using squats, because their somewhat weaker lower-back muscles fail partway through the set of squats, before the more powerful quadriceps and buttocks muscles have been trained to the limit. In this case, you should use pre-ex to pre-fatigue your quads to the point where the muscle group is relatively weaker than the spinal erector muscles. Then, you can really blast your legs with the heavy squats, although not with as heavy a weight as you might use without pre-exhausting the quadriceps.

"The simplest type of pre-ex superset for quads would be a compound of leg extensions and squats. But with considerable experimentation, I discovered that I needed to compound three movements. Trisetting leg presses, leg extensions, and squats, I found that the presses and extensions efficiently pre-exhausted the quads so completely that I could push them brutally hard with squats.

"I've seen experienced bodybuilders such as Kent Keuhn (Mr. North America) collapse on the floor after doing 10-15 reps each of leg

seconds, and 50% after about 15 seconds. So it should be obvious that you must rest minimally between these exercises when doing torso muscle groups:

- Pectorals (in general) = Flat-Bench Flyes + Bench Presses
- Upper Pectorals = Incline Flyes + Incline Presses

presses with 360 pounds, leg extensions with 150, and squats with only 185 pounds! With consistently hard training on such a triset, I was able to handle considerably heavier poundages on each of these movements."

As good as the Weider Supersets Training Principle is for a majority of serious bodybuilders, it doesn't bear fruit for some top men. Take *Ron Love* (National Heavyweight Champion and Pro World Champion) as an example of such an athlete: "I have experimented heavily with a variety of supersets in the past, and have finally concluded that I make my best gains doing only straight sets with heavy weights in my training sessions. But I still urge any young bodybuilders I coach to also experiment with the Weider Supersets Training Principle to discover if supersets will be a valuable addition to their training philosophies.

"In my own case, I go great guns with intense mental concentration on the first exercise in a superset. But in the rush to begin my second supersetted movement, I invariably lose concentration and just go through the motions. Since I was only benefitting from the first exercise of all my supersets, I eventually concluded I needed all straight sets in my own bodybuilding workouts. This is the only way I can maintain intense mental concentration for a full training session."

TRAINING TO FAILURE

If you are to successfully use such techniques as cheating, forced reps, burns, and descending sets with which you can push your muscles past failure, you must first understand the concept of training to failure. This involves literally pushing each post-warm-up set to the point where you can no longer complete a full repetition in strict form.

Hypermassive *Josef Grolmus* (German and World Light-Heavyweight Champion) explains his concept of training to failure: "The average, moderately successful bodybuilding champion probably takes most sets in a workout to approximately 90% of failure. With a bit of effort and maximum psychological drive, he could probably grind out another superdifficult rep in strict form. For a few bodybuilders, going to 90% of failure is enough to build large,

powerful, well-defined muscles; and going past 90% failure—to 100%—is actually pushing too hard, which can soon result in an overtrained condition.

"For a large majority of serious bodybuilders, going to 100% of failure on many or all post-warm-up sets will build Herculean muscular

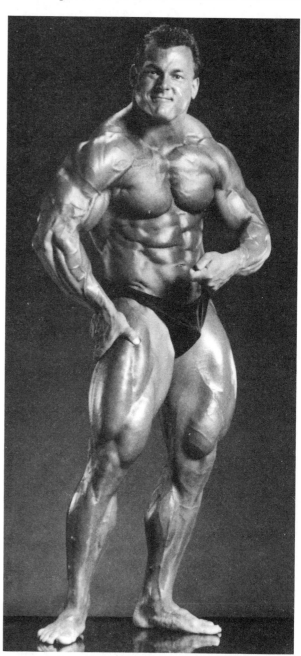

Tim Belknap, at the short height of only 5'3", won his Mr. America title at 21. But the real news is that Tim was the first great diabetic bodybuilder. In addition to Mr. America, he won Mr. World and Mr. Universe, and eventually opened a small one-on-one gym in Santa Monica, California, catering to entertainment figures and executives.

development far more quickly—and to a greater absolute degree of size—than training only to 90% failure, or to that point where the final repetition of a set is merely somewhat difficult to perform, not impossible to complete in strict form. Obviously, it takes a high level of mental drive and a relatively high pain threshold to consistently push your screaming muscles to do another repetition, and perhaps even another, until you literally can't complete more than a partial rep. But that is how you train to failure, as well as how you build huge, highly detailed muscles at the fastest rate of speed.

"For many bodybuilders, myself included, it

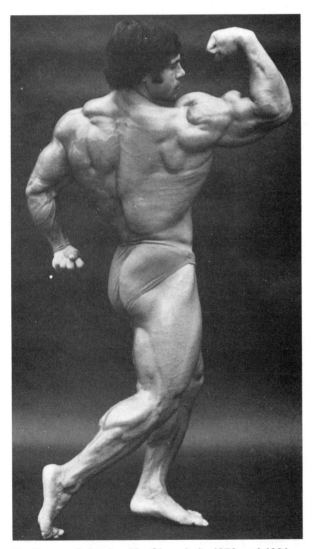

Dr. Franco Columbu, Mr. Olympia in 1976 and 1981, has his own chiropractic clinic in West Los Angeles, just south of the University of California, Los Angeles (UCLA). Franco has constantly improved both his mind and body since moving from Italy to America in 1970.

is best to push past the failure point with cheating reps, forced reps, burns, and/or descending sets. By bombing the skeletal muscles even more intensely than merely by training to failure, the ultimate degree of muscle mass and physical power can be reached."

Looking at Josef's huge muscles, it's easy to see why he is so in favor of training to failure, and frequently past failure. But there are some bodybuilders, such as hulking *Lou Ferrigno* (Mr. America and twice IFBB Mr. Universe), who overtrain if they attempt to consistently push sets past failure.

"I've tried to use forced reps several times in the past and always overtrained on them after only a few weeks," Ferrigno explains. "So I am now content to go to 90%–100% of failure in all of my bodybuilding sessions. No further. In this way, I avoid becoming overtrained, stale, or chronically injured, ensuring that I am always making good gains from my bodybuilding workouts."

CHEATING REPS

The most fundamental way to train past failure is using the Weider Cheating Training Principle, one of the first principles I added to the Weider System of Bodybuilding back in the late 1940s. With the Cheating Principle, you will first take a set of barbell curls, for example, to the point of failure in strict form. Then when you can no longer complete a strict repetition, you will cheat up the weight by imparting just enough torso swing to boost the bar past the point on its upward arc where it sticks and refuses to move any farther in a strict rep. The cheating curl is then completed in fairly strict form using your own biceps strength, then finally lowered in strict form while you powerfully resist the downward momentum of the barbell.

Cheating is an intermediate and advanced technique for pushing past failure, because novice bodybuilders invariably cheat to make a set easier. In contrast, more advanced trainees cheat only to extend a set past failure, thereby making the set considerably more difficult. When you do cheating reps correctly, the working muscles will burn like someone is playing a blow torch over them, a sign that the cheating reps are building new muscle mass.

There are many ways you can cheat on an exercise once you've gone to positive failure. Among the most common cheating methods are torso swing and/or backbend on all types of curls, back arching on bench presses and inclines, knee jerk on all types of overhead presses, and torso swing on various types of upright rows and bent rows. With a little time, you will learn how you can cheat a little on virtually any exercise. But be sure that you cheat only to extend a set past failure, not merely to make that set easier for your rapidly tiring muscles to complete.

The number of cheating reps that you do past the point of momentary muscular failure is important. Working with research exercise physiologists at the Weider Research Clinic, I have determined that you should do no more than 2–3 forced reps past failure on any one set. Anything more than that, and your fatigued muscles are so bushed that you will be doing virtually all of the work with body cheat rather than the power of the prime-movement muscles. In essence, any more than three cheating reps are worthless for building greater muscle mass.

FORCED REPS

"You can encounter one problem with cheating reps," notes *Dr. Franco Columbu* (Mr. World, Mr. Universe, and twice Mr. Olympia). "In cheating up the weight in barbell curls or some other bodybuilding exercise, you will find it difficult to impart just enough momentum to the bar to get it past the sticking point. Sometimes you will generate too much momentum, and the bar will virtually leap up to the finish point at your shoulders, requiring little or no biceps muscle contraction. Other times, you might impart too little momentum to the bar, and it will stall out just short of the sticking point, again yielding little or no meaningful biceps muscle contraction. The trick is to impart just enough momentum to the bar to squeeze it past the sticking point, after which you complete the movement solely with biceps strength rather than momentum.

"The best way to solve the problem with cheating reps is to remove just enough weight from the bar to allow completion of a repetition past failure. The Weider Forced Reps Training Principle is an excellent means of extending a set past momentary failure.

"To illustrate forced reps in action, load up a bar resting on the support rack of an incline bench, setting it with a poundage that allows you to complete no more than 7–8 full positive and negative reps in strict form. With your training partner standing by, take your grip on the bar, then have him assist you in taking the bar from the rack and bringing it to the starting point at straight arms' length directly above your chest. Start to grind out each repetition in perfect biomechanical form, doing full, solid reps to the point of failure.

"The moment you fail partway up on a repetition, your training partner should grasp the middle of the bar and pull upward with exactly the correct amount of force necessary to help you complete a forced repetition with the effectively lighter barbell. For the sake of illustration, you might have failed with 225 pounds, but still have sufficient strength and endurance to do a rep with 210, so your partner pulls up hard enough on the bar to allow the next forced rep.

"In the same manner, you can complete a second forced repetition, and in some cases a third one. Obviously, your pecs, front delts, and triceps will be growing progressively more fatigued with each succeeding forced rep, so your training partner will be forced to pull upward on the bar with progressively more force. Ultimately, after two or three of these forced reps, your chest, shoulder, and arm muscles will be so fatigued that you won't be able to force out any additional repetitions. At that point, you can terminate your set secure in the knowledge that you have pushed your working muscles far past the failure point, thereby generating a great deal of muscle hypertrophy."

DESCENDING SETS

If you have available two training partners, you can use a third means of pushing a set past failure, the Weider Descending Sets Training Principle. Also called "stripping sets" and used by Arnold Schwarzenegger, the immortal seven-time Mr. Olympia, descending sets are

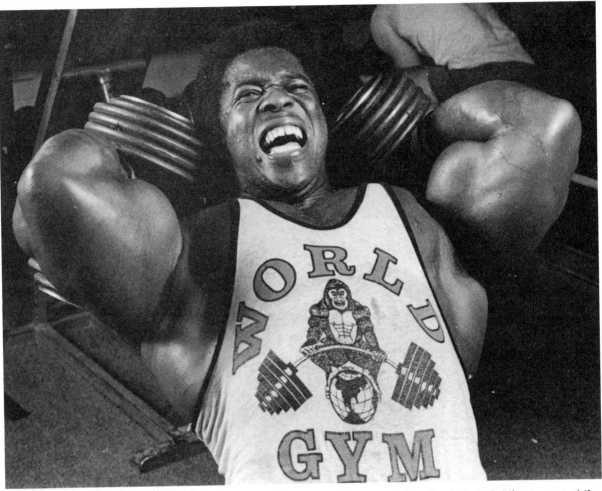

Noticing his awesome potential, Joe Weider brought England's Bertil Fox to America to train for three years at the Master Blaster's expense. Super powerful and hugely muscled, Brutal Bertil never quite lived up to his potential, his best pro placing being fifth in the 1983 Mr. Olympia competition in Munich.

started by loading up a barbell with many 10- and 5-pound plates, matching the configuration on each side, but leaving the collars off the bar. As you train to failure, your partners remove equal weights from the bar so you can continue to push. Because this can be dangerous to perform, I urge you to be very cautious and prudent in using this technique.

Let's use seated presses behind the neck as an illustration of descending sets, with humongous *Bertil Fox* as the subject of the exercise. I've often seen Foxy doing descending sets on this movement. First, Bertil would work up to 315 pounds on the movement, jumping slowly upward in 50-pound increments in order to thoroughly warm up his deltoid and triceps muscles. After doing a solid six reps at 315, he loads the bar to 335–355 pounds, the actual weight determined by how strong he feels dur-

ing his warm-up procedure. The crucial thing is that he has several 25-pound plates loaded on each side of the bar, plus 1–2 10-pound plates for stripping purposes.

With a training partner stationed at each end of the bar, Foxy sits on a bench with its incline board set at about 85 degrees, wedging his spine firmly against the back board. After Bertil takes his grip on the bar, his assistants lift it off the rack to a position resting across his trapezius muscles. Then a superstar descending set of presses behind the neck is begun.

With the heaviest poundage of the day, Bertil grinds out 6–7 full repetitions, a mighty effort in itself. As soon as the bar comes to rest on his traps behind his neck after the sixth or seventh repetition, his partners instantly strip either 40 or 70 pounds from the bar, depending on whether he is using 335 or 355 pounds. Then he instantly begins to grind out 5-6 more reps with this still impressive weight, a full 295 pounds. Another drop to 245 is made, and he does 5-6 more very hard reps, followed by another drop to 195 pounds for a final 5-6 super-hard reps.

"When I'm finished with this descending set," Bertil modestly muses, "my delts are nearly done in. But I still have many sets of lateral raises to the side, front, and out to the sides in a bent-over position to complete, as well as about five heavy sets of upright rows. And this is a primary reason why my deltoids are so huge and minutely detailed. The descending sets are great!"

Arnold Schwarzenegger offers a couple of ways in which you can do descending sets when you don't have training buddies handy: "With selectorized weight stacks, you can instantly move the pin up the stack each time you need to strip weight. Alternatively, you can go down the rack on various dumbbell movements, using successively lighter dumbbells each time you need a weight drop."

Despite Bertil Fox's prodigious efforts with descending sets, experience and research has convinced me that most bodybuilders make their best gains with descending sets when they do no more than 2-3 weight drops, always on basic exercises like bench presses and standing presses. Always stick to this formula, and you will reap great benefits from using the highly intense Weider Descending Sets Training Principle.

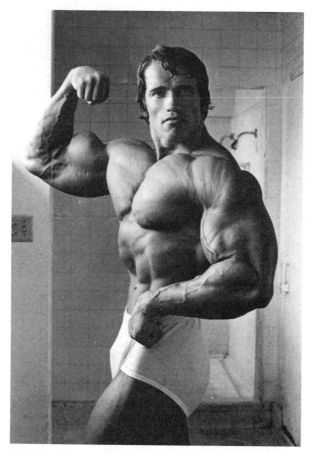

Despite his, uh, unconventional posing attire, Arnold Schwarzenegger shows off one of the greatest physiques in sports history. His picture was taken just prior to a Mr. Olympia contest in the early 1970s, either just before or just after Arnold's post-workout shower (you pick the answer). That arm measured 21 inches cold. Arnold's height of 6'1½" and competitive weight of about 238 pounds makes him the tallest Mr. Olympia.

BURNS

Forced reps require one training partner to spot you, while descending sets usually demand the use of two willing partners. But what can you do to push a set past failure if you happen to train alone in your basement or garage gym? Then you can use the Weider Burns Training Principle, which advocates the use of quick, short partial reps after a trainee can no longer complete an additional full repetition in strict form.

I will let *Andreas Cahling* (IFBB Pro Mr. International) tell you about how he incorporates burns into his own training program: "When I teach aspiring competitive bodybuilders how to do burns, I invariably first have

them do a set of standing calf machine heel raises to positive failure. When they can't take another rep more than about halfway up to the correct finish position, I have them lower a bit more quickly than usual to the bottom position of the movement when the calf muscles are maximally stretched. Then I have them rapidly bounce from this low position upward as high as possible, then back down for 8-12 burns. The heels probably move as little as 2-3 inches, but the calves are forced to continue working very hard past the point of normal failure.

"A rapid accumulation of lactic acid and other fatigue by-products will cause your calves to burn like the fires of Hades when you do burns on your standing machine calf raises, hence the name of this productive training

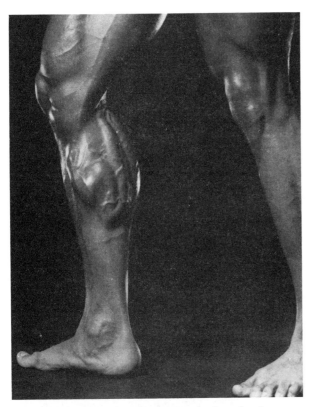

When Schwarzenegger first came to America from Europe in 1968, he had pitiful calves. But by cutting off the lower legs of all of his sweat clothing, he was reminded at every turn in the gym to see how really pathetic they were. He began to train them like a madman, until they became as good as any bodybuilder's of the era. Looks almost like writhing snakes when he flexes them!

technique. Ordinarily, the heavy fatigue pain in your calf muscles will ultimately cause you to terminate a set. But do no more than 12–15 of these quick, short movements; if you can do more than 15, I would suspect that you didn't reach true failure when doing your full repetitions, and you should push that part of your set a lot harder.

"While burns are most frequently performed in the starting position of an exercise, I have also used them quite effectively in the peak-contracted finish position of many movements. In this case, I push only to about 90% of failure before beginning my series of 10–15 burns each set in the top position of the exercise. Obviously, this variation of burns is best performed on peak contraction movements such as leg extensions, leg curls, various types of rows, chins, and variations of lat machine pulldowns.

"To give you an idea of how much benefit I received from incorporating burns into my routines as a means of pushing selected sets past failure, consider my progress during the year leading up to my Mr. International victory. A year before, I was not yet doing burns, and had cut out at 185 pounds. In none of the previous 3–4 years had I gained more than 3–4 pounds of solid new muscle mass. But after eight months of doing burns, I was up to 196 superhard pounds of dense muscle mass and won my biggest title!"

Historically, the first champion to extensively use burns was one of my greatest pupils, Larry Scott, victor in the first two Mr. Olympia competitions, plus winner of the Mr. California, Mr. America and Mr. Universe titles. As an example of how he trained using burns, the Great Scott would do a set of six full reps with a heavy barbell in preacher curls, then immediately do six burns in the bottom position before terminating his set. And Larry's arm development became legendary!

RETRO-GRAVITY REPS

Often referred to as negative reps, the reverse-gravity reps instantiated in the Weider Retro-Gravity Reps training Principle offer great rewards of increased muscle mass and physical power. Exercise physiologists during the 1960s conclusively demonstrated the proper application of the negative (lowering) phase of every repetition. Thus were retro-gravity reps added to the Weider System of Bodybuilding.

In pure retro-gravity training, you will require two sturdy training partners. After you have warmed up your pectorals, anterior deltoids, and triceps on a basic exercise like bench presses, a bar is loaded with approximately 130% of the amount with which you can do a single maximum bench press effort.

With you lying on your back on a flat exercise bench, your partners give you a chance to correctly place your grip on the bar, then lift it from both ends to straight arms' length above your shoulders. From there, you slowly lower the weight down to your chest, pushing mightily against it in an effort to slow down or even stop the descent of the heavy barbell.

After a rest interval of 30–60 seconds, you can do a second retro-gravity rep in exactly the

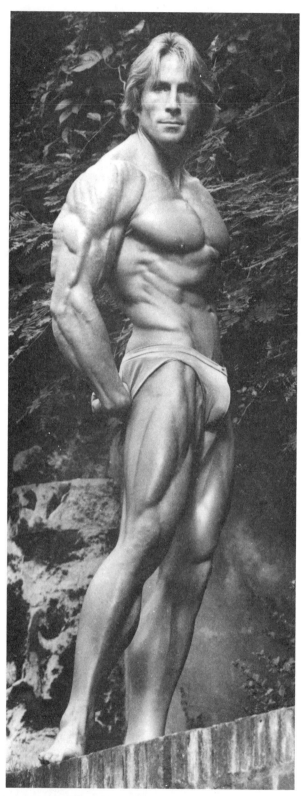

Lean and symmetrical Steve Davis won the IFBB Mr. World title, plus Mr. California prior to hanging it up competitively and getting into the gym business for several years. Having disappeared from the southern California muscle scene, Steve is rumored to be selling insurance or real estate over in the Palm Springs area.

same manner. Continue alternating rest intervals with single negative reps until you have completed 8–10 of them. This constitutes all of the negative reps you need do on a single basic exercise in order to reap great benefits from the Weider Retro-Gravity Training Principle.

I have discovered that doing retro-gravity reps every workout will soon lead to a badly overtrained condition. Therefore, I feel you should perform one negative-reps-only workout after every 3–4 normal bodybuilding sessions. Even training on negatives this infrequently will give you greatly accelerated gains in muscle mass, quality, and power.

OTHER FORMS OF NEGATIVE REPS

In practice, it is normally very difficult to incorporate pure retro-gravity reps into your training system, because it is very difficult to find two training partners willing to sacrifice their own bodybuilding workouts to assist you in your own. Therefore, I have developed several applications of retro-gravity reps that you can perform either by yourself or with a single training partner.

The most simple form of retro-gravity reps done on one's own is called "negative emphasis." With this method, you will simply slow down the negative cycle of each repetition so it takes twice as long as normal, thereby emphasizing the negative cycle of each repetition and increasing its potential benefit. If you usually raise a weight in three seconds and lower it in five, begin raising it in three and lowering it in 10 seconds.

The second type of negative reps can be performed only on various exercise machines. It is called "negative assisted reps." Using a standing machine calf raise to illustrate this method, you should start by choosing an exercise poundage with which you can perform about 15 normal, complete repetitions. Do 6–8 of these reps as a final warm-up, then continue your set by pushing up with both legs, lowering on only one while powerfully resisting the downward momentum of the movement, pushing up with two, and lowering on the opposite leg. Continue alternating lowering legs like this until you reach total failure, and you'll quickly learn that negative assisted reps can be

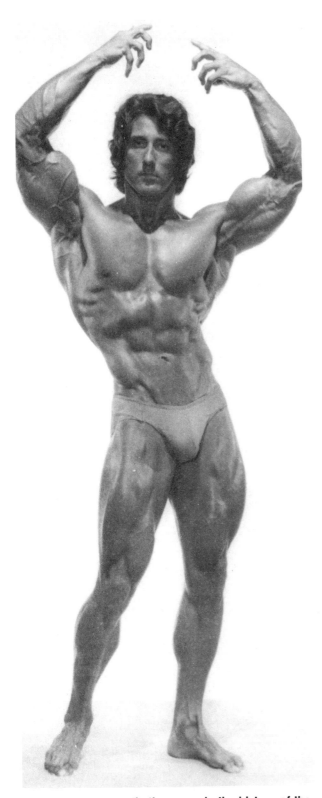

One of the most aesthetic posers in the history of the sport Frank Zane originally was a teacher in New Jersey, Florida, and California. Frank finally gave up teaching to pursue bodybuilding full-time. Now retired competitively, he is back teaching young bodybuilders his art at his learning center in Palm Springs, California.

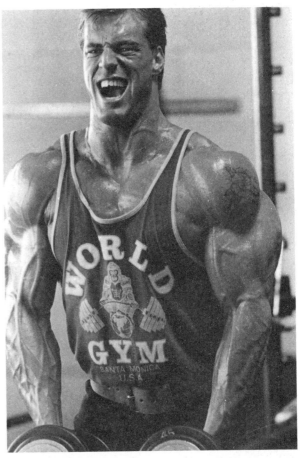

Muscular Dutchman Berry de Mey established himself as a legitimate star by winning the Mr. Europe title at the age of only 19. He has won the World Games Heavyweight Championship, and has been runner-up to many different Americans at the IFBB World Championships. He has placed sixth, fifth, sixth, and third in the Mr. Olympia shows of 1985–1988.

murder—productive murder, but murder nonetheless.

It should be obvious why negative assisted reps can be performed only on machine exercises, but I'm sure it will escape enough readers to warrant an explanation. It would obviously be possible to blast your delts using this method on a Universal Gym seated press station. But if you try to take one hand off of the barbell when doing standing barbell presses, the bar will fall very painfully on your tootsies, if you're lucky; on your head, if not so lucky.

The final type of retro-gravity reps, performed with the assistance of a single training partner, is called "forced negative reps." Let's use pec deck flyes to demonstrate this productive training method. Choose a weight with the selector pin sufficient to limit you to 6–8 full reps on your own, and station your training partner in front of you.

Start your forced negatives set with 6–8 reps to positive failure. As soon as you fail, your partner will give you a forced rep so you can press the pads together directly in front of your chest. Then in the forced negative part of the movement, he will actually push against the pads and force them apart and back to the starting position, with you exerting for all you are worth to slow—hopefully to stop—the movement of the pads.

With the extra resistance provided by your partner, you will effectively be doing a negative rep against tremendous resistance, which can only serve to increase muscle mass just that much more quickly. And you can use this forced negatives technique on most machine movements, as well as on many free-weight exercises. It's a bone crusher, but forced negatives really do build an incredible degree of muscle mass and quality. I sincerely hope you will give this variation of the Weider Retro-Gravity Training Principle a good trial in your own workouts, preferably when training your most stubborn body part(s).

A FORMULA FOR ULTRA-HIGH-INTENSITY TRAINING

Two of the hardest trainers in recent years formed the only brother tandem to win Mr. America titles, Mike (in 1976) and Ray (in 1979) Mentzer. Mike Mentzer also went on to win Mr. Universe, an IFBB Pro Grand Prix title, and his weight class in the '79 Mr. Olympia show. Both brothers were noted for huge muscle mass and awesome physical power.

By combining forced reps with retro-gravity reps, Mike and Ray developed a training system dubbed "Heavy Duty," which was of such high intensity that they seldom needed to perform more than 4–5 total sets for even the largest of muscle groups. Yet they still continued to grow huge muscles by leaps and bounds. What was their secret?

Let's take a close look at a set of barbell preacher curls as performed by the Mentzer brothers. With 185 pounds on the bar, Mike would drape himself over the bench and Ray would hand him the barbell with Mike's arms

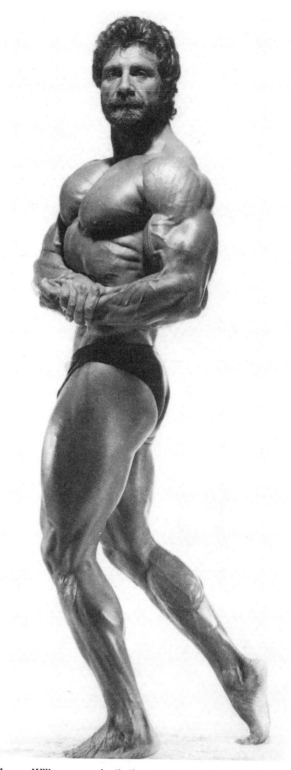

Jusup Wilkosz won both the amateur and professional versions of the IFBB World Championships, plus placed as high as third in Mr. Olympia in 1983. He and his wife Ruth own and operate a very successful soft- and hardcore gym in Stuttgart, West Germany. Jusup also does an odd film role from time to time on German television—you know, blacksmiths and the like!

running parallel to each other straight down the bench.

The first part of the set would be ordinary, if you feel that doing 6–8 strict preacher curls with an arm-shattering 185 pounds to be ordinary. When failure had been reached, Ray would give Mike 2–3 forced reps. Finally, he would give his brother 2–3 forced negative reps, concluding a set of mind-boggling intensity. And given this degree of workout intensity, it is easy to understand how Mike and Ray could both develop biceps measurements of 20+ inches on only 2–3 such sets per workout.

You can use this same ultra-high-intensity technique on virtually any basic exercise, but you should be careful to break in to the new program quite slowly and gradually. In this way, your skeletal muscle system and bony joints can be progressively strengthened, and you will run a minimal risk of either super-sore muscles or even outright injury, both of which will slow your progress toward developing an eye-popping physique. But use retro-gravity reps and forced reps correctly, and you will become Hercules reincarnated!

9
Building Mass
Through Exercise

When I asked him for some comments about mass-building, *Lee Haney* told me, "Every bodybuilder wants to develop huge, powerful muscles. In fact, that's usually the main reason why most of us started working out with weights in the first place—to build up a skinny frame so we could look huge and powerful. And no matter how massive a bodybuilder gets, he still wants to add a little more muscle mass to certain parts of his physique. I know that's the way I still feel about getting even more massive, and I'm sure I'll always feel that way."

At least half of the letters I receive from all over the world soliciting training advice pose the same question: How can I make solid muscle mass gains in the shortest possible amount of time? So, I have decided to devote an entire chapter to this interesting topic, presenting both my own ideas on the subject and those of some of the sport's most incredibly massive bodybuilders.

"If you never learn another thing about building muscle mass," notes Lee Haney, "you should etch this maxim on every barbell plate in the gym where you train: There is a direct correlation between how much weight you handle in strict form on a particular exercise and the relative mass of the muscles involved in that movement. In other words, you have to lift big to get big."

Therefore, the mass-building programs I will give you in this chapter will also drastically increase your strength levels. In fact, you will find that these routines have much in common with the training schedules of champion powerlifters. The primary difference is that bodybuilders not only do squats, bench presses, and deadlifts in their mass-building routines,

but also basic movements for all other body parts.

After plenty of scientific and practical experiments, I learned that the best repetition range for building muscle mass is 5–8. And if you happen to go below five repetitions, you might still build a certain amount of muscle mass, but

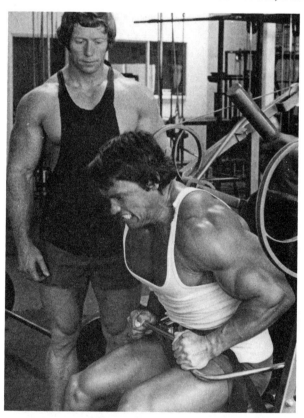

The former Emperor of Mass, Arnold Schwarzenegger, grinds out a final repetition of pullovers on an early design of the Nautilus machine. Arnold and Lee followed similar routes to the top—train hard, train consistently, and train heavy. Spotting Arnold is Kenny Weller, who won the IFBB Mr. Universe title (class and overall) in 1975 at Pretoria, South Africa.

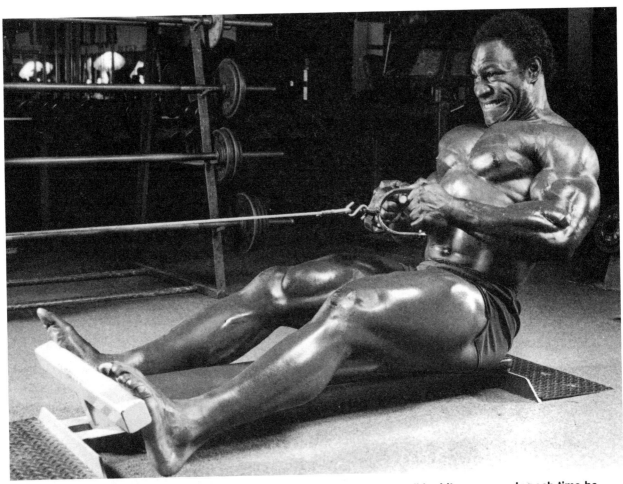

The current Emperor of Mass, Lee Haney is constantly blasting away to build a bit more muscle each time he goes into the gym. While Lee recognizes there is a direct relationship between the amount of weight a bodybuilder uses in an exercise and the relative mass of the muscles that move the weight, he's careful to always warm up thoroughly, keep his reps above five, and maintain consistently good exercise form, all in an attempt to make gains without getting injured.

you would primarily be increasing strength by developing stronger tendons and ligaments, plus improving muscle cell contractile power.

On the surface, you might think that most powerlifters train on relatively low reps—singles, doubles, triples—with maximum poundage. But in reality, these ultra powerful athletes have found that the risk of training injuries is vastly elevated when less than 5 max reps are performed for any set. So for most of the year, powerlifters train with reps in the range of 4-6, and perhaps as many as 8 on some sets. They only go down in reps to do triples or doubles—rarely any singles except at a competition—to gauge their strength levels in order to choose the correct starting poundages for each of the three lifts at a competition.

Bodybuilders would also be courting train-ing injuries if they attempted to lift maximum weights for relatively low repetitions. They would also probably injure themselves if they failed to warm up thoroughly and/or did not maintain perfect form on every set. I've person-ally known many potentially great bodybuild-ers who suffered career-ending injuries through poor warm-ups, bad biomechanics, and/or doing excessive, ego-building single at-tempts with massive exercise poundages.

The best way I have found of getting thor-oughly warmed up and then using the correct number of repetitions for mass building on any movement is to use a half pyramid system of poundages and repetitions, increasing the weight and reducing the reps on each succeed-ing set. A sample of this half pyramid pound-age-rep scheme follows for a squat workout (poundages have been arbitrarily selected merely for the sake of illustration):

Set Number	Weight (lbs.)	Repetitions
1	135	15
2	205	12
3	255	10
4	305	8
5	345	6
6	365	5

In the foregoing example, the first three sets can be considered a continuation of the basic warm-up taken prior to any heavy mass-building weight workout. And the last three sets, which fall within the range of mass-building repetitions are purely for increasing leg muscle mass.

BASIC EXERCISES

"A second major feature of mass-training routines is an extensive use of basic exercises," reveals massive *Tom Platz.* "I define basic exercises as movements which stress the largest muscle groups of the body—quadriceps, lats, pecs, etc.—usually in conjunction with one or more other smaller body parts.

"A typical thigh isolation movement would be leg extensions, which isolate stress on the quadriceps muscles. In contrast, squats—the best basic exercise for legs—work the quads in concert with the buttocks, hamstrings, lower-back, and upper-back muscles." You will find a list of Tom's favorite basic exercises in the figure on page 113.

"While isolation movements are excellent for shaping and adding detail to a muscle group," Platz continues, "the basic exercises are best for increasing general muscle mass and improving strength levels. As an aspiring bodybuilder, you should do virtually all basic movements in your mass-training program.

"Check over your current training schedule to see how many isolation movements have crept into it, even though you are attempting to build general muscle mass. If you are anything like other bodybuilders, you are probably doing many isolation exercises in a mass-training program.

"One of the biggest mistakes I see when I first look over the training program of someone whom I'm coaching is excessive use of isolation movements. If you are attempting to build up your muscle mass, you should be doing almost exclusively basic exercise, using maximum poundages on these movements in strict form."

Lee Haney concludes the discussion of basic exercises: "I personally didn't begin adding in isolation exercises until I had been training for three years and already weighed 210 pounds, so don't get carried away with too many concentration curls and cable side lateral raises early in your bodybuilding involvement."

AVOIDING OVERTRAINING

"The biggest road block to success in body-building is overtraining," believes *Mike Christian* (National and World Heavyweight Champion, third/Mr. Olympia). "A young, highly enthusiastic bodybuilder can often get carried away with doing more and more total sets, until he eventually overtrains. And once he has overtrained, he can expect few if any gains from even the hardest and most consistent workouts. In some extreme cases of overtraining, his mus-

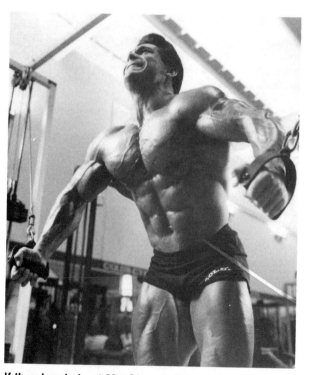

If they handed out Mr. Olympia titles on true grit alone, Rich Gaspari would have won several already. He's long been noted as one of the most fanatic trainers in the sport, and he'll get that Mr. O trophy one of these years.

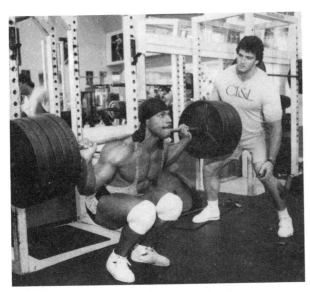

Mike Christian's oft-maligned legs get a heavy squat workout, with Mr. Los Angeles Christian Duffy (right) spotting. Heavy training on basic movements like squats, benches, barbell rows, overhead presses, and barbell curls, are the most proven route to achieving a highly massive physique in the shortest possible time.

ALTERNATIVE "A"

Monday-Thursday	Tuesday-Friday
Thighs	Back
Upper Arms	Chest
Forearms	Shoulders
Abdominals	Calves

ALTERNATIVE "B"

Monday-Thursday	Tuesday-Friday
Chest	Thighs
Shoulders	Back
Triceps	Biceps
Abdominals-Forearms	Calves

ALTERNATIVE "C"

Monday-Thursday	Tuesday-Friday
Chest	Shoulders
Thighs	Back
Biceps	Triceps
Calves-Forearms	Abdominals

cular development and strength levels might actually regress.

"The best way to avoid overtraining when mass-building is to limit the total number of sets you perform for each muscle group. If you have less than three months of steady training under your belt, you won't need to do more than 5-6 total sets for large muscle groups and 3-4 for smaller ones. Intermediates with up to 6-8 months of steady training behind them, should do no more than 6-8 sets for large body parts and 4-5 for smaller muscle groups. And advanced men should not perform more than 10-12 sets for large body parts and 5-7 for smaller ones. For the sake of definition, I consider the large muscle groups to include legs, back, chest, and perhaps shoulders; and smaller body parts are biceps, triceps, calves, abdominals, and forearms.

"If the foregoing ranges for total sets per muscle group seem a little too low to you, you are a perfect candidate for overtraining. But if they seem like enough work, you are sure to succeed in building up a high degree of muscle mass."

There are many ways in which you can split up your various body parts for a four-day split routine. Following are three alternative examples:

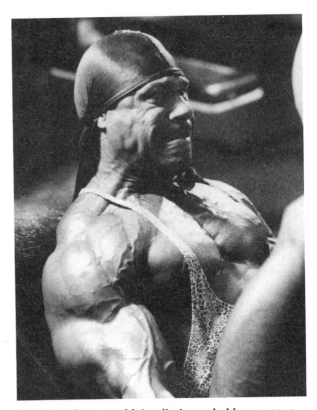

Christian gives equal intensity to angled leg presses in an effort to further expand his quadriceps muscles. Note the sublime expression of intensity on Mike's face as he fights off the pain and continues his set past the mythical pain barrier. Mike has won the NPC Heavyweight and Overall Nationals (1984) and IFBB Heavyweight World Championship (1984).

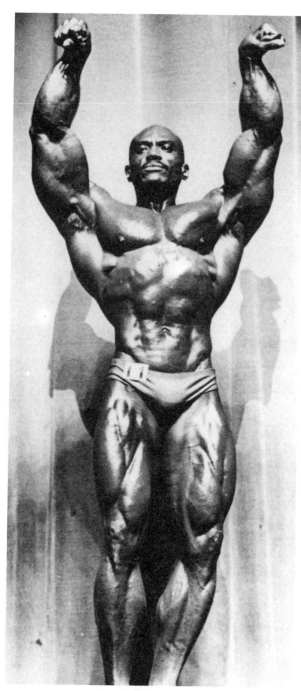

you follow a scheme in which the training sessions are grouped similarly to the alternatives presented.

PUTTING IT TOGETHER

I am well aware that the bodybuilders reading this book are not all super-advanced men like Lee Haney or Tom Platz. So I have given you two suggested mass-building routines. On page 113 (top), you will find a program that I recommend for bodybuilders with less than 4-6 months of steady training experience. And on page 113 (bottom), you will find a training schedule for bodybuilders with more than six months of training. Choose the one that suits

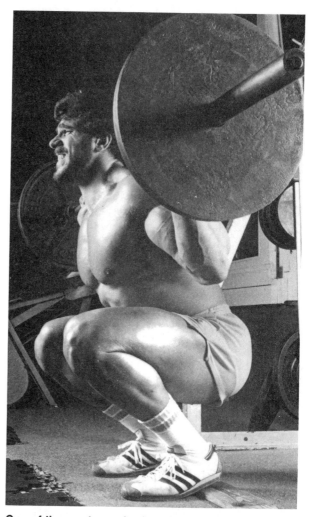

No bodybuilder has *ever* displayed this degree of muscle mass in this particular pose. Chicago cop (via Cuban defection in 1959) Sergio Oliva brings off the pose with elan. Sergio and his wife Arlene own and operate their own gym in Chicago.

Choose whichever of these alternatives you feel might work best for you, but don't be constrained by the workout days listed for each one. A lot of bodybuilders who have physically demanding jobs will find it best to get two heavy workouts in on the weekends and the other two at some time during the week. Just be sure that

One of the most massive bodybuilders of all time (285 pounds in hard shape at a height of 6'5") Lou Ferrigno earned his physique the hard way—by working for it with heavy basic movements. Notice in particular his perfect squat form, his torso held as erect as possible and his head up enough to keep from bending forward at the waist unnecessarily.

your experience level, and follow it religiously for at least 2-3 months, before switching to a different routine.

You should also follow these six workout performance rules when attempting to increase muscle mass:

- Always use spotters when doing heavy bench presses and squats.
- Go to within 95% of failure on your top sets of each exercise.
- Always maintain strict exercise form.
- Avoid doing forced reps on all but the final set of each movement.
- Once you can do five reps without assistance on your final set of each exercise, increase the training weights for that movement by 10–20 pounds.
- Never miss a scheduled workout for any reason other than illness.

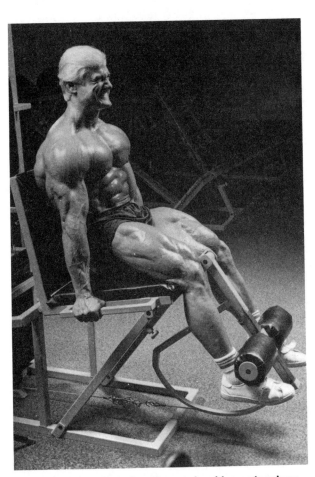

Even though in the relaxation cycle of leg extensions, Tom Platz mirrors the mental strain he's going through in order to complete his set. One of the most massive bodybuilders of all time, Tom won the IFBB Middleweight World Championships in 1977, and placed as high as third in Mr. Olympia in 1981.

ENTRY-LEVEL MASS-BUILDING ROUTINE
MONDAY–THURSDAY

Exercise	Sets	Reps
Incline Sit-Ups	2–3	15–20
Bench Presses	6	15–5*
Barbell Bent Rows	6	15–5*
Standing Barbell Presses	5	12–5*
Seated Calf Raises	5	15–6*
Barbell Reverse Curls	3	10–6*
Barbell Wrist Curls	3	10–15

TUESDAY–FRIDAY

Exercise	Sets	Reps
Hanging Leg Raises	2–3	10–15
Squats	6	15–5*
Stiff-Legged Deadlifts	4	12–6*
Standing Barbell Curls	4	12–6*
Close-Grip Bench Presses	4	12–6*
Standing Calf Raises	5	15–6*

Note: Pyramid all exercises marked with an asterisk.

ADVANCED-LEVEL MASS-BUILDING ROUTINE
MONDAY–THURSDAY

Exercise	Sets	Reps
Incline Sit-Ups	3–4	15–20
Incline Barbell Presses	6	15–5*
Parallel Bar Dips (weighted)	4	12–6*
Seated Pulley Rows	6	15–5*
Front Lat Pulldowns	4	12–6*
Seated Machine Front Presses	5	12–5*
Barbell Upright Rows	3	10–6*
Seated Calf Raises	6	15–6*
Barbell Reverse Curls	4	10–5*
Barbell Wrist Curls	4	10–15

TUESDAY–FRIDAY

Exercise	Sets	Reps
Hanging Leg Raises	3–4	10–15
Squats	6	15–5*
Angled Leg Presses	5	12–5*
Stiff-Legged Deadlifts	5	12–5*
Lying Leg Curls	3	10–6*
Barbell Preacher Curls	5	15–6*
Close-Grip Bench Presses	5	15–6*
Standing Calf Raises	5	15–6*

Note: Pyramid all exercises marked with an asterisk.

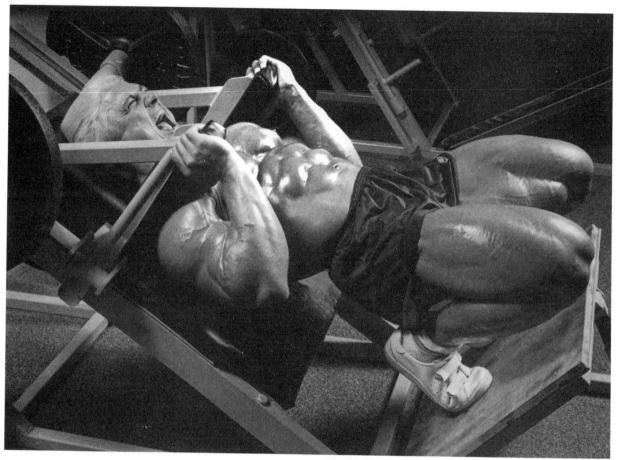

Platz at it again, showing an incredible degree of strength, flexibility, and true grit in a set of hack squats. His exceptional muscle mass is evident even in this casual workout photo.

MASS-BUILDING DIET

An entire chapter is devoted to mass-building diet elsewhere in this book. But I feel I should touch lightly on the subject in this chapter as well.

Each time you eat a meal, that meal should contain some complete protein foods—meat, fowl, fish, eggs and milk—or you won't be able to turn the dietary protein into muscle tissue. It is also important to note that the human digestive system can only digest and make ready for assimilation approximately 25–30 grams of protein foods per meal. And this fact leads experienced bodybuilders attempting to increase muscle mass to consume 5–6 small, protein-rich meals each day rather than the nor-mal three, relatively large meals most people consume.

Why? Simply put, anyone who can digest 30 grams of protein per meal can only make ready for assimilation 90 total grams of protein when consuming three meals per day. That's a math-ematical certainty. But when you eat six times per day, 30 grams of protein at each meal, you make ready for assimilation into muscle tissue 180 grams of protein, or twice as much.

Eating small, protein-rich meals actually makes the digestive system more efficient. You will digest and make ready for assimilation into muscle tissue much more complete protein when eating small meals than three large feasts.

10
Training Injuries

At one time or another, every serious body-builder experiences progress-stalling training injuries. Sometimes serious injuries actually end a promising bodybuilding career. So in a very real sense, successfully avoiding injuries and curing those injuries you do incur will have a marked effect on how successful you will ultimately be in the competitive arena.

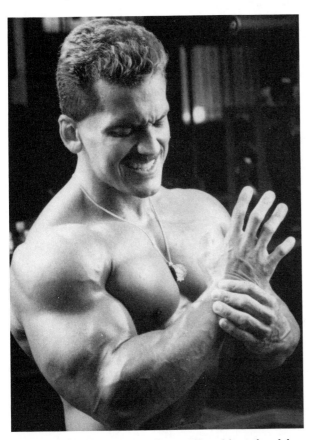

Minor training injuries, such as suffered here by rising pro Lee Labrada, can be home treated safely by using the suggestions outlined in this chapter. Lee has won the pro Night of the Champions and several other IFBB Pro Grand Prix competitions by carefully avoiding injuries, while training as hard and consistently as possible.

I will discuss two types of training injuries—relatively serious traumas, which involve some disruption of body tissues, severe enough that you will miss days, perhaps even weeks, of training while the injury heals; and the insidious, low-grade microtraumas, which will gradually accumulate over a long period of time, until a bodybuilder begins to experience long-term chronic joint pain. Each type of injury should be treated differently.

INJURY PREVENTION

Preventing injuries from occurring in the first place is the best solution you can possibly have to training injuries. And all you must do to prevent injuries is to always warm up thoroughly, and maintain correct body mechanics (form) as you execute every repetition of every set in your bodybuilding workout. I've said this earlier in the book, but can't emphasize these injury prevention rules strongly enough to keep all bodybuilders from mistakenly starting a workout before being properly warmed up, or standing around in the gym sufficiently to cool off, then using poor biomechanics to lift a heavy weight.

MICROTRAUMAS

Chronically sore joints are an occasional complaint among bodybuilders in their 30s (and older) who continue to train hard and enter bodybuilding competitions. A few bodybuilders are merely prone to having minor joint arthritis, but usually sore joints can be prevented completely, or at least minimized in severity.

There are three primary causes of joint, con-

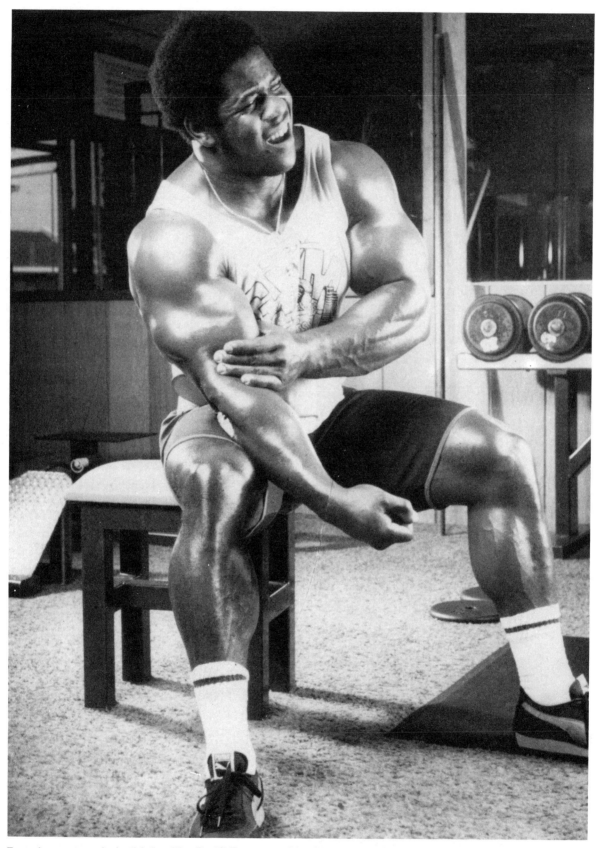

Even huge-muscled athletes like Bertil Fox are subject to occasional minor pains and strains from their workouts. Usually, simple rest does the trick, but the RICE method outlined on page 118 will help you treat anything short of severe injuries.

nective tissue, and muscle microtraumas. The first of these, as just mentioned, is failing to warm up thoroughly prior to each training session, or then failing to stay warmed up throughout your training session. The solution to this problem is obvious.

You also can prevent further microtraumas in weak joints by wrapping selected sore joints during each workout, particularly if you use neoprene rubber bands to cover the joint in question. These rubber wraps keep moist heat around the injury site, which is very beneficial and soothing.

The second cause of microtrauma is faulty biomechanics. In each workout, you must attempt always to maintain perfect body mechanics whenever lifting even light weights, but particularly when using heavy poundages. Consistently keep motionless all parts of your body save those which move to lift the weight, and carefully move the bar slowly over an exercise's complete range of motion.

You must particularly avoid doing any movements in a jerky fashion, rebounding the bar at the bottom of any movement. Rebounding the weight like this is particularly dangerous because it places much greater-than-normal stress on connective tissue. I know of several bodybuilders who have ruptured biceps tendons by bouncing the bar at the bottom of a rep of barbell preacher curls, for example. And many shoulder and chest injuries have occurred when a bodybuilder bounced the barbell heavily off his chest in the bottom position of bench presses.

Thirdly, you *can* eventually have sore joints if you train too frequently with maximum weights in any of your exercises. This will sound like heresy to some bodybuilders, but it's possible to go heavy too frequently in your workouts. A lot of bodybuilders jump from zero right up to their peak poundages in basic exercises, and the wear and tear on cold joints and connective tissue in such a case is much greater than would be the case when a bodybuilder warms up thoroughly prior to using maximum poundages. You definitely should use heavy weights in each exercise, but only after you have performed a succession of progressively heavier sets moving from a light weight to your max over at least 3–4 sets.

You will read in some bodybuilding books and magazines that you can only make optimum gains when training with maximum weights for only a few sets per body part. The Heavy Duty system is typical of this type of training, inasmuch as bodybuilders are expected to do fewer than five total sets for each muscle group, always with absolute maximum poundages.

Unfortunately, too few Heavy Duty advocates warm up thoroughly enough to prevent serious injuries in midworkout. And with the emphasis on constantly working with maximum weights, Heavy Duty trainers frequently use bouncing, heaving, or jerky reps in poor form. As a result, this type of training system makes bodybuilders much more prone to injury than bodybuilders training in more normal fashion.

Even if you don't feel obvious pain when training without a proper warm-up, using poor body mechanics, and/or bouncing the bar in the bottom position of an exercise, you are probably still absorbing the effects of microtraumas. And the accumulation of thousands of such small, microscopic injuries can eventually cause sore joints. Care must always be taken, or you might end up with a permanent shoulder or lower back injury.

If you do suffer from joint pain, there are several ways to minimize the pain and allow yourself to continue training hard for that upcoming competition. The first treatment is to ice the area for at least 30 minutes after each workout. This is a common throwing arm treatment among major league pitchers and NFL quarterbacks following games. But it's also used by many bodybuilders, including the great Larry Scott, who recently made a comeback at nearly 50 years of age.

Icing a joint prevents swelling in the area. This is beneficial, because swelling promotes—rather than minimizes—arthritic symptoms in a joint. The best way to ice a joint is to submerge it in a bucket or basin of ice-water.

If submersion is too cumbersome to accomplish, you should prepare for direct icing by freezing water in paper cups, preferably with a popsickle stick or tongue depressor propped in the middle of the cup. This way you can rub ice directly on the skin over the affected joint while holding the stick, or simply with a towel wrapped around some ice chunks. Alternatively, you can use commercially prepared, refreezable ice packs, which can be purchased at most sporting goods stores.

I also recommend taking a couple of aspirin tablets prior to each heavy workout, as well as immediately after a training session. Not only will the aspirin relieve pain, but it will also help to alleviate inflammations in the affected joint. Do not, however, take prescription pain medication just to get through a workout with a joint, muscle, or connective tissue injury. You can seriously injure a joint by blocking pain signals from the injury to your brain with such medication, signals that would alert you to shut down your set before the joint tears itself apart. The sensation of pain is important in injury prevention, and it should always be heeded rather than masked.

Many bodybuilders do take prescription antiinflammatories, such as Motrin, Nalfon, or Feldene, which can relieve the pain of minor arthritis or tendinitis. Ideally, you should always check with your family physician before taking such drugs, but the pain relief medication found in Motrin is also available in lesser strength in nonprescription pain medications containing ibuprofen (Advil and Mediprin are two such OTC drugs).

MAJOR TRAINING INJURIES

Truly major injuries—such as muscle tears, tendon ruptures, or joint dislocations—should *never* be home treated. You should immediately apply ice to the area, immobilize it, and rush to see your physician. You may consider seeing a sports medicine specialist if your physician is not so qualified. Ignoring such a serious injury can be disastrous, particularly if it is left to linger before treatment. I've known of major injuries left neglected which ended promising amateur and professional bodybuilding careers.

If the injury is less serious—a muscle strain or pull, a back sprain—your physician will advise you to follow the RICE rule for home treatment:

R = rest
I = ice
C = compression
E = elevation

When you incur one of the more serious injuries, the joint or muscle which has been injured should be rested completely. This is one reason why a physician will immobilize an injured area with a temporary cast, arm sling, or other type of restraint until it has had sufficient time to heal.

The length of time the injured area should be rested will depend on the severity of the injury. At a minimum, you should rest a more seriously injured joint or muscle complex for 7–10 days before beginning to rehabilitate the injury-weakened area. And in the case of a broken bone, or serious joint or connective tissue injury, you might be forced to rest the area for at least 2–3 months.

Icing an injured joint or muscle mass will limit the severity of the injury by inhibiting swelling and further injury due to muscle spasm at the injury site. The less the amount of swelling, the more quickly you can get back into the gym to train hard again.

Ice should be applied immediately after an injury occurs for up to 30 minutes, as already mentioned. But you should also ice the area for 10–15 minutes every waking hour or two for a minimum of 48 hours and up to 72 hours. Periodic icing and immobilization of the injured area are absolutely essential steps to take to limit the severity of the injury.

Compression of an injured area will also inhibit swelling and speed recovery. Compression can most easily be achieved by wrapping the injured area with an elastic bandage. Wrap the area tightly, and loosen the wrap for about five minutes every hour you are awake. Loosening the wrap will prevent loss of blood circulation in the injured area, while compression in conjunction with icing will minimize swelling.

Elevation is also intended to limit swelling at the injury site. In combination with icing and compression, elevation of the injury will effectively limit swelling and speed recovery from the injury.

INJURY REHABILITATION

After 72 hours of RICE, you should begin applying heat to the injury site for 5–10 minutes each 1–2 hours throughout the day. The easiest way to apply heat to an injured area is to wrap a hot water bottle in a damp towel, then hold the bottle over the injury site. Damp heat is much more efficiently conducted into the deep tissues at the injury site than is dry heat.

As an alternative, you can find heat pads at drug stores, and commercial heat packs at most sporting goods stores. Whatever the source of heat, the periodic heat treatments—*given only after swelling has abated*—will begin to speed the healing process. This heat should be applied for at least 2–3 days.

Once you have begun heat treatments, you should also begin gently moving the injured area to regain full mobility in the joint or muscle. But you should do your stretching and joint manipulation only *after* you have thoroughly warmed up the area with a heat application. And you should always back off on the intensity of this light exercise whenever you feel pain at the injury site.

After you have regained mobility in the injured area—usually after 7–10 days—you can begin to exercise it with very light weights. Do the weight workout for the injured muscle group or joint every other day, and only after a thorough warm-up with heat treatment and light stretching.

Again, you should let pain be your guide to training intensity. Whenever you feel pain, back off on the amount of weight you use. Then gradually increase the poundages, until you are back up to your normal level, a process that should not take more than 3–4 weeks to achieve. Only then can you consider the injured joint or muscle completely rehabilitated.

Throughout the rehabilitation phase, you should make haste slowly. Pushing too hard to ready yourself to get back to training with high intensity can set back your progress several weeks if you happen to reinjure the area.

TRAINING AROUND AN INJURY

Good bodybuilders are always able to find a way to train around an injury. This procedure allows you to heal a low-severity injury without having to take a layoff from training the balance of your body parts. And in some cases, a chronically injured joint will require the same treatment if you wish to make continued progress from your bodybuilding efforts.

I'll give you some examples of how experienced bodybuilders train around injuries.

LOWER BACK INJURY

With everything but a serious back injury, you can do most of your exercises while either lying or seated. You can do dumbbell lateral raises facedown on a flat exercise bench, or lying on one side on an incline bench. You can do leg presses and/or leg extensions rather than squats. And you can do incline dumbbell curls or seated triceps extensions for your arms.

SHOULDER INJURY

With a little experimentation, you can almost always find exercises for each of your torso muscle groups, which don't cause more than minor pain in an injured shoulder. You might not be able to do benches or inclines for your pectoral muscles, for example, but you can do pec deck flyes until your shoulder has healed. Similarly, you might be able to do cable upright rows for your delts when any type of overhead pressing aggravates the shoulder injury.

KNEE INJURY

While it may be impossible to do even light squats when you have a knee injury, you can often do relatively heavy leg presses for your quadriceps and buttocks. And when knee pain keeps you from doing leg curls for your hamstrings, you might still be able to do stiff-legged deadlifts or good mornings to intensely stress the same area.

Ultimately, you will learn how to train around most injuries through experience. Almost all high-level bodybuilders know how to do this. Just be sure to avoid any exercises which cause more than a mild pain in a joint, muscle, or connective tissue.

Experience will also teach you how to avoid serious injuries when in hard training, how to heal these injuries as quickly as possible, and how to rehab an injured part of your body. And experience will allow you to continually train hard enough to consistently make great gains from your workouts, despite nagging minor injuries.

11
Intermediate
Training Tips

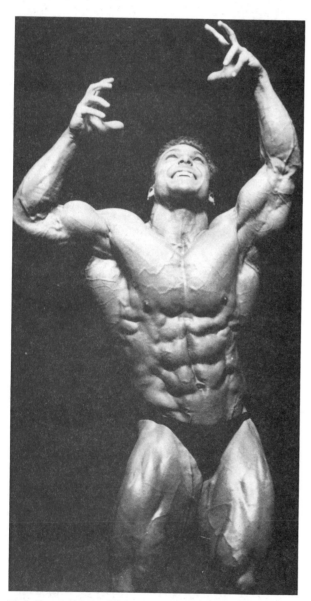

Rich Gaspari from Watertown, New Jersey, epitomizes the ultimate combination of maximum muscle and hypermuscularity. When you can see vascularity in the lower abs and obliques like Richie displays, you *know* **someone is as ripped-up as humanly possible.**

Every bodybuilder encounters sticking points, or times when they fail to make progress in building new muscle mass, regardless of how hard and consistently they train. The speed with which you vault past sticking points will dictate how quickly you become a champion bodybuilder.

Many sticking points are reached as a consequence of overtraining. So your first step when you encounter a sticking point should be to go through your checklist of overtraining symptoms. And if you *are* overtrained, take appropriate steps to remedy the problem. I can't place enough stress on the fact that you can't make any progress when overtrained.

Many other sticking points are a consequence of your body adapting to an overly consistent type of training program. This is an easy mistake to make. You forge consistently along in your workouts, constantly striving to add reps and resistance to each exercise in your training program. But somewhere along the way, you get too set in your ways, and are tempted to quit pushing with 100% intensity at all times.

When you get stuck in doing the same exercises, sets, and reps with the same training tempo, it's easy for your body and mind to go to sleep on you. That's when your muscles cease to increase in mass and strength, and you reach one of those dreaded sticking points. But you should not despair when you hit a sticking point, because it's possible to vault past one if you know how to recognize the need to do it.

How will you know when you reach a sticking point? Even at the best of times, it's difficult to see gains in muscle mass. But strength gains should come gradually and progressively.

When you have not made any gains in strength on even basic exercises for at least six weeks, you have definitive evidence that you have reached a sticking point.

The best attack when you reach a sticking point is to change your workout schedule. I recommend cutting back on training frequency and volume while concurrently increasing intraset training intensity. Go shorter, harder, and heavier for a few weeks, blasting away only four days per week. And to avoid adapting to the new program too quickly, constantly vary your routine from workout to workout.

MUSCLE CONFUSION TRAINING PRINCIPLE

The best tool you have for avoiding sticking points is the Weider Muscle Confusion Training Principle, which advocates constantly shaking up your routines. *Lou Ferrigno* comments on the Muscle Confusion Principle: "Whenever I stick to a routine too long, my mind grows bored with it, and my body becomes so perfectly adapted that I cease to make gains in muscle mass. So instead of changing to a new routine every 6–8 weeks like so many other bodybuilders, I switch off every day. And this method keeps the gains coming all the time, rather than in short spurts after routine bimonthly training program changes.

"There are several variables which you can change when using muscle confusion. Some of them are the number of days per week you work out, the times of day you train, the body part combinations each workout day, the relative poundages used, exercises included in your schedule, sets, reps, workout tempo, and training principles utilized. Since I'm able to work with this many variables, it's easy to see why I tell personal trainees that I can go an entire year without repeating a particular workout.

"This is a case when variety truly *is* the spice of life. The more variety you can inject into your workouts, the less chance you have of your mind and body adapting to your training program, thereby causing you to come up against a sticking point. By using what I sometimes call a 'non-routine routine,' you will be able to make almost continual progress from your training efforts."

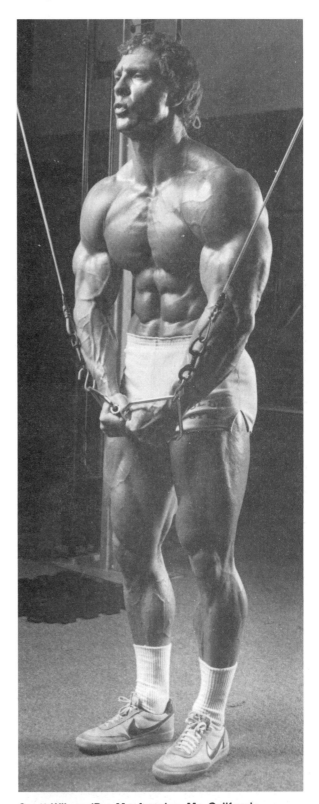

Scott Wilson (Pro Mr. America, Mr. California, Portland Pro Grand Prix Champion) knocks out a set of Cable Crossovers to etch even more striations across his pectorals. One of the best pro bodybuilders on the circuit at the present time, Scottie works as manager of the Gold's Gym in San Jose, California.

OTHER CAUSES OF STICKING POINTS

It's also a good idea to rededicate yourself to always using 100% effort in every workout. Everyone has a natural tendency over time to slack off a little in training sessions. Whenever you feel yourself losing workout momentum, vow to push the intensity of effort back up to a maximum level. This will be a constant battle, but one you must win over the long haul if you want to have any chance of reaching the top in competitive bodybuilding.

In addition to a physical and mental cause of sticking points, there is a nutritional variable which can cause them. Following a poor diet, or eating sporadically (missing meals), can also result in a progress stall, regardless of how mentally committed you are, or how hard and consistently you train. Whenever you are tempted to eat a pizza and drink a pitcher of beer, think about what that little slip will do to your progress. Maintain a good, nutritious diet year-round, and you'll be on the path to consistent gains in muscle mass and quality.

OUTDOOR TRAINING

In southern California, the climate is so great that bodybuilders can train out of doors virtually year-round. This is particularly true down at the beach where smog is seldom much of a problem. This is where you can find bodybuilders pumping iron at two well-known outdoor gyms—the old Muscle Beach weight pen, and Joe Gold's great World Gym outdoor section.

Training outdoors simultaneously gives you large muscles and a deep, healthy tan to show them off. So if you don't have access to an outdoor gym, but do have good weather, why don't you drag some home gym equipment out into your back yard? If you do, you'll quickly discover training outdoors to be a great change of pace. And you will soon be addicted to fresh-air training.

WORKOUT PARTNERS

There are several personal traits which will determine whether you will wish to utilize a training partner. Rugged individualists who are self-motivated, like three-time Mr. Olympia winner Frank Zane, can make excellent gains training alone. And even Zane has had a variety of training partners, including his wife Christine, for short periods through the years.

Bodybuilders who train either very instinctively, or use the Weider Muscle Confusion Principle, will also benefit from training alone. It's always difficult to find a training partner who wants to keep up with you when you tailor each new workout to unique physical requirements, or are simply shaking up your routines for variety's sake.

Approximately half of the great bodybuilders with whom I've worked over the years have preferred to have one or two training partners. A partner can act as an ever-present spotter. He can also be the one person who can drag you through a hard workout when your energy and/or mental drive are at an ebb. And you will usually develop a healthy competition to train harder among training partners, which in turn boosts the effectiveness of training partners as a team.

Bertil Fox prefers to work out with two training partners: "I train so heavily year-round that I need two strong partners to set up weights for me in a variety of exercises. For example, my heaviest set of incline presses requires a pair of 180-pound dumbbells which my mates hand to me while I'm lying back on an incline bench.

"During an off-season training cycle, I prefer two partners, because during that cycle, I am training both heavily and slowly. When three partners switch off on an exercise, rest intervals between sets are about 2–2½ minutes, which affords sufficient recovery time to go all out on my next heavy set.

"When it comes to peaking for a competition, however, I must train progressively faster in order to reach top physical condition. So about 10 weeks out from a show, I switch to using only one workout mate, which automatically speeds up my workouts. Then 4–5 weeks out—the length of time out from a show varying according to how quickly I am ripping up—I go it alone using more moderate poundages in each movement. This allows me to train more intensely at top speed. Add in a tight precontest diet, and speed training puts me into peak contest condition like nothing else."

Your first consideration when choosing a training partner should be finding one with a similar workout philosophy. He can be either stronger or weaker than you are, but he should be training the same number of days per week and doing a similar number of total sets for each body part. Incidentally, be prepared to compromise on your training style in order to meet a workout partner halfway—find a middle ground between his training approach and your own.

Pick a training partner who is dependable. It's of no value to you to sit for an hour in the gym waiting for someone to show up for a workout. You'll probably either miss your own training session, or go through it half-speed. Your partner should have the same commitment as you do to be in the gym every workout day in plenty of time to warm up for a heavy session with the iron. The camaraderie a training team can develop over the months and years can go a long way to turning you both into champs.

In recent years, more male-female training partnerships have developed, particularly between couples who are already involved with each other. I've concluded that such partnerships are valuable, because each sex has unique training talents which can help the other. Women have greater endurance and higher pain thresholds on average, which helps them to push men to longer and more intense workouts. And men are usually much stronger, which helps the women train heavier. So if a man and woman are compatible, they can effectively train together.

FREE WEIGHTS VERSUS MACHINES

Prior to 1970, there were very few training machines available that gave direct resistance to the working muscles. True, there were leg extensions/leg curl machines, and even some for doing biceps curls, but otherwise the world of bodybuilding revolved around free weights. Barbells and dumbbells were the norm.

Then at the 1970 Mr. America competition in Culver City, California, Arthur Jones unveiled the first of his revolutionary Nautilus machines. Since his machines were specifically

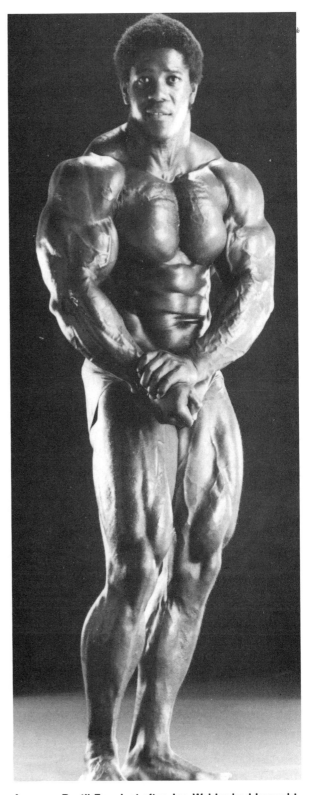

A young Bertil Fox, just after Joe Weider had brought the British athlete over from Europe and started to refine his incredible natural degree of muscle mass. Bertil routinely does eight reps in the Seated Press Behind Neck for deltoids with weights ranging from 340–375 pounds, the poundage depending on his relative energy levels on the day in question.

engineered to provide the ultimate in intensity every repetition, they quickly became popular with bodybuilders and the general public. Within a decade, it seemed that Nautilus machines were everywhere.

Following Nautilus's lead, a large number of manufacturers began turning out other resistance machines to take over the load once borne exclusively by free weights. Some of the better companies included Paramount, David, Flex, Icarian, Corbin-Pacific, and TK Star. My own engineers also developed a series of exercise machines, which became mainstays in the Weider line of gym equipment.

There are advantages and disadvantages to using machines and free weights. But before we get into them, I must state that no exercise resistance machine has ever been invented that produces any type of training effect that can't be duplicated by barbells, dumbbells, cables, benches, and various chinning/dipping bars.

The main advantages of machines are that they are easy to learn to use, and they are almost totally safe. Compared to learning the kinetics of pressing two heavy dumbbells upward while lying on an incline bench, it's ludicrously easy to learn how to use a Nautilus double-chest machine. And very few people have ever been seriously injured when training on machines.

A third advantage of resistance machine training is the superior type of resistance they place on working muscles. Almost all of them supply rotary resistance, which means the resistance is always directly against the working muscles throughout the full range of motion. That isn't the case with many barbell/dumbbell exercises, which provide natural resting points where little resistance is on the working muscle(s).

Because the resistance is rotary, machines also allow peak contraction effort on virtually every exercise. Again, this is better than a lot of free-weight movements, which frequently don't have any weight on the working muscles at all when they are fully flexed.

In addition to rotary resistance, some machines (notably Nautilus) provide balanced resistance by using a cam (pulley) with a varying radius. The radius has been calibrated by computer so greater weight is placed on the muscles in parts of the full range of movement when they are strongest. This is one function barbells and dumbbells can't duplicate, incidentally.

Now for the bad news. Machine manufacturers provide very few exercises for each major muscle group, frequently only one or two movements per body part. This can soon lead to boredom with your training program, since it will be totally static. While machines do supply superior resistance to working muscles, they are best used in conjunction with free weights. That's the way most bodybuilders make effective use of exercise resistance machines.

Cost is another very real problem with machines. A full line of Nautilus machines that works every part of your body costs tens of thousands of dollars. In contrast, a full home gym free-weight set-up can cost less than $400. Even memberships at spas that have a lot of exercise machines are higher than average, since the spa owners must amortize the cost of the machines.

Third, machines require a lot more maintenance than free weights and related equipment. Cables, bearings, hand grips, and foam/fabric components wear out constantly and must be replaced. A machine is down and unusable whenever it is under repair. By comparison how many times do you break a metal 10-pound plate?

BASIC VERSUS ISOLATION EXERCISES

Basic exercises are movements that work the larger muscle groups of your body, usually in combination with other smaller muscles. The best basic exercise for your lower body is the squat, which works the quads and buttocks in concert with the hamstrings, lower-back, and upper-back muscles. An upper-body equivalent to the squat, the bench press, primarily stresses the pectorals, but also involves the anterior-medial delts, triceps, and those upper-back muscles that impart rotational movement to the scapulae.

In contrast, isolation exercises limit stress to only one body part, or sometimes to only a section of a single muscle group. A good quadriceps isolation movement is the leg extension. And a good one for the pectorals is the cable crossover.

THE BEST BASIC AND ISOLATION EXERCISES.

Body Part	Basic exercises	Isolation exercises
Thighs-Buttocks	Squats, Leg Presses	Leg Extensions, Leg Adductions/ Abductions, Lunges
Hamstrings	Stiff-Legged Deadlifts	Leg Curls
Lower back	Deadlifts	Hyperextensions
Middle back	Barbell/Dumbbell/Cable Rows, Chins, Pulldowns	Bent-Arm Pullovers, Cross-Bench Pullovers, Stiff-Arm Pulldowns, Cable Crunches
Upper back	Barbell/Cable/Dumbbell Upright Rows	Barbell/Dumbbell/Cable Shrugs
Shoulders	Overhead Presses, Upright Rows	Front/Side/Bent-Over Laterals
Chest	Bench Presses, Incline Presses, Decline Presses, Parallel Bar Dips	Flat/Incline/Decline Flyes, Pec Deck Flyes, Cable Crossovers
Biceps	Reverse-Grip Chins, Standing Barbell Curls	Barbell/Dumbbell Concentration Curls, Cable Curls, Preacher Curls
Triceps	Parallel Bar Dips, Close-Grip Bench Presses	Pulley Pushdowns, Barbell/Dumbbell Triceps Extensions
Forearms	Reverse Curls	Barbell/Dumbbell Wrist Curls/Reverse Wrist Curls
Calves	Jumping Squats	Standing/Seated Calf Raises, One-Legged Calf Raises, Donkey Calf Raises, Calf Presses
Abdominals	Sit-Ups, Leg Raises	Crunches, Side Bends

A listing of the best basic and isolation exercises can be found above.

Basic movements are best used for building great muscle mass. Top bodybuilders usually concentrate their efforts in the off-season on basic exercises, because their main goal during an off-season training cycle is to increase general muscle mass. Using relatively low repetitions and very heavy weights on basic exercises, any bodybuilder can markedly increase his muscle mass during a four- to six-month off-season cycle.

Isolation exercises are intended more for shaping and ripping up each muscle group. While a champion bodybuilder will use about 20%–25% isolation exercises and 75%–80% basic movements in the off-season, this ratio shifts to about 50/50 during a peaking cycle. And some Olympians actually reach an 80/20 ratio of isolation-to-basic exercises.

HEAVY VERSUS LIGHT TRAINING

Exercise physiologists have done muscle biopsies on thousands of athletes and have discovered that there are two general categories of muscle cells. One such category is fast-twitch cells, which are involved in heavy, low-repetition movements, particularly when reps are performed explosively. The other category is slow-twitch cells which are involved in light, high-rep movements like distance running and cycling.

Generally speaking, you can develop your fast-twitch muscle cells by doing heavy, low-rep workouts. And you can develop slow-twitch cells by doing long, light, high-repetitions workouts. This dichotomy has produced two primary categories of bodybuilders, one who stresses heavy power training and another who does primarily light, high-rep, pumping workouts.

While both types of bodybuilders ultimately build large, high-quality muscles, I believe it is wrong to train exclusively on one or the other type of reps. When you train exclusively with heavy weights or only with light weights, you are developing only one of the two main types of muscle cells. From my own experiments over the years, this allows a bodybuilder to develop only a fraction of his ultimate potential degree of muscle mass and quality.

While the majority of exercise physiologists believe there are two main categories of muscle cells (slow- and fast-twitch), many others believe there are actually scores of subtypes ranging between the two extremes. So, why should a bodybuilder handicap himself by training to develop only one type of muscle cell, leaving the other type(s) relatively underdeveloped? If a bodybuilder is serious about winning major competitions, he should train to develop not only the two main cell types, but also the myriad of subtypes.

My answer to the eternal heavy-or-light question is the Weider Holistic Sets Training Principle. When training holistically, you should include set–rep–weight schemes in each routine that embrace both major muscle cell types, as well as the gradations between these distinct cell types. Only by training in this manner can you develop your full potential of muscle mass and quality.

In my experience, you can best train holistically on basic exercises for each muscle group. Assuming that you are doing squats, here is a typical holistic set–rep–weight progression (weights have been arbitrarily chosen merely for the sake of illustration):

Set Number	Repetitions	Poundage
1	20	135
2	15	205
3	12	255
4	10	295
5	8	325
6	6	350
7	4	370
8	1–2	385

As you can see from this example, you will do both high and low reps, plus many gradations of medium reps between these two extremes. And in this way, you can develop every possible type of muscle cell.

When you are doing isolation movements, you can also train holistically. But with isolation exercises, I feel it is best to vary your repetitions and training poundages from one workout to the next, rather than within one training session. Over a one-month period of time, then, you can perform high, low, and medium reps of dumbbell side laterals, for instance, which will develop every possible cell type in your medial deltoids.

SPLIT ROUTINES

It should become obvious to you that your workouts will eventually become so long and involved when training your whole body in one session that it becomes impossible to work every muscle group with the highest possible degree of intensity. The body parts early in a full-body training session are bombed very intensely, while those toward the end of your workout receive less intensity than they could handle.

Once your full-body training sessions are hours long, you should begin to follow a split routine in which you divide your body parts into two relatively equal groups and work out four or more days per week, doing only part of your body each workout day.

The most fundamental split routine involves four workouts per week, two for each major muscle group. There are several ways in which you can divide your body parts up into two equal groups. Since you are still allowing a minimum of two full rest days between sessions for each muscle group, you can safely train more than three days per week when following a split routine. Several examples of four-day split routines can be found on page 127.

After you have been following a four-day split routine for 4–6 months, you might wish to step up intensity by following a five-day split. With a five-day split routine, you still divide your body parts up into two relatively equal groups. The first week, you do one group on Mondays, Wednesdays, and Fridays, and the other on Tuesdays and Thursdays, resting over the weekend. And the next week, you reverse the body part groupings. An example of a five-day split routine (designating parts of your body either "A" or "B") is on page 127.

A few more months down the road, you may wish to switch to the more intense three-on, one-off program used by a majority of top bodybuilders during the off-season. In this case, you divide up your body parts into three groups. Day one you do Group "A"; day two, Group "B"; and day three, Group "C." Day four is a rest day, and on day five you begin to repeat the cycle. This type of split routine will screw up a lot of your weekends, but it fosters much better recovery than any of the six-day split routines once used by top bodybuilders. An example of the three-on, one-off split routine can be found on page 127.

EXAMPLE OF A THREE-ON, ONE-OFF SPLIT ROUTINE

Day 1	Day 2	Day 3	Day 4
Calves	Abdominals	Calves	Rest
Chest	Thighs	Shoulders	
Back	Forearms	Upper Arms	

EXAMPLES OF FOUR-DAY SPLIT ROUTINES
ALTERNATIVE 1

Monday-Thursday	Tuesday-Friday
Abdominals (hard)	Abdominals (easy)
Chest	Thighs
Shoulders	Arms
Back	Calves

ALTERNATIVE 2

Monday-Thursday	Tuesday-Friday
Calves	Abdominals
Chest	Thighs
Shoulders	Back
Triceps	Biceps
Forearms	

ALTERNATIVE 3

Monday-Thursday	Tuesday-Friday
Abdominals (hard)	Calves
Thighs	Back
Chest	Shoulders
Biceps	Triceps
Forearms	Abdominals (easy)

EXAMPLE OF A FIVE-DAY SPLIT ROUTINE

	Monday	Tuesday	Wednesday	Thursday	Friday
Week 1	A	B	A	B	A
Week 2	B	A	B	A	B
Week 3	A	B	A	B	A
Week 4	B	A	B	A	B

Note: "A" and "B" designate rival halves of the body.

EXAMPLE OF A SIX-DAY SPLIT ROUTINE
Each Major Muscle Group Trained Twice per Week

Mon-Thurs	Tues-Fri	Wed-Sat
Calves	Abdominals	Calves
Shoulders	Thighs	Chest
Upper Arms	Forearms	Back

EXAMPLE OF A SIX-DAY SPLIT ROUTINE
Each Major Muscle Group Trained Three Times per Week

Mon-Wed-Fri	Tues-Thurs-Sat
Abdominals (hard)	Abdominals (easy)
Chest	Thighs
Shoulders	Lower Back
Upper Back	Upper Arms
Calves	Forearms

The most intense type of split routine involves six workouts per week and one day of rest. The six-day split comes in two variations. The less intense of the two involves two workouts per week for each major muscle group. An example of this type of six-day split routine can be found on page 126-128. The more intense form of six-day split routine involves three workouts per week for each major muscle group. You can find an example of this type of six-day split routine on page 127.

Six-day split routines are highly intense, so only the most advanced bodybuilders should train six days per week. And the better athletes tend to follow the less intense form of six-day split in the off-season and the more intense type for only 6–8 weeks prior to a competition when attempting to bring out optimum muscularity.

BELTS AND WRAPS

"The heavier you train, the more you will need to rely on a lifting belt and joint wraps," says massive *Mike Christian*. "Most bodybuilders, myself included, use a weightlifting belt buckled firmly around their waists whenever they are doing squats, overhead pressing movements, and heavy back exercises such as deadlifts, barbell rows, and T-bar rows. The belt adds stability to the middle of your body, protecting your lower back and abdomen from injury.

"You can purchase weightlifting belts in many sporting goods stores, or through advertisements in *Flex, Muscle & Fitness,* and other bodybuilding magazines. They come in two types, one with a back four inches wide and the other with a back six or more inches wide. The

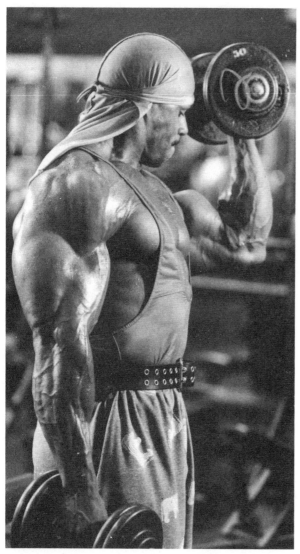

Sartorial splendor notwithstanding, Mike Christian gets in a super-intense set of Alternate Dumbbell Curls with a pair of 50-pounders. Actually, dress for comfort and non-restriction of movement, and you're halfway there. Let style take care of itself.

narrow-backed belt is only for weightlifting and powerlifting competitions, so be sure to purchase the wide-backed training belt. You should expect to pay $25 for a low-quality belt and about $60 for one with a quality suede backing."

There's quite a bit of debate about the value of joint wraps. *Tom Platz* (Mr. Universe) feels they are a detriment to proper training: "Whenever I've worn knee wraps when squatting, I began to rob the working muscles of much of the stress they should be feeling in a heavy set. With wraps on my knees, the legs tend to become very efficient levers for moving the weight upward. So in my seminars, I always recommend not using joint wraps."

Other bodybuilders feel that joint wraps can protect a joint weakened by previous injuries. Typical of this group is *Rich Gaspari*, who says, "Wraps can protect an old injury site, or prevent you from getting injuries in the first place. The wraps come in two types, neoprene rubber tubes, which can be fitted over a joint, or elastic fabric strips, which can be wrapped around a joint. Expect to pay something in the range of $5-$15 for the rubber wraps and about $6-$10 for good-quality fabric wraps.

"Rubber wraps are excellent for keeping damp heat around the injured joint. They can be used around the knee or elbow, as well as around the waist when a back injury is acting up. But rubber wraps provide very little actual support to an injured joint.

"If you need to add support to a previously injured knee, or some other joint, you should use fabric wraps. The best type is called a Superwrap. It's the same type of elastic fabric wrap used by powerlifters who are squatting hundreds of pounds more than most bodybuilders. Superwrap has elastic which will bounce back from full stretch literally hundreds of times without losing elasticity.

"When wrapping a joint, first take a couple of turns around the limb 4–6 inches above or below the joint, wrapping over the first turn of fabric to anchor one end of the wrap. Then wrap upward or downward in spirals, being sure that the wrap overlaps itself enough so you always have two layers of fabric over the joint. When you finish the wrap, tuck the loose end of the fabric under one or two of the coils to anchor it securely."

When a knee has been injured repeatedly— particularly in violent contact sports like football—osteoarthritis can occur. In this case, the joint will always be at least slightly sore. You can still do relatively heavy squats with this condition, however. What you should do to protect the joint from pain or further injury is first slip a rubber tube wrap over the joint. Over the tube, you can slide your warm-up pants. And then over the tube and pants, wrap the joint conventially with a Superwrap.

The combination of rubber and fabric wraps is very therapeutic, because the heat kept around the joint will sooth any long-term injury. And the additional support given by a fabric wrap will allow you to continue squatting or doing heavy leg presses without further injuring your knee.

PERSONALIZED TRAINING PROGRAMS

When a bodybuilder becomes involved in the sport, he invariably starts training on routines suggested by the author(s) of books and/or

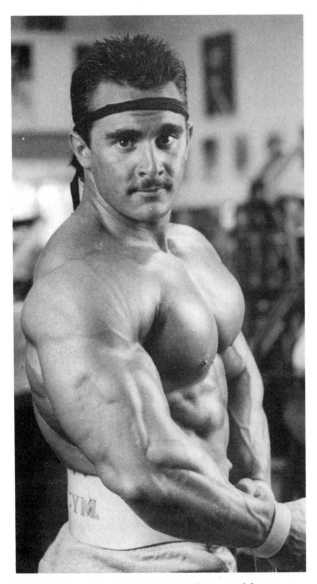

Young Shane Dimora, who recently moved from Florida back up to his hometown, Rochester, New York, won the NPC National Middleweight Championship at age 19 in 1986. He's since done quite well, thank you, in several IFBB pro competitions.

magazine articles on proper training procedures. For a few months, a novice bodybuilder can continue to follow progressively more intense training programs outlined by such authors. But eventually he must learn to formulate routines perfectly tailored for his unique physical structure and physiological abilities. This occurs because he will both outgrow set routines and will respond better to personalized programs.

It's possible to learn this process simply by reading every available champion's training schedules. Within a few years, you will probably become adept at recognizing most of the patterns that the top men in the sport use in making up their own personalized training programs. However, you can much more easily learn to make up your own routines by following the simple rules outlined in this chapter.

Body Part Sequencing

One of the first rules you must accept is that body parts should be trained in a particular sequence. They should be worked in order from the largest in mass down to the smallest. Large muscle groups require a much greater energy expenditure to train with optimum intensity than do smaller muscle groups. And you probably already know it is much easier to face a short biceps workout when your energy reserves have been nearly depleted than a leg training session consisting of the same number of sets.

Whether you are working your entire body in one session, or following a split routine in which you train only a part of your body each workout, this is the hierarchy of body parts from largest to smallest:

- Legs (including buttocks)
- Back
- Chest
- Shoulders
- Calves
- Upper arms
- Forearms
- Abdominals

Notice that I haven't included the neck in this body part hierarchy. The reason for this seeming oversight is the fact that very few top bodybuilders ever need to train their necks directly. The neck muscles invariably grow by leaps and bounds simply as a by-product of hard training for the upper chest, shoulders, and upper back.

Within the foregoing hierarchy, there are three subrules. The first of these is that upper-arm work should always be scheduled after exercises for the torso muscle groups (chest, shoulders, and back). Why?

The torso muscle groups are much larger and stronger than either biceps or triceps. As a result, the arm muscles are relative weak links when you perform such basic torso exercises as bench presses, overhead presses, upright rows, chins, pulldowns, and various types of bent-over rows. Since the weaker arm muscles fatigue and fail before the corresponding torso groups, it just stands to reason that you should strictly avoid training biceps or triceps first, making them even weaker and thereby aggravating the problem.

The second subrule is that you should always train calves *after* thighs. *Shane DiMora*, who had an unbelievably sensational competitive year in 1986 while still a teenager (he won the Teenage National, Junior National, and National Championships at the age of 19), comments on this rule: "Like all bodybuilders, I've tried working my calves prior to doing a heavy squat workout, and I found that my legs vibrated so badly as a result that I couldn't do either squats or leg presses with anything higher than mid-range poundages. So, I didn't get a very good leg workout. But by avoiding early calf work—by scheduling calves on either a different day altogether, or during a different half of a double-split—I no longer have a problem training either thighs or calves."

Despite the body part hierarchy presented earlier in this chapter, many bodybuilders seem to prefer doing calves first in their routines, as either a warm-up for the rest of a training schedule, or because calves are a muscle group which needs specialized training to bring it up to the level of the remainder of the body. Due to the leg vibration problem, you must make a point of training calves first only on non-leg days, or at a time separate from the rest of your workout.

Third, many bodybuilders prefer to train abdominals at the start of a workout as either a warm-up for the rest of the body parts, or because the abdominals might also require specialized training to bring them up to the rest of your body parts. In either case, you should feel free to violate the rule which says to do the midsection work last in your program.

PRIORITY BODY PART SCHEDULING

You've already learned about the Weider Muscle Priority Training Principle, and you *must* adhere to it when you are making up a new training program. That's the only way you can hope to become a superstar in the sport. Whenever you are giving priority to a weaker body part, you must schedule it either first in your program each workout day, or on a completely separate day.

RELATIVE WORK LOAD

I keep coming back to relative work load, because scheduling too many total sets for each body part into your program will cause you to overtrain. And that, in turn, will prevent you from making good gains from your workouts. The number of sets you can safely perform for each muscle group depends solely on your relative level of experience in the sport, and the efficiency of between-workout recovery ability generated by such experience.

One general rule for work load which I keep coming back to is *always do less total sets than you think your body needs for each muscle group*. It's much better to consistently *under*train than consistently *over*train when it comes to building huge, highly detailed muscles.

Contest-level bodybuilders should attempt to stay within the guidelines I have set for advanced bodybuilders whenever they are training in an off-season building cycle. But when a competition approaches—particularly if a bodybuilder is using anabolic steroids to help him peak out—up to 15-20 total sets can be done for each body part for a time limit of no more than 6-8 weeks each peak.

PART III
ADVICE TO
ADVANCED
BODYBUILDERS

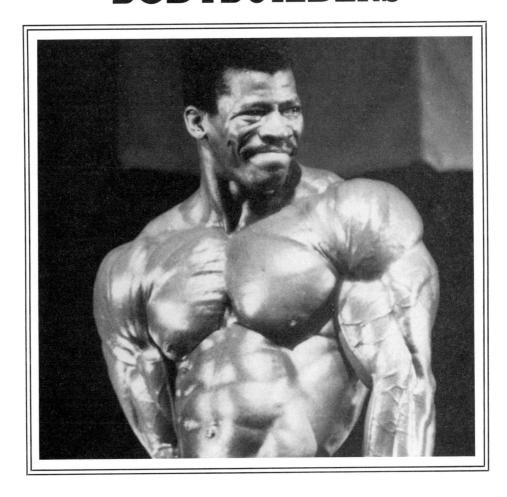

12
Advanced
Training Techniques

This is the last chance I have to introduce you to several of the more high-intensity Weider Training Principles. The rest of the book is concerned with nutrition and bodybuilding psychology. So in this chapter, I'll teach you to use these Weider Principles:

- Trisets and Giant Sets
- Double-Split System
- Staggered Sets
- Peak Contraction
- Continuous Tension
- Quality Training
- ISO-Tension
- Rest-Pause

All of the foregoing Weider Training Principles—with the possible exception of Rest-Pause and Trisets and Giant Sets—are most applicable when you are peaking for a competition.

I'll conclude this chapter with a brief discussion of the ethics of using various bodybuilding drugs. Some authors actually suggest precise drug programs. But since the IFBB has taken a firm stand against drug usage in bodybuilding, I will confine my brief discussion to the ethical question of bodybuilding pharmacology.

In Part II, I described how to use supersets (combinations of two movements with no rest between exercises and a normal rest interval between supersets) to increase training intensity by reducing the average length of rest interval between sets. And I described two types of supersets—a less-intense variation in which movements are compounded for antagonistic body parts such as biceps and triceps, and a second, more-intense type in which exercises for the same muscle group are supersetted. As an advanced bodybuilder, you can now take this method further.

TRISETS AND GIANT SETS

There are several more ways you can use compounded sets to take additional steps up the ladder of training intensity. The first of these is to do trisets, or a series of three movements for the same body part, with no rest between movements and a normal rest interval between trisets. These trisets are used on body parts with three or more segments, such as the deltoids, concentrating on the anterior, medial, and posterior heads. One movement is chosen for each aspect of that muscle complex.

A sample triset for deltoids, with exercises specifically chosen for each deltoid head (in this chapter, brackets will enclose exercises to be compounded into trisets and giant sets) would look like this:

{
Dumbbell Bent Laterals (posterior head)
Seated Presses Behind Neck (anterior head)
Standing Dumbbell Side Laterals (medial head)
}

Following are other trisets for the chest and back muscles, which you can insert into your training program:

Chest

{
Incline Dumbbell Presses (upper pecs)
Decline Flyes (lower–outer pecs)
Bench Press to Neck (middle–outer pecs)
}

Back

{
Front Chins (lat width)
Stiff-Arm Pulldowns (lower lats)
Pulldowns Behind Neck (upper lats)
}

There are many gradations of training intensity when using giant sets, which are compounds of four, five or six movements, with no

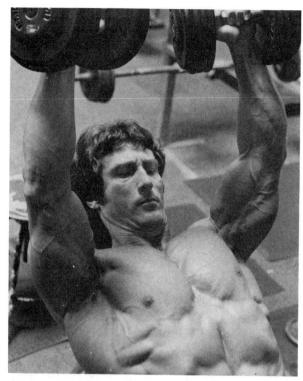

One of the most introspective and intuitive trainers of all time was Frank Zane. He was constantly monitoring every possible piece of biofeedback data in an effort to determine more precisely just what his physique required in the way of training on a particular workout day.

rest between exercises and a more normal rest interval between giant sets. The least intense type of giant set consists of four movements, the next most intense involves five movements, and the most intense type of giant set consists of six exercises.

Among four-movement giant sets, the least intense type includes movements for two antagonistic body parts. Here is an example of that type of giant set:

{
Bench Press (middle-outer pecs)
Chins Behind Neck (upper lats)
Incline Flyes (upper pecs)
Barbell Bent Rows (mid-back thickness)
}

Another step up the intensity ladder, you will find four-movement giant sets with exercises chosen for a single muscle group. Here is an example of this type of giant set:

{
Barbell Shrugs (traps)
Front Lat Pulldowns (lower-middle lats)
Hyperextensions (lower back)
Seated Pully Rows (lat thickness)
}

Among five-exercise giant sets, the least intense form includes movements for two antagonistic muscle groups, three movements for one body part and two for the other. Here is an example of this type of giant set:

{
Squats (general quadriceps mass)
Lying Leg Curls (mid-lower hamstrings)
Leg Extensions (quadriceps cuts and shape)
Seated Leg Curls (mid-upper hamstrings)
Angled Leg Presses (lower quadriceps)
}

Moving up another rung on the intensity ladder, we come to five-movement giant sets for a single muscle group. Following is an example of such a giant set:

{
Incline Barbell Presses (upper pecs)
Cross-Bench Dumbbell Pullovers (serratus-general pecs)
Decline Dumbbell Presses (lower-outer pecs)
Cable Crossovers (lower-inner pecs)
Pec Deck Flyes (inner-general pecs)
}

Among six-exercise giant sets, the least intense consists of exercises alternated for antagonistic muscle groups. Here is a sample of such a giant set:

{
Bench Presses (lower-outer pecs)
Pulldowns Behind Neck (upper lats)
Incline Cable Flyes (upper-inner pecs)
Seated Pulley Rows (lat thickness)
Cable Crossovers (lower-inner pecs)
Stiff-Arm Pulldowns (lower lats-serratus)
}

And the final step up the ladder of training intensity using compound sets is a six-movement giant set consisting of exercises for a single, complex muscle group. Here is such a giant set:

{
Front Chins (lower lats)
Barbell Shrugs (traps)
Seated Pulley Rows (lat thickness)
Hyperextensions (lower back)
Barbell Bent Rows (mid-back thickness)
Stiff-Arm Pulldowns (lower lats-serratus)
}

In the same way the Weider Supersets Training Principle is a considerable step up in intensity from straight sets, the Weider Trisets Training Principle is a big leap upward in intensity from supersets, and the Weider Giant Sets Training Principle is a significant series of

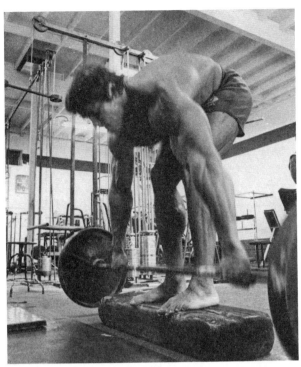

Arnold Schwarzenegger performs a heavy set of Barbell Bent-Over Rows while standing on a block for a greater range of motion. This dramatic, mid-workout photo was taken at the original Gold's Gym on Pacific Avenue in Venice, California, about 1971. In 1974 the gym was moved briefly to a location at Second and Broadway Streets in Santa Monica. And in 1977 it took residence at its present site, 360 Hampton Boulevard in Venice, California.

fornia in 1973, until about 14 years later, I had experienced a great deal of trouble isolating my upper-arm muscles, which are naturally quite powerful, from my lat movements. As a result, I had very poor latissimus dorsi development.

"I finally learned how to isolate my lats by doing trisets of mid-back exercises, typically compounding barbell bent rows, lat machine pulldowns to the front of my neck, and T-bar rows. By arching my spine, thinking the movement into the working latissimus dorsi muscles, and pushing every set as far past the failure point as possible, I was able to triset my mid-back muscles up to a level I'd given up hoping

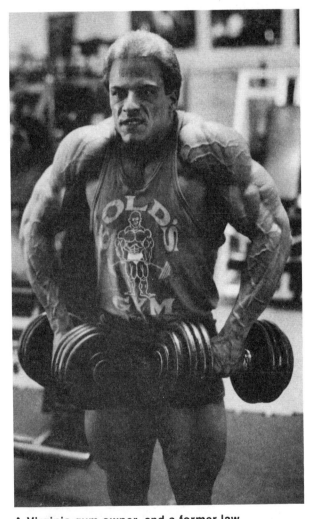

A Virginia gym owner, and a former law enforcement officer whose back injury put him on permanent disability, John Hnatyschak has successfully trained around his injuries and reached fantastic shape. He's a former NPC National Middleweight Champion and IFBB World Middleweight Champion, as well as a successful pro, who placed third in the highly competitive IFBB Chicago Pro Grand Prix in 1988.

additional upward steps in training intensity from trisets. As a result, you should only work upward in intensity gradually, perhaps taking six months or more to break in to full trisets training for a relatively stubborn muscle complex, and perhaps another six months or more to jump up to four-movement giant sets.

As I hinted in the above paragraph, I believe that trisets and giant sets should be best used for specializing on a lagging muscle group. Indeed, only 3–4 trisets or 2–3 giant sets for a weaker muscle group should give it a considerable growth boost in just a few weeks. And within 6–8 months, trisetting or giant setting should bring even the most stubborn body part up to par with the balance of your physique.

Massive *Scott Wilson* (Pro Mr. International and the IFBB Portland Pro Grand Prix Champion) is typical of a top bodybuilder who has used trisets to bring up a weak muscle group: "My back was always a weak area, until just the last year or so. From the time I won Mr. Calito achieve. And for my money, the key to all of this was using the Weider Trisets Training Principle."

For a top bodybuilder who solved a weak body part problem using giant sets, listen to what super-symmetrical *John Hnatyschak* (National and World Middleweight Champion) has to say: "Prior to winning my national and international titles in 1984, my back had been a weak area. But while reading an article on giant setting in *Flex* magazine, I learned the secret of bringing up my back musculature, so it balanced out my physique. And I immediately won my NPC National Championship and IFBB World Championship, both in the middleweight division.

"My solution for weak back development was to giant set my back exercises one workout per week, and do the other back training session with straight sets. On my giant-setting day, I would do 3–4 giant sets of 8–10 reps on these movements: front chins, bent-over dumbbell laterals, pulldowns behind neck, seated pulley rows, and stiff-arm lat pulldowns. My lats and mid-back muscles were the lagging parts of my back, so that's what I giant setted. Traps and erectors were trained in normal straight-sets fashion.

"I simply couldn't believe how quickly my lats and mid-back musculature came up once I began bombing them with much greater intensity using the Weider Giant Sets Training Principle. These back muscles expanded in mass and ripped up almost overnight. I can't recommend giant sets enough if you have a weak point. They're a tough row to hoe, but they bring results!"

DOUBLE-SPLIT ROUTINES

When peaking for a major national or international competition, highly experienced bodybuilders take split routines another step up the ladder of training intensity by using the Weider Double-Split System Training Principle. When double splitting, each day's split routine workout is further subdivided into two parts, with half of the workout done in the morning and the rest of it done in the late afternoon or evening.

Let's put double-split training into simpler terms. Assuming that you might be blasting two muscle groups per day (say chest and back, for the sake of illustration) on your split routine, you would do only chest in the morning when double-splitting, and only back in the evening.

Double-split routines work great during a peaking cycle, when your energy reserves have been depleted more than usual by a strict pre-contest diet and the significantly greater volume of training normally undertaken during a peaking phase. When your energy is low, you can usually still do a 30- to 45-minute workout for only one major muscle group in the morning with relative ease. Then after 6–8 hours of rest, you can usually bounce back enough to hit a second body part quite intensely that evening. Eight or nine hours of sleep that night will then allow you to recover sufficiently to repeat the process the next day, blasting other muscle groups.

Physiologists have determined that each workout—whether with weights, or aerobically—elevates a bodybuilder's basal metabolic rate (BMR) significantly for 2–3 hours after the session. So by training twice per day—perhaps three times a day when including aerobics—you keep your metabolism high, and it's much easier to get ripped up for a competition. Indeed, this is one of the main reasons some top bodybuilders follow a double-split routine when peaking for an important competition.

Albert Beckles explains how he personally husbands and expends energy when double-splitting: "I normally sleep 8–9 hours each night, which restores my workout-depleted energy reserves by morning. After eating, I get into the gym for a light abdominal session and 25–30 total sets for a major muscle group. That's about all of the training I have enough energy to complete when I'm dieting strictly.

"I return home after my workout, eat, and take a good nap for 2 hours. That refreshes me and replenishes my energy reserves. I take care of any pressing business problems, before again having a light meal. Then at night I'm back in the gym for another tough 25–30-set workout for a major body part. Because I have most of my energy back following my lengthy nap and two light protein-and-carbohydrate rich meals,

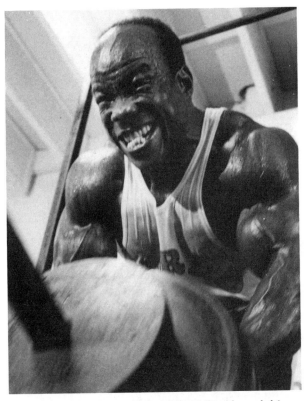

At 57 it stands to reason that Albert Beckles might not have that many more good competitive years left. So, he spends it with some of the hardest, wildest, heaviest training sessions you've ever seen, coupled with a diet so strict that a large house cat might not be able to survive it.

I can train that muscle group with the same high level of intensity as I displayed in the morning training session.

"After the second workout of my double-split, I return home, have a good high-protein meal, and relax for an hour or two before retiring for the night. I sleep soundly for 8–9 more hours, recover all of my energy reserves, and bounce out of bed the next morning eager to repeat my two daily workouts.

"There are two keys to successful double-splitting: sleep and food. As long as I get sufficient sleep and maintain a healthy, high-carbohydrate/high-protein diet, I am able to make excellent gains training with very high intensity twice a day."

EASING INTO A DOUBLE-SPLIT REGIMEN

As with split routines, there is a hierarchy of intensity levels. Experience coaching thousands of the sport's biggest stars over the years

has shown me conclusively that the best way to break into double-split training is to do a morning workout for whatever major muscle groups have been scheduled that day, then come back in the late afternoon or evening to do scheduled abdominal, calf, and/or forearm work. This mild form of double-split program is only a half step up the intensity ladder from normal split-system training, but it still allows you to attack every body part with more energy than is available when doing the entire body in one session.

I'll let *Robby Robinson* tell you about this less intense type of double split: "I've almost always followed a modified double-split program year-round. I think of it as a half-double-split routine. On Mondays, Wednesdays, and Fridays, I'll actually double-split my program, doing two sessions on those days. But on Tuesdays, Thursdays, and Saturdays, I'll train only once, in the morning. This type of double-split routine allows me optimum recovery time, and I've always made great gains when using it."

Here's how Robby divides up his body parts for his modified double-split schedule:

Mon-Wed-Fri (AM)	Mon-Wed-Fri (PM)
Abdominals (hard)	Calves (hard)
Chest	Back
Biceps	Triceps
Forearms	Neck (if it needs it)

Tues-Thurs-Sat (AM)
Abdominals (easy)
Thighs
Deltoids
Calves (easy)

A word of caution: double-split routines should be used only by highly experienced bodybuilders, and then only during the last 4–6 weeks of a competitive preparation cycle. A double-split program will elevate your metabolism so high that you will find it difficult to maintain your body weight. Only a handful of superstars, such as Lee Haney and the ageless Albert Beckles, can profitably use a double-split schedule during the off-season.

After you've peaked once or twice using Robby's modified double-split routine, you can give a full double-split a trial for your next peaking cycle. The first time you use a full double-split,

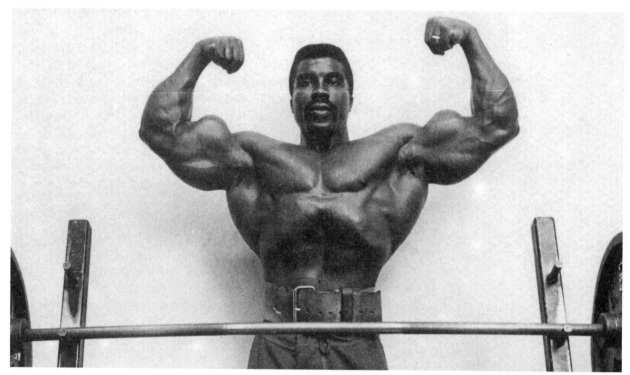

One of the most devastating front double-biceps shots in the sport belongs to the Black Prince of Bodybuilding, Robby Robinson, who has won too many pro titles to list accurately. At 41 years of age, he is a legend in the sport and a full-time pro bodybuilder living in Venice, California, and trains at Gold's Gym.

try one in which you train each major muscle group twice per week. This is the least intense form of double-split routine. And after you have peaked once or twice with the less-intense double-split, go ahead and experiment with all-out double-split training in which you bomb major body parts three times per week.

Following are examples of both types of full double-split routines:

FULL DOUBLE-SPLIT ROUTINE

(Body Parts Twice a Week)

Mon-Thurs (AM)	Mon-Thurs (PM)
Abdominals (hard)	Calves (hard)
Chest	Middle Back
Forearms (hard)	Triceps

Tues-Fri (AM)	Tues-Fri (PM)
Abdominals (easy)	Traps
Thighs	Lower Back
Forearms (easy)	Calves (easy)

Wed-Sat (AM)	Wed-Sat (PM)
Abdominals (hard)	Calves (hard)
Deltoids	Biceps
Neck	Forearms (hard)

FULL DOUBLE-SPLIT

(Body Parts Three Times a Week)

Mon-Wed-Fri (AM)	Mon-Wed-Fri (PM)
Abdominals (hard)	Calves (hard)
Chest	Deltoids
Biceps	Traps

Tues-Thurs-Sat (AM)	Tues-Thurs-Sat (PM)
Abdominals (easy)	Calves (easy)
Thighs	Mid Back
Lower Back	Triceps
Neck	Forearms

A few bodybuilders, such as massive Lee Haney, actually triple split—do *three* workouts per day—prior to a competition. But this type of program is very fatiguing, and only the *creme de la creme* of the sport can use it for the final 4–6 weeks prior to a competition.

Again, be careful you don't overtrain when following a double-split program. The only way to succeed with one is to nap between workouts and keep your calories up. Even then, you will need superior recovery ability to productively use a double-split.

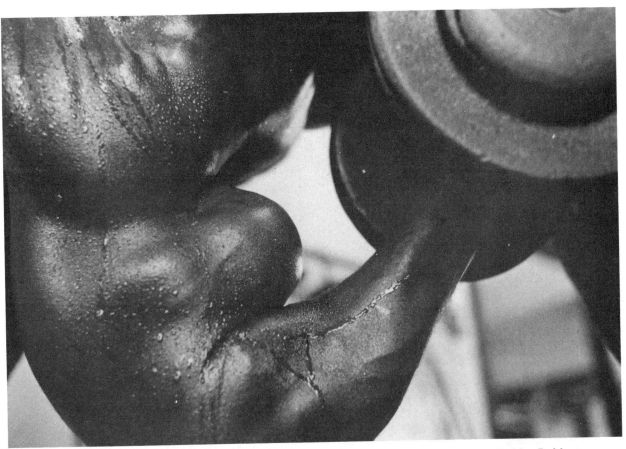

One of the greatest arms on earth in action doing a heavy concentration curl. When Robby Robinson trains arms, even the most jaded bodybuilding fans put down their own weights and observe every movement of the Black Prince, hoping they might learn a little from him that will help them build their own arms up to maybe about 60% of the size and development Robby has achieved.

STAGGERED SETS

At the advanced level of competitive bodybuilding, you may wish to use the Weider Staggered Sets Training Principle. I'll let *Ron Love* tell you about staggered sets: "The closer a champion gets to a scheduled competition, the more he has to do boring sets of abdominal training each day in order to have a strong, tightly muscular midsection onstage.

"The Staggered Sets Principle alleviates the boredom of doing large numbers of sets of abdominal work by interspersing them—I like to say intersetting them—between sets for other body parts. And when you use this technique, you can perform more than 20 sets of ab work almost without realizing you've done it.

"Let me give you an example of how staggered sets work. You might have 15–20 sets of midsection work to perform with your chest and back workout. Start your warm-up sets of bench presses, then do a set of hanging leg raises after every two sets of benches. Do the same after inclines, dips, and pec-deck flyes, as well as after every two sets of back work if you have a lot of abdominal sets to complete.

"Since it doesn't take much energy to do a set of any type of abdominal work, you won't affect your chest or back routine. Nor will the chest or back work hurt your abdominal session. And you'll get your abdominal schedule completed with strong intensity and very little boredom."

PEAK CONTRACTION

Most of the techniques discussed so far have involved sets and reps, now let's look at a technique that involves the biomechanics of an exercise. In order to understand the Weider Peak Contraction Training Principle, you must first understand how muscles contract to move a barbell. And to understand muscle contraction, you need to learn a little about skeletal muscle anatomy at the microscopic level.

The basic unit of all skeletal muscles is a *muscle cell*. These cells are strung end to end to form a *muscle fiber*. And fibers are bundled together to form a skeletal muscle. Within your

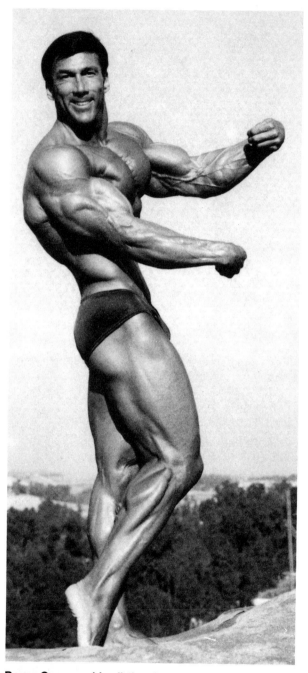

Boyer Coe near his all-time best, just days before he placed third in the 1980 Mr. Olympia competition in Sydney, Australia. So many photos of the better bodybuilders have been taken in this setting by the Editor-in-Chief of *Flex* magazine that it's become known as "Reynolds' Rocks."

biceps muscle, or any other skeletal muscle complex, are literally hundreds of thousands of muscle cells which contract to pull against the weight you are using in a particular bodybuilding movement.

Physiologically speaking, there are no partial muscle cell contractions. A muscle cell either contracts completely (and shortens when contracted), or it doesn't contract at all. Exercise physiologists call this the "all or nothing" model of muscle contraction.

I'll give you a simplified model for the way muscle cells contract to shorten a muscle fiber. Imagine a long series of woolen stockings sewed end to end. Each stocking is a muscle cell, and the entire string of them is a muscle fiber.

When you wet and then quickly dry a woolen stocking, it will shrink. This shrinking effect is analogous to a muscle cell contracting and shortening in length. Finally, imagine a squirt gun with which you can wet each stocking. The squirt gun represents a nerve, which enervates a muscle cell to cause it to contract.

In a mild muscle contraction, perhaps one in 20 stockings shrinks. Each contraction shortens the length of the string of stockings, regardless of where that shrunken stocking is placed in its end-to-end string. As you shrink more and more stockings, the contraction intensity becomes greater and the overall length of the stocking string shortens.

An actual skeletal muscle contraction works in the same way. As you slowly flex your arm when doing a standing barbell curl, more and more cells shrink, until the maximum number of cells is contracted. Then your arm is completely bent. And, in a kinesthetic sense, your biceps are significantly stronger when your arm is fully bent and the maximum number of muscle cells has been contracted.

It's only logical that you can receive the most benefit from each repetition when you have a heavy weight pulling against the working muscle when it is completely contracted. In point of fact, this is the entire object of the Weider Peak Contraction Training Principle: to heavily load each muscle in its fully contracted position. And as such, peak contraction greatly enhances muscle mass and density.

Unfortunately, many exercises do *not* place a

PEAK CONTRACTION EXERCISES

Body Part	Exercises
Quadriceps	Leg Extensions, Leg Adductions/Abductions
Hamstrings	Lying, Seated, and Standing Leg Curls
Lats	Chins, all variations of Pulldowns, all variations of Bent-Over Rows
Traps	Shrugs, Upright Rows
Spinal Erectors	Hyperextensions
Pecs	Pec-Deck Flyes, Cable Flyes at various angles
Delts	Front Raises, Side Laterals, Bent-Over Laterals
Biceps	Machine Curls, Barbell Concentration Curls
Triceps	Barbell and Dumbbell Kickbacks
Forearms	Standing Barbell Wrist Curls
Calves	All types of Calf Raises and Calf Presses
Abs	Hanging Leg Raises, all types of Crunches

load on the muscles they are intended to stress when those muscles are fully contracted. The barbell curl is a good example of such a movement, because there is little or no weight on the biceps in the top position where the arm is completely flexed (bent). Then, only the shoulder-girdle muscles are feeling any type of load.

When using Peak Contraction, you must carefully select exercises which *do* stress each muscle group when the maximum number of its muscle cells is contracted. Rather than doing barbell curls for your biceps, you can do either machine curls or bent-over barbell concentration curls, both of which provide peak contraction emphasis.

Actually, virtually all machine exercises do provide peak contraction. And there are many free-weight exercises which also give a peak contraction effect. In the figure above, you will find a list of the best peak-contraction movements for each body part.

The Weider Peak Contraction Training Principle can be used year-round, but it's most valuable during a contest peaking cycle. Combined with the Weider Slow, Continuous Tension Principle described next, Peak Contraction will etch the deepest possible striations across each muscle group.

CONTINUOUS TENSION

Bar momentum robs most inexperienced bodybuilders of part of the stress their muscles should be given in an all-out set. This is particularly true when you use cheating form on some of your reps. Your muscles get much more benefit, and become much stronger, when you take pains to *feel* the resistance over an exercise's complete arc of movement.

The object of the Weider Slow, Continuous Tension Training Principle is to slow down each rep and build maximum tension into the working muscles as you move the weight, so you can build plenty of quality muscle mass. Continuous tension, particularly when combined with Peak contraction, gives your muscles a great degree of muscle density and intramuscular detail.

Mike Quinn (Mr. USA, Mr. Universe) tells you how he uses Continuous Tension in his own workouts: "For many years, I trained with maximum poundages, primarily on basic exercises, in order to increase general muscle mass. This formula worked well because I was able to get as big as a house. But I eventually learned that I needed to add more detail to my muscles in order to further my professional career.

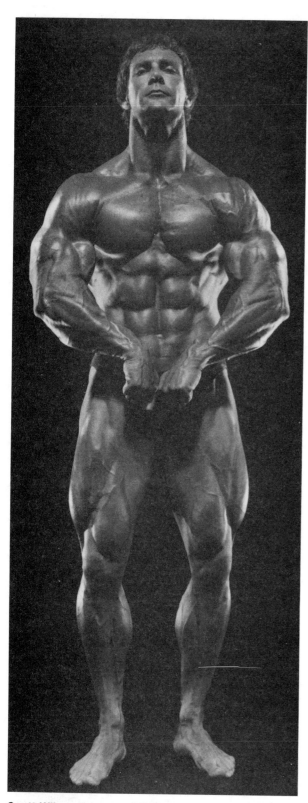

Scott Wilson has one of the most overlooked great physiques of all time. He's also very powerful, having squatted 750 pounds, benched 580, and deadlifted 735 in open powerlifting competition while weighing within the 242-pound weight limit. Scott, his wife Vi, and all of their various kids live in the San Jose, California area.

"One mainstay of my muscle-detail program was Continuous Tension, a technique which worked admirably in increasing the striations over each muscle mass. I'll tell you how I used Continuous Tension on my quads using leg extensions. Using a weight about 70% of my normal exercise weight, I move it slowly over the full range of motion of the exercise. The speed at which I move the weight is about half of normal, that is, it takes me twice as long as normal to complete the full cycle of each repetition.

"Merely moving the weight slowly increases the value of a set, but there's more to the Weider Slow, Continuous Tension Training Principle. While moving the weight slowly, I consciously keep both the working quads and the antagonistic biceps femoris muscles tensed to the max. This makes each repetition gruelling, which is the main reason why I have to use a lighter-than-normal weight. In fact, I could probably get a hell of a lot out of a Continuous Tension set using less than 50% of normal on an exercise."

QUALITY TRAINING

It takes more than just a tight diet during a peaking cycle in order for a bodybuilder to achieve optimum muscularity. It also takes more than a consistent aerobics program and tight diet to get a man's physique contest ready. He also must train faster than in the off-season using the Weider Quality Training Principle.

I'll let National Champ *Tom Terwillger* tell you about Quality Training: "As you probably know, there are three ways in which you can increase training intensity. First, you can increase the number of reps you do with a particular weight. Second, you can increase the amount of weight you use for a certain number of reps. And third, you can do the same sets and reps with a fixed weight, but take less rest between sets. This third method is the crux of Quality Training.

"You have to work harder than ever before whenever you are using Quality Training, because you need to constantly fight to keep your exercise weights up while reducing rest intervals. That is a tough row to hoe—particularly when you're dieting—but every successful champion guts it out. He has to, or he doesn't stand a chance of winning. Despite the diet and reduced rest intervals, you should fight against dropping poundages more than about 20%–25%.

"There's no fixed rule for how little time you should be resting between sets when at peak Quality Training intensity. I can tell you how I do it, however. In the off-season, I rest 60–90 seconds between sets, with the longer rest intervals between sets for large muscle groups like back and legs. Over a 6–8-week period, I gradually cut rest intervals down to half of normal, or to 30–45 seconds' rest between each set. Combined with a low-calorie diet, this type of Quality Training, largely accomplished through pure guts and supersets, rips me to doll rags."

ISO-TENSION

One thing I teach all of the champs is how to correctly use the Weider ISO-Tension Training Principle to harden up their muscles for a competition. This technique consists of tensing each muscle group as hard as possible for 8–10 seconds, followed by about 10 seconds of rest and more "reps" of contracting that muscle group. As many as 30–40 reps can be performed for each muscle group, utilizing many different poses for that body part.

ISO-Tension should be used only when peaking, and then it should be done every day. You can either utilize ISO-Tension in the gym between sets, or at home between normal weight sessions. Using this technique consistently for 6–8 weeks prior to a competition will greatly increase your control over each muscle group when posing onstage, which in turn will make your muscles appear harder than they would under normal circumstances.

REST-PAUSE

One of the best methods for increasing muscle mass and power is the Weider Rest-Pause Training Principle. The best exponent of Rest-Pause in recent years is *Mike Mentzer*. He discusses the topic: "Looking back over my career and analyzing the methods that yielded the best results, I can readily state that rest-pause training (RPT) was one of the most productive. I learned about it from Bob Gajda [a former Mr. America and Mr. World] and Tony Garcy [a former National Weightlifting Champion] at Gajda's Sports Fitness Institute in Chicago in late 1978. I began using RPT when I was preparing for my first professional bodybuilding competition, the Southern Professional Cup, held in Miami, Florida, in early February of 1979.

"I started training for the show on December 4, 1978, and incorporated RPT with a couple of variations. In some workouts I used weights that allowed two or three reps in succession without using RPT; in others I used a weight in RPT fashion, including added resistance after the positive cycle of the rep, for a maximum or near-maximum negative repetition. There was no pattern to these variations; I performed them as experiments or merely as whims.

"While my weight didn't change much after starting RPT, my appearance altered dramatically. On December 4, I was a smooth 217 pounds and was not on steroids. But on December 11, I wrote in my journal, 'There has been no weight gain, but no loss either. And my muscles seem rounder, with more cuts. Something is happening!'

"By January 1, 1979, I was on steroids in preparation for the Southern Pro Cup five weeks later. I competed at 213 pounds and won the competition in convincing fashion over Robby Robinson. So while I actually lost four pounds, it was obvious that I had replaced considerable fat with quite a bit of muscle mass. I had reached the best condition of my life up to that point using RPT.

"I'd been using my Heavy Duty workout methods like pre-exhaustion and forced-rep training for several years. I had made excellent gains, having gone from 195 to 210 pounds in hard contest condition. But I'd grown so strong and my ability and willingness to generate maximum effort was so dramatically improved that each repetition of a normal six-rep set was too intense and severe.

"What I needed at that point was a new training method that would allow more sustained, intense contractions while simulta-

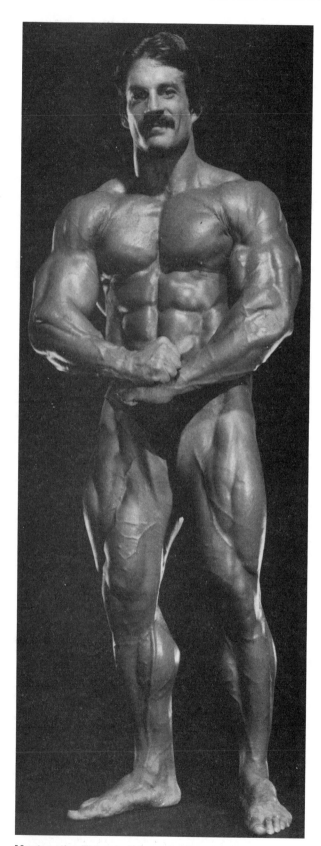

Mentzer the Elder, in this case Mike, has become a successful bodybuilding writer. He lives and works in the heartland of international bodybuilding, Venice, California.

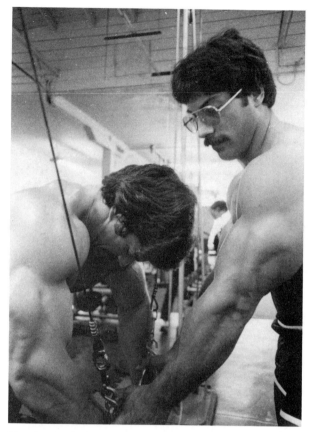

It's nice having a training partner, particularly when he's your brother. In this photo, Ray Mentzer gives his brother Mike a couple of forced reps at the end of a set of Cable Crossovers. Very few men have ever trained as consistently hard—set-to-set—as the Mentzer brothers.

neously slowing the onset of oxygen debt and build-up of waste metabolites such as lactic acid. This view was corroborated by authors Edington and Edgerton in their fine textbook of exercise physiology, *The Biology of Physical Activity*:

> 'Muscle contractions can become so intense that blood flow to the muscle is decreased. . . . In effect, not enough time between contractions is permitted for the vasculature to fill before the onset of the subsequent contractions. Blood flow to the working muscles does not decrease at high work intensities when the duration of the contractions is short enough and the duration of relaxation is long enough. . . .'

"I didn't think there was much I could do to shorten the duration of the contractions without also compromising the effort I wanted to generate. But who says you have to perform two or more reps in rapid succession or that an exercise poundage allowing 6–10 repetitions is best?

"With my version of RPT only one rep is performed in strict style before taking a rest–pause. Maximum weight requires maximum effort, so intensity is high. Putting the weight down for 10 seconds after each rep allows normal blood flow through the muscles, so a bodybuilder can continue with another maximum effort following the 10-second rest-pause.

"After the second rep another 10-second rest–pause interval is allowed to elapse before performing the third repetition. But by the third rep your strength will have diminished, and you will either have to decrease the weight by 20% or have your partner give you enough of a forced-rep assist for you to complete it. The third rep should be followed by a 15-second rest–pause rather than 10 seconds because fatigue will have increased so much that a longer interval will be needed to assure a maximum-effort fourth repetition.

"I believe four rest–pause reps are best because you will probably not have enough energy left for more. I personally started out trying six reps per set but found it to be too much.

"I increased the intensity another step by adding a maximum negative to each of the four repetitions I was performing. After each rep of incline presses, for instance, my training partner would apply extra downward pressure to the bar so the negative aspect of the movement was as close to maximum as possible.

"I experimented with several other methods of increasing normal RPT intensity. The one that worked best for me was doing four reps in normal RPT fashion, followed by three ultra-intense negative repetitions in succession.

"After another couple months of pure RPT, I found myself yearning for some of my previous Heavy Duty methods, specifically forced and pre-exhaustion reps, so I combined them with RPT. For one thing, performing several reps in succession provides muscle pump. And while a pump is not necessarily indicative of growth stimulation, it has an important psychological effect that shouldn't be overlooked.

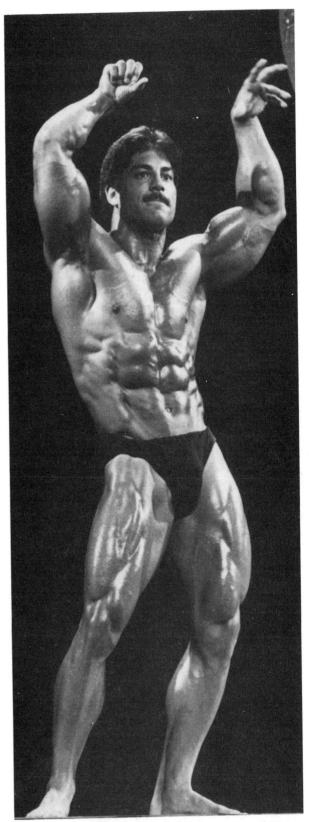

Mentzer the Younger, brother Ray, had a reasonably successful pro career before retiring in 1983. After having lived in Australia for several years, he's back in southern California and is planning a competitive comeback.

"The sustained effort of RPT will eventually drain you physically and psychologically if you do it exclusively for extended periods of time. I find it best to use RPT for no more than 4–6 weeks at a time, with periods of my normal Heavy Duty training interspersed.

"Precisely how you combine RPT with other types of training isn't too important, as long as your intensity remains high and you keep your workouts short. My best gains from RPT came when I rested 10 seconds between reps and performed 12 or fewer sets per session. Any more rest or any more sets, and my progress slowed dramatically.

"Since rest-pause is a very intense form of training, I don't recommend it to beginners. A beginning bodybuilder will develop larger muscles using conventional routines that emphasize basic exercises such as squats, rows, standing presses, bench presses, curls, and so forth, for a few sets of 6–12 reps performed on three nonconsecutive days a week.

"The effort generated in rest–pause training would be overkill for a beginner. And the amount of learning and confidence, which comes only with years of experience, needed to produce such sustained effort won't be present.

"Intermediate bodybuilders with one to two years of steady, intense training might benefit from occasionally doing single workouts or parts of workouts in RPT fashion. Those still climbing the ladder of training intensity and those who are still not highly developed will make excellent gains using pre-exhaustion, forced, and negative repetitions.

"The only bodybuilders who should consistently use RPT are those who have been training hard for at least three years and have attained rather heavy muscular development. Even then RPT should be used in combination with other Heavy Duty methods, or exclusively for short periods of no more than 4–6 weeks. Advanced bodybuilders have consistently exposed themselves to high-intensity training stresses and will need this unusually intense stimulus to induce continued muscle growth."

Mike recommends this rest-pause routine for advanced bodybuilders.

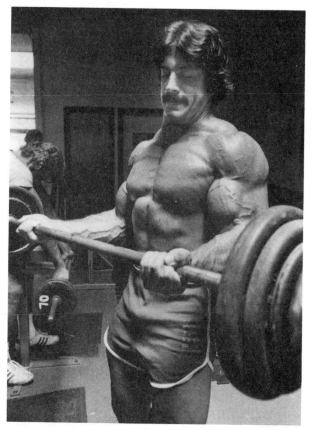

Mike Mentzer was the leading proponent of the Weider Rest–Pause Training Principle, in which he'd do a few hard reps with a heavy weight, set the weight down for about 10 seconds, pick it up for a few more super-difficult reps, take another 10–15 second rest-pause, and then grind out a few more super-intense reps of the same movement.

MONDAY-THURSDAY

Legs

Leg Extensions: 1 set

Leg Curls: 1 set

Squats*: 2 sets, 6-10 reps

Seated Toe Raises: 1 set

Back

Nautilus Pullovers: 1 set, or . . .

Stiff-Arm Lat Machine Pulldowns: 1 set

Barbell Bent Rows*: 2 sets, 5-7 reps

Under-Grip Lat Pulldowns: 1 set

Barbell Shrugs: 2 sets

Stiff-Legged Deadlifts*: 2 sets, 5-7 reps

Note: Exercises marked with an asterisk are performed in normal fashion.

TUESDAY-FRIDAY

Chest

Nautilus Flyes, Pec-Deck Flyes, or Dumbbell Flyes: 1 set

Nautilus Bench Press or Barbell Incline Press: 1 set

Parallel Bar Dips (negative style only): 1 set, 5 reps

Delts

Nautilus Lateral Raises or Dumbbell Side Laterals: 1 set

Nautilus Press or Barbell Presses Behind Neck: 1 set

Arms

Concentration Curls: 1 set

Standing Barbell Curls: 1 set

Nautilus Triceps Extensions, or Pulley Pushdowns: 1 set

Parallel Bar Dips (torso erect): 1 set

No direct abdominal or forearm work needs to be done, because these areas are indirectly stressed by the suggested routine.

PHARMACOLOGY

I'm sure that you probably expected a long discussion of bodybuilding drugs in a book of this scope. But I can't give you such a discussion because the IFBB has moved to make anabolic drug use an illegal aid to bodybuilders. They test for drug use at all major national and international meets, and severe penalties are meted out to bodybuilders who are caught using proscribed drugs.

I'm ecstatic about the IFBB's move. While there is little doubt steroids work, they have serious, dangerous side effects. And it is unethical to use an artificial aid to defeat another bodybuilder who isn't also using it. The IFBB is cleaning up the sport and showing all bodybuilders that they can build incredible physiques the natural, healthy way. Go for it without drugs!

13
Other Advanced
Training Topics

In this chapter I will discuss advanced-level training principles and topics—layoffs, more details about the Heavy Duty system of training, weightlifting and powerlifting as a part of bodybuilding, and stress management.

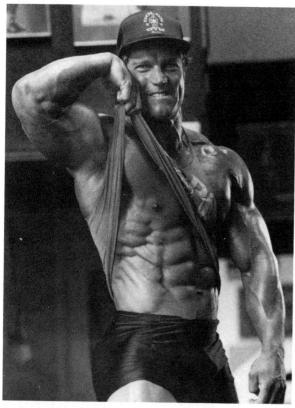

One of the fastest rising stars of the sport in the past three years has been Gary Strydom, a transplanted South African, who lives with his wife Alyse in Marina del Ray, California. Strydom first made waves by winning the heavyweight class at the US Championships in 1984, his class and the overall title at the NPC Nationals two years later, the Night of the Champions pro show in 1987, and placed fifth in Mr. Olympia in 1988. Not a bad career so far, and he's been training specifically for bodybuilding now for only five years.

LAYOFFS

I'm all for hard, consistent training. It's what builds big, impressive muscles. But I'm also in favor of programmed layoffs as a means of preventing overtraining, because these layoffs also build muscle mass.

Scott Wilson talks about layoffs and overtraining: "I'm one of the many victims of overtraining. After I won my Portland Grand Prix title, I decided that that taste of success made me want more competitive successes very badly. So I more or less doubled up on my training.

"If 15–18 hard sets per body part gave me the type of muscle mass and quality necessary to win one pro show, then 30–40 sets would most certainly give me even more muscle mass and quality, and I'd win a bigger pro competition. If 4–5 workouts a week, two sessions for each major muscle group did the trick in Portland, then 6–7 days per week of training, three times for each major muscle group would be better. If 30–60 minutes of aerobic training three times per week was good, then 2–3 hours daily would be much better.

"It doesn't take an expert to realize that all of this work was causing me to overtrain. But it's difficult to see that when you're actually training and thinking it's working. In reality, however, I was inexorably grinding myself down to dust, slowly and steadily sinking into a complete overtrained state in which I was actually losing muscle mass and tone with each workout.

"Finally, I had to face reality. I was overtrained, and I wasn't going to start improving again unless I completely changed my approach to bodybuilding training. So I cut back drastically on my workout frequency and vol-

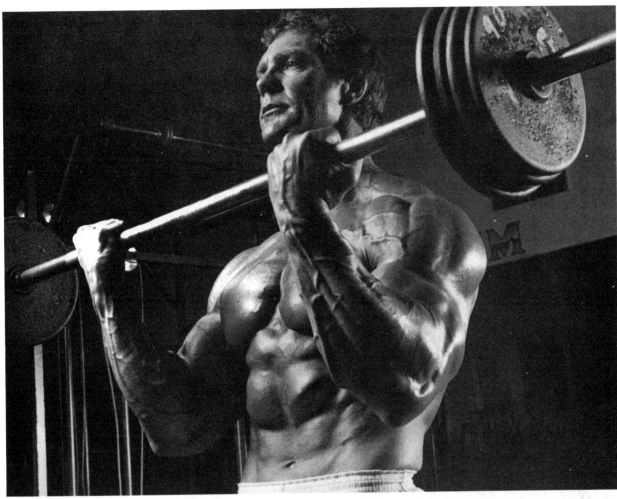

Scott Wilson makes his 20-inch upper arm measurement a bit larger with an intense set of Standing Barbell Curls. Barbell Curls have long been the favorite builder of biceps and forearm flexor muscles for virtually all top bodybuilders throughout the long history of the sport.

ume, and I completely quit doing aerobics. I trained very hard and very fast, getting into and out of the gum in only 60 minutes per workout. And I began to program in short layoffs from time to time. The approach worked wonders, because I am now making better gains than at any other time in my bodybuilding career."

Preprogrammed layoffs? "Every two weeks, I'd take the entire weekend off from training. Each month I'd take 4–5 days off training to completely refresh my system. And every three months, I would take a two-week layoff to accomplish the same purpose. Each time I got back into the gym, my minor injuries would be healed, my enthusiasm for my workouts would be higher than ever, and I'd begin making excellent gains right away.

"Obviously, you lose a little ground every time you take a layoff, but by the time I'd done a week of hard workouts again, I'd be back on top and ready for some fantastic gains. And I credit these regular layoffs for much of my success. They allow my body to fully recover from the rigors of highly intense training, which I'd never be able to do if I trained through the time I would have taken off. I suggest this technique to everyone in the sport, everyone who is really serious about making good gains."

HEAVY DUTY TRAINING

One of my greatest pupils, Mike Mentzer, originated and popularized a system of high-intensity training which featured past-failure training on a limited number of total sets per muscle group (usually only 2-4 per body part). He

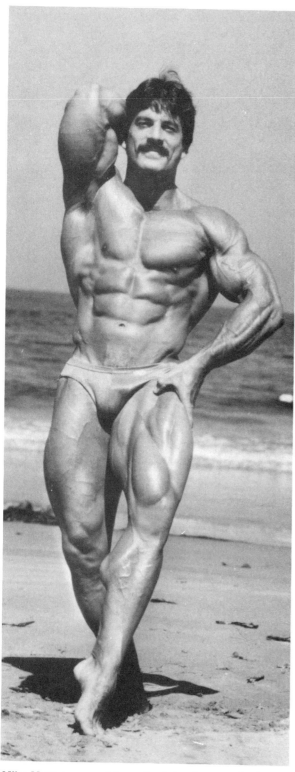

Mike Mentzer, near his peak of development in the late 1970s or early 1980s, was winning virtually every title in sight. He lost only two major contests—the 1979 Mr. Olympia to Frank Zane, and the 1980 Olympia to legendary Arnold Schwarzenegger. Shortly after losing to Arnold, Mike retired from competition and took up the pen, writing a wealth of controversial and informative bodybuilding articles. Truly, he was a bodybuilding Renaissance Man.

christened this amalgam of Weider Training Principles the Heavy Duty System of Training.

When Heavy Duty was in vogue, Mike had thousands of bodybuilders world-wide training with his system, and he sold countless thousands of courses detailing how to train the Heavy Duty way. But like many fads, Heavy Duty has run its course and is no longer popular. Few bodybuilders train in the Heavy Duty manner nowadays, and there seems to be little promise that the system will regain its former popularity.

The Heavy Duty System featured the following Weider Training Principles:

- Forced Reps
- Retro-Gravity Reps
- Rest Pause
- Pre-Exhaustion

By pushing each set as far past failure as humanly possible, Mike Mentzer was able to make great gains from only 2–3 sets on smaller muscle groups and 3–4 on larger body parts. But there are some drawbacks to this system.

First, many bodybuilders have been seriously injured using Heavy Duty. Usually they failed to warm up properly, used heaving, jerking form to get the weight moving, and normally trained so far past failure that they pushed their nervous systems to the point of collapse.

Second, very few bodybuilders can actually generate the type of energy and mental drive necessary to get sufficient stimulation from so few sets. They go at less than 100% effort, and as a result get less than 100% success.

And third, bodybuilders who followed the Heavy Duty system often had difficulty in achieving the type of intramuscular striations and other details necessary to win top titles. They'd come into shows very big and very hard, but lacking the fine details which *made* the great champs like Frank Zane and Arnold Schwarzenegger, who both defeated Mentzer in various Mr. Olympia shows.

If you want to try the Heavy Duty system, keep these failings firmly in mind. If you don't, you probably will be injured, and if you aren't, you won't make the type of gains you have been promised. With normal bodybuilding training, you *will* make great gains, and you probably won't incur any serious injuries in the process.

WEIGHTLIFTING AND POWERLIFTING

When I got involved in bodybuilding during the middle 1930s, every bodybuilder was also a weightlifter, myself included. We were just *expected* to lift heavy weights, preferably competitively, and do some bodybuilding shaping movements on the side. If we happened to end up well-built in addition to strong, that was great. But not many weightlifters actually did end up having great physiques.

There's a lot to be said for training heavy for either Olympic weightlifting or powerlifting at one phase of your bodybuilding career. The heavy training builds a foundation of strength that translates into an ability to train with much heavier-than-normal weights in your actual bodybuilding movements. And that, in turn, gives you greater muscle mass and quality than if you were forced to train with baby weights.

Very few bodybuilders these days do much Olympic lifting, but a lot of them train for powerlifting at one time or another, and some of them stay powerlifters. We've lost some very good bodybuilders to powerlifting. But powerlifting has given us many other great bodybuilders, and it's certainly improved the physiques of many serious bodybuilders who have dabbled in the heavy sport.

It *is* possible to train for both powerlifting and bodybuilding at the same time, specializing in either sport for 8-10 weeks prior to competing in it. But it is difficult to be truly good at both sports simultaneously. Eventually, you'll need to specialize in one sport or the other. I hope it will be bodybuilding that occupies the major part of your competitive efforts in future years. But you have to make the choice yourself.

A good program for combining powerlifting and bodybuilding training is presented here:

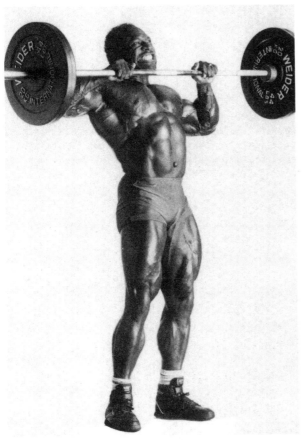

The current King of the Hill, Lee Haney, demonstrates his form in the Power Clean, a great exercise for the trapezius and other upper-back muscles. Attention to little details like traps and rhomboids is one thing that has made Haney essentially unbeatable. In both 1987 and 1988, he won the Olympia with perfect scores, not a single black mark by any judge on any score sheet.

MONDAY–THURSDAY

Exercise	Sets	Reps
Hanging Leg Raises	3-5	15-20
Bench Presses	6-8	5
Incline Dumbbell Presses	3-4	5
Seated Machine Front Presses	5-6	5
Barbell Upright Rows	3-4	6-8
Barbell Incline Triceps Extensions	5-6	6-8
Seated Calf Raises	5-7	8-10
Barbell Wrist Curls	3-4	8-10

TUESDAY–FRIDAY

Exercise	Sets	Reps
Incline Sit-Ups	3-4	15-20
Hyperextensions	2-3	10-15
Squats	8-10	5
Deadlifts (once every 2-3 weeks only)	4-6	5
Barbell Bent Rows	5-7	5
Barbell Shrugs	3-4	10-15
Standing Barbell Curls	4-5	5
Barbell Reverse Curls	2-3	8-10
Standing Calf Raises	5-7	10-15

Note: On all exercises for which five reps are listed, you should stick with that number of reps and jump upward each set by 30-50 pounds, until you reach a limit weight for five or less repetitions. As soon as you can do five reps with the top weight, increase it by 10-20 pounds, and again work at getting the full five reps.

STRESS MANAGEMENT

If you had a problem coping with everyday stress prior to taking up systematic bodybuilding training, you probably no longer have a stress problem. This is due to the fact that regular exercise, whether it be heavy weight work or lighter aerobic sessions, is one of the best stress reducers known to man.

Some bodybuilders place a lot of stressful pressure on themselves during the training and dietary cycle leading up to an important competition, however, and this type of negative stress can have a harmful effect on your onstage physical condition. Therefore, you should learn about other means of reducing stress, so you won't choke up at your next competition.

In general, stress is considered to be any type of mental or physical demand placed on your mind and body. Stress can be either good (a long hike on mountain trails) or bad (the tension of driving in heavy rush-hour traffic). The object of stress management, then, is to decrease all possible bad stress in your life, while simultaneously increasing as much as possible all good stress.

The late *Hans Selye*, an Austrian-born physician who conducted extensive research on stress at the University of Montreal, became the leading world authority on stress. He noted, "You should not and cannot avoid stress, because to eliminate stress would mean to destroy life itself. If you make no more demands on your body, you are dead."

Both positive and negative stress elicit the same physiological reactions—increased pulse and respiration rate, elevated blood pressure, increased blood sugar, and heightened glandular response. Whether the stress is negative or positive depends entirely on how your mind perceives it.

Following are 20 possible symptoms of stress-related illness:

- Chronic fatigue
- Grinding of teeth (especially while sleeping)
- Insomnia, nightmares, restless sleeping
- Depression
- Irritability
- Migraine or tension-related headaches
- Anxiety
- Sexual dysfunction

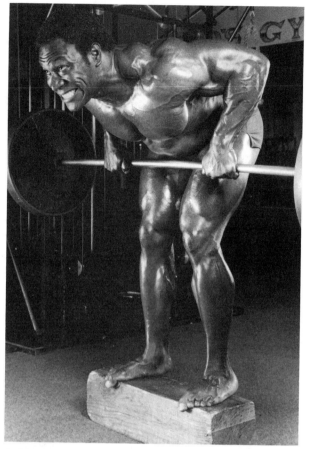

Going at 'em! Lee Haney's bodybuilding philosophy is simple: "If it works, why fix it?" And heavy basic movements like Barbell Bent-Over Rows (for the lats, traps, rear delts, brachialis, biceps, and forearm flexors) have always formed the core of his workouts.

- Impulsive, irrational behavior
- Neck, shoulder, and back pain
- Over- or undereating
- Apathy
- Lack of concentration ability
- Indigestion
- Tachycardia (racing, irregular pulse rate)
- Spontaneous sweating
- Frequent body infections, cold, flu
- Increased drug or alcohol use
- Dependence on tranquilizers
- Slurred speech

If you exhibit two or more of the foregoing symptoms of stress-related illness when peaking for a competition, you should begin to limit negative stressors (things or situations that produce negative stress). Most probably, your negative stressors will be related to the approaching competition, but they could also exist in work, family, and/or social situations.

METHODS FOR STRESS REDUCTION

You won't have much trouble identifying negative stressors, because to most bodybuilders they are rather easy to identify. But you should make a written list of them for future reference when you attempt to limit the negative stressors from your life.

Once you have identified and written down all of your negative precontest stressors, you should take each one in turn and plan how to eliminate it. Most problems have solutions, or half solutions, which will either totally or partially eliminate the stressor agent. This technique sounds simple, and it is, but it's also very effective in reducing precontest stress.

Possible examples of precontest stressors are worry about forgetting your posing routine onstage, anxiety over how high you will place, and uncertainty about what music to choose for your free-posing program. The best way to reduce this type of negative precontest stress is to resolve each of the uncertainties. If you're worried about forgetting your posing routine, practice it 50 times per day if that's what it takes to be sure you will remember it. Forget about how high you *might* place, because you can't do anything about your final placing except by entering the show perfectly prepared both physically and mentally for the competition. And if you're uncertain about what music to choose, enlist the aid of a more musical friend.

In addition to the foregoing technique, there are several other external factors and techniques that can be employed to limit stress. The first of these is having a friend with whom you can discuss your problems. If you don't have a wife or girlfriend available to serve this function, you should attempt to enlist one of your closer friends. Talking out your problems is a very effective technique for reducing negative stress in your life. If you feel you have serious psychological problems, consider talking to a psychologist or psychiatrist and don't think of them as behavioral judges, but merely friends you must pay to talk to.

There are many relaxation techniques available, such as meditation and fractional relaxation, both of which are discussed in detail in Part VII. You can employ these techniques to good effect in relaxing your mind and body, so you drain away harmful stress before it can have a deleterious affect on you.

Frequent, regular exercise, as mentioned earlier, is one of the best ways of reducing stress. With all of the extra training and heavy aerobics you'll be involved in prior to a show, you probably will be too tired and relaxed to even think about negative stress. But you can also program in a relaxing walk with a spouse, girlfriend, or other friend if you are feeling too keyed up.

A final stress-reduction method is getting involved in a hobby outside of bodybuilding. This could be as simple as putting together model airplanes or getting involved in a regular discussion group. You can spend a little money on your hobby, or a lot; and you can spend a little time on it, or a lot. This all depends on your tastes and inclination.

The object of a hobby is to do something that involves your hands while letting your mind roam relatively free. This is the most efficient way to drain off stress without actually getting

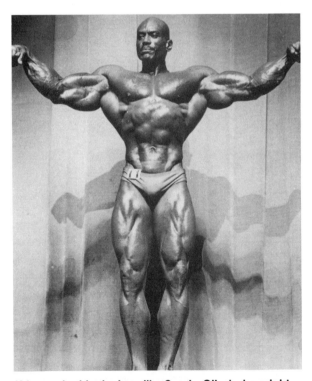

If Icarus had had wings like Sergio Oliva's, he might have been able to do away with the feathers and wax, and flown safely out of captivity. As it is, Oliva's lat spread—and phenomenal difference between chest-shoulder and waist-hip measurements—belongs in a museum of some sort, perhaps the National Aeronautics Museum.

out and running 20 miles around a lake, or walking until your toes peek through the holes in your shoes.

What I'm really suggesting to you as a means of reducing precontest negative stress is involving yourself in extra activities that will make you a more well-rounded individual. The guys who really crack up when precontest stress builds up are the ones who have nothing in their life but bodybuilding. When they have nothing else, they end up feeling they *have* to win each competition, or else they have no self-worth. And that can really build up negative stress levels.

A well-rounded man, on the other hand, has his family, friends, job, hobbies, and other pursuits to fall back on if he happens to lose his next show. I'm not saying you should *lose* your next competition on purpose, because you definitely should try as hard as possible to win every time you step onstage for a prejudging. What I am saying instead is that you won't feel as much pressure prior to your next competition if you understand that you have much more in your life than pumping iron and competing for some trophies.

When you can look at your bodybuilding as a valuable addition to your life rather than your life itself, you will feel very little negative stress, regardless of how big and important your approaching competition might be. And *that* automatically improves your chances of winning every competition you enter.

14
Aerobics and Bodybuilding

Aerobic training began to gain in popularity during the early 1980s, until now it is an integral part of the training philosophies of most bodybuilders. Aerobics has become particularly popular during a peaking cycle, when it's a means of burning body fat, which reveals the underlying musculature with such bold detail that it looks like a bodybuilder's skin is as thin as tissue paper.

To achieve optimum health and physical fitness you must do three types of training: weight workouts (for strength, muscle mass, and muscle tone), aerobic sessions (for cardiovascular fitness), and stretching (for flexibility). These three types of exercise are like the legs of a tripod supporting a heavy brick of gold called physical fitness. If one leg of the tripod is weakened or removed, physical fitness will topple into the mud, perhaps to be lost forever.

"When you are training with heavy weights in the gym," notes *Berry de Mey* (European and World Games Champion) "you are doing anaerobic work. This is a type of training so intense that it takes place at an energy and intensity level well above your body's ability to supply sufficient oxygen to the working muscles. As such, anaerobic work results in an oxygen debt which must be paid back with several minutes of intense breathing. Anaerobic training burns glycogen, the sugar found in your muscles, liver, and blood stream, to supply its energy requirements. It does not reduce body fat stores.

"Aerobic training, such as running, cycling, swimming, mountain hiking, takes place at an intensity low enough that your body can supply sufficient oxygen to carry on the activity. Aerobic training burns primarily body fat to supply its energy needs. As a result, most bodybuilders do a lot of aerobic work when peaking, in order to metabolize all visible fat between the skin and muscles. Combined with a tight diet, aerobics will lean you out to the point where you are *super* ripped, rather than just cut up."

The most popular form of aerobic training among top bodybuilders is stationary cycling.

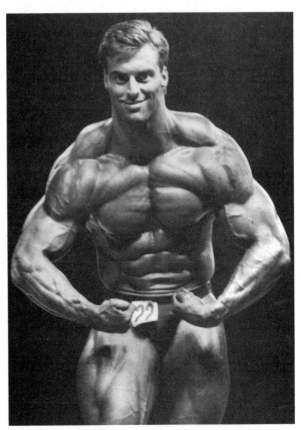

Exciting Dutchman Berry de Mey has consistently moved up in the pro standings over the years, first qualifying for the Mr. Olympia event in 1985. In his most recent effort, 1988, he placed a strong third behind Lee Haney and Rich Gaspari. For a 6'2" athlete, Berry can get as cut-up as any lightweight bodybuilder.

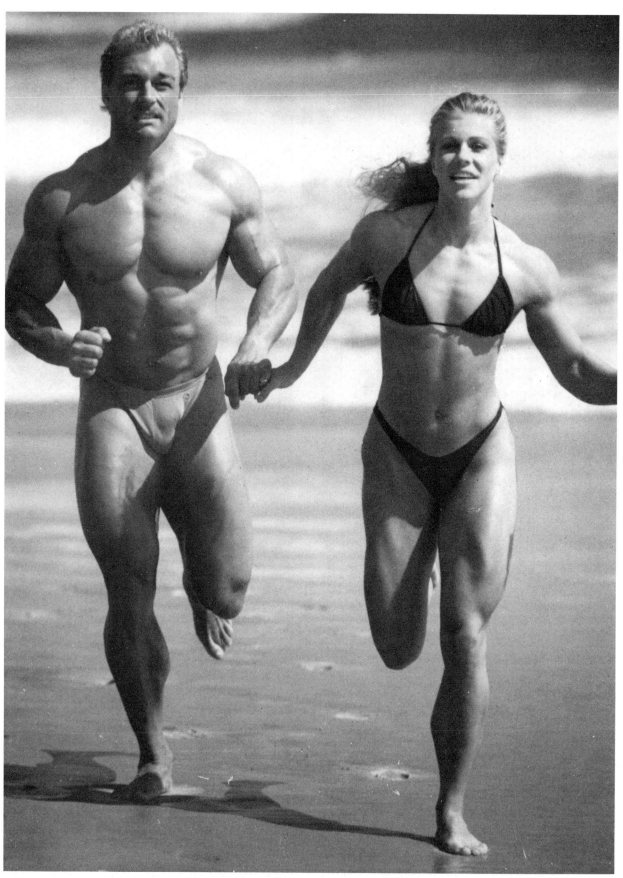

Gunter Kuhni, former German Champion and current IFBB pro runs with Anja Langer, the 1988 second-place finisher in Ms. Olympia.

Indeed, many of the top men have exercise cycles in their homes or apartments, so they can do their aerobics at the most convenient time, whether that is in the morning, evening, or middle of the night. A lot of the champs will ride an exercise bike in front of the television, keeping track of time by watching a favorite 30- or 60-minute program on the tube.

I'm in favor of stationary bikes that have computer programs that automatically vary the intensity of each ride at intervals of a few minutes each. I have one of them in my own completely equipped home gym.

Quite a few champs have gotten on the bandwagon for a new type of stationary bike in which you can recline on your back while you do the workout. These recumbent cycles have models in which resistance can be adjusted, and they tend to be a lot less expensive than the sit-up type of bike.

Actual ballistic cycling is also popular and effective for fat-burning purposes. It is somewhat dangerous, however. At the worst, there are several cases of serious injuries, and at least one death among competitive bodybuilders, in vehicle-bicycle accidents. And you can even fall over and skin up the side of an arm or leg only a few days before a competition. So if you are interested in cycling, try to stay off busy streets and *be careful.*

Rowing machines have become popular in recent years. They provide a less-expensive, but still effective, alternative to cycling. Weider sells an excellent rowing machine for less than $250, and there are scores of brands of machines available at sporting goods stores. Rowing works the upper body as well as the legs, which can be an improvement on cycling or running.

Swimming also uses the upper body, and it is very effective in helping rip up your body for a competition. *Gary Strydom* swims at least once a week when peaking. "It also helps to keep my shoulder joints loose and free from injury," he says.

Walking is growing in popularity as an aerobic activity, particularly when it can be done up flights of stairs and/or at a relatively quick pace. *Mike Quinn* says, "I've given up on all forms of aerobics save walking up an extremely long flight of stairs in Santa Monica, California, right near Gold's Gym, for up to 30–40 minutes at a clip," Mike reveals. "Climbing

stairs has also been beneficial for my calves, which get pumped up very quickly when I'm climbing."

Some champion bodybuilders also like to take organized aerobic dance classes, although I'm not sure whether they do it for the aerobic

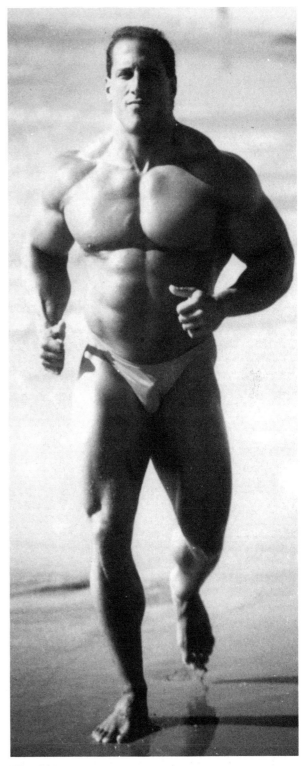

Mike Quinn

benefit or to look at all of the foxy women who invariably populate such classes. Such dance-aerobics classes can be quite effective at burning off unwanted body fat.

Running on the flat or up stairs is extremely popular as a means of burning calories from body fat stores. But running is a badly misunderstood activity, which can lead to chronic injuries if done incorrectly. I personally enjoy and benefit from running 30 minutes three or

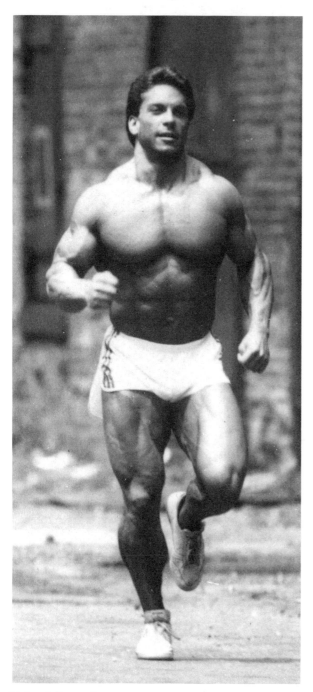

Richard Gaspari

four times per week. But I'm deeply concerned that the current running revolution is literally running millions of healthy men and women into the ground.

PROS AND CONS OF RUNNING

Since running has become America's favorite aerobic activity, I want to discuss the safe and sane way to achieve aerobic conditioning through running. By using my sensible guidelines, you'll be able to avoid the pitfalls that waylay so many runners.

Since Frank Shorter won the 1972 Olympic marathon (a marathon distance is 26 miles, 385 yards), there's been a boom in marathon running in America. Newsstand racks are jammed with running and triathlon magazines, and there are more than 100 marathons conducted each year in the United States alone. Some of the classic marathon races—specifically those held at Boston, Chicago, and New York City—attract more than 10,000 runners per event.

This love affair with running 26.2 miles has seduced millions of men and women into taking daily (and sometimes even twice-daily) runs of 6-10 miles. Running to such extremes—particularly for a person with limited background and no monetary payback in the sport—doesn't allow the body enough time to recover adequately between training sessions. The resulting fatigue leads to overuse injuries.

Thousands of runners subject their feet, ankles, leg muscles, knees, hips, and lower back to relentless pounding day after day. As a result, most serious runners train with at least one minor, but persistent, joint or muscle injury. And an injury that may seem minor today can have major repercussions when you reach your fifties, sixties, and seventies.

At the start of a marathon, you'll notice that the runners usually aren't discussing their competitive times, their training methods for the race, or even the weather. Instead, they all seem to be discussing their *injuries*. "Yeah," says one, "I've had a lot of chondromalacia lately, but I've kept running."

Runners who train to extremes suffer from a bewildering array of injuries. Here are some of the most common injuries (almost all of them are related to what physicians call "overuse syndrome"):

- Achilles tendinitis or rupture
- Shin splints
- Heel bone damage
- Bursitis (usually under the kneecap, in the hips, in the toes, or between the Achilles tendon and the heel bone)
- Stress fractures
- Knee chondromalacia
- Strained or torn muscles
- Spinal compression (and related sciatica)
- Leg muscle pulls and tears
- Muscle cramps
- Blood in the urine
- Chronic dehydration
- Sprained ankles, knees, hips
- Inflamed ligaments
- Foot arch problems
- A chronically overtrained state (and related colds, flu, etc.)

Runner's World magazine surveyed its readers and found that the most common overuse injuries runners suffered affect the knees (18%), Achilles tendons (14%), shins (usually shin splints) (11%), foot arches (7%), and ankles (6%). Virtually all runners who train to extremes suffer from such injuries.

Tragically, many runners prefer to ignore pain, nature's warning that they are injured. They try to "run through" an injury, often making that injury much more serious than it would have been had they rested. I know of a veteran long-distance runner, who began to notice mild sciatica pain in his hip. By attempting to run through the injury, he further compressed the spinal vertebrae, ended up flat on his back in excruciating pain for several days, and spent hundreds of dollars on chiropractic treatment. Clearly, no one should ever try to "run through" any running-related overuse injury.

Another persistent habit among runners is to insist that running is the perfect form of exercise. It's true that running, done correctly, is a superior means of developing cardiorespiratory (heart-lung) fitness. However, running actually decreases body flexibility, builds little or no strength, and it doesn't develop a well-toned, muscular body. To attain all of these qualities, you must be on a regular exercise program that

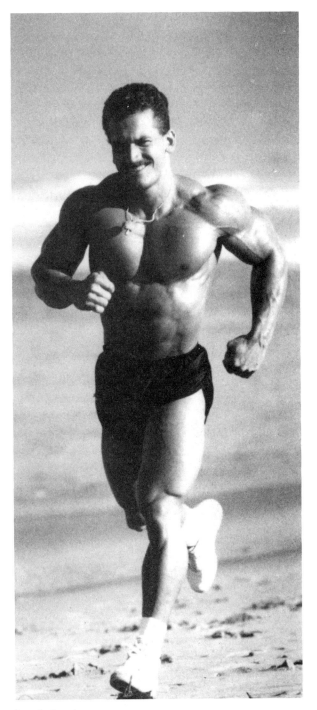

Lee Labrada

includes all three legs of the fitness tripod I mentioned before: weight training, aerobic conditioning, and stretching.

Exercise physiologists determine the aerobic effectiveness of a type of exercise by measuring an athlete's ability to consume and efficiently process oxygen. To do this, they use what is called an "oxygen uptake test." In terms of oxygen uptake, champion cross-country skiers consistently score higher than champion long-distance runners. And there are many other types of aerobic activities that are also very effective while inflicting far fewer injuries. These activities include cycling, swimming, circuit training with weights, and rowing.

So far I suppose I've painted a rather bleak picture of running. However, as I've said, done correctly, running does have far-reaching benefits. And running—unlike cross-country skiing, rowing, or cycling—does not require special equipment or facilities and is not dependent on weather conditioning. Therefore, running is certainly a more convenient method of achieving a superior level of aerobic conditioning.

Obviously, running strengthens the heart and circulatory system, helping to prevent cardiac disease, arteriosclerosis, strokes, and a host of other heart, lung, and circulatory diseases. A good indication of this is the lowered pulse rate runners achieve; a low pulse rate indicates superior heart and circulatory efficiency.

Running melts away excess body fat and can dramatically lower blood cholesterol and triglyceride levels. In short, if done correctly, running can make profound, and often life-prolonging, changes in the body, Therefore, I think that everyone should give running a fair trial as an aerobic conditioning method.

GUIDELINES FOR RUNNING

Based on my own extensive experience with running, coupled with my many years of research, I have developed the following 11 rules that promote sane running.

1. Always combine running with weight training and stretching. As I've mentioned, running falls far short of being the perfect form of exercise. Always be conscious of your physical fitness tripod. Don't let it topple by undercutting one of the legs.

2. Never run two days in a row. The reason why runners develop overuse injuries in the first place is that they run nearly every day and don't allow themselves time to recover. *Dr. Kenneth Cooper,* the father of aerobics, believes that running three miles a day three days per

week will give most men and women adequate aerobic fitness. I agree with him. If you feel that you need more aerobic training, try cycling or swimming on the days you aren't running.

3. Buy good-quality running shoes. Running shoes that cushion and support the feet cost about $30–$60 per pair, and they're worth every penny. Top-quality running shoes are specifically engineered to prevent running injuries, and they do a good job of it. Running in cheap sneakers is inviting trouble.

4. Never try to run through an injury. If you experience pain while running, switch to swimming or cycling until your discomfort abates. Then return to running.

5. Don't run on an uneven surface. As long as you wear high-quality running shoes, it's often better to run on concrete than on grass. Grass surfaces can be uneven, and every depression you step into increases the stress on your legs. Also be careful not to run on the slanted shoulder of a road, since this puts enormous strain on your legs and lower back. And don't do too much running up and down hills.

6. Run within your capabilities. Never overextend yourself, either in the speed or the duration of a run. To keep from doing this, run according to time, not distance. For example, run for 20 minutes, not for two miles. Timing yourself over a certain distance automatically causes you to push yourself, because you naturally want to beat your record for the distance. It's best to run easily and fluidly until you're comfortably fatigued, then stop.

7. Progress slowly. In the next section of this chapter, I'll suggest some running programs. Advance slowly and easily with them, and don't overextend yourself. When running, you needn't induce great pain or fatigue to achieve aerobic conditioning.

8. Run in a relaxed manner to minimize jarring. Running will be more enjoyable and less stressful if you relax during your workouts. If you feel tension in any part of your body, especially in your thighs, chest, neck, or shoulders, slow to a more comfortable pace.

Many people believe that jogging is harmful but running is not, so they try to run faster than is good for them. In fact, jogging is just slow, rhythmic, relaxed running. A jogging pace is an excellent way to start out your running program. Then as your conditioning improves, you may want to increase your speed.

9. Dress for the weather. If you dress appropriately, you can run in very cold weather. And if you consume sufficient liquids (particularly electrolyte replacement drinks), you can run in hot weather with no ill effects. Wear a minimum of clothing when it's hot, and sufficient clothing when it's cold. In cold weather, several thin layers of clothing provide much better insulation than one or two thick layers.

10. Make running an enjoyable habit. Like weight training or any other form of exercise, running is more beneficial when it's done regularly. So make running a pleasant habit. If you don't enjoy it, don't run. Exercise should be something you look forward to doing each day.

11. Forget about racing. Racing is one of the most destructive things you can do as a runner. The thought of competition immediately causes everyone to train to excess, which leads to overuse injuries. Run for the pleasure of running and for the aerobic fitness it provides, not for a T-shirt with the name of some obscure race printed on it.

If you've been physically inactive for a long period of time, walk before you run. Spend two or three weeks walking every other day, going a littler farther or a little faster each session. Then mix walking with short stretches of jogging. Gradually, you'll condition your body until you can run steadily—albeit slowly—for 15 consecutive minutes. Then you'll be ready for a regular running program.

I personally run every other day, which means I'm on the road three days one week and four the next. For most health- and fitness-conscious men, however, it's easier to run only three days per week, alternating days of running with days of weight training. Keeping the

fitness tripod in mind, you should do a stretching workout every day.

A RUNNING PROGRAM

I don't think you need to run more than 30–40 minutes at a time to reach optimum aerobic conditioning. To work up to this level, use a gradual progression. Here is a sample program. Remember to run within your limits. If aerobic conditioning is new to you, be sure you do a lot of walking before you start a running program.

Week One

Tuesday	15 minutes
Thursday	20 minutes
Saturday	15 minutes
Weekly Total =	50 minutes

Week Two

Tuesday	20 minutes
Thursday	15 minutes
Saturday	20 minutes
Weekly Total =	55 minutes

Week Three

Tuesday	15 minutes
Thursday	25 minutes
Saturday	20 minutes
Weekly Total =	60 minutes

Week Four

Tuesday	20 minutes
Thursday	25 minutes
Saturday	20 minutes
Weekly Total =	65 minutes

Week Five

Tuesday	25 minutes
Thursday	20 minutes
Saturday	25 minutes
Weekly Total =	70 minutes

Try to progress slowly and gradually, staying well within your limits of strength and endurance. And don't be a slave to the schedule I've just outlined. Use it only as a guide.

Running and serious bodybuilding are very compatible. By including regular running and stretching in your bodybuilding workout program, you'll ultimately build a better body. You'll have greater endurance for your workouts, and your body fat levels will remain lower throughout the year. Running or some other type of aerobic activity will make it easier for you to cut up for a competition. So I heartily recommend a running program for bodybuilders as long as the guidelines for sensible running are followed.

AEROBIC BODYBUILDING

If you've read much about contest peaking in bodybuilding magazines, you already know that virtually all of the champs do plenty of aerobic training on a daily basis when preparing for a competition. And they do so primarily because aerobics is the most efficient way to burn off excess body fat.

It is possible to train aerobically with weights, and I recommend doing so for 2-3 months if you feel you have a significant weight problem. The method you can use to aerobicize your weight workouts is called circuit training. And circuit training is very effective when combined with diet and normal aerobic workouts.

CIRCUIT TRAINING

Circuit training consists of setting up a series of stations (anything between 10-20 stations) consisting of 2-3 exercises each for the entire spectrum of body parts each circuit. Then you run through the entire series of stations, doing 8-10 reps per movement, and resting as little as possible between stations. Ideally, you should work up to training almost nonstop, breaking between sets only long enough to walk to the next station. During each workout, you can go through your circuit as many as 3-5 times.

Circuit training can be brutally hard if you aren't in good cardiorespiratory (heart–lung) condition before initiating a circuit training program. So, you should start out by resting 45-60 seconds between each station of your circuit the first couple of times through. Then you can progressively decrease your rest intervals between stations, systematically improving cardiorespiratory fitness, until you are down to the absolute minimum amount of rest between stations.

You will find a sample circuit training pro-

gram in the figure in page 163, which you can give a trial in your own workouts.

You may find it difficult to set up your circuits in a public gym during peak attendance hours, so you'll probably need to restrict yourself to early morning or late evening workouts when circuit training. It's also difficult to circuit train in some home gyms due to limited equipment. But with a little ingenuity, you shouldn't have much difficulty in setting up a workable circuit.

It's important when you set up a circuit that you choose exercises in a sequence that skips around your body. Doing two or three movements in a row for a single muscle group will pump that area up, and muscle pump is actually something you should avoid during circuit workouts. But even though you won't be pumping up much during a circuit training session, your muscles will still receive great benefit from the workout.

PHA TRAINING

There is a specialized short circuit called PHA (peripheral heart action) training, which enjoyed a vogue during the late 1960s and early 1970s. The system was popularized by *Bob Gajda* (Mr. America and Mr. World) via articles in various bodybuilding magazines. It was used most successfully by Gajda, but was also used by Bob's training partner, Sergio Oliva, for a few months. Oliva at the time was about two years from winning the first of his three Mr. Olympia titles.

While studying for his Ph.D. in exercise physiology, Bob Gajda learned about how peripheral heart action assisted in blood circulation. The heart itself is a very powerful organ, but it is not sufficiently strong to pump several quarts of blood around many miles of arteries, veins, and capillaries. If you had to depend solely on the action of your heart, you would eventually die from a pooling of blood in the lower extremities.

Nature has provided more than 600 auxiliary "hearts" in the form of skeletal muscles. When a skeletal muscle contracts, it milks blood past one-way valves in the circulatory system. And the more voluntary skeletal muscle contrac-

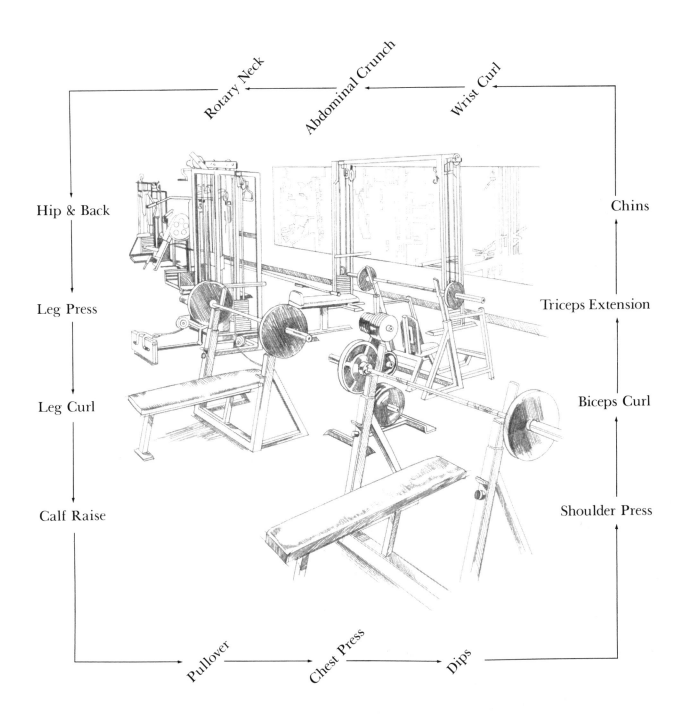

Rotary Neck — Abdominal Crunch — Wrist Curl

Hip & Back

Chins

Leg Press

Triceps Extension

Leg Curl

Biceps Curl

Calf Raise

Shoulder Press

Pullover — Chest Press — Dips

Example of a PHA Training Circuit

tions, the better your overall blood circulation.

The peripheral heart action also allows a bodybuilder to perform a terrific number of total sets each workout, because the body releases buffers to cleanse the blood of fatigue toxins when circulation is at a peak during a workout. Gajda himself often did 35–40 total sets for each workout, resting no more than 20–30 seconds between sets.

Gajda set up his PHA programs so that he would be moving to exercises by skipping around the body from one muscle group to another. And he was able to not only train very quickly, but also extensively, which developed both great muscle mass and terrific muscle quality. In fact, Gajda was several years ahead of most bodybuilders in the type of muscularity he exhibited onstage. His physique would be competitive even 20 years later.

I have given you a sample three-day-per-week PHA program, which any intermediate bodybuilder can follow at right. If you plan to use use this routine, however, remember to break slowly into the system, giving your body a chance to adapt to the higher intensity of PHA workouts.

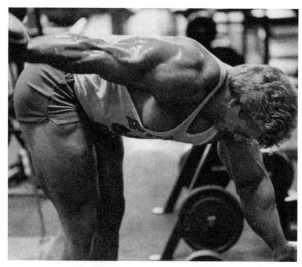

One of the tragic figures of the sport, Cincinnatian Matt Mendenhall placed a close second in the heavyweight class (behind overall winner Lee Haney no less!) at the 1982 Nationals. Then in several other attempts to win the same title, he placed second one more time, made the top five a couple of times, and was out of the top 10 twice more. Matt's usual downfall has been deficient onstage muscularity.

For more advanced bodybuilders, I have presented an advanced split routine PHA program below. Again, break in slowly.

Bob Gajda used the PHA system year-round, but most bodybuilders who have stuck to the system tend to use it only in an 8–10 week peaking phase. For the rest of the year, a more normal three-on, one-off split routine is followed, concentrating on basic exercises for low reps with very heavy weights.

SAMPLE INTERMEDIATE-LEVEL PHA ROUTINE
MONDAY-WEDNESDAY-FRIDAY

Series 1	Series 2
Bench Presses	Seated Pulley Rows
Calf Presses	Pulley Pushdowns
Lat Machine	Hanging Leg Raises
Pulldowns	Barbell Wrist Curls
Incline Sit-Ups	Lying Leg Curls
Angled Leg Presses	

Series 3	Series 4
Leg Extensions	Barbell Incline
Seated Machine	Presses
Presses	Barbell Reverse Curls
Incline Dumbbell	Dumbbell Side
Curls	Laterals
Seated Calf Raises	Incline Barbell Triceps
Standing Barbell Wrist	Extensions
Curls	Bent-Arm Pullovers

Do 3–4 cycles through each series, with minimal rest between exercises and no more than 2–3 minutes between series.

SAMPLE ADVANCED-LEVEL PHA SPLIT ROUTINE
MONDAY-THURSDAY

Series 1	Series 2
Incline Dumbbell Presses	Seated Pulley Rows
Hanging Leg Raises	Parallel Bar Dips
Vertical Leg Presses	Dumbbell Concentration
Barbell Preacher Curls	Curls
Smith Machine Front	Barbell Shrugs
Presses	Seated Leg Curls
Seated Calf Raises	Lying Barbell Triceps
	Extensions

Series 3	Series 4
Barbell Upright Rows	Lat Machine Pulldowns
Barbell Reverse Curls	Calf Presses
Leg Extensions	Hyperextensions
Flat-Bench Flyes	Dumbbell Bent Laterals
Dumbbell Side Laterals	Stiff-Arm Pulldowns

TUESDAY-FRIDAY

Series 1

Squats

Crunches

Bench Presses

Cable Side Laterals

Standing Leg Curls

Series 2

Angled Leg Presses

Front Chins

Incline Leg Raises

Leg Extensions

Standing Barbell Wrist
   Curls

Series 3

Sissy Squats

Cable Upright Rows

Incline Sit-Ups

Pulley Pushdowns

Series 4

Stiff-Legged Deadlifts

Dumbbell Preacher Curls

Lungs

Alternate Dumbbell
   Presses

Do 3–5 cycles of each series, completing 8-15 reps in each set.

I personally prefer to put top bodybuilders on a more conventional type of workout, but have nothing against the PHA program. I urge you to give this system a good trial during an off-season cycle, perhaps also in combination with a moderately strict diet if you need to lose weight. Experiment with the PHA system for 8–10 weeks, evaluate it, and decide whether you will want to include the system in your overall training philosophy.

15
Flexibility and the Bodybuilder

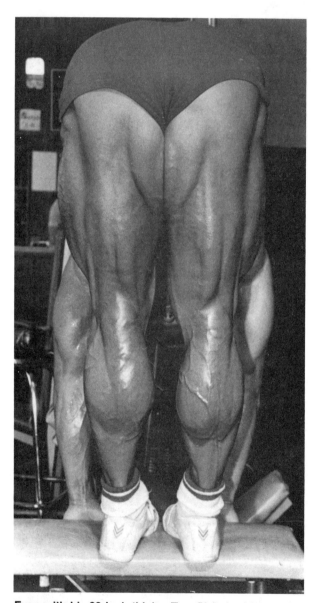

Even with his 28-inch thighs, Tom Platz is able to demonstrate tremendous flexibility in his lower body. Here he displays his thigh biceps to great effect, holding his legs straight and pulling down with his hands on the edge of the bench. Tom is also capable of doing full splits.

There are six basic reasons why every bodybuilder should do regular stretching workouts:

- *Stretching improves appearance.* Stretching lengthens the muscles, giving you the long, lean, well-toned look onstage.

- *Stretching improves health and fitness.* In concert with bodybuilding training and aerobic workouts—running, cycling, swimming, rowing, etc.—stretching gives you the ultimate in health and physical fitness.

- *Stretching prevents injuries.* Most everyday injuries and bodybuilding training injuries are caused either by trauma (a fall, a car crash, the plates sliding off one end of the bar, etc.) or by overextension of a joint, muscle, or connective tissue (muscle pulls, sprains, strains). Athletes who follow regular and progressive stretching programs suffer at least 50% fewer overextension injuries than those who don't.

- *Stretching is a good warmup before or cooldown after other types of training sessions such as bodybuilding.* But above and beyond this, a preworkout stretching program improves neuro-muscular coordination. And after a workout, stretching will prevent soreness, as well as promote faster physiological recovery.

- *Stretching is a good warm up or cooldown after other types of training sessions such as bodybuilding.* But above and beyond this, a preworkout stretching program improves neuromuscular coordination. And after a workout, stretching will prevent soreness, as well as promote faster physiological recovery.

- *Done correctly, stretching is enjoyable.* Have you ever awakened in the morning and, still in bed, slowly stretched your entire body? It felt great, didn't it? Well, that same superbly sensual feeling can be yours every day of the week.

WHO SHOULD STRETCH?

Every man and woman can benefit enormously from following a regular and progressive program of stretching exercises. And there are no age limits. Senior citizens can stretch often when orthopedic problems prevent them from doing other forms of exercise. Even toddlers can stretch along with Mom and Dad.

Obviously, all athletes should include stretching in their conditioning programs. Many NFL teams now employ a flexibility coach, so what is good for the football players is good for bodybuilders as well.

The best book illustrating and describing stretching programs for all sports is Bob Anderson's *Stretching*, which can be found in most book shops. If you don't find it on the shelves, the shop can usually get it for you in less than a week.

Some individuals are more adept at stretching than others. Generally speaking, women will be more flexible than men, and children will be far more flexible than adults.

WHY BODYBUILDERS SHOULD STRETCH

During the past few years, many champion bodybuilders—notably Tom Platz (Mr. Universe), Boyer Coe (World Pro Grand Prix Champion), and Lee Haney (four times Mr. Olympia)—have discovered that stretching is an excellent supplement to bodybuilding training.

"It builds bigger, better-quality muscles," *Boyer Coe* notes. "The first time I seriously used stretching workouts was prior to an Olympia, and everyone there said I'd improved 25%-30% since the previous Mr. O. I'm convinced by that experience that stretching is a superior adjunct to bodybuilding training."

Lee Haney chips in, "I've remained almost completely injury-free over the many years I've been bodybuilding. I am convinced that one of the main reasons why I avoid injuries so successfully is my preworkout stretching program.

It keeps me loose and supple, which effectively prevents training injuries."

WHEN TO STRETCH

Having been a bodybuilding coach to thousands of the best men and women in the sport, I have developed some very definite conclusions about stretching. First, anyone who is serious about improving his or her flexibility, health, appearance, and athletic performance should stretch every day for at least 10–15 minutes. Stretching 3–4 times per week will slowly im-

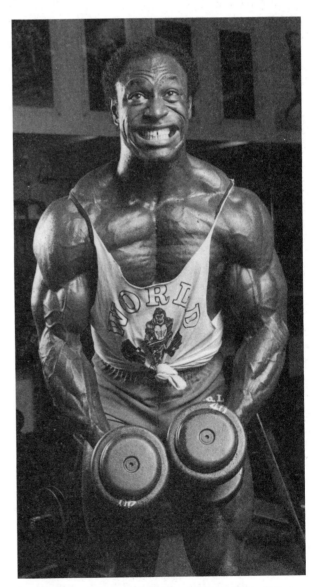

A man on a mission, Lee Haney, who now has five consecutive Mr. Olympia victories and is aware of Arnold's records: six straight and seven overall. My money is on Large Lee from Atlanta to eventually obliterate all of Arnold's records.

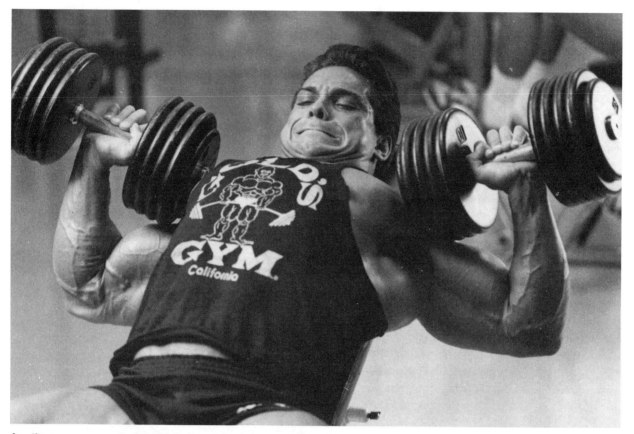

Another man on a mission, Rich Gaspari, who would give his eye teeth to finally defeat his old training partner, Lee Haney. The pair has met annually at the Mr. Olympia since 1985, with Rich third then and second ever since. Gaspari's bad dreams must all be about the man from Atlanta.

prove joint and muscle flexibility, but daily stretching will increase flexibility 4–5 times more quickly. And I've gotten tremendous results with some very experienced bodybuilders by putting them on a twice-a-day stretching program.

If you participate in some other form of exercise, the best time to stretch is as a warm-up, for that activity. Many men and women do this subconsciously. You've no doubt seen a runner briefly stretch his calves before setting out for a run, or a basketball player quickly stretch his hamstrings before going into a game. Such an abbreviated stretching session does very little for the athlete, however.

To be effective as a warm-up, such a stretching session should last 10–15 minutes and include flexibility exercises for every part of the body. Done in this sane manner, a stretching workout also acts as an excellent cooldown following a game or workout. You'll be truly amazed at how quickly you can recuperate if you do 10–15 minutes of stretching after each workout.

If you don't stretch prior to a workout, the best time is in the late evening before you go to bed. This will relieve all the tensions you've built up during the day and give you a stretcher's "high" akin to a runner's high, or the pump a bodybuilder experiences. After an evening stretching workout, you'll be relaxed and will sleep peacefully.

HOW TO STRETCH

I'm totally amazed at the abusive ways some men and women do their stretching exercises. They stretch too hard or they bounce into a stretch, losing much of the value of the exercise in the process. Correctly applied, stretching is a gentle form of exercise, and unless you pursue it gently you will lose most of the benefits it can give you.

Because it's easy to injure yourself by overextending the range of motion of a joint or muscle, nature has provided your body with two protective mechanisms. Both are specialized types of neurons (nerve endings). One type senses when a muscle is being overstretched and signals this fact by sending pain signals back to the brain.

The second type of neurons is part of a protective mechanism called the "stretch reflex." When a stretch is sensed by the second type of neurons to be progressing too quickly, the mind reflexively begins to contract the stretched muscle. And this acts as a shock absorber, slowing, then halting the stretch before the muscle or its tendons can be injured. This is somewhat like the way your thigh muscles flex to absorb the shock of landing when you jump off a table onto the floor.

When you stretch a muscle group ballistically (that is, in a bouncing manner), the stretch reflex is activated and the muscle shortens to stop the stretch. So while it may seem logical to some that bouncing would intensify a stretch and bring faster results, such ballistic stretching actually has the opposite effect. Because of the stretch reflex, the stretched muscles actually shorten and you come up far short of reaching a fully stretched position.

To fully stretch a muscle (or joint), you must *slowly ease into the stretch.* In order to circumvent the stretch reflex, take 30–40 seconds to move slowly into a stretch to the point where you just begin to feel slight pain in the stretched muscle. This is the maximum point to which you should stretch. Stretching experts call this the "pain edge." And if you stretch much past this point, you can actually begin to pull tiny muscle fibers apart, injuring the muscles.

So now you have enough physiological information to understand my description of the perfect stretch. Regardless of the flexibility movement you use, take 30–40 seconds to ease into it. Then once you encounter the pain edge, back off until the pain has just disappeared. Once you've reached this "stretching zone," hold the stretch in that position for 30–60 seconds, gradually working up to two minutes in each stretch. Breathe shallowly, although with normal rhythm, when holding a stretched posi-

tion. Finally, relax the stretch and repeat it a minute later, or move on to another stretching movement.

If you are to receive the maximum benefit from this exercise, you must discover your personal stretching zone. It's only while holding a flexibility exercise in this zone that you will derive the greatest benefit from a program of stretching.

STRETCHING PROGRESSION

Anyone who has never undertaken a stretching program—even if that person has been physically active—should begin very slowly on the program outlined at the end of this chapter. You can actually injure your muscles and become very sore if you push too hard. Proper stretching is virtually effortless, and yet you will slowly gain flexibility from even the easiest program.

Beginners should back far away from the pain edge in their first stretching efforts and hold each stretch for only 20–30 seconds. They should also do only one repetition of an exercise for each muscle group. From this point, *slowly* add to the duration of each stretch (until you can hold it for a full two minutes) and then relax. For our purposes, however, I recommend doing a 1–2-minute stretch in one exercise for each body part, a workout you'll be able to complete in 10–15 minutes.

RELATED ACTIVITIES

Yoga is one of the best forms of stretching. Many professional athletes have turned to yoga for stretching. Some of the best yoga books on the market, in case you wish to learn more about this activity, are B. K. S. Iyengar's *Light On Yoga* (New York: Shoken Books, 1979), Sandra Jordan's *Yoga With a Partner* (New York: Areo Publishing Co., 1980) and Bikram Choudhury's *Bikram's Beginning Yoga Class* (Los Angeles: J. P. Tarcher, Inc., 1978).

Classic and jazz ballet classes also place a premium on flexibility, and therefore develop a flexible body. In addition to the flexibility benefits, dance classes will also help you to formulate an outstanding free-posing routine.

YOUR STRETCHING EXERCISES

By comparing the photos in this chapter with the following exercise descriptions, you'll have no trouble learning every movement perfectly.

Torso Stretch

Emphasis—This movement stretches primarily the front abdominals, but also the muscles of the chest, hips, and thighs.

Starting Position—Assume the starting position you would take for a push-up, your hands set shoulder width apart on the gym floor, your arms straight to support your upper body, and your body straight so your torso and legs form one long, unbroken line. Keeping your arms and legs straight, flex your body at the waist and push your hips up as high as possible from the floor.

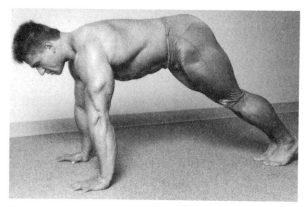

Torso Stretch

Stretched Position—Keeping your arms and legs straight, lower your hips as close to the floor as comfortably possible. Hold this stretched position for the required number of seconds.

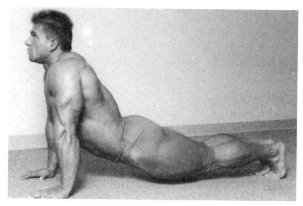

Torso Stretch (finish)

Hamstrings Stretches

Emphasis—This exercise and its variations stretch the hamstrings muscles at the backs of your thighs, buttocks, and lower-back muscles.

Starting Position—Place your feet about 6-8 inches apart on the gym floor, stand erect, lock your legs for the duration of the exercise, and extend your arms straight upward from your shoulders.

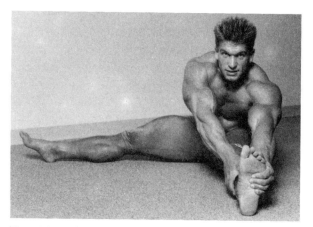

Hamstrings Stretch

Stretched Position—Keeping your legs straight, bend forward and touch your hands to your feet. As you become more flexible, you will be able to lay your torso against your thighs in this position.

Variations—Two variations of this exercise exist. In the first, the legs are spread and you bend over to grasp your legs individually with your arms. In the second, you bend slightly to the side and grasp the ankle of one leg and pull gently with both hands to pull your torso downward and more intensely stretch your hamstrings.

Standing Side Stretches

Emphasis—This exercise directly stretches the muscles at the sides of your waist and torso.

Starting Position—Place your left hand on your hip and extend your right arm overhead. Your feet should be set about shoulder width apart, and you should keep your legs relatively straight throughout the exercise.

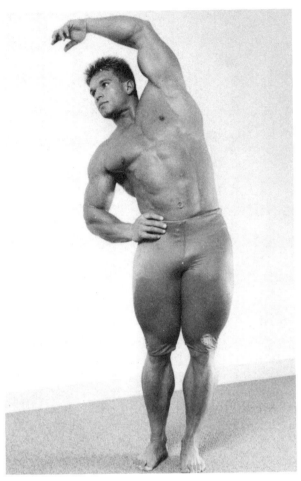

Standing Side Stretch

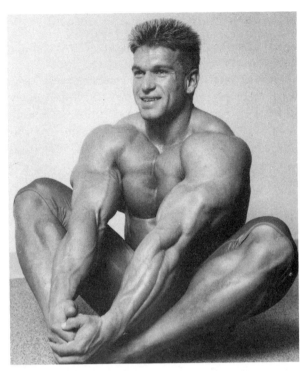

Seated Groin Stretch (start)

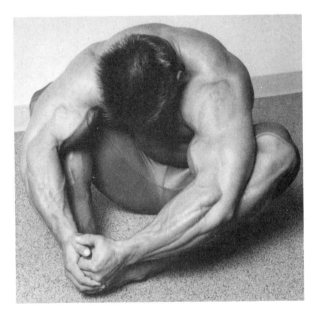

Seated Groin Stretch (finish)

Stretched Position—Bend at your waist directly to the side as far as comfortably possible. Hold this position for the required number of seconds. Reverse body position and repeat in the opposite direction.

Seated Groin Stretches

Emphasis—This exercise stretches all of the muscles of the groin and inner thighs.

Starting Position—Sit down and grasp your toes, bending your legs as completely as possible (ideally, your heels should be right up against your pelvic structure). Switch your grip to grasping your knees. Be sure to keep your torso erect throughout the movement.

Stretched Position—Use your hands to slowly push your knees apart until they are as close to the floor as comfortably possible.

Hurdler's Stretch

Emphasis—This exercise stretches both the hamstrings and groin muscles.

Starting Position—Sit on the floor. Extend your right leg forward and lock it straight throughout the movement. Your left leg should be bent at a 90-degree angle and lying flat on the floor behind your body. Your torso should be upright and your arms extended directly forward, parallel to the floor.

Stretched Position—Bend slowly forward over your right leg and grasp your ankle to gently pull your torso down to a position as close to your leg as comfortably possible. After stretching with your right leg forward, do an equal amount of stretching with your left leg extended forward.

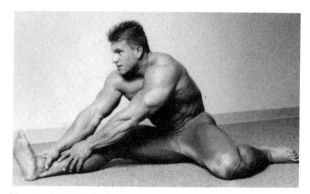

Hurdler's Stretch (start)

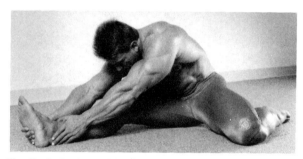

Hurdler's Stretch (finish)

Lying Hip Stretches

Emphasis—This exercise stretches and tones the hip girdle, upper leg, and midsection muscles.

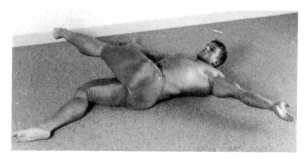

Lying Hip Stretch (start)

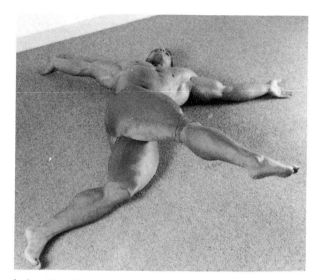

Lying Hip Stretch (finish)

Starting Position—Lie on your back on the gym floor. Place your legs roughly parallel to each other as you lie on the floor, and extend your arms directly out from your shoulders, forming a rough crucifix with your torso. Keep your arms motionless on the gym floor throughout the exercise.

Stretched Position—Keeping your right leg in contact with the floor, raise your left foot upward and to the side until your foot (left leg is held straight) touches the floor about halfway between your hip girdle and your right hand. Hold this stretched position for the required period, return to the start, and repeat the stretch to the opposite side.

Thigh Stretches

Emphasis—This exercise strongly stretches the quadriceps muscles on the front of your thighs.

Starting Position—Stand erect and balance on your left foot with your leg held straight throughout the stretch. Reach behind and grasp your right ankle with your right hand as illustrated. You can balance your body by grasping a sturdy upright with your free hand.

Stretched Position—Pull gently upward on your ankle to stretch your thigh muscles.

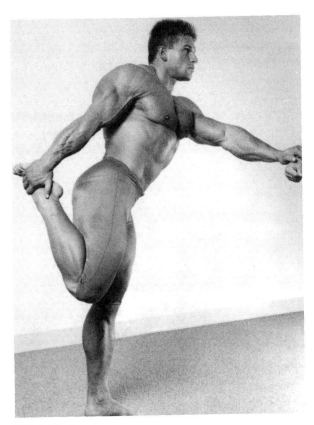

Thigh Stretch

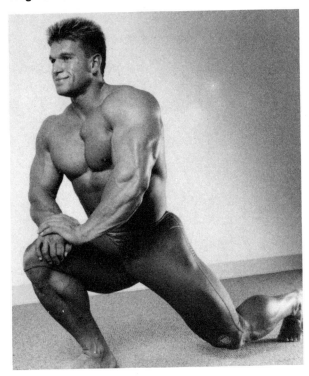

Lunging Stretch

Lunging Stretches

Emphasis—This movement stretches the muscles of the hips, buttocks, and front thighs.

Starting Position—Stand erect, hands on hips, feet set about shoulder width apart.

Stretched Position—Step forward with either leg and bend it fully while keeping the other leg straight. Hold this position for the required length of time and then repeat the movement with the other foot forward.

Calf Stretches

Emphasis—This exercise stretches and tones all of the muscles at the back of your lower legs.

Starting Position—Face a wall and place your hands on the wall at shoulder height. Move your feet backward until your right leg, torso, and arms make one straight line. Your left leg should be bent to take weight off of it.

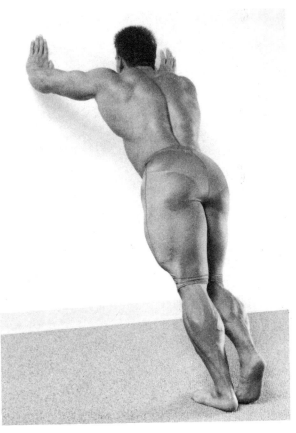

Calf Stretch

Stretched Position—Gently press your heel down to the floor. If you can comfortably place your heel flat on the floor, put your foot back another 4-6 inches to intensify the stretch. Be sure to do an equal amount of stretching for each leg.

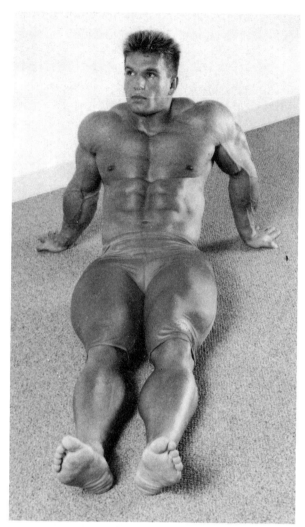

Chest/Shoulder Stretch

Chest/Shoulders Stretches

Emphasis—This movement strongly stretches the pectoral and deltoid muscles.

Starting Position—Sit down and bend your legs slightly, placing them on the floor for balance. With your arms held straight throughout the exercise, lean backward and place them on the floor.

Stretched Position—Slowly move your hands more and more to the rear to gently stretch the chest and shoulder muscles.

Wrist Stretches

Emphasis—This exercise stretches all of the muscles and joints of your fingers and wrists.

Starting Position—Stand erect and place the tips of your fingers together with your palms facing inward. As an alternative, you can place your fingers together with your palms facing outward.

Stretched Position—Press your wrists gently toward each other. Hold the stretched position. Repeat.

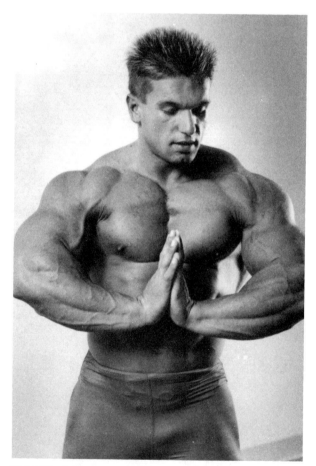

Wrist Stretches

Neck Stretches

Emphasis—These stretches influence all of the neck muscles. They are particularly good for relieving job-related stress.

Starting Position—Stand erect with your hands on your hips. Maintain this position with your legs, arms, and torso throughout the movement.

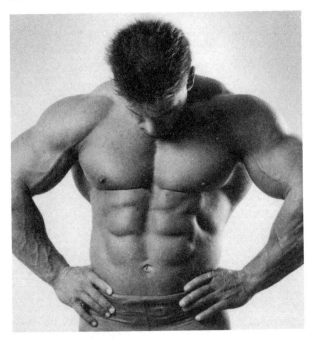

Neck Stretching (one)

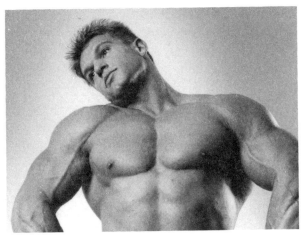

Neck Stretching (two)

Stretched Position—Tilt your head as far forward as possible and hold this position. Then tilt your head as far backward as possible and hold that position. Next tilt your head as far to the right side as possible and hold that position. And finally tilt your head as far to the left side as possible and hold that position.

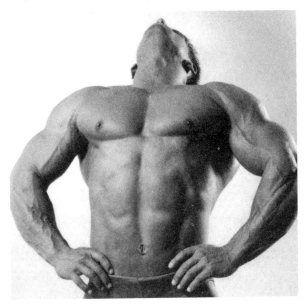

Neck Stretching (three)

SUGGESTED STRETCHING ROUTINE

Do each of the stretching exercises in the listed order, going through the cycle one time. Shoot for 30-60 seconds in each stretched position. Slowly work the program upward until you are doing two series with as much as two minutes in each stretch.

PART IV
BODY PART
TRAINING REGISTER

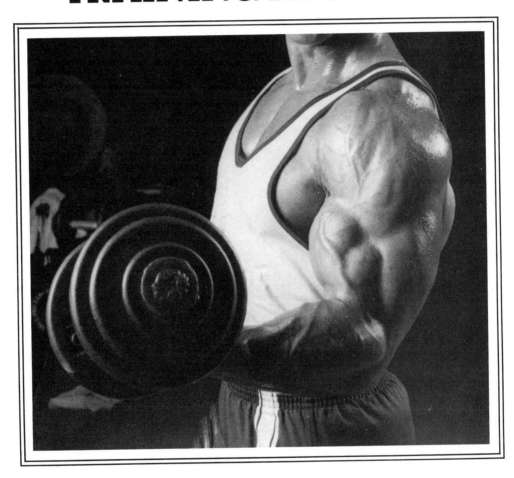

16
Developing
Awesome Abdominals

The muscle groups that give complete development to your midsection are among the most important in your physique. One reason they are important is that they contribute to health and the integrity of your lower back and abdomen. Many lower-back injuries are a result of weak abdominals rather than underdeveloped spinal erectors.

John Hnatyschak has developed a set of super-impressive abdominals, which also ease a sore back condition. According to Hnatyschak, "I was injured in a car accident that severely wrenched my lower back and damaged a couple of the fibrous discs between my vertebrae. During the nine months after the injury, I had quite a few days in which my lower back was incredibly painful. The only natural way I could relieve my spinal pain was to get into the gym after my doctor gave me the okay to work out, then rebuild my abdominal strength and midsection muscle tone. Now that I have achieved this, I have virtually no lower-back pain."

The abdominals are also important to competitive bodybuilders. A tightly muscled midsection is a sure signal to the judging panel that you are in optimum physical condition for a show. In contrast, a flabby and weakly developed midsection is a sure sign that you are underprepared.

There is also great psychological impact of having great abdominals when you are onstage, in terms of both the judges who will evaluate your physique and the audience which will respond to your efforts. The human eye is invariably drawn first to the middle of a large object such as a bodybuilder's physique. In this case, judges and audience will first look at your midsection when you initially step onstage.

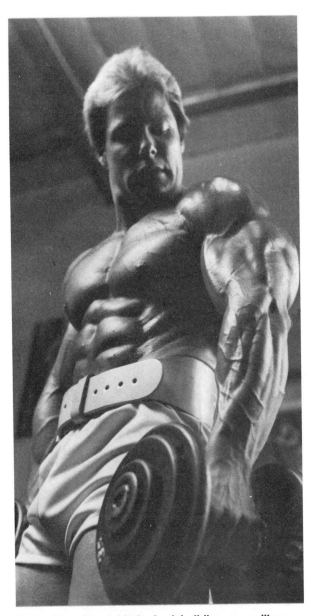

Young Dave Hawk hit the bodybuilding scene like a meteor in 1985 by winning the Light-Heavyweight/ Overall US Championships, and soon after the IFBB World Games Light-Heavyweight Championship. He has recently made a conversion to bicycling racing.

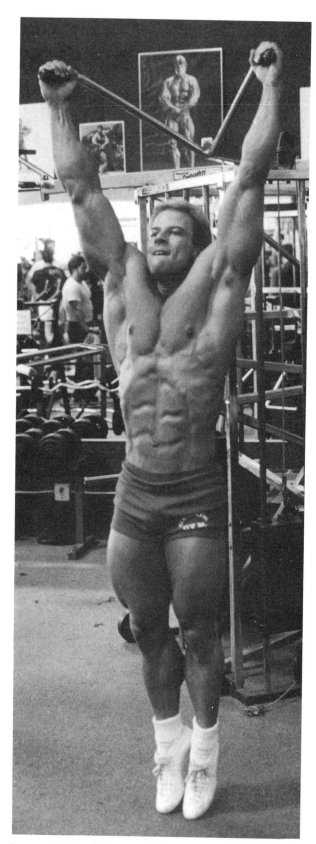

Long noted for his supremely developed abs, John Hnatyschak can even display a few lines across his rectus abdominis when his body is at full stretch hanging down from a chinning bar.

And if your abdominals are thickly muscled and tightly defined, a favorable first impression can lead the judges and audience to look favorably on you throughout the rest of the prejudging and evening show.

ABDOMINAL ANATOMY AND KINESIOLOGY

Many muscles make up your midsection anatomy, and they are located in a manner which allows you to twist your torso in relation to your hips, bend forward to flex your torso at the waist, bend directly to either side, or combinations of these three types of movements.

The most obvious abdominal muscle group is the *rectus abdominis*, a large, flat muscle wall covering almost the entire front of your abdomen between lower ribcage and hip girdle. This muscle contracts to flex your body at the waist, as in a sit-up or leg raise movement. It also contracts to pull your shoulders toward your hips when your spine is relatively straight, such as during a crunch movement.

Some bodybuilders feel that sit-up movements tend to isolate stress on the upper abdominals, while leg raising movements tend to stress primarily the lower part of the rectus abdominis. In actual practice, this is only true when you concurrently focus your mental attention on the section of the front abdominals you wish to develop. All sit-ups and leg raises, however, stress the entire rectus abdominis, and merely place a degree or two more stress on the section you are attempting to isolate.

At the sides of your waist is a complex muscle group called the *external obliques*, which contract to both rotate your torso in relation to your hip structure and bend your torso directly to either side. Actually, the external obliques consist of three muscle groups, the *internal obliques*, *transverse obliques*, and *external obliques*, each layer of muscle having a separate function, and in concert the three types of obliques allow a large number of torso flexions and twists.

Running diagonally down the sides of the upper part of your midsection (below the ribcage) are the *intercostals*, muscles which both help flex your body at the waist and pull your torso forward and to the side simultaneously.

This is a very impressive muscle group, which can only be seen in bold relief when a bodybuilder has taken the time to develop it completely and has also dieted down to a low percentage of body fat.

ABDOMINAL TRAINING TIPS

Lee Haney discusses the importance of sharp abdominal development for big men: "A dozen years ago, contest judges really didn't expect heavyweight bodybuilders—those men weighing over 200 pounds in contest condition—to have sharply delineated abdominal muscles. The bigger men could get away with having plenty of muscle mass to complement their lofty stature, qualities which invariably set the heavyweights apart from lightweights and middleweights with their sharp abdominals. Today, it's a whole other matter.

"Today, men competing at body weights up to 250 pounds or so as I do, all of the taller bodybuilders, must now have total abdominal development, with thick ridges of muscle in the front abs, obliques, and intercostals, plus deep grooves between the major abdominal groups

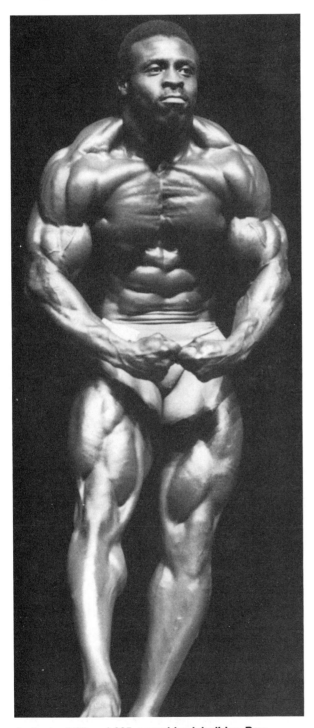

A stocky 5'8" and 225-pound bodybuilder, Roy Callender (a former Pro Mr. Universe winner and amateur World Champion) still displays the sharp abdominal formation of an athlete almost 50 pounds lighter.

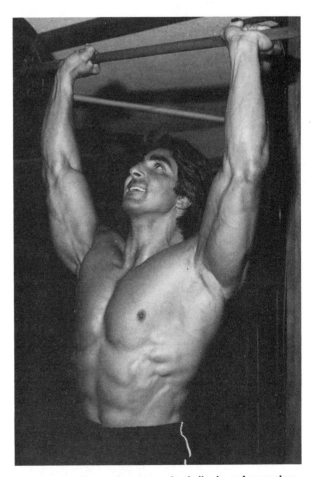

Another totally unchoreographed display of superior abs is given by Dennis Tinerino (winner of several Mr. Universe titles) as he completes a repetition toward the end of a set of heavy Standing Barbell Presses for his shoulders and triceps.

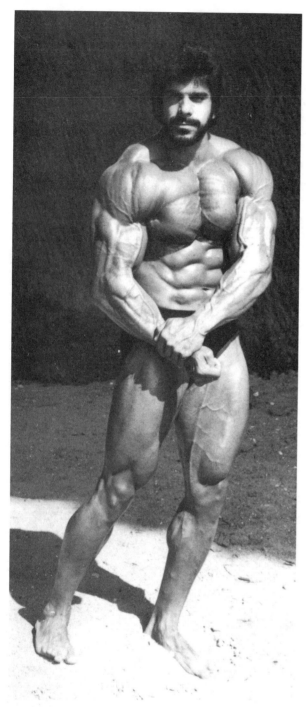

Great abs on an athlete as tall as 6′5″ Lou Ferrigno are rare, but Louie pulls off his midsection display with the best of them.

and even cross striations within each abdominal muscle complex. I was able to bump off all of the competition throughout my amateur competitive career, but once I became a pro bodybuilder, I knew I had to bear down on abs to bring them up to the level of the rest of my physique.

"My training approach was to hit my abdominals hard during both off-season and pre-contest cycles until I had them up to par. I used the Weider Muscle Priority Training Principle by bombing abdominals first in my routine when I was totally fresh and had maximum mental and physical drive. Within a couple of years, my abdominals were up to the level I had set, at which point I could back off somewhat on the length and intensity of my abdominal training sessions. And after another year, my abs were so good that I could even reduce the frequency with which I trained them in the off-season. Then I could kick in high-intensity abdominal training and a tight precontest diet for 10–12 weeks prior to an Olympia and bring my abdominals up to their current high level of development."

John Hnatyschak uses a reverse of the Muscle Priority Principle: "My abdominals have been at a very high standard from about the second or third year of steady, systematic training. So, I generally save my ab routine for the end of my workout, devoting my early workout time and energy to blasting whatever body part I feel is weak. But if my abdominals *were* a weak point, I'd absolutely be working them first in each training session."

Hnatyschak continued his discussion by debunking one myth of abdominal training: "Many so-called bodybuilding authorities will tell you that doing too much abdominal training will widen your waistline. I don't believe a word of it! At least, I don't believe it will happen if a bodybuilder has a genetically narrow waistline. And it also won't happen unless you do heavy side bends, which will rapidly enlarge the obliques. I've even used weight on such movements as Roman chair sit-ups without making my waist look wider.

"You must make abdominals both a physical and mental priority. The first thing I say when coaching a bodybuilder who has weak abdominal development is first to work on getting more in touch with the muscle complex mentally. This involves working on mental concentration every time you train abdominals, forcing your mind back on the muscle group whenever it strays off to some other subject.

"When you are training abdominals correctly, you should feel a heavy growth burn in

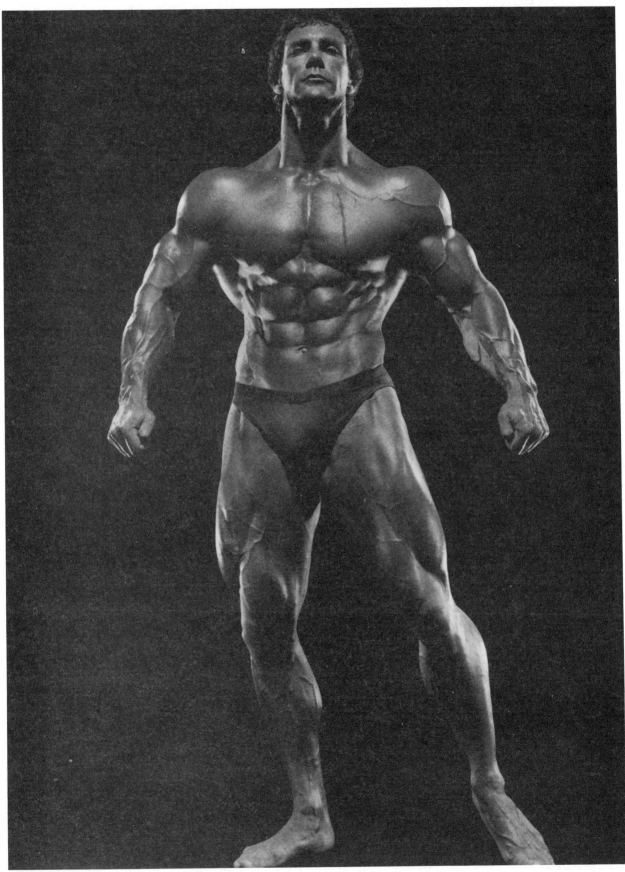

Massive Scott Wilson sets off his highly competitive pro physique with sharp abdominal development, particularly in the rectus abdominis and intercostals.

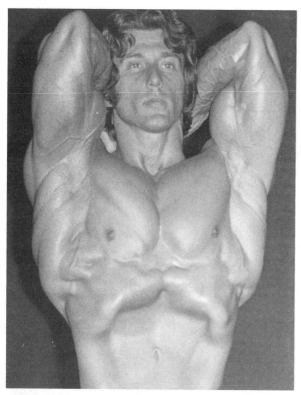

One of the best abdominal vacuums in the sport has long been done by three-time Mr. Olympia Frank Zane. Frank has often called this one of his two or three favorite poses.

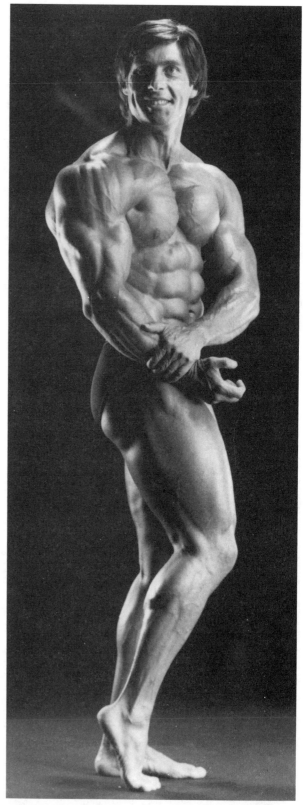

Frenchman Jacques Neuville won the IFBB World Light-Heavyweight World Championships in 1981 in Cairo, Egypt. A gym owner, he is particularly noted for his great upper-body development and sharp abdominals.

the muscle group during each set. And after you have completed your ab routine, the muscle group should be pumped up, just the same as the biceps, delts, or back muscles would be after a tough workout.

"I've found it's best to have a novice bodybuilder, or one who isn't making gains in abdominal development, practice keeping his abdominals under powerful tension throughout each set of a midsection workout. In this way, he can build up his concentration ability, and the continuous tension on the abdominals can be very beneficial for developing the body part."

A bodybuilder with weak abs should also experiment with the widest possible variety of exercises, movement sequences, rep schemes, and so forth, until he discovers what works best for him.

Jacques Neuville talks about the importance of using the Weider Giant Sets Training Principle for abdominal development: "When I first started to get serious about competing, I began to use a lot of trisets, followed by a normal rest interval of 1–2 minutes before launching into another triset for abdominals. A typical triset would consist of hanging leg raises, Roman chair sit-ups, and crunches. This principle really gave me a lot of abdominal development, but after a couple of years I hit a progress sticking point and discovered that I needed to increase my abdominal training intensity somehow.

"While reading a copy of Joe Weider's first training book, *Bodybuilding: The Weider Approach*, I learned about giant sets. These giant sets are compounds of 4–6 exercises for the same muscle group, with an absolute minimum of rest between movements and a normal rest interval at the end of each giant set. After reading about this training principle, I decided to try it out on abdominals.

"My first giant sets consisted of four movements, and my abdominals started making progress again after several months [of being] stalled. But after about 7–8 months, I reached another midsection sticking point, at which time I initiated a program of five-exercise giant sets. Again, after about a year, I reached another midsection sticking point. Then I took up six-movement giant sets for abdominals, and I've never again hit a sticking point for abdominal development.

"I definitely recommend compound sets and a variety of exercises for abdominal training. I'd suggest starting out with trisets, like I did, then gradually progress through four-, five-, and six-exercise giant sets as a means of incrementally increasing abdominal training intensity. In this way, you should always be improving your midsection development."

Rich Gaspari tells us about the contrast between off-season and precontest abdominal training: "Unless your abdominals are a weak point, you will not have to work them that intensely during an off-season training cycle. I think three midsection workouts per week will be sufficient for maintenance of abdominal muscle tone. A total of 10–12 quick sets will be sufficient in the off-season.

"As a competition approaches, however, you must increase both the frequency and intensity of your abdominal workouts. Most champion bodybuilders gradually add to the number of weekly midsection sessions, usually peaking

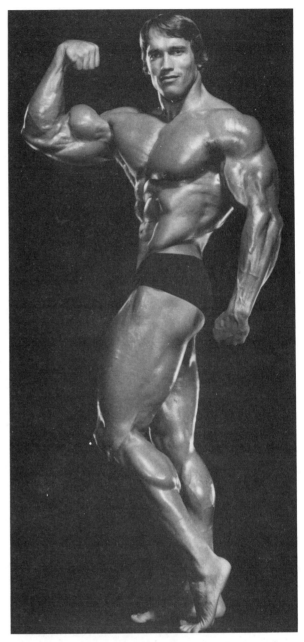

With no discernable weak points in his physique, it comes as no surprise that Arnold Schwarzenegger also possesses a highly detailed midsection.

out at one 15–20-minute midsection workout each day. I've even known of a few top bodybuilders who actually blast away at their abdominals twice a day, 6–7 days a week.

"The volume of your workouts should also increase as a means of augmenting training intensity. It's not at all uncommon for a champion bodybuilder to get in 20 or more sets of direct abdominal training, often using trisets and giant sets in a midsection workout. And you can increase intensity by using weight or raising the end of your inclined abdominal board to make your sit-ups and leg raises more difficult to perform.

"When you have a large number of abdominal sets to do prior to a competition, you should look into using the Weider Intersets Training Principle. With this method, you will interject one set of abdominal work between each 2-3 sets of training for a major muscle group. In other words, you might do two sets of benches, a set of sit-ups, two more sets of benches, another set of sit-ups, two sets of inclines, a set of sit-ups, and so forth until you have completed your entire midsection training program right along with the program for whatever other major muscle group you have scheduled.

"The beauty of the intersets technique is that you almost won't notice how many sets you perform of your abdominal work. You might have done 20 total sets of midsection work, but when you don't do all of these sets together, you will find that you are not bored during your abdominal training session. I've personally used this technique and endorse it for use by all competitive bodybuilders."

ABDOMINAL EXERCISES

As you know from the kinesiology discussion earlier in this chapter, the abdominal muscles contract to force the shoulders toward the hip girdle, flex the torso at the waist, or bend and twist the torso to the sides. There are only 14 major abdominal movements in this chapter, but with variations on each exercise, you will have more than 25 total midsection exercises to work into your bodybuilding programs.

Sit-Ups

Emphasis—This is the most basic of all bodybuilding exercises for the midsection. It works the entire rectus abdominis muscle wall, with somewhat more stress placed on the upper half of that muscle wall than the lower half. When performed while twisting alternately from one side to the other, sit-ups can also involve the intercostals and even the obliques.

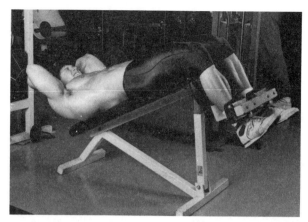

Sit-Ups (start)   Model: Gary Strydom

Starting Position—Lie on your back on an abdominal board and hook your toes and insteps under the roller pads or looped strap provided at the foot end of the board. (Alternatively, you can lie on your back on the floor and hook your feet under a heavy piece of furniture.) Bend your knees about 30 degrees to remove potentially harmful stress from your lower back, and keep them bent in this position throughout your set. Place your hands behind your neck and interlace your fingers to keep them in this position as you do your set.

Movement Performance—Slowly curl your torso off the bench by raising first your head, then successively your shoulders, upper back, and lower back. Keep sitting forward until your torso reaches a position perpendicular with the gym floor. While holding this position, reverse the movement and slowly return to the starting point. Repeat the movement for the suggested number of repetitions.

Training Tips—Never jerk your torso from the abdominal board. You can do this movement twisting your torso about 30 degrees to the right and left as you do the movement. My favorite system of twisting is to do one straight forward, one twisting to the right, one straight forward again, one twisting to the left, one straight forward, and so forth until you have done the required number of repetitions. To add resistance to your sit-ups, you can either incrementally raise the foot end of the bench, hold a loose barbell plate or two behind your head, or both.

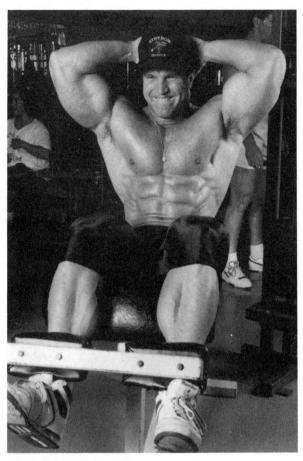

Sit-Ups (finish)

Roman Chair Sit-Ups

Emphasis—This is one of the newer abdominal exercises, one which has only been done universally in the sport since about 1975. Roman chair sit-ups place stress on the entire rectus abdominis muscle wall, with more stress on the upper half of this muscle complex than the lower half. When performed twisting to each side, Roman chair sit-ups can also place significant stress on the intercostals and somewhat less intense stress on the obliques at the side of your lower waist.

Starting Position—Sit on the Roman chair seat and hook your toes beneath the restraint bar down near the floor. Cross your arms over your chest and keep them in this position throughout your set.

Movement Performance—Moving only at your hips, incline your torso backward until it is

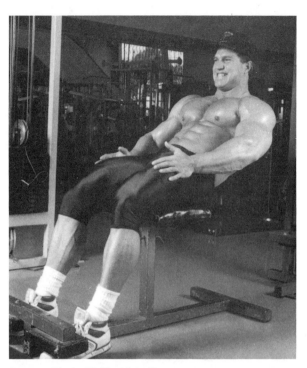

Roman Chair Sit-Ups (start)

about 6–8 inches above a position parallel with the floor. Then rock forward until you feel tension coming off your abdominal muscles. Crunch forward and downward with your torso in this position, then relax and return to the position in which your torso is 6–8 inches above, parallel with the gym floor. Continue rocking back and forth over this short range of motion, until you have completed the stated number of repetitions.

Training Tips—Be sure to do this movement slowly and deliberately; momentum should be totally eliminated from Roman chair sit-ups. You can also twist from side to side when you do your Roman chair sit-ups, a movement that involves the muscles at the sides of your waist more intensely. You might also experiment with placing the front end of the Roman chair upon a thick block of wood (4×4-inch and 6×6-inch pieces are good), which will intensify the stress placed on the abdominal muscles when you perform this movement. Another way to add resistance to Roman chair sit-ups is to place the apparatus so you are facing away from a floor pulley, pass a rolled-up towel through a loop handle attached to the end of

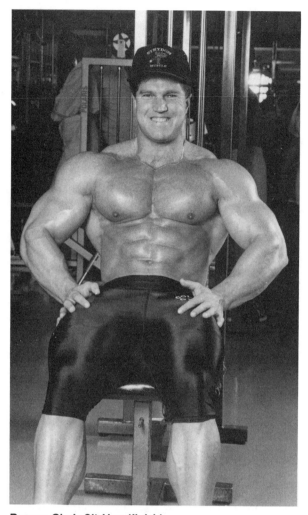

Roman Chair Sit-Ups (finish)

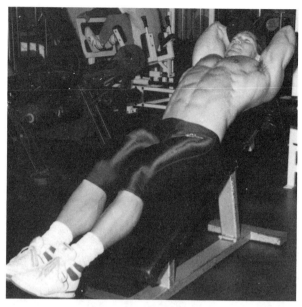

Leg Raises (incline variation—start)

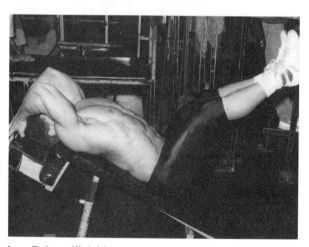

Leg Raises (finish)

the cable, and sit on the seat with one end of the towel over each shoulder, grasping an end in each hand while doing the movement.

Leg Raises

Emphasis—This fundamental abdominal exercise places primary stress on the rectus abdominis muscle wall, with a larger share of that resistance on the lower half of the muscle wall than on the upper half. Minor secondary stress is also placed on the intercostal muscles at the sides of your waist.

Starting Position—Lie on your back on an inclined abdominal board with your head toward the upper end. Grasp either the roller pads or looped foot restraint to keep your upper body from moving as you do your set.

(Alternatively, you can lie on your back on the floor and restrain your upper body by grasping either a heavy piece of furniture or a loaded barbell resting on the gym floor.) Bend your legs about 15-20 degrees in order to remove potentially harmful stress from your lower back, and keep them bent like this throughout your set.

Movement Performance—Use front abdominal strength to raise your feet in a semicircular arc from the bench to a position directly above your hips. Immediately return your feet back along the same arc until they are just clear of the bench, then repeat the movement for the required number of repetitions.

Training Tips—To increase resistance on the abdominals, you can incrementally raise the head end of the bench. Alternatively, you can wear iron boots on your feet, or hold a light dumbbell between your feet as you do the movement.

Bench Leg Raises

Emphasis—As with leg raises, this movement places primary stress on the rectus abdominis muscle wall, with a larger share of that resistance on the lower half of the muscle wall than on the upper half. Secondary stress is also placed on the intercostal muscles at the sides of your waist. When you do bench leg raises rather than normal leg raises, you are achieving a longer range of motion during the exercise, which improves the quality of stress you place on your abdominal muscles.

Starting Position—Lie on your back on a flat exercise bench with your hips at the end of the bench. Reach back and grasp the edges of the bench behind your head to restrain your upper body on the bench as you do the movement. Press your legs together and bend your legs about 15-20 degrees for the entire movement. Raise your feet just clear of the gym floor.

Movement Performance—Use abdominal strength to raise your feet upward and to the rear in a semicircular arc, until your feet are directly above your hips. Slowly return your feet back along the same arc to the starting point, and repeat the movement for an appropriate number of repetitions.

Training Tips—Be sure that you don't start swinging the movement, using muscle rebound at the bottom to accelerate the exercise cadence. You should always do bench leg raises—indeed, all abdominal movements—with a slow and deliberate cadence.

Hanging Leg Raises

Emphasis—This is a highly intense movement for placing stress on the rectus abdominis, particularly on the lower half of the muscle wall. Significant secondary stress is on the intercostals.

Starting Position—Jump up and take an overgrip on a chinning bar with your hands set about shoulder width on the bar. Hang your body straight downward from your hands, and bend your leg about 15-20 degrees for the entire movement.

Movement Performance—Use abdominal strength to raise your feet forward and upward in a semicircular arc until they are slightly above the level of your hips. Hold this peak-contracted position for a moment, then slowly lower back to the starting position. Repeat the movement for the correct number of repetitions.

Training Tips—You can also raise your feet up to the level of your hands on the chinning bar, a movement which is even more intense than normal hanging leg raises. You will find that with practice you can time your leg raises to prevent your body from swinging backward

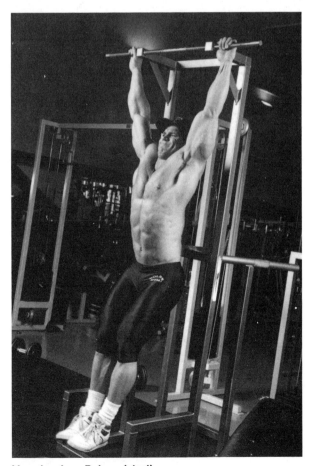

Hanging Leg Raises (start)

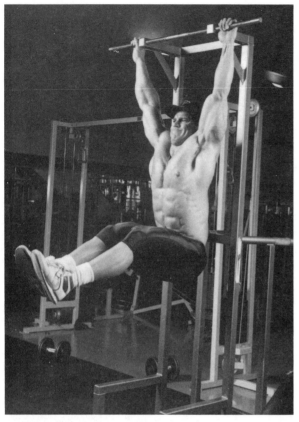

Hanging Leg Raises (finish)

and forward from your hands. Alternatively, you can have your training partner hold the sides of your hips to keep you from swinging beneath the bar.

Parallel Bar Leg Raises

Emphasis—This is a slightly less intense movement than hanging leg raises, but more intense than either normal leg raises or bench leg raises. As with all of these variations of leg raises, primary stress is on the rectus abdominis muscle wall, particularly the lower half of the muscle group. Secondary stress is on the intercostals at the sides of your waist.

Starting Position—Grasp the parallel bars and jump up to support yourself on straight arms with your hands set on the parallel bars with palms facing each other. Press your legs together and bend your legs about 15-20 degrees for the movement.

Movement Performance—Use abdominal strength to move your feet forward and upward in a semicircular arc to about the level of your

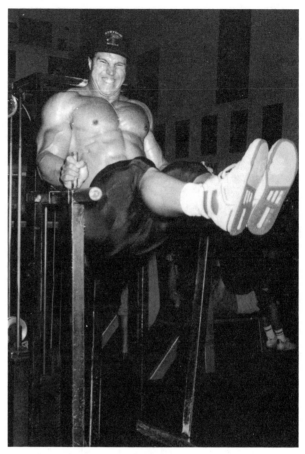

Parallel Bar Leg Raises (midpoint)

hips. Hold this peak-contracted position for a moment, then return to the starting point. Repeat for a moment, then return to the starting point. Repeat the movement for the suggested number of repetitions.

Training Tips—You can more intensely affect the working abdominal muscles if you pull your feet even higher, perhaps to the level of your eyes.

Knee-Ups

Emphasis—When performed without additional resistance, this movement is a relatively easy one for stressing the rectus abdominis, particularly the lower part of the muscle wall. Secondary stress is placed on the intercostals at the sides of your waist.

Starting Position—Sit at the end of a flat exercise bench and brace your torso at a 45-degree angle with the bench by grasping the edges of the bench. Extend your legs straight downward

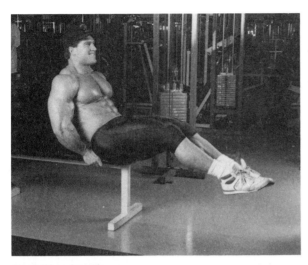

Knee-Ups (start)

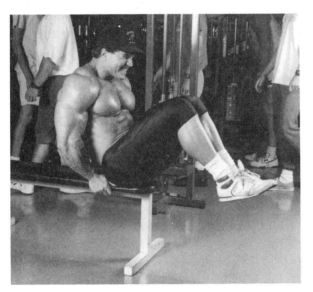

Knee-Ups (finish)

at an angle, so your body makes one long line at a 45-degree angle with the floor. In the correct starting position, your heels should be just clear of the gym floor.

Movement Performance—Use front abdominal strength to pull your knees up to your chest while simultaneously bending your legs completely. Hold this peak-contracted position for a moment, then slowly lower back to the starting point. Repeat the movement for an appropriate number of repetitions.

Training Tips—There are two ways in which you can add resistance to this movement. One is to strap a cable running through a floor pulley to your feet while seated at the end of a

flat exercise bench, and the other is to sit at the end of a leg extension machine and hook your toes and insteps under the lower set of roller pads, then do the movement. When using a cable to add resistance, you can also do the exercise while lying on your back on the gym floor, your feet toward the pulley. This variation is a favorite of John Hnatyschak, who has sensational abdominal development.

Hanging Frog Kicks

Emphasis—This is a somewhat more intense version of knee-ups, performed while hanging from your hands at a chinning bar. It places the most intense stress on the rectus abdominis, particularly the lower section of the muscle wall. Significant secondary stress is placed on the intercostals at the sides of your waist.

Starting Position—Jump up and take an over-grip on a chinning bar, your hands set about

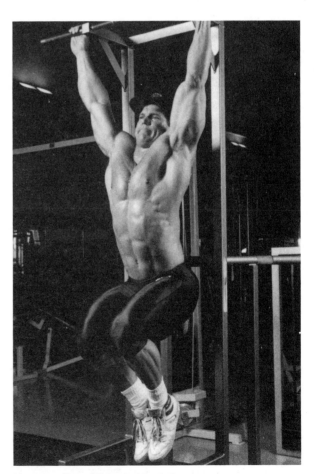

Hanging Frog Kicks (midpoint)

shoulder width on the bar. Hang your body straight downward from the bar.

Movement Performance—Moving only your legs, pull your knees up to your chest while simultaneously bending your legs completely. Hold this peak-contracted position for a moment, then slowly lower back to the starting point. Repeat the movement for the correct number of repetitions.

Training Tips—If you have trouble swinging under the bar, have a training partner hold the sides of your hips to restrain you. You can also do this movement twisting to each side on successive reps, a movement which involves the intercostals more intensely.

Crunches

Emphasis—This is a very intense isolation exercise for the entire rectus abdominis muscle wall, equally distributing stress from top to bottom on this muscle group. Minor secondary emphasis is on the intercostals.

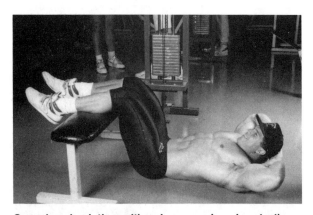

Crunches (variation with calves over bench—start)

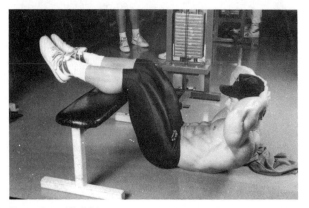

Crunches (finish)

Starting Position—Lie on your back with your lower legs draped across the surface of a flat exercise bench in such a position in which your thighs are perpendicular to the gym floor. Place your hands behind your head and interlace your fingers to restrain them in this position throughout your set.

Movement Performance—You must perform the following four tasks simultaneously: 1) use lower-abdominal strength to pull your hips from the gym floor; 2) use upper-abdominal strength to raise your shoulders and upper back from the floor; 3) force your shoulders toward your hips, effectively shortening your torso; and 4) forcefully exhale all of your breath. When you correctly perform these four tasks, you will feel a very powerful contraction along the entire length of your rectus abdominis muscle wall. Hold this peak-contracted position for a slow count of two, lower back to the starting point, and repeat the movement for the suggested number of repetitions.

Training Tips—You can also do this movement with your feet pressed flat against the gym wall, upper legs held perpendicular to the gym floor, and lower legs held parallel to the gym floor. Regardless of the variation employed, be sure that you don't pull your hips away from the floor using hamstrings strength; the movement must originate from the lower-abdominal muscles.

Nautilus Crunches

Emphasis—Primary emphasis in this movement is on the entire rectus abdominis muscle wall, with secondary stress on the intercostal muscles at the sides of your waist and lower ribcage.

Starting Position—Adjust the seat height so when you are sitting in it, your toes rest under the roller pads beneath the seat. Sit down and hook your toes and insteps under the roller pads. Reach upward and backward to grasp the padded handles of the machine. Allow the handles to pull your torso upward, stretching the front abdominal muscles.

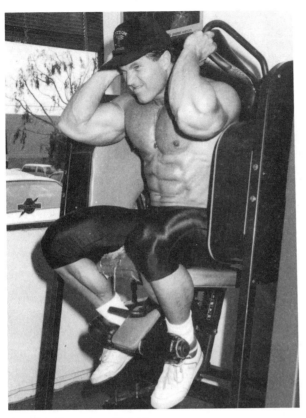

Nautilus Crunches (finish)

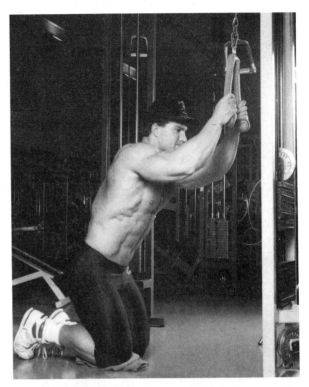

Pulley Crunches (start)

Movement Performance—Use front abdominal strength to curl your shoulders forward and downward, intensely contracting all of the abdominal muscles. Hold this peak-contracted position for a slow count of two, then return slowly to the starting point. Repeat the movement for the desired number of repetitions.

Training Tips—If you don't have access to a Nautilus machine of this type, you can substitute normal floor crunches and/or pulley crunches.

Pulley Crunches

Emphasis—This movement places primary stress on the entire rectus abdominis muscle wall. Strong secondary stress is on the lower lats and the serratus muscles at the sides of your ribcage.

Starting Position—Attach a rope handle to the end of a cable running through an overhead pulley. Grasp the two ends of the ropes and kneel down about 1-1½ feet back from the cable. Extend your body and arms directly upward toward the pulley.

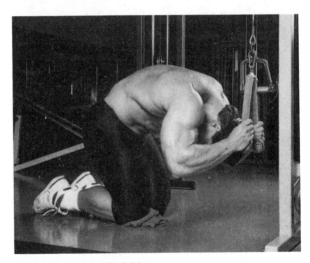

Pulley Crunches (finish)

Movement Performance—Simultaneously bend forward at the waist and perform a small pullover motion with your hands, forcefully exhaling your breath at the same time, and touch the gym floor about 3–5 inches ahead of your forehead with your hands. Hold this peak-contracted position for a slow count of two, then slowly return to the starting point. Repeat the movement until you have done a full set.

Training Tips—If you want greater involvement from the serratus and intercostal muscles, you should do this exercise with one arm at a time. I personally recommend doing one set with the left arm, one with the right arm, and one with both arms. And of course, you can do multiples of this exercise triad.

Side Bends

Emphasis—This is the premier exercise for directly bombing the obliques at the sides of your waist.

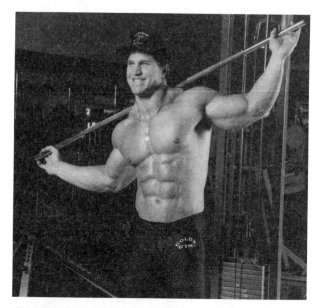

Side Bends (with bar—to right)

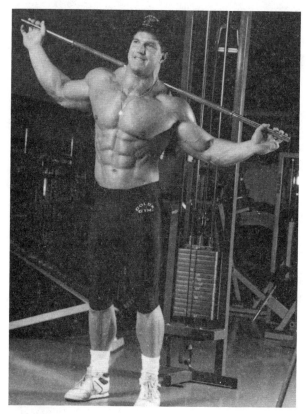

Side Bends (with bar—to left)

Training Tips—You can also do side bends with light dumbbells held in both hands, or with an unweighted bar held across your shoulders behind your neck, grasped at each end of

Starting Position—Grasp a light dumbbell in your left hand, set your feet a comfortable distance apart, place your right hand behind your neck, and stand erect. Allow the weight to pull your torso as far as comfortably possible directly to the left.

Movement Performance—Slowly move your torso as far to the right as possible, bending only at the waist. Return slowly to the starting point and repeat the movement for a minimum of 25-30 repetitions. Be sure to do an equal number of sets and reps with the dumbbell held in each hand.

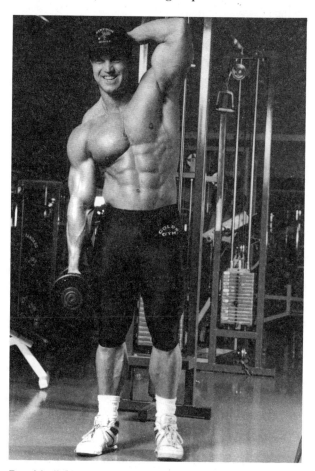

Dumbbell Side Bends (hand behind neck)

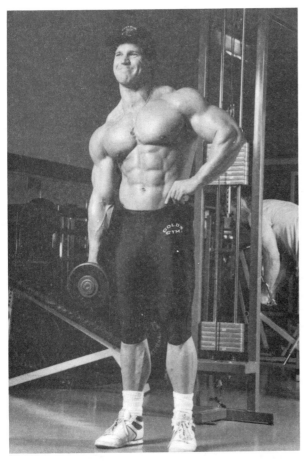

Dumbbell Side Bends (hand at side)

bench to restrain your body on the bench. Place an unweighted barbell handle or broomstick across your shoulders behind your neck. Wrap your arms around the bar throughout your set.

Movement Performance—Twist forcefully as far as you can to the left, then immediately back to the right. Continue rhythmically twisting from side to side until you have performed the suggested number of repetitions to each side.

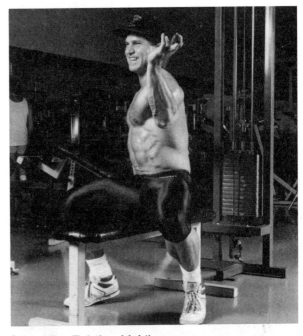

Seated Bar Twisting (right)

the bar to keep it in position. You must be careful to avoid using heavy weights and low reps (under 10–15), because the external obliques can be built up in mass very quickly. And once they are thickly developed, they detract from the marked difference between shoulder breadth and waist width, which judges look for.

Seated Twists

Emphasis—This exercise is designed to add tone to the transverse obliques, under the external obliques. It is reputed to have benefit in trimming the waistline, although I personally don't believe that contention. This is also a good movement for use at the beginning of your warm-up as a means of loosening your lower-back vertebrae.

Starting Position—Sit in the middle of a flat exercise bench, your legs straddling the bench. Brace your feet around the upright legs of the

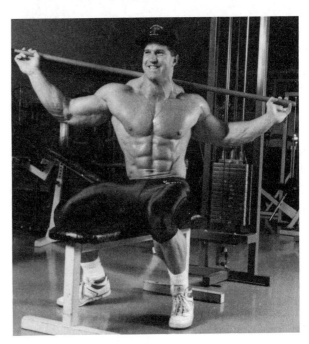

Seated Bar Twisting (left)

Training Tips—Many bodybuilders do this movement standing erect with their feet set 6–8 inches wider than their shoulders. But this movement is difficult to perform correctly, since the hips are difficult to restrain from moving as you do your set.

Standing Bent-Over Twists

Emphasis—Often referred to as bent twists, this movement has a very similar effect to seated twists. It tones the transverse obliques and lower-back muscle groups.

Starting Position—Place a broomstick or unweighted barbell bar across your shoulders and wrap your arms around it to keep it in position. Set your feet about 6–8 inches wider than your shoulders and stand erect. Bend forward at the waist until your torso is parallel with the floor.

Movement Performance—Twist as far as possible to the left, then as far as possible to the right. Rhythmically twist from one side to the other until you have completed the required number of repetitions to each side.

Training Tips—Never do less than 25–30 repetitions on this or any other twisting movement.

SUGGESTED ABDOMINAL ROUTINES

In this section I will give you three progressively more intense midsection training schedules which you can use for 6–8 weeks each before moving up to the next level of intensity. And once you have finished 6–8 weeks on the third of these routines, you will be in sufficiently good condition to try one of the routines presented in the concluding section of this chapter.

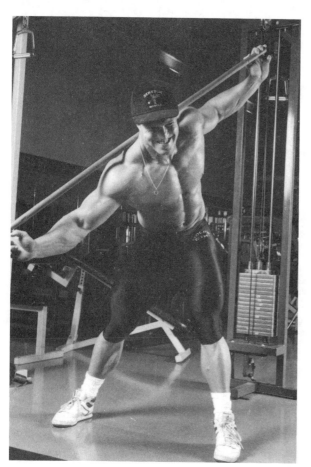

Standing Bent-Over Bar Twisting

BEGINNING LEVEL

(2–3 Times per Week)

Exercise	Sets	Reps
Sit-Ups	2–3	20–30
Leg Raises	2–3	20–30

INTERMEDIATE LEVEL

(3–4 Times per Week)

Exercise	Sets	Reps
Bench Leg Raises	2–3	20–30
Roman Chair Sit-Ups	2–3	20–30
Rope Crunches	2–3	20–30

This routine is performed as a triset, with minimum rest between exercises and a more normal rest interval of 2–3 minutes between trisets.

ADVANCED LEVEL

(3–4 Times per Week)

Exercise	Sets	Reps
Hanging Leg Raises	2–3	10–15
Roman Chair Sit-Ups	2–3	25–30
Side Bends	2–3	50–100
Crunches	2–3	25–30

This routine is performed as a giant set, with the minimum possible rest between exercises and a more normal rest interval of 2–3 minutes between giant sets.

MIDSECTION ROUTINES OF THE CHAMPIONS

I am giving you 15 sample routines of top NPC and IFBB bodybuilders. They should give you some solid idea of how you should formulate your own advanced abdominal training programs.

Unless you are a seasoned, nationally ranked bodybuilder you should not attempt the high-level abdominal routines presented in this section. You would invariably overtrain your abdominals and begin to lose muscle tone in your midsection. You might be encouraged, however, to learn that it's easier to work up to an Olympian-level abdominal routine much more quickly than you can for any other muscle group.

Lee Haney

ROUTINE "A"

Exercise	Sets	Reps
Roman Chair Sit-Ups	3–4	40–50
Side Bends	3–4	50–100
Crunches	3–4	25–30

ROUTINE "B"

Exercise	Sets	Reps
Hanging Leg Raises	3–4	15–20
Pulley Crunches	3–4	24–30
Incline Leg Raises	3–4	20–30

Peter Hensel

Exercise	Sets	Reps
Roman Chair Sit-Ups	3–4	25–40
Bench Leg Raises	3–4	25–40
Incline Sit-Ups	3–4	20–30
Side Bends	3–4	50
Crunches	3–4	25–30

All five exercises are giant setted, taking the minimum possible rest between exercises and a more normal rest interval of 2–3 minutes between giant sets.

Tim Belknap

Exercise	Sets	Reps
Incline Sit-Ups	5	20–30
Cable Bench Leg Raises	5	20–30
Side Bends	5	30–50

Lou Ferrigno

Exercise	Sets	Reps
Roman Chair Sit-Ups	3–4	50
Crunches	3–4	25
Hanging Leg Raises	3–4	20
Pulley Crunches	3–4	30

Danny Padilla

WORKOUT "A"

Exercise	Sets	Reps
Roman Chair Sit-Ups	4	25–50
Seated Twists	4	50–100
Hanging Leg Raises	4	15–20
Side Bends	4	50–100
Crunches	4	25–30

WORKOUT "B"

Exercise	Sets	Reps
Incline Sit-Ups	4	25
Seated Twists	4	50–100
Bench Leg Raises	4	25–30
Side Bends	4	50–100

John Hnatyschak

Exercise	Sets	Reps
Roman Chair Sit-Ups	2–3	50–100
Leg Raises	2–3	50–100
Rope Crunches	2–3	20–30
Knee-Ups (with resistance)	2–3	30–50

Richard Baldwin

Exercise	Sets	Reps
Roman Chair Sit-Ups	3	30–50
Hanging Leg Raises	3	15–20
Crunches	3	25–30
Rope Crunches	3	25–30

Gary Strydom

Exercise	Sets	Reps
Incline Sit-Ups	3–4	20–30
Bench Leg Raises	3–4	20–30
Roman Chair Sit-Ups	3–4	30–50
Crunches	3–4	20–30
Rope Crunches	3–4	20–30

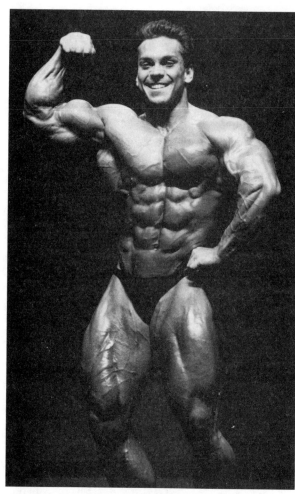

Rich Gaspari struts his stuff at the 1986 Mr. Olympia, where he placed second to Lee Haney for the first time. It's difficult to believe that a physique this great can be beatable, but Haney had only one second-place vote (and everything else first-place votes) against his old training partner and roommate, Gaspari. If you ever want to know the definition for the word "ripped," just think about this photo of Richard Gaspari in top physical condition.

Ron Teufel

Exercise	Sets	Reps
Incline Sit-Ups	1-2	100
Roman Chair Sit-Ups	1-2	100
Bench Leg Raises	1-2	100

Mike Christian

Exercise	Sets	Reps
Hanging Leg Raises	4-5	15-20
Roman Chair Sit-Ups	4-5	25-40
Crunches	4-5	25-30
Side Bends	4-5	50-100

Mike Mentzer

Exercise	Sets	Reps
Roman Chair Sit-Ups	2	12
Hanging Leg Raises	2	maximum
Side Sit-Ups	2	12

On the first and third exercises the first set is very heavy, while the second set is performed with less resistance.

Josef Grolmus

WORKOUT "A"

Exercise	Sets	Reps
Hanging Leg Raises	3	15-20
Incline Sit-Ups	3	25-30
Crunches	3	25-30

WORKOUT "B"

Exercise	Sets	Reps
Bench Leg Raises	3	30-40
Roman Chair Sit-Ups	3	40-50
Rope Crunches	3	25-30

Dennis Tinerino

Exercise	Sets	Reps
Roman Chair Sit-Ups	3-4	50-100
Hanging Leg Raises	3-4	15-25
Twisting Crunches	3-4	25-30
Seated Twists	3-4	100

Jacques Neuville

Exercise	Sets	Reps
Hanging Leg Raises	3-5	20-30
Incline Sit-Ups	3-5	20-30
Dumbbell Side Bends	3-5	20-30
Bench Leg Raises	3-5	20-30
Crunches	3-5	20-30
Rope Crunches	3-5	20-30

Ron Love

Exercise	Sets	Reps
Incline Sit-Ups	4-5	20-30
Incline Leg Raises	4-5	20-30
Pulley Crunches	4-5	25-30
Roman Chair Sit-Ups	4-5	25-30
Side Bends	4-5	40-50

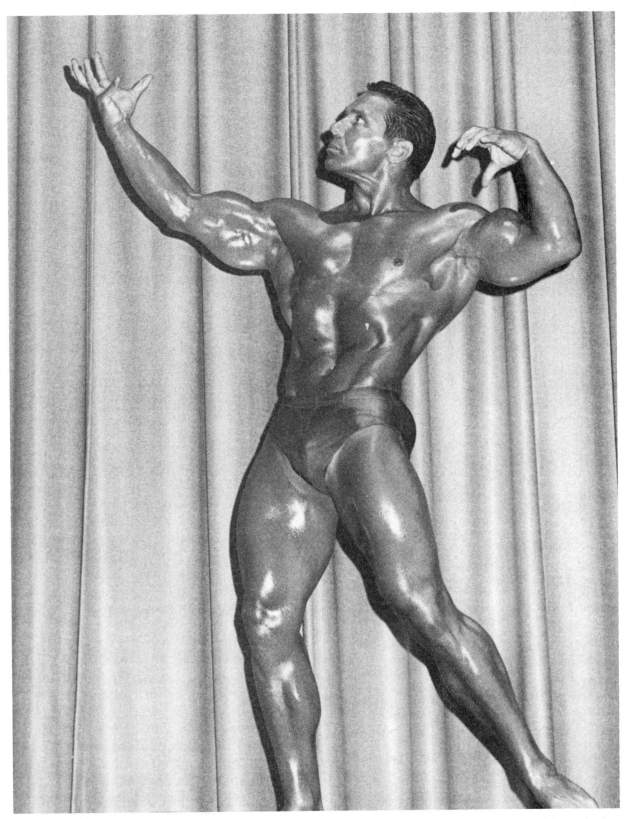

The originator of the V-spread latissimus dorsi conformation so widely imitated since Bill Pearl used it to win the 1953 Mr. America and Mr. Universe titles. Incidentally, this outstanding photo was taken of Pearl at the age of 53, as he guest posed on the 30th anniversary of his Mr. America win. Bill is in the wholesale gym equipment sales business near Grant's Pass, Oregon, and is one of a handful of successful vegetarian bodybuilders.

17
Big Back Bombing

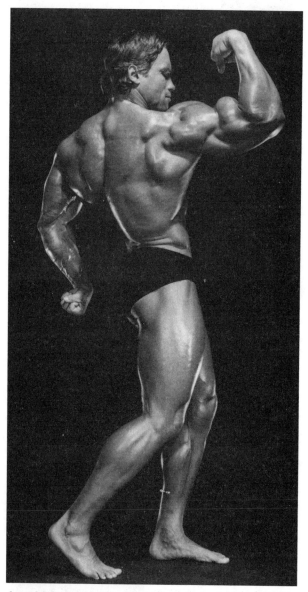

Arnold Schwarzenegger's legendary back took him to seven Mr. Olympia titles, six of them consecutively. The money he made from the sport was so wisely invested that he reaps millions of dollars in real estate income yearly. And the charisma he learned onstage helped him enormously in his film career.

At the national and international level of competitive bodybuilding, a bodybuilder's relative degree of back development often causes him to either win or lose the titles he goes after. I've frequently seen otherwise superbly developed bodybuilders turn around in the contest line-up and virtually disappear. Incredibly muscular when viewed from the front and either side, they have so little back development that they actually look like different bodybuilders—and not very good ones—when they turn their backs to the judges.

One reason why many bodybuilders fail to achieve great back development is laziness. Next to the thighs and buttocks, the back muscles are the largest in the body, and it takes great energy reserves to train your back as hard as you should. No one has ever trained the back without becoming very breathless between sets. And many who have never trained the back hard end up barfing the first time they get into the gym and really pound their lats, traps, and erectors the way they should be trained.

Due to the large energy expenditures and oxygen consumption that occurs when training the back hard, you will find that you must learn to crash past the pain barrier nearly every set. Merely going to the pain threshold and then backing off will give you a minimum of back development, and I think this is the reason why there are many potentially great bodybuilders languishing in local and state competitions because of inferior back development.

Another reason why many bodybuilders have weak back development is that they fail to realize that the back is really *three* body parts: trapezius, latissimus dorsi, and erector spinae. They spend a lot of time blasting away on their showy lats, which can be seen even in front poses, and almost totally neglect traps and erector training.

If you feel you want to train all three back muscle groups in one session, go ahead and do so. But I personally lean toward training lats by themselves, traps as part of the shoulder workout, and erectors as part of the leg session. For instance, you will often do upright rows for deltoids—the movement is also excellent for the trapezius muscles. And your lower back muscles come strongly into play when you do squats and other primary leg movements, as well as stiff-legged deadlifts for your hamstrings. And when you do lats as a major workout, you can easily pair it up in your split routine with biceps.

Over the years virtually every Mr. Olympia winner has had superb back development. Larry Scott (1965–66) started it off with one of the widest lat flares and thickest upper back developments of all time. A former Olympic lifter, Sergio Oliva (1967–69) had what was probably the best V-shape of any bodybuilder, with a very tiny waist-hip structure and awesome lat flare. And Oliva's back thickness was legendary.

Arnold Schwarzenegger (1970 through 75 and 1980) dominated the 1970s with a back displaying both width and thickness, but with a type of muscular definition that had not been seen on bodybuilders up to his era. Arnold's sidekick, Franco Columbu (1976, 1981) had such incredible lats that his back spread looked like the hood of a cobra jacked up for attack. Frank Zane (1977–79) redefined the word muscularity, in as much as his back was as ripped up as any bodybuilder before or after him. Zane never had awesome muscle mass; but his proportions, symmetry, and muscularity were unparalleled.

Chris Dickerson (1982) won his Mr. Olympia title with a physique reminiscent of Zane's. Chris's back was, for his structure, both remarkably broad and thick, plus very muscularly dense. Samir Bannout (1983) also had superior back development, and many aficionados of the sport feel that his back had the greatest muscular detail of any in the modern era of the sport.

My personal favorite "Best Back" Mr. Olympia winner is Lee Haney (1984–1987). Lee is certainly one of the most massive and muscular men the sport has ever produced, weighing a ripped-up 248 pounds at just under six feet in height. You've never seen more raw muscle under tension than Lee displays whenever he does his patented lat spread show from either the front or back. And the cuts and density in traps, lats, and erectors is *nonpareil* whenever he does a back double-biceps pose.

ANATOMY AND KINESIOLOGY

The trapezius is a large kite-shaped muscle mass situated in the upper back area. The points of the kite are at the base of the skull, near the points of the shoulders, and about halfway down the spine. The primary function—and the one which you will most frequently work in a back training session—is to

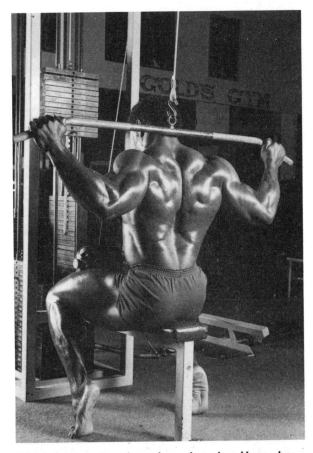

With a back as broad as a barn door, Lee Haney has swept to five Mr. Olympia victories in six tries. (He had to settle for third place behind winner Samir Bannout and runner-up Mohamed Makkawy in his first attempt at Munich, West Germany, in 1983.) Since 1984, it's been all Haney, and all of his victories have been largely dependent on his sensationally broad, thick, and ripped-up back.

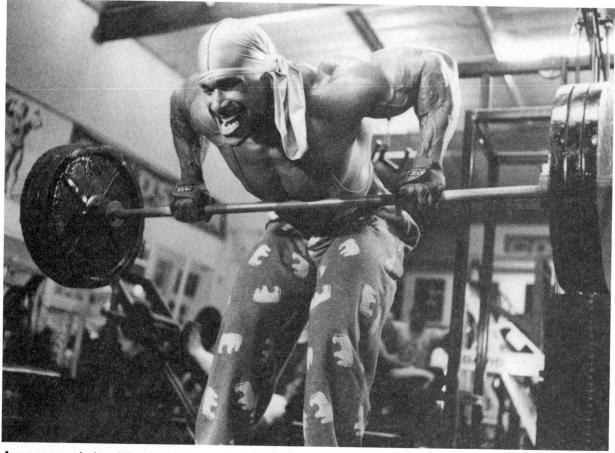

A man on a mission, Mike Christian won the US Pro Championships and IFBB World Pro Championships in early 1988, expecting the momentum he developed to improve his previous best Mr. Olympia placing, third in 1987. Unfortunately, illness prevented him from even entering the Big O in 1988.

pull the shoulders upward and backward. Secondarily, the trapezius muscles also contract to help arch the back.

The latissimus dorsi is a large mid-back muscle group. It appears like two large slabs of muscle when viewed from the front, in that it gives your torso a maximum V-shaped taper. From the back, it appears more like two bands of muscle below the traps. The primary function of the lats is to pull the upper arm bones downward and backward. Secondarily, the lats help to arch the back.

The erector spinae are two large, thick columns of muscle on either side of the spine, running from just above the hips to a point about halfway up the back. The spinal erectors contract to straighten the spine from a fully bent position. The erectors also are the major muscle group most responsible for arching the spine.

TRAINING TIPS

Massive *Mike Christian* gives aspiring bodybuilders this tip: "The keys to building great lats are using the longest possible range of motion on each back exercise, plus being sure that your spine is arched in the finish position of every latissimus dorsi exercise. You won't be able to fully contract your lats when your back is straight. So remember when training lats to always perform a full movement on every rep and be sure your back is arched in the finish position of every repetition."

Rich Gaspari reveals the difference between width and thickness back exercises: "If you're after width in your lats, the best exercises for stimulating it are various types of chins, various types of pulldowns, and pullovers. And for thickness, you should stick to all types of barbell, dumbbell, and machine rowing movements. If you could only do one exercise for your lats, I'd pick seated low-pulley rows, which tend to build both width and thickness, to say nothing of some trapezius and spinal erector development."

Casey Viator talks about traps: "One of the best ways to work traps is using the Weider Pre-Exhaustion Training Principle. This involves doing a superset of barbell or dumbbell shrugs followed immediately by a set of upright rows. Since the traps are a very strong muscle group, they need to be fatigued as much as possible before you do a trap exercise with arms, such as upright rows. This way, your traps are temporarily stronger than your arms and you can push them to the limit with the upright rows. But be sure to rest no more than 3–4 seconds between the two exercises, then for a normal rest interval of 1–1½ minutes between supersets."

Young *Dave Hawk* (USA and World Games Champion) does personal coaching and has a remedy for his pupils who want to train around a sore lower back: "You can often do noncompression erector movements like hyperextensions even with a sore back, but you'll need to avoid deadlifts and other back exercises which tend to compress your lower back. You'll also need to avoid any exercises for other body parts which cause back pain. Combine these tips with plenty of stretching, and you will soon find that your sore back is history."

BACK EXERCISES

There are more than 30 back exercises described and illustrated in this chapter. Counting the variations on each movement, the exercises presented in this section will give you more than 60 good trapezius, latissimus dorsi, and erector spinae movements for use in your own training programs.

Barbell Power Cleans

Emphasis—This excellent exercise places at least a little stress on virtually every muscle group in the body. But you will do it primarily for back development, and it is excellent for building up the traps, spinal erectors, and other mid-back muscle groups. Significant sec-

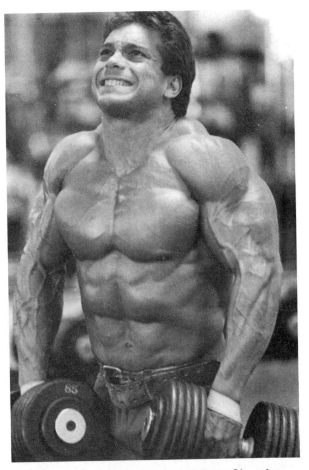

Despite placing second in the past three Olympias, Rich Gaspari is still only 24 years of age in a sport where athletes often mature in their late 30s and early 40s. Great things are expected of him, and he's sure to have sensational traps if he faithfully keeps doing his dumbbell shoulder shrugs with maximum weights.

ondary stress is on the biceps, brachialis, forearm flexor, buttock, and thigh muscles.

Starting Position—Place a moderately weighted barbell on the gym floor. Step up to it so your shins are touching the bar and set your feet about shoulder width apart, your toes pointed directly forward. Reach down and take a shoulder-width overgrip on the barbell. Keeping your arms straight, flatten your back and bend your knees so you assume a starting position in which your back is at an approximate 45-degree angle with the floor, your shoulders are above the level of your hips, and your hips are above the level of your knees.

Movement Performance—Initiate the pull from the floor by first straightening your legs.

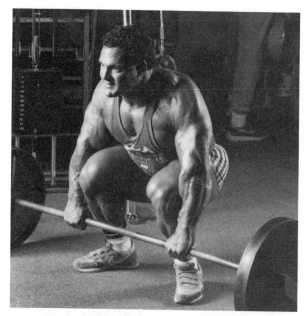

Barbell Power Clean (start)   Model: Tim Belknap

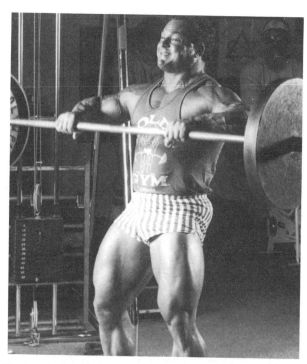

Barbell Power Clean (near finish)

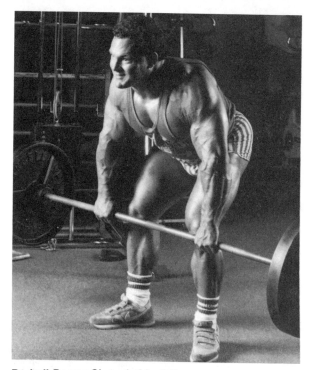

Barbell Power Clean (midpoint)

Follow this movement by an extension of your torso, bringing it to a vertical position. Finally, pull with your arms and then whip your elbows under the bar to fix it at your shoulders. As a shock absorbtion technique, you should bend your knees and dip your body about six inches as you whip the bar up to your shoulders. Lower the bar back to the floor by revers-

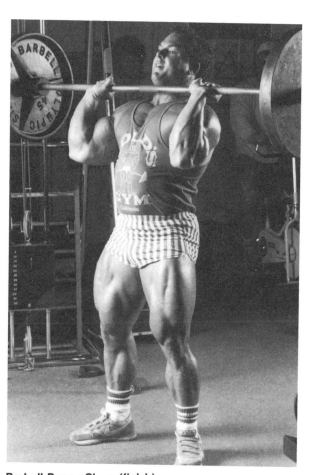

Barbell Power Clean (finish)

ing the instructions I just gave you for lifting the weight upward. Repeat the movement for the required number of repetitions.

Training Tips—With heavier weights, you will probably want to reinforce your grip with straps. I also recommend use of a lifting belt when doing all heavy back exercises, and particularly so when doing power cleans. You can also do power cleans while holding two moderately heavy dumbbells in your hands.

Barbell High Pulls

Emphasis—As with power cleans, this movement stresses virtually every skeletal muscle group in the body. But you will do it primarily as a trapezius and lower back exercise. Strong secondary stress will be placed on your biceps, brachialis, forearm flexor, thigh, and buttock muscles.

Starting Position—Place a moderately weighted barbell on the gym floor. Step up to it so your shins are touching the bar and set your feet about shoulder width apart, your toes pointed directly forward. Reach down and take a shoulder-width overgrip on the barbell. Keeping your arms straight, flatten your back and bend your knees so you assume a starting posi-

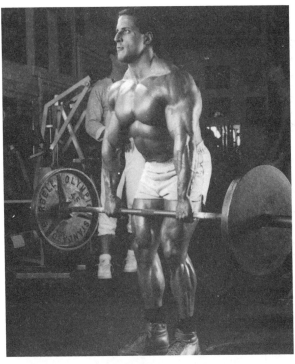

Barbell High Pull (midpoint)

tion in which your back is at an approximate 45-degree angle with the floor, your shoulders are above the level of your hips, and your hips are above the level of your knees.

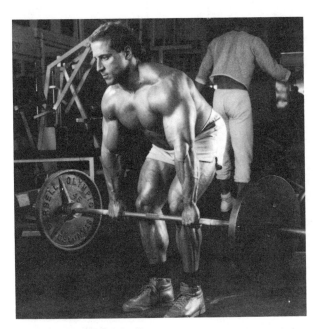

Barbell High Pull (start)

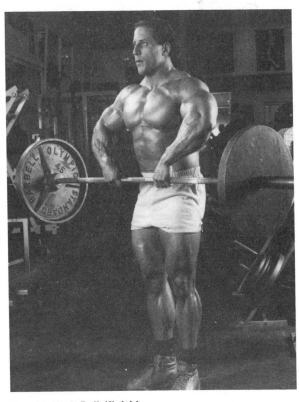

Barbell High Pull (finish)

Movement Performance—Initiate the pull from the floor by first straightening your legs. Follow this movement by an extension of your torso, bringing it into a vertical position. Finally, pull with your arms to raise the barbell to the level of your lower chest, shrugging your shoulders upward to help finish the pull. Slowly return the weight to the floor and repeat the movement for the suggested number of repetitions.

Training Tips—You will probably be able to use 25%–30% more weight in high pulls than in power cleans. As with power cleans, you can do high pulls with a pair of heavy dumbbells. Whether using a barbell or two dumbbells, you should reinforce your grip with straps and protect your lower back by wearing a weightlifting belt tightly cinched around your waist.

Barbell Shrugs

Emphasis—This is a good movement for isolating stress on your trapezius muscles. Secondary stress is borne by the forearm flexors and upper pectorals.

Starting Position—Take an overgrip about shoulder width apart on a moderately heavy barbell. Set your feet about the same distance apart, toes forward, and shins up to the bar. Flatten your back and dip your hips to assume the basic pulling position described for power cleans and high pulls. Straighten your legs and then your back to lift the weight up to a position across your upper thighs. Keep your body motionless and arms straight throughout the set. Allow the weight to pull your shoulders forward and downward as far as comfortably possible.

Movement Performance—Use trapezius strength to shrug your shoulders upward and to the rear as high as possible. Hold this peak contracted position for a moment, then slowly return to the starting point. Repeat the movement for the suggested number of repetitions.

Training Tips—To conserve strength for the actual shrugging movement, you can place the bar on a rack with the pins set 3–4 inches below

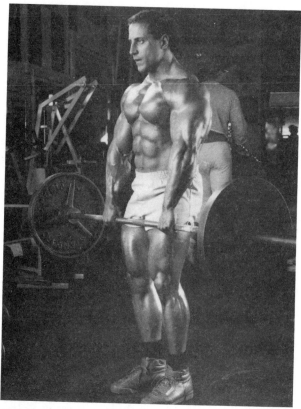

Barbell Shrugs (start)

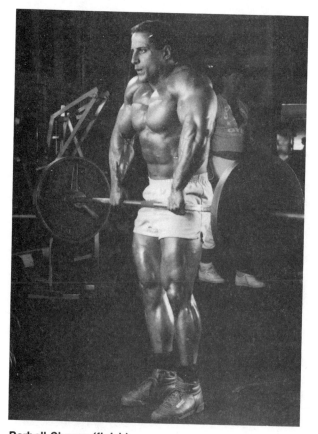

Barbell Shrugs (finish)

the position the bar would be when held across the upper thighs, then load up the bar for your set. You should wear lifting straps and a weightlifting belt when utilizing heavy weights for this movement. For different effects on your traps, you should experiment with varying grip widths.

Dumbbell Shrugs

Emphasis—As with barbell shrugs, this is an excellent way to isolate stress on your trapezius muscles. Secondary emphasis in on the forearm flexors and upper pectorals.

Starting Position—Grasp two moderately heavy dumbbells lying on the floor, set your feet about shoulder width apart between the dumbbells, assume the correct pulling position, and lift the weights upward to hang at straight arms' length at the sides of your thighs as you stand erect. Allow the weights to pull

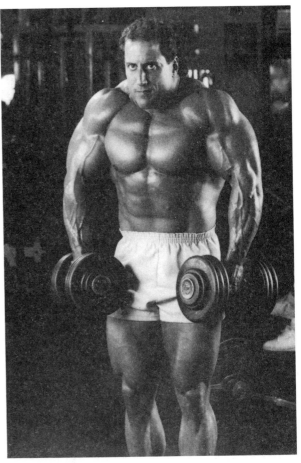

Dumbbell Shrugs (finish)

your shoulders as far downward and forward as possible.

Movement Performance—Use trapezius strength to shrug your shoulders as high and as far to the rear as possible. Hold this peak-contracted position for a moment, then lower the dumbbells back to the starting point. Repeat the movement for an appropriate number of repetitions. Return the weights to the gym floor at the end of your set.

Training Tips—Use straps and a lifting belt when using maximum poundages. You can also do a movement with dumbbells called rotating shoulder shrugs. In this exercise you start in the same position, but shrug your shoulders straight upward as high as possible, then move them directly to the rear, then lower them directly downward, and finally move them forward to the starting point. You can also move the dumbbells in reverse when doing rotating shoulder shrugs.

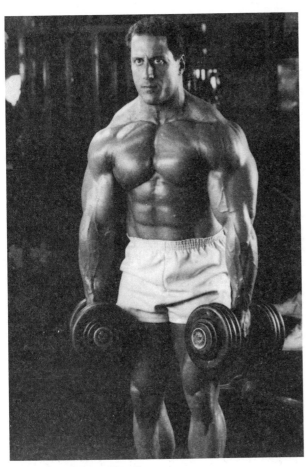

Dumbbell Shrugs (start)

Universal Shrugs

Emphasis—As with all types of shrugs, this is a good way to isolate stress on your trapezius muscles. Secondary emphasis is on the forearm flexors and upper pectorals.

Starting Position—Stand between the handles of the bench press station of a Universal Gym, facing toward the weight stack. Keeping your arms straight throughout your set, reach down and take an overgrip on the middle of each handle. You will have to bend a bit forward at the waist to do this. Stand erect and allow the weight to pull your shoulders downward and forward as far as possible.

Movement Performance—Use trapezius strength to shrug your shoulders as high and as much to the rear as possible. Return to the starting point and repeat the movement for the required number of repetitions.

Training Tips—If you are relatively short in stature, you may need to stand on a block of wood when you do this movement. You can perform Universal shrugs facing away from the weight stack as well, and you should wear a lifting belt and straps when using maximum poundages.

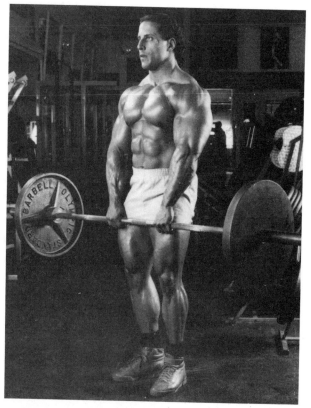

Barbell Upright Row (start)

Barbell Upright Rows

Emphasis—All types of upright rows are the best exercise for developing trapezius–deltoid tie-ins. Upright rows are an excellent trapezius muscle stressor and also place direct stress on the medial and posterior deltoids. Secondary emphasis is on the anterior delts, biceps, brachialis muscles, and forearm flexors.

Starting Position—Load a barbell lying on the gym floor with a moderate weight. Take a narrow overgrip in the middle of the bar (4–6 inches of space should be showing between your index fingers). Set your feet about shoulder width apart and stand erect with your arms straight down at your sides and the barbell resting in your hands across your upper thighs.

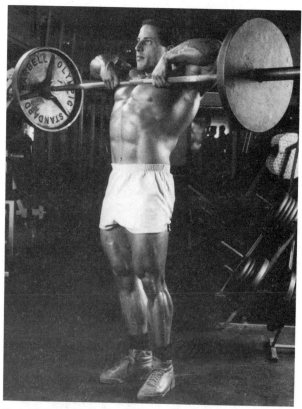

Barbell Upright Row (finish)

Movement Performance—Keeping your elbows above the level of your hands throughout the movement, slowly pull the barbell straight upward 1-2 inches away from your torso until the backs of your hands touch the underside of your chin. Your shoulders should be pulled back in the finish position, and your elbows *must* be well above the level of your hands. Slowly reverse the movement to return the barbell to the starting position. Repeat the movement for the desired number of repetitions.

Training Tips—You can vary the width of your grip on the bar, the wider your grip, however, the less the movement stresses the traps, and the more it bombs the medial delts.

Cable Upright Rows

Emphasis—As with barbell upright rows, this is a great movement for building trap-delt tie-ins. Primary stress is on the trapezius and medial-posterior deltoids. Secondary stress is placed on the anterior delts, biceps, brachialis muscles, and forearm flexors.

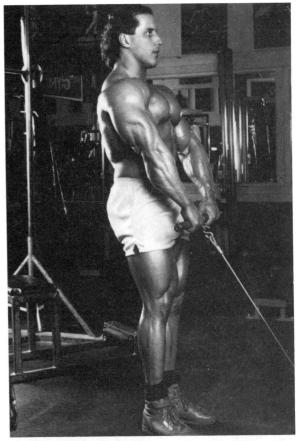

Cable Upright Row (start)

Starting Position—Attach a straight bar handle to the end of a cable running through a floor pulley. Take a narrow overgrip on the handle (4-6 inches of space should be showing between your index fingers), set your feet about shoulder width apart, and stand erect with your arms straight down at your sides and the bar resting in your hands across your upper thighs. Your toes should be about six inches from the pulley when you are in the correct starting position.

Movement Performance—Being sure that your elbows are above the level of your hands at all times, slowly pull the pulley handle directly upward 1-2 inches from your torso until the backs of your hands touch the underside of your chin. At the top point of the movement, your shoulders should be rotated to the rear and your elbows *must* be well above the level of your hands. Reverse the procedure to slowly return the handle to the starting point. Repeat the movement for the suggested number of reps.

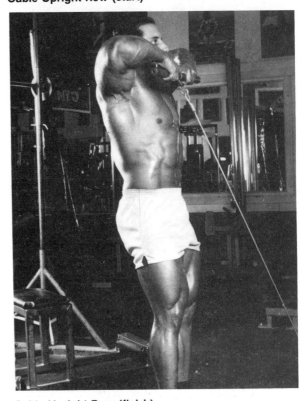

Cable Upright Row (finish)

Training Tips—Never allow the weight in any type of upright row to fall quickly back to the starting point, because that will cause you to miss out on about 50% of the benefit the movement should be giving you. On cable upright rows, you can experiment with various grip widths on the pulley handle.

Dumbbell Upright Rows

Emphasis—As with barbell and cable upright rows, this is a great movement for building trap-delt tie-ins. Primary stress is on the trapezius and medial-posterior deltoids. Secondary stress is on the anterior delts, biceps, brachialis muscles, and forearm flexors.

Starting Position—Grasp two moderately heavy dumbbells, set your feet about shoulder width apart, and stand erect with your arms straight down at your sides. Move the dumbbells to a position across your upper thighs, your palms facing toward the rear.

Movement Performance—Keeping your elbows above the level of your hands throughout the movement, slowly pull the dumbbells directly upward to shoulder level. Reverse the movement and slowly lower the weights back to the starting point. Repeat the movement for the correct number of repetitions.

Training Tips—You can pull the dumbbells upward along a wide variety of arcs, each of which hits your traps and delts a bit differently. This is an advantage when you have some minor shoulder soreness, because you can pick the arc that yields the least pain.

Dumbbell Bent Laterals

Emphasis—Although most bodybuilders do this movement for their posterior deltoids, it is also an excellent exercise for the entire trapezius muscle complex.

Starting Position—Grasp two light dumbbells, set your feet about shoulder width apart, and bend over so your torso is held parallel to the floor throughout your set. In the starting position, your arms should be hanging downward from your shoulders, your hands rotated so your palms face each other. Bend your arms a few degrees and keep them rounded like this throughout your set. Press the dumbbells together directly beneath your chest.

Movement Performance—Use shoulder and upper back strength to raise the dumbbells slowly in semicircular arcs directly out to the sides until they are slightly above the level of your shoulders. Reverse the movement and slowly return the weights to the starting point. Repeat the movement for the suggested number of reps.

Training Tips—You can also do this exercise with two floor pulleys, the cables crossed beneath your torso. Whether using a pair of dumbbells or the floor pulleys, be certain that you raise your arms directly to the sides. Raising the weights even a couple of inches to the rear will decrease stress on the posterior delts and trapezius and increase involvement of the latissimus dorsi muscles.

Deadlifts

Emphasis—This is one of the best movements for building terrific back muscle mass and overall body power. Direct stress is placed on the spinal erectors, buttocks, quadriceps, forearm flexors, and trapezius muscles. Secondary stress is on virtually every other skeletal muscle group, but particularly the remaining muscles of the back and the hamstrings.

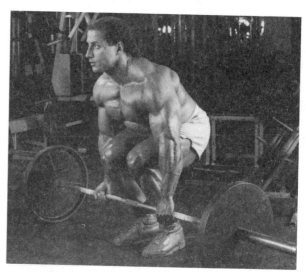

Deadlift (start)

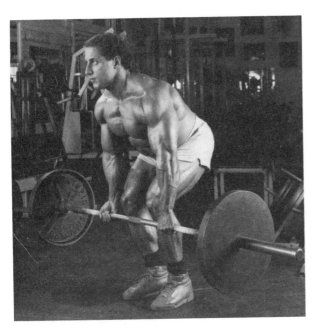

Deadlift (midpoint)

Starting Position—Load up a heavy barbell lying on the gym floor. Set your feet about shoulder width apart, toes pointing straight ahead and shins touching the bar. Bend over and take a shoulder-width overgrip on the bar. Keep your arms straight throughout the movement. Flatten your back and dip your hips to assume the correct pulling position in which your shoulders are above the level of your hips and your hips above the level of your knees.

Movement Performance—Lift the barbell from the floor to a position resting across your upper thighs by first straightening your legs and then extending your torso, so you are standing erect with your arms straight down at your sides and the bar across your upper thighs. Reverse the movement to slowly return the barbell back along the same arc to the floor. Repeat the movement for the desired number of reps.

Training Tips—With heavy weights, you should wear a lifting belt. You can either reinforce your grip with straps, or reverse your grip on the bar (hold it with one palm facing the rear and one facing forward). Be sure your shoulders are pulled back when you are in the top position of the movement. You can also do deadlifts while holding a heavy pair of dumbbells in your hands.

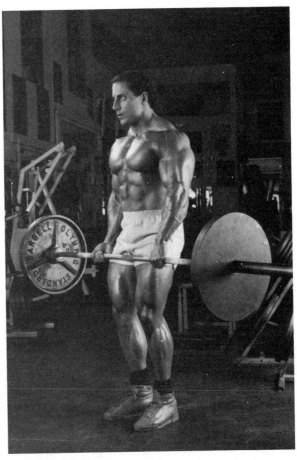

Deadlift (finish)

Stiff-Legged Deadlifts

Emphasis—This great all-around exercise places direct stress on the hamstrings, glutes, and spinal erectors. Strong secondary stress is on the remaining back muscles and the forearm flexors.

Starting Position—In order to increase the range of motion, this exercise is normally performed while standing on a flat exercise bench or thick block of wood. Your feet should be placed fairly close to each other, toes pointed directly forward. Take a shoulder-width overgrip on the barbell. Stand erect and keep both your arms and legs completely straight throughout the movement.

Movement Performance—Slowly bend forward at the waist and lower the barbell down until it touches either your toes or the bench/block right in front of your toes. Reverse the procedure and slowly return to the starting

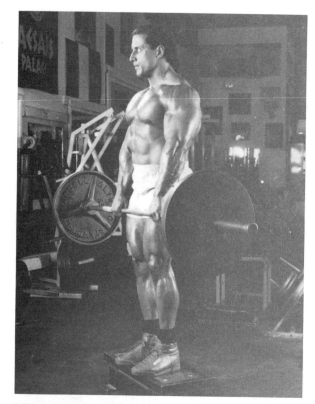

Stiff-Legged Deadlift (start)

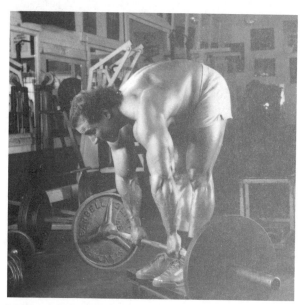

Stiff-Legged Deadlift (finish)

will be inconvenient to wear a lifting belt when doing this exercise, but you can reinforce your grip with straps if you feel it necessary. As with deadlifts, you can do stiff-legged deadlifts with a pair of heavy dumbbells held in your hands.

Hyperextensions

Emphasis—This exercise places direct stress on the hamstrings, glutes, and spinal erectors. Minimal secondary stress is placed on the other back muscles.

Starting Position—Stand in the middle of a hyperextension bench facing the large pad. Lean forward and place your hips on the pad, allowing your heels to come to rest beneath the smaller pads behind you. Keep your legs

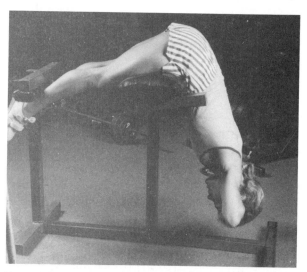

Hyperextensions (start)

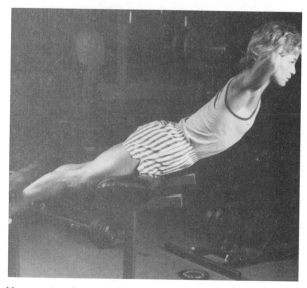

Hyperextensions (finish)

point. Repeat the movement for the desired number of repetitions.

Training Tips—When using an Olympic bar, the plates will be so large that they will touch the gym floor too early and terminate the movement short of the fullest possible range of motion. This is why you must stand on a bench or block of wood when you do the exercise. It straight for the entire set. Place your hands behind your head and neck. Allow your torso to hang directly downward from your hips.

Movement Performance—Use back, glute, and hamstrings strength to raise your torso upward in a sort of reverse sit-up, until your torso is above an imaginary line parallel with the floor. Return slowly to the starting point and repeat.

Training Tips—If you don't have a hyperextension bench, you can still do this movement with the help of a training partner. Simply lie with your legs across a high exercise bench or your kitchen table. Your partner can restrain your legs by pushing down on your ankles, allowing you to do the exercise. For added resistance, you can hold a loose barbell plate or two behind your head and neck as you do the movement.

Good Mornings

Emphasis—This movement stresses the spinal erectors, glutes, and hamstrings, with minimum stress on the other back muscles.

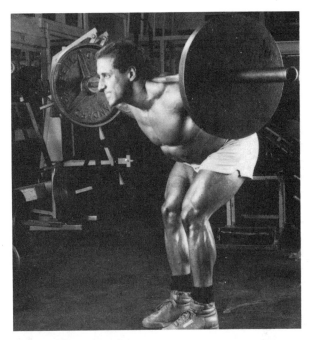

Good Mornings (finish)

Starting Position—Lift a light barbell up to a position across your shoulders behind your neck, and balance it in this position by grasping the bar out near the plates. Set your feet about shoulder width apart, toes angled straight ahead, and stand erect. Hold your legs straight throughout the movement.

Movement Performance—Slowly bend forward at the waist until your torso is slightly below a position parallel with the floor. Slowly reverse the procedure and return to the starting point. Repeat the movement for the required number of repetitions.

Training Tips—If you feel that the bar is cutting into your spinal bones behind your neck, you should pad the bar with a towel.

Barbell Bent Rows

Emphasis—This exercise places major stress on the lats, traps, posterior, deltoids, biceps, brachialis, and forearm flexor muscles. Secondary stress is borne by the remaining back muscles.

Starting Position—Take a shoulder-width overgrip on a barbell, set your feet about shoulder width apart, bend your legs slightly, keep your arms straight, and arch your back up

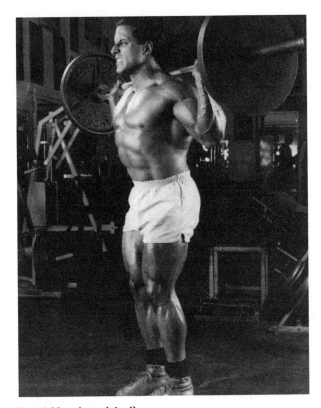

Good Mornings (start)

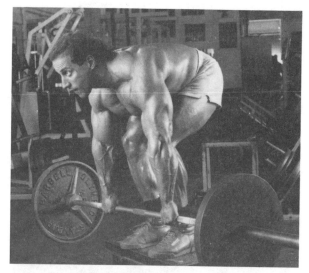

Barbell Bent Rows (start)

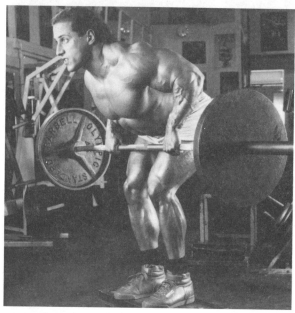

Barbell Bent Rows (finish)

sufficiently to raise the barbell just clean off the floor.

Movement Performance—Keeping your elbows back, slowly pull the barbell from straight arms' length directly upward to touch your lower ribcage. Reverse the movement to slowly return the barbell to the starting position. Repeat the movement for the suggested number of repetitions.

Training Tips—When you are using an Olympic bar, you might need to stand on a flat exercise bench or thick block of wood to foster a

complete range of motion on the exercise. This movement can also be performed resting your head on a high exercise bench, a variation particularly valuable when you are experiencing some lower-back soreness. Regardless of the variation, you can vary the width of your grip from one as narrow as having both hands touching in the middle of the bar to one as wide as the length of the bar will permit.

Bench Rows

Emphasis—Very similar to barbell bent rows, this movement places intense stress on the lats, traps, rear delts, biceps, brachialis muscles, and forearm flexors.

Starting Position—Lie facedown on a high, flat exercise bench and take a shoulder-width undergrip on a moderately heavy barbell. (You might need a training partner to hand the bar to you.) Straighten your arms, being sure that the bench is high enough to allow the plates to be clear of the floor in the correct starting position.

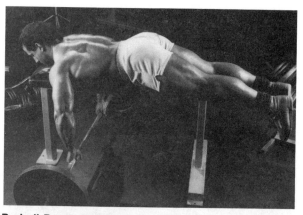

Barbell Bench Rows (start)

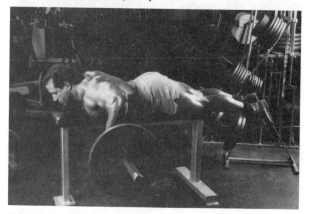

Barbell Bench Rows (finish)

Movement Performance—Keeping your elbows back, slowly pull the barbell from straight arms' length directly upward until it touches the under side of the bench just beneath your lower ribcage. Reverse the movement to slowly return the barbell to the starting point. Repeat the movement for an appropriate number of repetitions.

Training Tips—To involve a bit more trapezius action, you can raise the head end of the bench a few inches. You should also experiment with various grip widths.

Dumbbell Bent Rows

Emphasis—Bent rows performed with dumbbells place intense stress on the lats, traps, rear delts, biceps, brachialis, and forearm flexor muscles. Secondary stress is placed on the remaining back muscles.

Starting Position—Grasp two moderately weighted dumbbells, set your feet about shoulder width apart, unlock your legs slightly, and bend over until your torso is parallel with the floor. Your arms should be dangling straight down from your shoulders, your palms facing either the rear or inward toward each other.

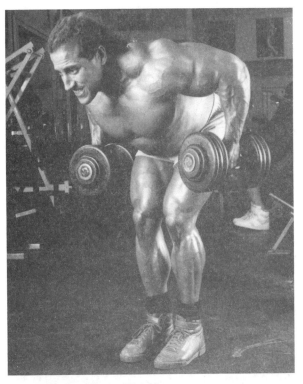

Dumbbell Bent Rows (finish)

Movement Performance—Keeping your elbows back, slowly pull the dumbbells directly upward until the inner plates of each dumbbell contact the sides of your torso. Reverse the movement to slowly lower the dumbbells back to the starting point. Repeat.

Training Tips—You can brace your head on a high, flat exercise bench to relieve stress from your lower back. You might also experiment with pulling the dumbbells upward along different arcs.

One-Arm Dumbbell Bent Rows

Emphasis—As with most rowing movements, one-arm dumbbell bent rows place direct stress on the lats, traps, rear, delts, biceps, brachialis, and forearm flexor muscles. Secondary stress is on the rest of the back muscles.

Starting Position—Place a moderately heavy dumbbell on the gym floor next to a flat exercise bench. Grasp the weight in your left hand and place your right hand on the bench to brace your torso in a position parallel with the floor throughout your set. Place your right foot for-

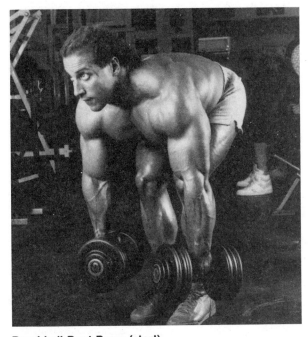

Dumbbell Bent Rows (start)

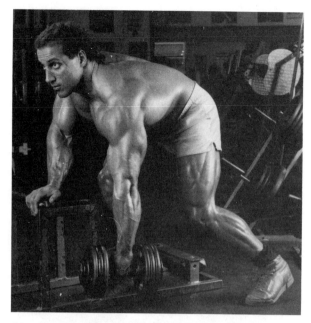

One-Arm Dumbbell Bent Rows (start—note alternative position in which both feet rest on floor)

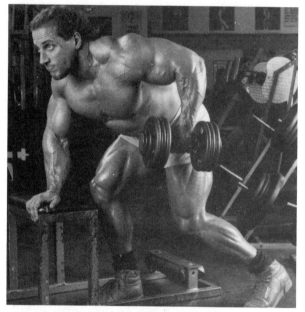

One-Arm Dumbbell Bent Rows (finish)

ward and left foot to the rear, straighten your arm, and raise the dumbbell one or two inches from the floor.

Movement Performance—Keeping your elbow back, slowly pull the dumbbell upward until its inner plates touch the side of your torso. In this position, you should rotate your left shoulder upward. Reverse the movement and return the dumbbell slowly to the starting point. Repeat the movement for the suggested number of

repetitions. Be sure to reverse your body position and do an equal number of sets and reps with your right arm.

Training Tips—Many bodybuilders currently prefer to perform this movement with the knee of the inside leg set on a bench. You can also do one-arm dumbbell bent rows without the bench, merely placing your nonexercising hand on its corresponding knee.

T-Bar Rows

Emphasis—This is one of the best full-back exercises in that it places direct stress on the traps, lats, and erectors in conjunction with the rear delts, biceps, brachialis, and forearm flexor muscles.

Starting Position—Stand on the small platforms provided on either side of the T-bar. With your legs slightly bent to remove stress from

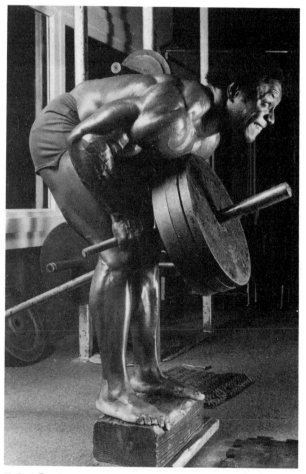

T-Bar Rows

your lower back, bend over and grasp the handles of the T-bar. (There are several different types of handles, and the one that provides a parallel-hands grip is better than one on which you must take an overgrip.) Arch your back sufficiently enough so that the bar and its plates are free from the floor when your arms are held straight.

Movement Performance—Without allowing your torso to cheat upward, slowly bend your arms and pull the T-bar up until either it or its plates touch your chest. Lower slowly back to the starting point, and repeat the movement for the desired number of repetitions.

Training Tips—On many T-bar apparati, it is best to use small-diameter plates, which increases the range of motion of the exercise. If you don't have a T-bar, you can improvise one by placing the end of a bar (unloaded) in the corner of a gym, loading up the other end, and grasping the loaded end of the bar with your fingers interlaced.

Seated Pulley Rows

Emphasis—This is another great full-back exercise. It places direct stress on the traps, lats, erectors, biceps, brachialis, and forearm flexor muscles.

Starting Position—There are several different types of handles which you can attach to the end of a cable running through a floor pulley. The best one allows a parallel-hands grip with your hands relatively close together. Grasp the handle, place your feet against the stop bar at the end of the machine seat toward the pulley, and sit down on the seat. Your legs should be slightly bent throughout your set to keep harmful stress off your lower back. Straighten your arms completely and lean toward the pulley to completely stretch your lats.

Movement Performance—Simultaneously sit erect and pull the handle toward your lower ribcage, being sure to keep your elbows in close to your sides. As the handle touches your lower ribcage or upper abdomen, be sure to arch your back to fully contract your lats. Slowly reverse

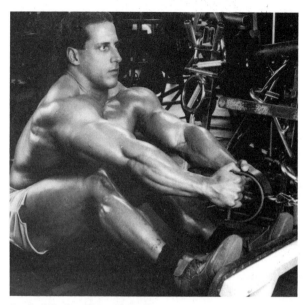

Seated Pulley Rows (start)

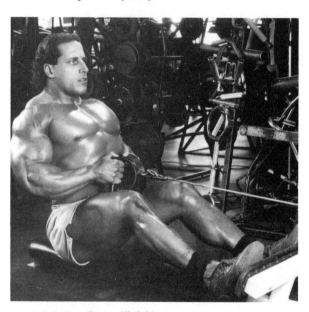

Seated Pulley Rows (finish)

the procedure and return to the starting point. Repeat the movement for an appropriate number of repetitions.

Training Tips—There is also a handle which allows you to take a shoulder-width, parallel-hands grip, as well as a straight bar handle on which you can assume an overgrip or undergrip. While most bodybuilders tend to prefer a low pulley for this movement you will also find a high pulley (one set at 3-4 feet from the floor) to be quite beneficial when used to develop your back muscles.

Standing One-Arm Low-Pulley Rows

Emphasis—This is a good exercise for the lower lats, which are ordinarily difficult to build up. The exercise stresses the lats, rear delts, biceps, brachialis, and forearm flexor muscles.

Starting Position—Attach a loop handle to the end of a cable running through a floor pulley. Grasp the handle in your right hand and step back 2½–3 feet from the low pulley. Extend your right leg toward the pulley and bend it at about a 30-degree angle. Extend your left leg away from the pulley and keep it relatively straight. Rest your right hand on your right knee and extend your left arm toward the pulley.

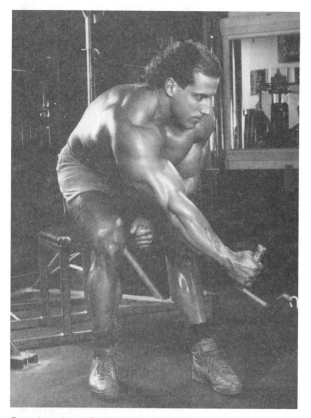

One-Arm Low-Pulley Rows (start)

Movement Performance—Starting with your palm facing the floor, slowly pull your hand in to touch the side of your waist, simultaneously rotating your hand so your palm is facing upward at the end of the movement. Reverse the movement and slowly return the handle to the

starting point. Be sure that you do an equal number of sets and repetitions with each arm.

Training Tips—You can also do this movement with two hands at once in a standing position, facing directly toward the pulley and grasping the handle with both hands, fingers interlaced.

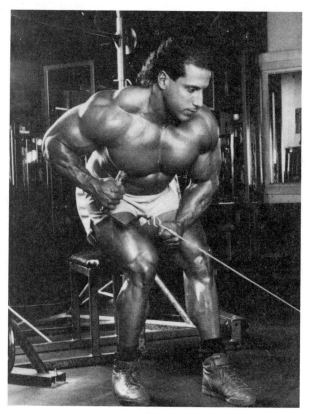

One-Arm Low-Pulley Rows (finish)

Nautilus Rowing Machine

Emphasis—This is a good isolation movement for the lats and lower traps, as well as for the rear deltoids.

Starting Position—Sit in the machine facing away from the weight stack, and force your arms between the vertical roller pads, arms parallel with the floor. The outsides of your forearms should be resting against these pads.

Movement Performance—Use back and deltoid strength to move your elbows (and hence the roller pads) directly to the rear in as complete a motion as possible. Hold the peak-contracted position for a moment, then return slowly to the starting point. Repeat.

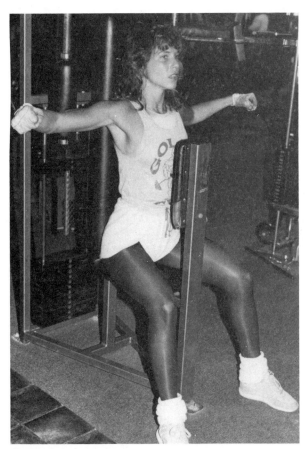

Nautilus Row Machine

Training Tips—This movement can also be performed with one arm at a time, a practice that fosters somewhat more complete mental concentration on the working muscles.

Nautilus Pullover Machine

Emphasis—This movement places intense stress on the lats and other upper back muscles which impart rotational stress to the scapulae. Significant secondary stress is placed on the pectorals, deltoids, and upper abdominals.

Starting Position—Sit in the machine and adjust the height of the seat so that your shoulder joints are on the same level as the rotational centers of the machine's pulley cams. Fasten the seat belt over your lap. Push down on the foot pedal to bring the lever arm forward enough so you can place your elbows against the pads attached to it. You can grasp the metal part of the lever arm with your hands to keep them occupied. Release the pedal and allow the

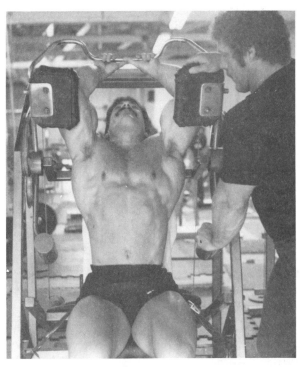

Nautilus Pullover (start)

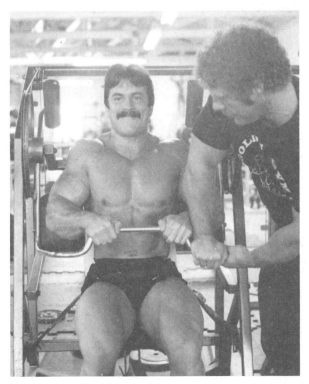

Nautilus Pullover (finish)

weight of the machine to pull your elbows upward and backward as far as is comfortably possible. Release the pedal. Use torso strength to push with your elbows against the pads, moving the lever arm in a large semicircular arc until its crossbar contacts your waist. Hold this peak-contracted position for a slow count of two, then slowly return back along the same arc to the starting point. Repeat the movement for the listed number of repetitions.

Training Tips—You can easily give yourself forced reps by pushing with your feet on the pedal just enough to boost yourself past a normal sticking point toward the end of the downward path of the machine lever arm.

Nautilus Behind Neck Machine

Emphasis—This unique machine isolates intense stress on the lats and other upper back muscles which impart rotational stress to the scapulae. Secondary stress is borne by the deltoids, particularly the posterior head of the muscle complex.

Starting Position—Adjust the seat height so your shoulder joints are at the same level as the pivot points of the cams when you sit in the seat. Sit down and fasten the lap belt around your waist. Extend your arms straight upward and force them between the two horizontal roller pads. Your elbows should be against the pads and your palms should be facing forward throughout your set.

Movement Performance—Use upper-back-muscle strength to push with your elbows

against the pads, moving them outward and downward in semicircular arcs to as low a position as humanly possible. Hold this peak-contracted position for a moment, then return slowly back to the starting point. Repeat for the desired number of repetitions.

Training Tips—If you really want to strengthen your lats, try doing burns in the finish position of the movement, doing reps about 6–8 inches long toward the bottom point of the exercise.

Chins

Emphasis—This is the most basic exercise for adding width to the lats. It places intense stress on your lats, posterior deltoids, biceps, brachialis, and forearm flexor muscles.

Starting Position—Jump up and take an overgrip on a chinning bar with your hands set 3–5 inches wider on each side than your shoulders. Straighten your arms completely to stretch your lats. Bend your legs at 90-degree angles and cross your ankles.

Movement Performance—Use latissimus dorsi and arm strength to pull yourself slowly upward until your chin is above the level of the bar. Be sure that you concentrate on pulling your elbows both downward and to the rear on each rep. And it is essential that you arch your back as much as possible in the top position of the movement. Slowly lower yourself back to the starting point, and repeat the movement for an appropriate number of repetitions.

Training Tips—The movement just described is usually called front chins, and it stresses the lower and middle lats most intensely. You can also do chins behind the neck, in which you pull yourself up to touch the bar to your traps behind your neck, and this movement stresses the upper lats most intensely. You can use a wider or more narrow grip on your chins, but the wider grip actually reduces the range of motion of the movement, thereby robbing you of some of the stress you should be receiving from the exercise.

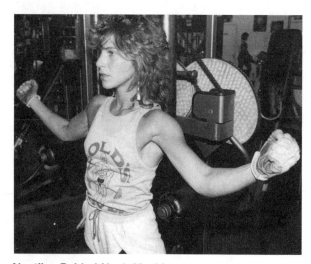

Nautilus Behind Neck Machine

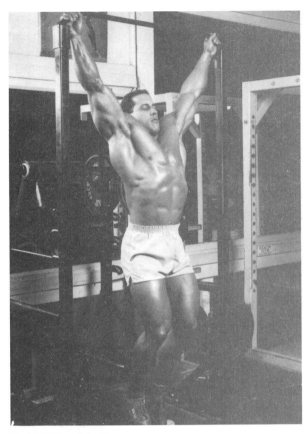

Front Chins (start)

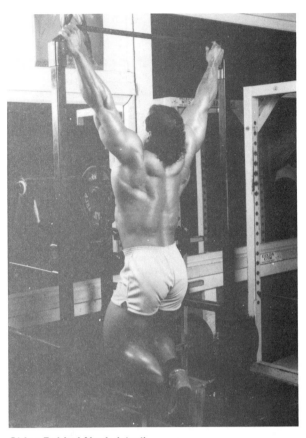

Chins Behind Neck (start)

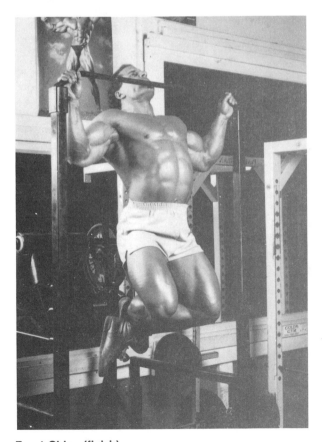

Front Chins (finish)

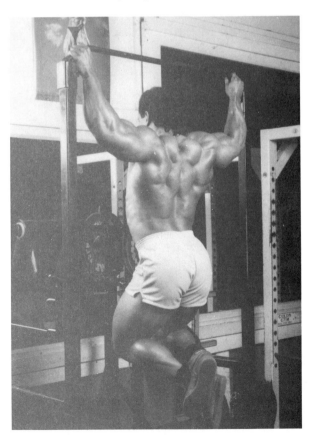

Chins Behind Neck (near finish)

V-Bar Chins

Emphasis—Often called close-grip chins, this movement is excellent for stressing the whole latissimus dorsi complex, particularly the upper part of the muscle group. Strong secondary stress is borne by the posterior and medial deltoids, biceps, brachialis, and forearm flexor muscles.

Starting Position—Place the V-bar over the middle of a chinning bar. This apparatus allows you to take a narrow parallel-hand grip for your chins. Jump up and take your grip on the handles of the V-bar. Straighten your arms completely to fully stretch your lats. Bend your legs at 90-degree angles and cross your ankles.

Movement Performance—Lean back throughout the movement and slowly pull yourself up to the bar, touching your chest to the handle with your back completely arched. Lower slowly back to the starting point and repeat the movement for the suggested number of repetitions.

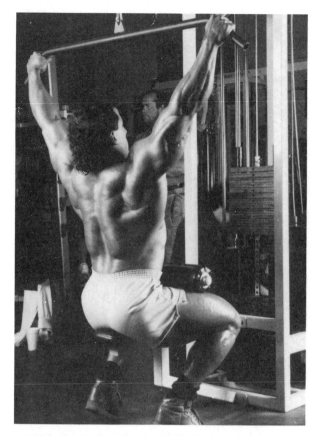

Lat Machine Pulldowns (start for both front and behind-neck variations)

Lat Machine Pulldowns

Emphasis—This movement is very similar to chins, in that it places intense stress on the lats (particularly in terms of width enhancement), rear delts, biceps, brachialis, and forearm flexor muscles.

Starting Position—There are several different types of handles which you can attach to the end of a cable running through a floor pulley. The narrow, parallel-hands handle used for pulley rows can also be used for pulldowns, as can the handle which gives a shoulder-width parallel-hands grip. But for purposes of this exercise description, let's use a long bar handle. Take an overgrip on the handle with your hands set 3–5 inches wider than your shoulders on each side. Straighten your arms fully and wedge your knees under the restraint bar provided. If there is no such bar, you can either sit or kneel on the gym floor and have a training partner restrain your body by pushing down on your trapezius muscles on either side of your head.

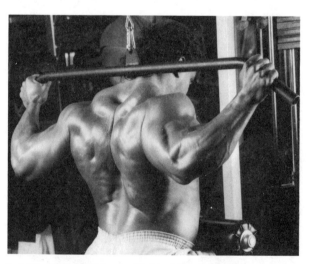

Lat Machine Pulldowns Behind Neck (finish)

Movement Performance—Arching your back and being sure to keep your elbows back during the movement, slowly pull the bar down to touch the upper part of your chest. Slowly return the bar to the starting point and repeat the movement for the desired number of repetitions.

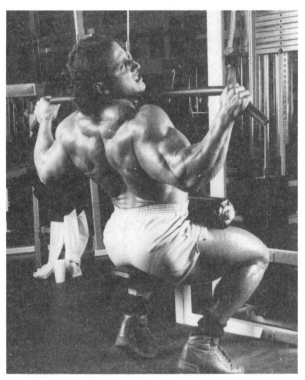

Lat Machine Front Pulldowns (finish)

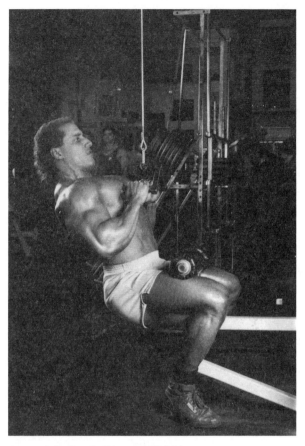

Close-Grip Lat Pulldowns (finish)

Training Tips—As with chins, you can do pulldowns behind your neck. You should also experiment with every available handle to attach to the end of the cable. If you use every available variation of this movement, you will actually have more than 10 distinct exercises.

Bent-Arm Pullovers

Emphasis—This is a very direct latissimus dorsi exercise which also places intense stress on the pectorals and serratus muscles. Secondary stress is on the other upper-back muscles which impart rotational force to the scapulae, plus the deltoids, particularly the posterior aspect of that muscle group.

Starting Position—Take a narrow overgrip in the middle of the barbell handle (there should be about six inches of space showing between your index fingers). Lie back on a flat exercise bench with the bar resting across your chest and your head hanging off the end of the bench.

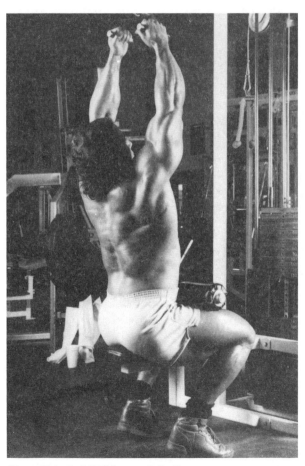

Close-Grip Lat Pulldowns (start)

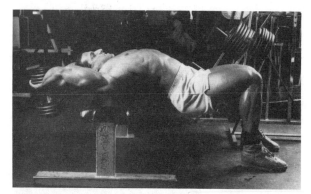

Bent-Arm Pullovers (bottom position)

Movement Performance—Keeping your elbows as close to each other as possible throughout the movement, slowly lower the barbell to the rear and downward in a semicircular arc to as low a position as possible. Return slowly back along the same arc to the starting point, and repeat the movement for the required number of repetitions.

Training Tips—With heavy weights you will find it difficult to stay on the bench. If this is the case, you should have a training partner restrain you by pushing down on your knees as you do a heavy set. Be very careful that you never allow your elbows to flare out to the sides as you do this movement, because this will put you in a weak mechanical position and you could easily injure your shoulder.

Cross-Bench Dumbbell Pullovers

Emphasis—Like bent-arm pullovers, this movement places direct and intense stress on

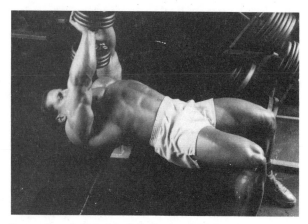

Cross-Bench Dumbbell Pullovers (start)

the lats, pecs, and serratus muscles. Secondary stress is on the other upper back muscles which impart rotational force to the scapulae, plus the deltoids, particularly the posterior aspect of that muscle group.

Starting Position—Place a moderately heavy dumbbell on end at the end of a flat exercise bench. Lie on your back across the bench, with your upper back and shoulders in contact with the bench surface. Your feet should be set a comfortable distance apart on the gym floor to balance your body on the bench. Reach over and place your palms against the underside of the top set of plates, being careful to encircle the dumbbell handle with your thumbs. Raise the dumbbell up to straight arms' length above your chest.

Movement   Performance—Simultaneously bend your arms about 20 degrees and lower the dumbbell in a semicircular arc to the rear and downward to as low a position as is comfortably possible. Return the dumbbell back along the same arc to the starting point, then repeat the movement. You should inhale as you lower the weight and exhale as you raise it back to the starting point.

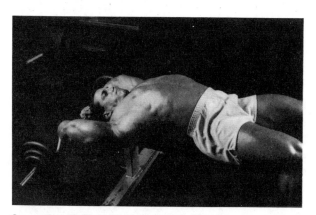

Cross-Bench Dumbbell Pullovers (finish)

Training Tips—To get a longer range of motion, you should dip your hips 4–6 inches as the dumbbell reaches the bottom point of the exercise. You can also do this dumbbell pullover lying lengthwise on the bench, but that isn't quite as good a movement as the cross-bench version.

Stiff-Arm Lat Pulldowns

Emphasis—The effect of this exercise is similar to that of the various pullover movements just discussed. Direct and intense stress is placed on the lats, pecs, and serratus muscles. Secondary stress is on the other upper-back muscles which impart rotational force to the scapulae, plus the deltoids, particularly the posterior aspect of that muscle group.

Starting Position—Attach a bar handle to the end of a cable running through an overhead pulley. Take a narrow overgrip on the handle (your index fingers should be about 6 inches apart). Set your feet about shoulder width apart 1–1½ feet back from the pulley. Bend your arms

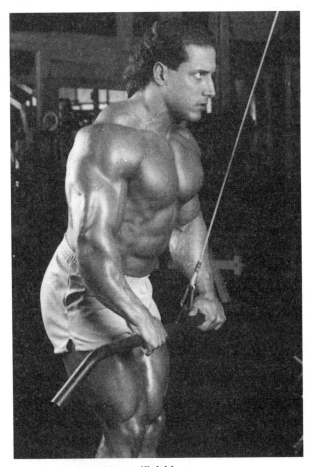

Stiff-Arm Lat Pulldown (finish)

about 10 degrees and hold them rounded like this throughout the movement. Bend slightly forward at the waist and maintain this torso lean throughout your set. At the start of the movement, your arms should be extended upward toward the pulley and at least at a 45-degree angle with the floor (ideally, however, they should be vertical at the starting point of the movement).

Movement Performance—Use torso muscle strength to move the handle forward and downward in a semicircular arc, until your hands and the bar touch your upper thighs. Return the bar slowly back along the same arc to the starting point. Repeat the movement for the correct number of repetitions.

Training Tips—You can also use a rope handle, short bar handle, or webbing-loop handle for this movement. You can also do the exercise while kneeling on the floor of the gym.

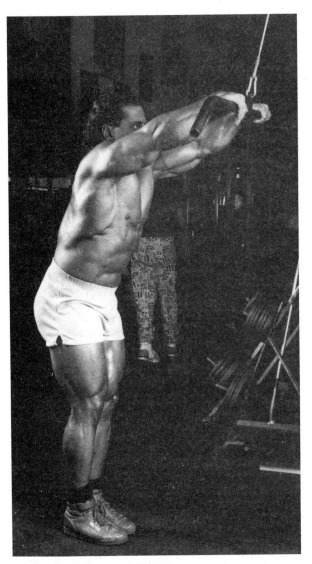

Stiff-Arm Lat Pulldown (start)

Pulley Crunches

Emphasis—As a back movement, this exercise stresses the lower lats very intensely and the remainder of the upper-back muscles which impart rotational force to the scapulae. Primary stress is also borne by the pectorals, serratus, intercostals, and rectus abdominis muscles.

Starting Position—Attach a rope or webbing-loop handle to the end of a cable running through a floor pulley. Grasp the handle with your hands parallel to each other. Kneel down about 1½–2 feet back from the pulley and extend your arms directly up toward the pulley.

Movement   Performance—Simultaneously bend forward at the waist, execute a small pull-over motion with your hands, and exhale forcefully. In the bottom position of the movement, your forehead should touch the floor and your fists should be touching the floor about 4–6 inches in front of your head as well. Return slowly to the starting point and repeat the movement for the suggested number of reps.

Training Tips—This exercise can also be executed twisting alternately from one side to the other, an exercise which places more intense stress on the intercostals. You can also do pulley crunches with one arm at a time, being sure to do the same number of sets and reps with each arm. (This exercise was illustrated on page 193).

SUGGESTED BACK ROUTINES

Virtually anyone who has read this far in the book will be well past the beginning and intermediate stages of development and training experience. Still, there will be a few less-experienced trainees reading this chapter, so I have included a series of routines in this section, which can be used by beginners, intermediates, and more advanced bodybuilders. Be sure to change to the next highest routine after you have spent 4–6 weeks on the current program.

BEGINNING ROUTINE

Exercise	Sets	Reps
Barbell Bent Rows	2–3	8–12
Front Lat Pulldowns	2–3	8–12

I don't recommend doing direct trapezius or spinal erector movements to beginners.

LOW-INTERMEDIATE ROUTINE

Exercise	Sets	Reps
Barbell Shrugs	2–3	10–15
Seated Pulley Rows	3	8–12
Pulldowns Behind Neck	3	8–12

HIGH-INTERMEDIATE ROUTINE

Exercise	Sets	Reps
Upright Rows	3	8–12
Hyperextensions	2–3	10–15
One-Arm Dumbbell Bent Rows	4	8–12
Parallel-Grip Front Pulldowns	3	8–12

LOW-ADVANCED ROUTINE

Exercise	Sets	Reps
{ Good Mornings	3–4	10–15
{ Rotating Dumbbell Shrugs	3–4	10–15
Front Chins	3	8–12
Nautilus Rows	3	8–12
Seated Pulley Rows	3	8–12

First two exercises are supersetted.

HIGH-ADVANCED ROUTINE

Exercise	Sets	Reps
{ Universal Shrugs	4	10–15
{ Stiff-Legged Deadlifts	4	10–15
Chins Behind Neck	4	8–12
Seated Pulley Rows	4	8–12
Nautilus Pullovers	2–3	10–15

OFF-SEASON CONTEST-LEVEL ROUTINE

Exercise	Sets	Reps
Barbell Shrugs	4–5	10–15
Stiff-Legged Deadlifts	4–5	10–15
V-Bar Chins	4	8–12
One-Arm Dumbbell Bent Rows	4	8–12
Pulldowns Behind Neck	3	8–12
Bent-Arm Pullovers	2–3	8–12

PRECONTEST CONTEST-LEVEL ROUTINE

Exercise	Sets	Reps
{ Barbell Shrugs	2-3	10-15
{ Cable Upright Rows	2-3	10-12
Deadlifts	5	10-12
{ Chins Behind Neck	4	10-12
{ Cross-Bench Dumbbell Pullovers	4	10-12
Seated Pulley Rows	4	10-12
Front Pulldowns	4	10-12

BACK ROUTINES OF THE CHAMPS

I am giving you nearly 40 back training programs of the world's top bodybuilders as examples of how you should train this powerful and massive body part. Feel free to modify your favorite superstar's back routine to meet your unique recuperative ability between workouts. Beginning bodybuilders should do no more than 4-6 total sets of back work; intermediates, 6-8; and advanced men, 10-12 total sets.

Lee Haney

Exercise	Sets	Reps
Barbell Bent Rows	4-5	12-6
Front Lat Pulldowns	3-4	8-10
Seated Pulley Rows	3-4	8-10
Dumbbell Shrugs	3-4	10-15

Arnold Schwarzenegger

Exercise	Sets	Reps
Wide-Grip Front Chins	4-5	8-10
Pulldowns Behind Neck	4-5	8-10
Barbell Bent Rows	4-5	8-10
T-Bar Rows	4-5	8-10
Seated Pulley Rows	4-5	8-10

Samir Bannout

Exercise	Sets	Reps
Pulldowns (warm-up)	3	15-20
Seated Pulley Rows	4	15-8
Barbell Bent Rows	4	15-8
Front Chins	4	8-12

Sergio Oliva

Exercise	Sets	Reps
Wide-Grip Chins	4-6	10
Close-Grip Chins	4-5	10
{ Wide-Grip Pulldowns	4	6-8
{ Close-Grip Pulldowns	4	6-8
{ Wide-Grip Pulley Rows	3-4	6-8
{ Close-Grip Pulley Rows	3-4	6-8
{ Wide-Grip Pulldowns	3-4	6-8
{ Narrow-Grip Pulldowns	3-4	6-8
{ Deadlifts	3-4	6-8
{ Good Mornings	3-4	6-8

Frank Zane

Exercise	Sets	Reps
Top Deadlifts	5	8-10
Pulldowns Behind Neck	4	10-12
Front Lat Pulldowns	4	10-12
Seated Pulley Rows	4	10-12
One-Arm Dumbbell Bent Rows	4	10-12

Mike Mentzer

Exercise	Sets	Reps
Nautilus Behind Neck Machine	2	6-8
Lat Pulldowns	2	6-8
Seated Pulley Rows	1-2	6-8
Deadlifts	1	8-12
Hyperextensions	1	8-12
Barbell Shrugs	2	6-8

Tim Belknap

Exercise	Sets	Reps
Wide-Grip Chins	2	10
Wide-Grip Front Pulldows	3	12-15
Seated Wide-Grip Pulley Rows	3	12-15
Narrow-Grip Seated Pulley Rows	3	12-15
Nautilus Pullovers	3	10-12
Stiff-Legged Deadlifts	3	10-12
Hyperextension	3	15-25

Berry de Mey

Exercise	Sets	Reps
Wide-Grip Chins	4	8
T-Bar Rows	4	6-10
One-Arm Dumbbell Bent Rows	3	6-8
Barbell Bent Rows	3-4	6-10
Pulldowns Behind Neck	3-4	8-10

Albert Beckles

Exercise	Sets	Reps
Barbell Bent Rows	5	10–12
T-Bar Rows	5	10–12
Parallel-Grip Front Pulldowns	5	10–12
One-Arm Dumbbell Bent Rows	5	10–12
Seated Low Pulley Rows	5	10–12

Tony Pearson

Exercise	Sets	Reps
Chins	6–8	10–12
T-Bar Rows	5	8
One-Arm Dumbbell Bent Rows	5	8
Hyperextensions	3–6	10–15

Roger Walker

Exercise	Sets	Reps
{ Chins Behind Neck	5	10–12
{ Barbell Bent Rows	5	10–12
{ Seated Pulley Rows	5	10–12
{ Front Lat Pulldowns	5	10–12
T-Bar Rows	5	10–12
One-Arm Dumbbell Bent Rows	5	10–12

Chris Dickerson

TRAPEZIUS ROUTINE

Exercise	Sets	Reps
Upright Rows	3	10–12
Dumbbell Shrugs	2	12–15
Barbell Shrugs	2	10–12

LATISSIMUS DORSI ROUTINE

Exercise	Sets	Reps
Front Chins	5	10–15
One-Arm Dumbbell Bent Rows	4–6	8–10
Pulldowns Behind Neck	4	8–10
One-Arm Pulley Rows	4	8–10
Seated Pulley Rows	4	8–10

Charles Glass

Exercise	Sets	Reps
Front Chins	4–5	10–12
One-Arm Dumbbell Bent Rows	4–5	10–12
Chins Behind Neck	4–5	10–12
T-Bar Rows	4–5	10–12
Narrow Grip Lat Pulldowns	4–5	10–12
Seated Pulley Rows	4–5	10–12

Bertil Fox

Exercise	Sets	Reps
Pulldowns Behind Neck	6	8–12
Front Lat Pulldowns	6	8–12
One-Arm Dumbbell Bent Rows	6	8–12
{ Front Chins	6	8–12
{ Cross-Bench Dumbbell Pullovers	6	8–12
T-Bar Rows, or . . .		
Seated Pulley Rows	6	8–12

Tom Platz

Exercise	Sets	Reps
Wide-Grip Front Chins	8–10	10–15
T-Bar Rows	4–5	10–15
Seated Pulley Rows	4–5	10–15
Barbell Bent Rows	4–5	10–15
Cross-Bench Dumbbell Pullovers	4–5	10–15
Deadlifts	4–5	6–10

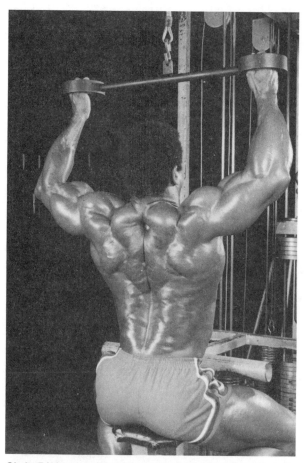

Chris Dickerson (Mr. Olympia 1982) built a great deal of width in his lats laboriously by doing thousands of sets of Lat Machine Pulldowns with a parallel-hands grip on the bar.

Lou Ferrigno

Exercise	Sets	Reps
Chins Behind Neck	4-5	10-15
Close-Grip Barbell Bent Rows	4-5	8-10
Front Chins	4-5	8-10
Seated Pulley Rows	4-5	8-10
Close-Grip Lat Pulldowns	4-5	8-10
Barbell Shrugs	4-5	10-15

Dr. Franco Columbu

Exercise	Sets	Reps
Wide-Grip Front Chins	6	10-15
T-Bar Rows	4	10
Seated Pulley Rows	4	10
{ One-Arm Dumbbell Bent Rows	3	10
{ Close-Grip Chins	3	10

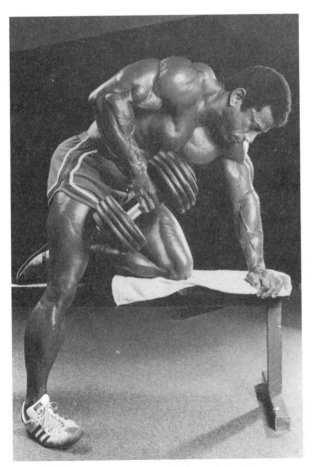

For width, Dickerson relied on all forms of Bent Rows, including the one-arm dumbbell variation. In recent years, it has become fashionable to place the knee opposite the exercise arm on the flat bench when doing the exercise. Chris is careful to keep his upper arm in close to his side in order to assert full force on his lats.

Robby Robinson

Exercise	Sets	Reps
Barbell Bent Rows	4	8-10
Seated High Pulley Rows	4	8-10
Chins Behind Neck	4	8-10
Cross-Bench Dumbbell Pullovers	4	10-15

Bronston Austin, Jr.

Exercise	Sets	Reps
Seated Pulley Rows	5-8	5-8
T-Bar Rows	5-8	5-8
Barbell Bent Rows	5-8	5-8
One-Arm Dumbbell Bent Rows	5-8	5-8
Nautilus Pullovers	5-8	5-8
Pulldowns Behind Neck	5-8	5-8

Andreas Cahling

Exercise	Sets	Reps
Front Chins	3	12-15
Pulldowns Behind Neck	2	8-12
Narrow-Grip Front Pulldowns	2	8-12
Wide-Grip Front Pulldowns	2	8-12
Reverse-Grip Pulldowns	2	8-12
Machine Rows	2	8-12

Roy Callender

Exercise	Sets	Reps
Bent-Arm Pullovers	8-10	8-10
Chins Behind Neck	6-8	8-10
Front Chins	6-8	8-10
V-Bar Chins	6-8	8-10
T-Bar Rows	6-8	8-10
One-Arm Dumbbell Bent Rows	6-8	8-10
Seated Pulley Rows	6-8	8-10

Bob Jodkiewicz

Exercise	Sets	Reps
{ Wide-Grip Chins Behind Neck	3-4	20-25
{ Cross-Bench Dumbbell Pullovers	3-4	20
{ T-Bar Rows	3-4	8-12
{ Front Lat Pulldowns	3-4	8-12
{ Seated Low Pulley Rows	3	10-12
{ Close-Grip Chins	3	10-12
Pulley Crunches	2	10-12
Barbell Shrugs	6	10-15
Hyperextensions	3	10-15
Good Mornings	3	10-15

Tony Emmott

Exercise	Sets	Reps
Barbell Shrugs	3	8-10
Hyperextensions	4	10-15
Front Chins (weighted)	4	6-8
Seated Pulley Rows	4	6-8
Pulldowns Behind Neck	4	6-8

Casey Viator

Exercise	Sets	Reps
Deadlifts	4-6	8-5
Nautilus Pullovers	4-6	10-15
Pulldown Behind Neck	4-6	10-15
One-Arm Dumbbell Bent Rows	4-6	10-15
Chins Behind Neck (weighted)	6-8	10-15
Front Chins (weighted)	6-8	10-15
Barbell Shrugs	6-8	15-20

Greg DeFerro

Exercise	Sets	Reps
{Wide-Grip Front Pulldowns	3	8-12
{Bench Rows	3	8-12
{Medium-Grip Front Pulldowns	3	10
{T-Bar Rows	3	10
Seated Low Pulley Rows	3	10
Seated High Pulley Rows	3	10
Hyperextensions	4	10-12

Steve Davis

Exercise	Sets	Reps
Wide-Grip Front Chins	5	12
Seated Pulley Rows	5	12
Cross-Bench Dumbbell Pullovers	3-4	15

Steve Michalik

Exercise	Sets	Reps
Seated Pulley Rows	10	8-10
Close-Grip Pulldowns	8-10	8-10
Nautilus Pullovers	8-10	8-10
Parallel-Grip Front Pulldowns	8-10	8-10
Seated Close-Grip Pulldowns	8-10	8-10
Dumbbell Bent Laterals	8-10	8-10

Scott Wilson

Exercise	Sets	Reps
Deadlifts	5	5
Barbell Bent Rows	5	6-8
T-Bar Rows	5	6-8
Behind Neck Pulldowns	5	8
One-Arm Dumbbell Bent Rows	5	8
Barbell Shrugs	5	8
Upright Rows	5	8

Rory Leidelmeyer

Exercise	Sets	Reps
Incline Dumbbell Pullovers	4	12
Medium-Grip Front Chins	4	max
Barbell Bent Rows	4	7-8
Seated Pulley Rows	3	7-8
Behind Neck Pulldowns	4	15

Ray Mentzer

Exercise	Sets	Reps
Seated Pulley Rows	2-3	5-8
Nautilus Behind Neck Machine	2-3	5-8
Nautilus Pullovers	1-2	5-8

Ralf Möller

Exercise	Sets	Reps
Front Chins	5-7	10-15
Seated Pulley Rows	4-5	10-15
Pulldowns Behind Neck	4-5	10-15
T-Bar Rows	4-5	10-15
One-Arm Dumbbell Bent Rows	4-5	10-15

Gary Leonard

Exercise	Sets	Reps
Wide-Grip Front Chins (warm-up)	3	15-20
{Barbell Bent Rows	4	8-10
{Pulldowns Behind Neck	4	8-10
{Seated Pulley Rows	3	8-10
{Nautilus Pullovers	3	8-10
{Close-Grip Front Pulldowns	2-3	8-10
{Hyperextensions	3-4	15-20
Dumbbell Shrugs	3-4	15-20

Jusup Wilkosz

Exercise	Sets	Reps
{ Barbell Bent Rows	5	10-12
{ Machine Pullovers	5	10-12
{ Front Chins	5	10-12
{ Stiff-Arm Pulldowns	5	10-12
Barbell Bent Rows	5	10-12
Behind Neck Pulldowns	5	10-12

Matt Mendenhall

Exercise	Sets	Reps
Front Chins (weighted)	5	8-10
Seated Pulley Rows	5	6-10
Parallel-Grip Front Pulldowns	4	6-10
One-Arm Dumbbell Bent Rows	4	6-10
Nautilus Pullovers	3	10-15

John Terilli

Exercise	Sets	Reps
Front Chins	4-5	10-15
Barbell Bent Rows	3	8-10
Behind Neck Pulldowns	3	8-10
Seated Pulley Rows	3	8-10

18
Biceps Blasting

Without a doubt, biceps building is the favorite subject of virtually all bodybuilders. Of all the mail we receive from advanced-level readers of *Muscle & Fitness* and *Flex* magazines, nearly 50% is concerned with how to develop more massive, high-peaked, and ripped-up biceps muscles. Everyone is out to bust the mythical 20-inch barrier for upper-arm measurements.

Actually, the biceps muscles make up only about 35% of your upper-arm mass. The triceps

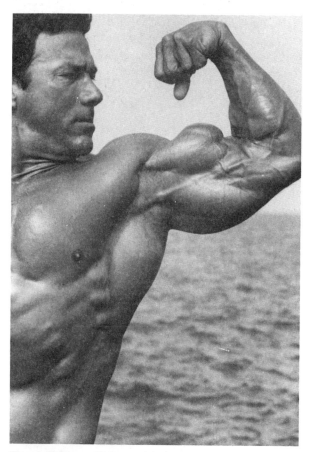

The definition of biceps development—Boyer Coe, the Ragin' Cajun, shows a *real* biceps, large, peaked, well-shaped, and ripped to the bone.

are significantly larger in mass than the biceps, and the brachialis muscles beneath the biceps also contribute a bit to the magnitude of your upper-arm measurement. But everyone still likes to train biceps as hard as humanly possible, enlarging them to the point where they appear like softballs surgically inserted under the skin.

The first of bodybuilding's big-arm superstars was John C. Grimek, who won the Mr. America title in 1940 and 1941. An Olympic Weightlifting Team member, Grimek trained his arms with a wide variety of exercises, *a la* the Weider Muscle Confusion Training Principle. John would pick 8–12 biceps movements for each workout, and then do only one or two sets of each exercise. Many of his favorite biceps movements were actually indirect arm exercise, movements like chins performed with a narrow reverse grip.

Virtually every Mr. America winner since Grimek has had exceptional biceps development. But one man, Steve Reeves (Mr. America in 1947), had special biceps development. His biceps were long and full—albeit not as high-peaked as those of some great bodybuilders—and his upper-arm measurements pushed toward the 19-inch barrier.

Reeves had a favorite biceps movement, dumbbell incline curls, which you probably should include in your biceps routines from time to time. To keep the exercise ultra strict, Steve attached a bar crosswise to the bench, on which he rested his triceps when he did the incline curls. This movement, then, was somewhat like today's preacher curls performed with dumbbells.

The first man to crack the 20-inch upper-arm barrier was an upper-body specialist named John McWilliams. John didn't have what could be called world-class legs, but his upper body was very impressive. And his 20-inch guns were very well defined and featured superior muscle density. McWilliams built this huge arm muscle mass through very heavy training, particularly on basic movements such as standing barbell curls and seated dumbbell curls.

During the 1950s, two of my pupils from northern California, Jack Dellinger and Clancy Ross, epitomized the big-arm tradition. Both men had won Mr. America titles, and Dellinger also added the Mr. Universe trophy to his collection, while Ross won Mr. USA.

Dellinger had only average arm development for much of his career, but by the time he entered and won his last competition, Mr. Universe, in 1956, his upper arms were sensationally well developed. Jack's secret was consistent training, and he only built his arms up to more than 19 inches through consistently hard training over a long period of time.

Clancy Ross became known as the King of Bodybuilders, and his upper arms were always quite good. I often trained with him, and he was one of the first exponents of the Weider Cheating Training Principle. Using a bit looser form than some of the super-strict trainers of his era, Ross could do 10 reps in standing barbell curls with 185–205 pounds on the bar. And his biceps showed remarkable mass and muscle density as a result of such heavy training.

Moving into the 1960s, Bill Pearl bore the standard of the big-arm kings. His 20-inchers helped him to win four Mr. Universe titles. Bill favored a wide variety of biceps movements, changing his training programs every six weeks. He also did quite a few more total sets for biceps than most of his contemporaries, usually something in the range of 20 sets. Now in his middle 50s, the Pearl of the Universe retains spectacular biceps development.

During the middle 1960s, Larry Scott, winner of the first two Mr. Olympia titles (1965 and 1966), set the standard for contemporary upper-arm development. His football-sized biceps boosted his upper-arm measurement to nearly 21 inches at a height of 5'8" and competitive body weight of 210 pounds. Larry's biceps development was largely a result of preacher

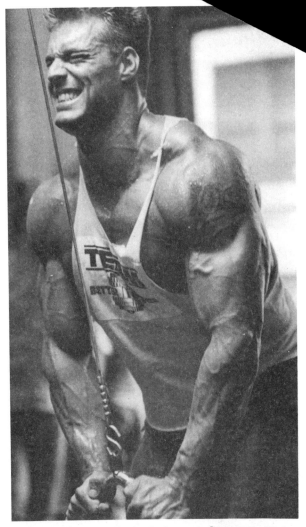

With his typical go-for-broke intensity, Berry de Mey has carved out a physique worthy of international admiration. At the 1988 Mr. Olympia, de Mey moved up three spots to third place for his efforts.

curls using barbells and dumbbells. Indeed, many bodybuilders now call this exercise "Scott curls" in his honor.

In recent years, I think that Arnold Schwarzenegger (seven times Mr. Olympia) has displayed the best pair of biceps. They peak up like the Matterhorn and have all of the cuts and muscle density you would ever expect to see with a man of the Austrian Oak's reputation. Schwarzenegger's unique training secret was the Weider Descending Sets Training Principle, in which he would reduce the weights two or three times within each set, continuing to grind out rep after painful rep with the progressively lighter poundages.

What type of biceps development will you have? Will your arm development win you

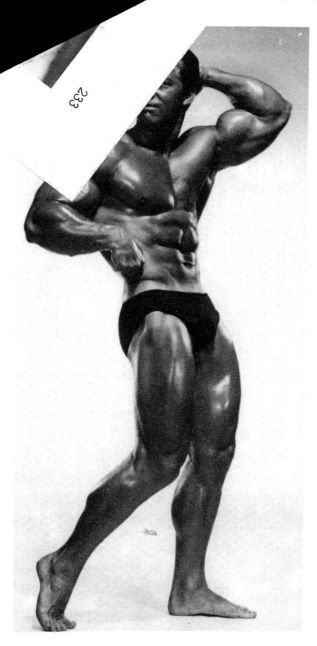

233

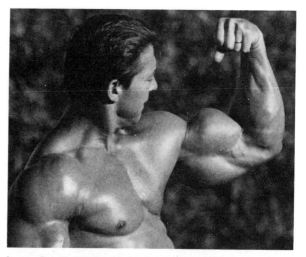

Larry Scott, at age 25, had won his second consecutive Mr. Olympia trophy and was on top of the world. Nearly 25 years after winning his last Olympia, Scott has retained the physique depicted here, including 20-inch upper arms on a 5'8" frame. What man in his late 40s wouldn't want to look like this?

some major physique titles, perhaps even Mr. or Ms. Olympia? Only time will answer these questions for you. But be sure that you train consistently, never missing workouts. That's the only way you will be able to maximize your biceps development and approach your ultimate potential for upper-arm mass, cuts, and density.

ANATOMY AND KINESIOLOGY

There are two muscle groups located at the front of the upper arm, and they both contract to flex the arm fully from a straight position. The smallest of these muscles is called the bra-

chialis, and you can see it as a thin band of muscle between the biceps and triceps when you display your upper arm from the rear. The brachialis muscle runs only about halfway up the humerus bone above the elbow. It can best be contracted when you have your palm toward the floor doing barbell reverse curls. But, as you may have noted from the Emphasis paragraphs in Chapter 17, it also comes strongly into play when you do many basic back exercises—chins, rows, and pulldowns.

The biceps are much larger in mass than the brachialis muscles, and it is the primary muscle group responsible for bending the arm. With an origin near the shoulder joint and insertions on the forearm bones, the biceps can contract to fully bend the arm from a straight position. Virtually all bodybuilders understand this function of the biceps muscles, but only a few of the more enlightened athletes realize that the biceps have a second function.

The other important function of biceps contraction is to supinate the hand. Bend your right arm so your forearm is parallel with the floor; this is called a *pronated* hand position, and the act of rotating your hand is called *pronation*. Next, rotate your wrist so your palm is facing upward; this is called a *supinated* position, and the act of rotating your hand to this position is called *supination*. Su-

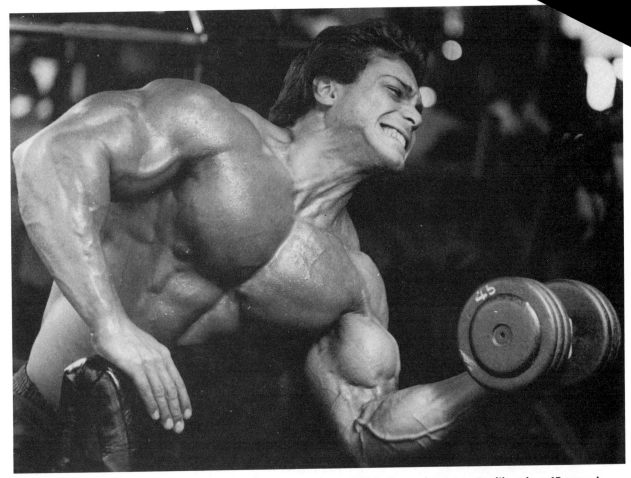

Shaping his biceps with One-Armed Dumbbell preacher curls, Richie Gaspari warms up with only a 45-pound dumbbell, a far cry from the 75-pounder he uses for his peak weight. Little wonder his arms are so sensationally developed!

pination, of course, is the second function of your biceps.

If you think about this supination process, you'll realize that doing standing curls with an EZ-curl bar has less of an effect on biceps development than ordinary standing barbell curls. This is due to the fact that your hands are many degrees off from a fully supinated position when you use the cambered bar, but almost fully supinated in standing barbell curls.

Taking this supination function a bit farther, you will be able to supinate your hands even more completely when you do dumbbell curls. In such a movement, you start each repetition with your palms facing inward toward your legs, a position halfway between full supination and full pronation. Then as you curl the dumbbells upward—actually about a third of the way up in the full range of motion—you rotate your hands into a supinated position

while still curling the weights upward. You finish the movement with your hands completely supinated, and then pronate your hands partway down to the finish position of each repetition. Thus, you work both biceps functions with a single exercise.

TRAINING TIPS

Shane DiMora, the sensational young bodybuilder who won the Teenage, Junior, and Open Nationals as a middleweight at only 19 years of age reveals, "I used to have very weak biceps and triceps, so my upper arms lagged behind the rest of my body and spoiled my proportional balance. After analyzing my training philosophy and the routines I was using to develop my arms, I concluded that I was going too heavy in my biceps exercises. Just by cutting back about 25% on my biceps

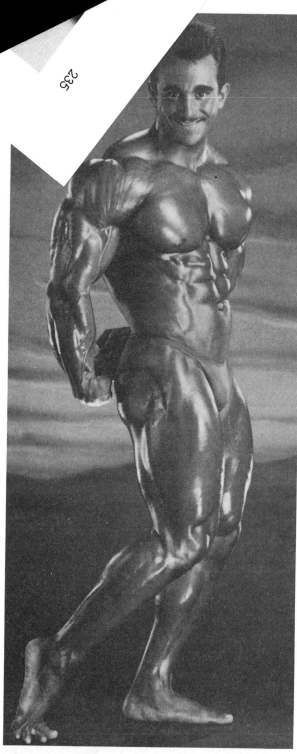

235

Young Shane DiMora, winner of the 1986 National Middleweight Championship at the tender age of 19, was placing in national teenage events at the young age of 15. His other titles include Teenage Mr. USA, Teenage Mr. America, Junior National Champion, and second place in an IFBB Pro Grand Prix event. Not bad for a kid standing only 5'2½" tall, who initially wanted only to put on a little muscle mass to normalize his appearance and keep neighborhood kids from harassing him.

movement weights and concentrating harder on each set, I was able to blast my arms up to the point where they are now in perfect harmony with the remainder of my physique."

National and World Champion *Lee Labrada* notes, "It's really easy to overtrain your arms. The biceps come strongly into play when you do most lat exercises, while the triceps are strongly contracted when doing pressing movements for your chest and shoulder muscles. Also, the biceps are very small in comparison to the torso muscles. So, I have found that I make my best progress in developing upper arms when I do about half the total number of sets I'm doing for larger body parts like chest, back, and thighs. And I think that any young bodybuilder will benefit from following the same philosophy when working upper arms."

Mike Christian says, "One of my favorite biceps training strategies is to do 21s with standing barbell curls. This is a very intense way of doing any exercise, and is particularly stressful when used with standing barbell curls. When doing 21s, you do seven half reps, starting from the bottom point of the movement, then seven more half reps on the upper part of the movement. Finally, you finish with seven full repetitions of barbell curls. If this doesn't set your biceps to burning, you might want to think about trying another sport. I've been able to push my upper arms to over 21 inches using this type of training technique. I'm sure it will work for everyone who tries it!"

Dr. Franco Columbu tells young bodybuilders, "Stick to the basic movements for at least a couple of years before switching over to isolation exercises for biceps. Spend lots of time on standing barbell curls, preacher curls, and seated or standing dumbbell curls with plenty of stress on full supination each repetition. Save the concentration curls and cable curls for the peaking phase just before a bodybuilding competition."

BICEPS EXERCISES

There are more than 40 biceps exercises described and illustrated in this chapter. Counting the variations on each movement, the exercises presented in this section will give you more than 75 good upper-arm movements for use in your own routines.

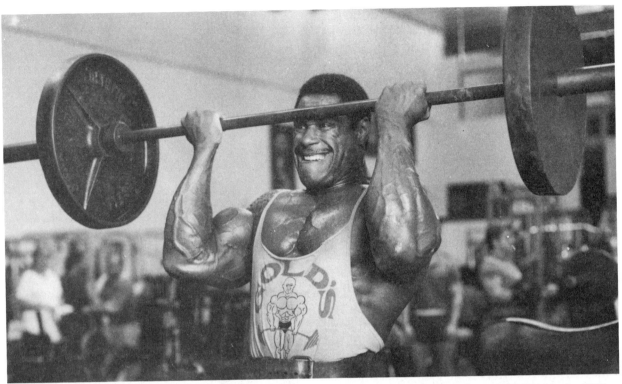

This is one way a pair of 21-inch upper arms is built on a 6'1" frame, as Mike Christian does the honors. In 1979, Mike had considered giving up the sport, but set as a goal winning the 1982 California Championship to prove whether he had what it took genetically to become a champion. He won that show, plus Nationals and the World Championships in 1984. During 1988, he won both the US Pro Championships and IFBB World Pro Championships, to go with a top-three placing in one recent Mr. Olympia.

Standing Barbell Curls

Emphasis—This is the most basic of biceps movements. It places primary stress on the biceps muscles and secondary emphasis on the brachialis and forearm flexor muscles.

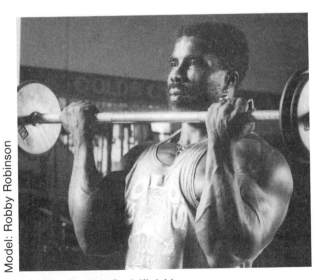

Model: Robby Robinson

Standing Barbell Curl (finish)

Starting Position—Place a moderately heavy barbell on the gym floor at your feet. Bend over and take a shoulder-width undergrip on the bar (palms facing away from your body). Stand erect with your arms straight down at your sides and the barbell resting across your upper thighs. Your feet should be set a comfortable distance apart, and you should avoid swaying your torso forward and/or backward to help you move the weight upward. Press your upper arms against the sides of your torso and keep them in this position throughout your set.

Movement Performance—Use biceps strength to curl the weight upward in a semicircular arc to a position just beneath your chin. You should hold your wrists relatively straight during the movement. Hold the top position for 3–4 seconds, powerfully contracting your biceps muscles, then slowly lower back to the starting point. Repeat the movement for the desired number of repetitions.

Common Mistakes—Torso movement during the exercise is cheating, and it robs your biceps muscles of some of the stress they should receive. Allowing your elbows to move outward to the sides away from your torso is also cheating.

Training Tips—If you have difficulty avoiding torso swing, you can alleviate the problem by wearing one of my Weider Arm Blaster units. This inexpensive piece of equipment effectively restricts any movement of the upper arms and torso as you do all types of barbell curls and dumbbell curls either standing or seated at the end of a flat exercise bench. Alternatively, you can avoid torso swing by doing barbell curls with your back pressed against the gym wall or the upright member of any exercise machine. Regardless of how you do the movement, you should experiment with different grip widths. Arnold Schwarzengger did most of his barbell curls with a relatively wide grip, his hands set 6–8 inches wider than his shoulders on each side, and his biceps are terrific. Rick Wayne (Mr. World and Pro Mr. America), on the other hand, favored a more narrow grip, his hands only 4–6 inches apart in the middle of the bar, and his biceps are also extremely impressive. Try using a wide variety of grip widths in an effort to discover which one works best for you.

Cheating Barbell Curls

Comment—This is the same movement as standing barbell curls, but with some body english added. At the beginning of the movement, when the bar is down across your thighs, you should incline your torso a bit forward at the waist. Then to start the bar's upward momentum, you shift your torso backward quickly as you pull hard with your biceps. This should swing the bar about halfway up the full range of motion. From there, you finish the movement solely with biceps strength. Slowly lower back to the starting point while resisting the downward force of the barbell. Usually, advanced bodybuilders start off a set with 5–6 strict reps in standing barbell curls to failure, followed by 3–4 cheating barbell curl repetitions to really blast the biceps muscles into oblivion.

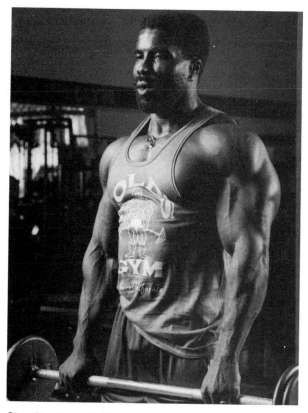

Standing Barbell Reverse Curl (start)

Barbell Reverse Curls

Emphasis—This movement is often used strictly as a forearm developer, because it strongly stresses the powerful supinator muscles of the forearms. Strong secondary stress is placed on the biceps and brachialis muscles.

Starting Position—Place a moderately weighted barbell on the gym floor at your feet. Bend over and take a shoulder-width overgrip on the bar (palms facing your body). Stand erect with your arms straight down at your sides and the barbell resting across your upper thighs. Your feet should be set a comfortable distance apart, and you should avoid swaying your torso forward and/or backward to help you move the weight upward. Press your upper arms against the sides of your torso and keep them in this position throughout your set.

Movement Performance—Use upper- and forearm strength to curl the weight upward in a semicircular arc to a position just beneath your chin. You should hold your wrists straight during the movement. Hold the top position for

3-4 seconds, powerfully contracting your arm muscles, then lower back to the starting point. Repeat the movement for the desired number of repetitions.

Training Tips—If you have trouble keeping your upper body motionless when doing reverse curls, you should perform the movement with your back pressed against the gym wall. Alternatively, you can do reverse curls while wearing your Weider Arm Blaster unit. You might find that you get more out of your reverse curls when you use a narrow grip with your index fingers set about 4-6 inches apart in the middle of the bar.

Barbell Slide Curls

Emphasis—Occasionally called drag curls, slide curls stress the biceps muscles from an entirely different angle than any other biceps movement. Secondary stress is placed on the forearm flexor muscles.

Starting Position—Place a moderately weighted barbell on the gym floor at your feet. Bend over and take a shoulder-width undergrip on the bar. Stand erect with your arms straight down at your sides and the barbell resting across your upper thighs. Your feet should be set a comfortable distance apart, and you should avoid swaying your torso forward and/ or backward to help you to move the weight upward.

Movement Performance—Allowing your elbows to travel directly to the rear, slowly bend your arms and slide the barbell up your abdomen to as high a point as possible. You probably won't be able to slide the bar upward much higher than the bottom edge of your pectorals, but even such a short-range movement will intensely stress the biceps muscles. Slowly reverse the movement to return the bar to the starting point. Repeat.

Training Tips—You can try varying the width of your grip on the bar.

Kneeling Barbell Curls

Emphasis—Doing barbell curls while kneeling on the floor powerfully stresses your biceps

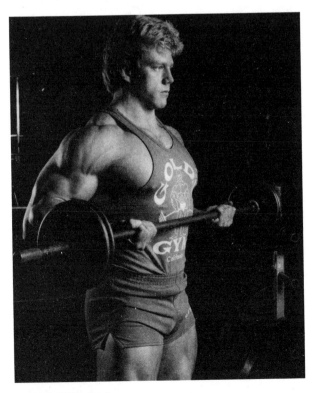

Barbell Slide Curl

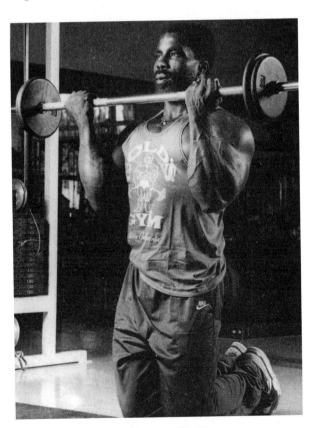

Kneeling Barbell Curl (top position)

muscles. Secondary stress is on the forearm flexors.

Starting Position—Kneel on the gym floor with your knees a couple of inches away from a moderately weighted barbell lying on the floor. Take a shoulder-width undergrip on the barbell handle and kneel erect with your arms down at your sides and the barbell resting across your upper thighs. Press your upper arms against the sides of your torso and keep them in this position throughout your set.

Movement Performance—Moving only your forearms, slowly bend your arms using biceps strength and curl the weight forward and upward in a semicircular arc to a position directly beneath your chin. Hold this finish position for a moment while powerfully contracting your biceps muscles. Reverse the movement and slowly return the barbell back along the same arc to the starting point. Repeat the movement for the suggested number of repetitions.

Training Tips—Doing barbell curls in a kneeling position makes the movement much more strict than the standing variation. Try both wide and narrow grips on this movement.

Barbell Concentration Curls

Emphasis—This movement is excellent for adding height to the peak on your biceps muscles. Secondary stress is placed on the forearm flexors.

Starting Position—Set your feet about shoulder width apart and bend over to take a narrow undergrip on a light barbell, your hands set 4–6 inches apart in the middle of the barbell handle. Keeping your legs only slightly bent, bend forward at the waist until your torso is parallel to the floor. Keep your torso motionless in this position throughout your set. Dangle your arms straight downward from your shoulders and keep your upper arms motionless in this position throughout your set.

Movement Performance—Using biceps strength with body momentum, slowly curl the barbell forward and upward to as high a posi-

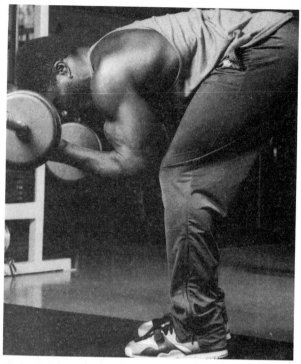

Barbell Concentration Curl (near finish)

tion as possible along a semicircular arc. Hold this peak-contracted position for a slow count of two before lowering the bar back along the same arc to the starting position. Repeat the movement for the desired number of repetitions.

Training Tips—This was a favorite biceps movement of superstar Robby Robinson. You can experiment with different grip widths when doing barbell concentration curls. You can also use a reverse grip, a movement which places proportionately more stress on the forearm supinator muscles.

Prone Barbell Curls

Emphasis—This movement is very similar in effect to barbell concentration curls. It is excellent for adding height to the peak on your biceps muscles. Secondary stress is placed on the forearm flexors.

Starting Position—Place a moderately weighted barbell on the floor at one end of a high, flat exercise bench. Lie facedown on the bench with your head off the end toward the barbell. Reach down and take a narrow undergrip on

Biceps Blasting

semicircular arc to as high a position as possible. Hold this peak-contracted position for a moment, then lower the weight back along the same arc to the starting position. Repeat the movement for the desired number of repetitions.

Training Tips—Try using a wider grip, with your elbows set in a position more narrow than your grip width on the bar. You can also experiment with a more narrow grip width, as well as with a reverse grip on the bar.

Barbell Preacher Curls

Emphasis—This is an excellent mass builder which especially adds mass to the lower section of your biceps down near the elbow.

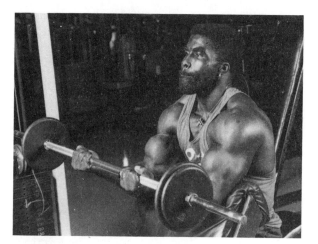

Barbell Preacher Curl (halfway)

Starting Position—Take an undergrip on a barbell with your hands set about 4-6 inches wider than your shoulders on the bar. Lean over a preacher bench with your upper arms running parallel to each other down the angled surface of the bench. The upper edge of the preacher bench should be set firmly under your armpits. Fully straighten your arms.

Movement Performance—Use biceps strength to curl the barbell upward in a semicircular arc until it reaches a point just beneath your chin. Lower slowly back along the same arc to the starting point, and repeat the movement for the required number of repetitions.

Training Tips—It's essential on all types of

preacher curls that you lower the weight slowly back to the starting point on each repetition. Several top bodybuilders have suffered biceps tendon injuries when doing this movement ballistically, attempting to bounce the weight in the bottom position of the exercise. You can experiment with a variety of grip widths on this movement, as well as with a reverse grip.

Barbell Preacher Reverse Curls

Emphasis—This movement places almost equal stress on the biceps, brachialis, and forearm supinator muscles.

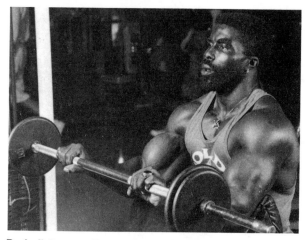

Barbell Reverse Preacher Curl (halfway)

Starting Position—Take a shoulder-width overgrip on a moderately weighted barbell. Lean over a preacher bench with your upper arms running parallel to each other down the angled surface of the bench. The upper edge of the bench should be wedged securely beneath your armpits. Fully straighten your arms.

Movement Performance—Use arm strength to curl the barbell upward in a semicircular arc to a position just beneath your chin. Lower slowly back to the starting point and repeat the movement for the suggested number of repetitions.

Training Tips—Experiment with various grip widths.

Incline Barbell Curls

Emphasis—This interesting short-range movement is an excellent one for adding to biceps muscle mass and density.

Starting Position—Take a shoulder-width undergrip on a moderately heavy barbell and lie back on a 30- to 45-degree incline bench with the barbell resting across your upper thighs. Press your upper arms against the sides of your torso and keep them motionless in this position throughout your set.

Movement Performance—Use biceps strength to curl the weight upward from the starting point in a semicircular arc to a position beneath your chin. Lower slowly back to the starting point, and repeat the movement.

Training Tips—Try using various grip widths.

Prone Incline Barbell Curls

Emphasis—This is an excellent movement for adding to the height of your biceps peak. Secondary stress is placed on the forearm flexor muscles.

Starting Position—Take a shoulder-width undergrip on a moderately weighted barbell and lie facedown on a 45-degree incline bench, the barbell hanging downward at straight arms' length from your shoulders. Be sure that you keep your upper arms motionless throughout your set.

Movement Performance—Use biceps strength to curl the weight forward and upward in a semicircular arc to as high a position as possible. Hold this peak-contracted position for a moment, then lower slowly back along the same arc to the starting point. Repeat the movement for the desired number of repetitions.

Training Tips—Vary the width of your grip on the barbell from time to time.

Standing Dumbbell Curls

Emphasis—Like barbell curls, this dumbbell movement places very intense stress on the biceps and lesser stress on the brachialis and forearm flexor muscles. But you will be able to supinate your hands using dumbbells, which gives you a better biceps contraction than is

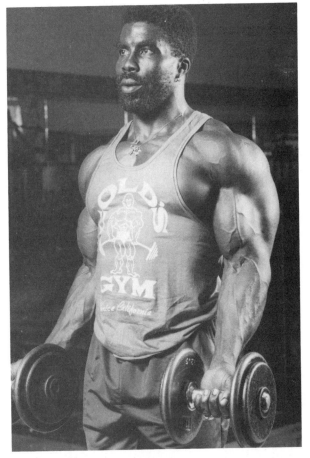

Standing Dumbbell Curl (bottom)

possible with barbell curls. The functions of your biceps are to flex your arm *and* to supinate your hand.

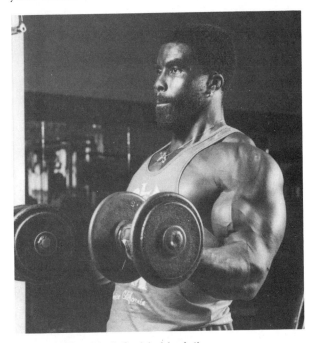

Standing Dumbbell Curl (midpoint)

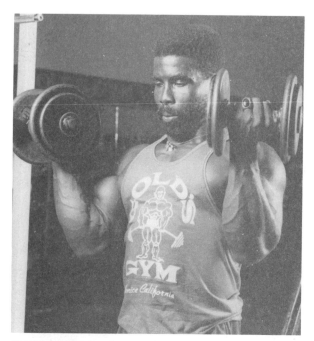

Standing Dumbbell Curl (top)

Starting Position—Grasp two moderately weighted dumbbells, set your feet about shoulder width apart, and stand erect with your arms hanging straight down at your sides, your palms facing toward your legs. Press your upper arms against the sides of your torso and keep them in this position throughout your set.

Movement Performance—Use biceps strength to simultaneously curl the dumbbells forward and upward in a semicircular arc to the shoulders. As the dumbbells reach the halfway point, rotate your wrists so your palms are facing upward during the second half of the movement. This wrist twist is called *pronation*. Lower the dumbbells slowly back along the same arcs to the starting point, and repeat the movement. As the dumbbells reach the halfway point back to the finish position, rotate your wrists again so your palms are facing inward toward each other for the second half of the lowerling movement. This wrist twist in the opposite direction from pronation is called supination.

Training Tips—To make this movement somewhat more strict, you can sit at the end of a flat exercise bench with your feet set flat on the floor to balance your body in position. As with barbell curls, you can do dumbbell curls while using either a Weider Arm Blaster unit or with your back pressed against the gym wall. With all variations of dumbbell curls, you can experiment with curling the weights a little out to the sides rather than directly forward on each repetition. You can also do alternate dumbbell curls in which you curl the weights in seesaw fashion, one weight coming down as the other is raised.

Standing Alternate Dumbbell Curls

Emphasis—This excellent movement places very intense stress on the biceps muscles, with secondary emphasis on the brachialis and forearm flexor muscles.

Starting Position—Grasp two moderately weighted dumbbells, set your feet a comfortable distance apart, and stand erect with your arms hanging down at your sides, your palms facing inward toward each other. Press your upper arms against the sides of your torso and keep them motionless in this position throughout the movement.

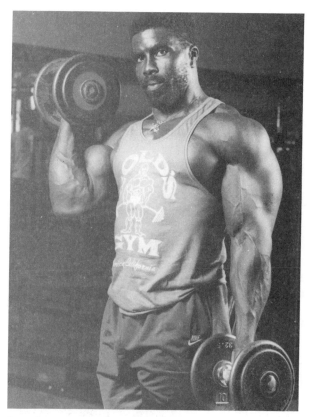

Standing Alternate Dumbbell Curl

Movement Performance—Use the strength of your left biceps to slowly curl the dumbbell in your left hand forward and upward in a semi-circular arc to shoulder level. As you begin to lower the dumbbell in your left hand back along the same arc to the starting point, slowly begin curling the weight in your right hand up to your shoulder. Continue curling the dumbbells in seesaw fashion like this until you have performed the correct number of repetitions with each arm.

Training Tips—When you do alternate dumbbell curls, the movement is automatically more strict than when you are curling the dumbbells upward and downward simultaneously. You can do alternate dumbbell curls while seated at the end of a flat exercise bench. On all variations of dumbbell curls you should experiment with curling the weights somewhat out to the sides rather than merely straight forward.

Standing Hammer Curls

Emphasis—While hammer curls do work the biceps quite intensely, they are primarily intended as a brachialis and forearm supinator exercise.

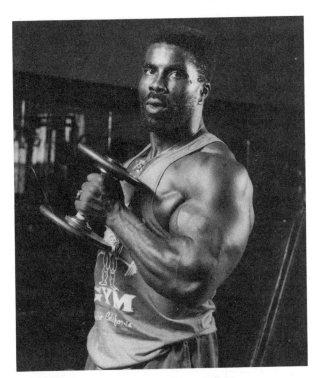

Hammer Curl (one-arm variation—finish)

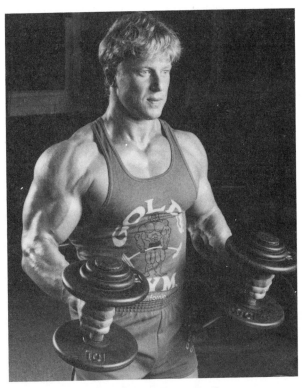

Hammer Curl (two-arm variation—start)

Starting Position—Grasp two moderately weighted dumbbells, set your feet a comfortable distance apart, and stand erect with your arms hanging down at your sides, your palms facing inward toward each other. Your palms should be facing each other throughout the set. Press your upper arms against the sides of your torso and keep them motionless in this position throughout the movement.

Movement Performance—Use arm strength to simultaneously curl the two dumbbells forward and upward in semicircular arcs to shoulder level. Hold this peak-contracted position for a moment while intensely contracting your upper arm muscles, then slowly lower the dumbbells back to the starting point. Repeat the movement for the suggested number of repetitions.

Training Tips—You can also do this movement while seated at the end of a flat exercise bench. The seated variation can be done with one arm at a time. Whenever you do a curling movement with one arm at a time, you are automatically able to concentrate more intensely on the working muscle(s).

Standing Zottman Curls

Emphasis—This excellent, all-around arm movement places stress on the biceps, brachialis, forearm supinator, and forearm flexor muscles.

Starting Position—Grasp two moderately weighted dumbbells, set your feet a comfortable distance apart, and stand erect with your arms hanging down at your sides, your palms facing toward each other. Press your upper arms against the sides of your torso and keep them motionless in this position throughout your set.

Movement Performance—This exercise is a bit complicated, since each arm will be doing something different at the same time while you are alternatively curling the dumbbells upward and downward. Start the movement by curling the dumbbell in your left hand upward with your palm facing up. When your left hand gets to the top point, reverse the movement by first rotating your wrist so your palm is facing downward as the weight is lowered. The moment you begin to lower the dumbbell in your left hand, you must begin curling the weight in your right hand upward with your palm facing up. Lower the weight in your right hand with your wrist rotated so your palm is down as the weight descends. Continue in this fashion until you have performed the required number of repetitions with each arm.

Training Tips—If you have trouble remembering what to do, try your first few sets using only one arm at a time rather than curling the weights alternately. And keep in mind, "Weight going up, palm up; weight going down, palm down."

Seated Dumbbell Curls

Emphasis—This popular exercise places intense stress on the biceps muscles and secondary stress on the brachialis and forearm flexor muscles.

Starting Position—Grasp two moderately weighted dumbbells and sit erect at the end of a flat exercise bench, your feet flat on the floor to balance yourself in position. Your arms should be hanging down at your sides, your palms facing inward toward each other. Press your upper arms against the sides of your torso and keep them in this position throughout the movement.

Movement Performance—Use upper arm strength to simultaneously curl the dumbbells forward and upward in semicircular arcs to shoulder level. Hold this peak-contracted position for a moment, then slowly lower the weights back along the same arcs to the starting point. Repeat the movement for an appropriate number of repetitions.

Training Tips—You can also curl the dumbbells alternately. You can also experiment with curling the dumbbells upward along various arcs out to the sides more than directly forward.

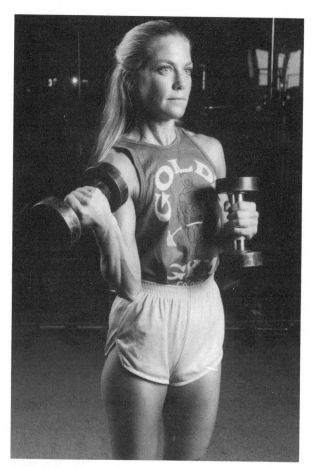

Zottman Curl

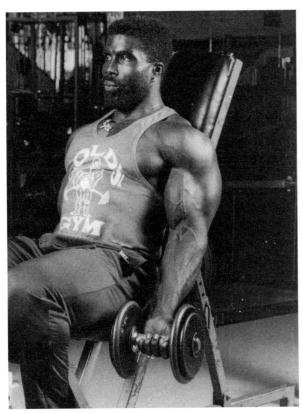

Seated Dumbbell Curl

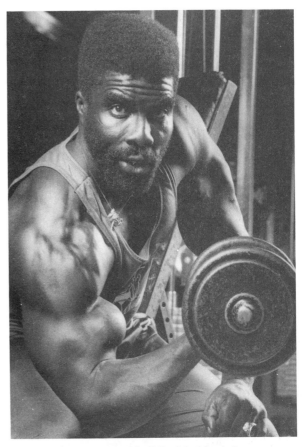

Seated One-Arm Dumbbell Curl (midpoint)

Seated One-Arm Dumbbell Curls

Emphasis—A favorite biceps exercise of Frank Zane, seated one-arm dumbbell curls place intense stress on the biceps muscles and secondary stress on the brachialis and forearm flexor muscles. Whenever you do curls with one arm at a time, you need not split your mental focus between both arms, which automatically gives you better concentration on the working muscles.

Starting Position—Grasp a moderately heavy dumbbell in your right hand and sit down at the end of a flat exercise bench. Your arm should be hanging down at your side, your palm facing inward toward your leg. Press your upper arm against the side of your torso and keep it motionless in this position throughout your set.

Movement Performance—Use biceps strength to slowly curl the dumbbell forward and upward in a semicircular arc to shoulder level. Supinate your hand about halfway up in the movement so you finish each repetition with

your palm facing upward. Reverse the movement to lower the weight back to the starting point, pronating your hand halfway down. Repeat the exercise for the required number of repetitions. Be sure to do an equal number of sets and repetitions with each arm.

Training Tips—This movement could also be done in the hammer curl position, your thumb facing upward throughout the movement.

Seated Alternate Dumbbell Curls

Emphasis—This variation of seated dumbbell curls places intense stress on the biceps and secondary emphasis on the brachialis and forearm flexor muscles.

Starting Position—Grasp two moderately weighted dumbbells and sit down at the end of a flat exercise bench, your feet flat on the floor. Sit erect with your arms hanging down at your sides, your palms facing each other. Press your upper arms against the sides of your torso and keep them motionless in this position throughout your set.

Movement Performance—Use upper-arm strength to curl the weight in your left hand up to your shoulder, being sure to supinate your hand halfway up in the movement. Immediately start to lower it back to the starting point, pronating your hand halfway down. The moment you begin lowering the dumbbell in your left hand, start to curl the weight in your right hand up to your shoulder. Continue alternately curling the dumbbells until you have completed the correct number of repetitions with each arm.

Training Tips—As you know from the text a few pages back, this movement can be performed curling both dumbbells simultaneously. As with all dumbbell curls, you can also experiment with curling the weights somewhat out to the sides rather than merely straight forward and upward.

Incline Dumbbell Curls

Emphasis—This exercise is excellent for adding both mass and peak to your biceps. Since your biceps muscles are under a partial stretch at the beginning point of the movement, you will find that incline dumbbell curls can actually be a more effective biceps builder than either standing barbell curls or dumbbell curls.

Starting Position—Grasp two moderately heavy dumbbells and lie back on a 30- to 45-degree incline bench. You can sit down if your bench has a seat. Allow your arms to hang straight downward from your shoulders, and rotate your wrists so your palms are facing forward at the beginning of the movement. Be sure to hold your upper arms motionless throughout your set.

Movement Performance—Use biceps strength to curl the dumbbells directly forward and upward to shoulder level. Hold this peak-contracted position for a moment while intensely tensing your biceps, then slowly lower back along the same arcs to the starting point. Re-

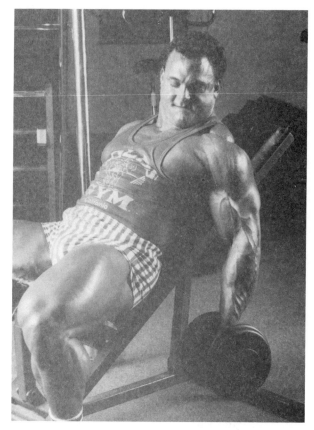

Incline Dumbbell Curl (start)

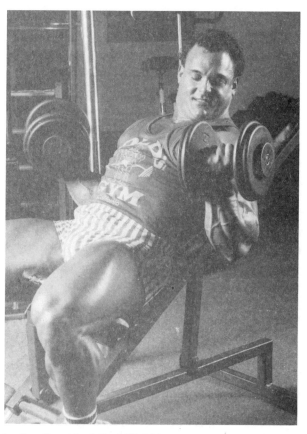

Incline Dumbbell Curl (finish)

peat the movement for the desired number of repetitions.

Training Tips—You will find this to be a very strict movement, because it is almost impossible to cheat when you are lying on your back on an incline bench. Be sure to try curling the weights somewhat out to the sides as well as straight forward. If you can curl the weights directly to the sides on an incline bench, you will find that you work your outer biceps head more intensely than is possible in any other manner.

Prone Incline Dumbbell Curls

Emphasis—A favorite biceps exercise of Boyer Coe, prone incline dumbbell curls help to both add mass to your biceps and enhance the peak on the muscle group.

Starting Position—Grasp two moderately weighted dumbbells and lie facedown on a 30- to 45-degree incline bench, your arms hanging

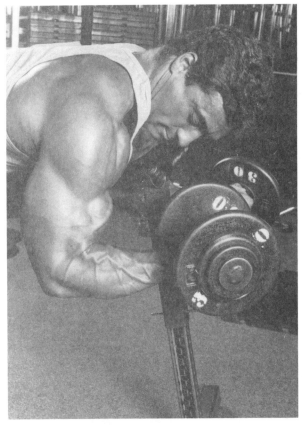

Prone Incline Dumbbell Curl (finish)

straight downward from your shoulders. Rotate your wrists so your palms are facing forward throughout the movement. Be sure to hold your upper arms as motionless as possible throughout your set.

Movement Performance—Use biceps strength to curl the dumbbells directly forward and upward in semicircular arcs to shoulder level. Hold this peak-contracted position for a moment while intensely tensing your biceps. Slowly lower back along the same arcs to the starting point.

Training Tips—Be sure that you don't allow your elbows to splay outward or move to the rear as you do this movement. You should also experiment with curling the dumbbells a bit out to the sides on some of your sets. Each change of arc will stress your biceps somewhat differently, and the accumulation of many types of arcs will contribute readily to optimum biceps development.

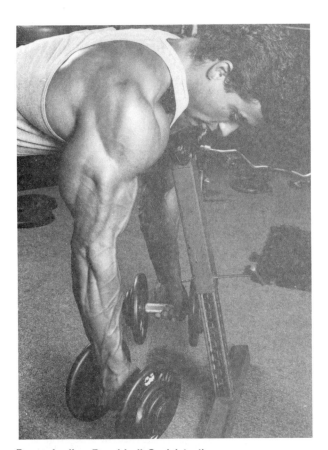

Prone Incline Dumbbell Curl (start)

Prone Dumbbell Curls

Emphasis—As with the prone incline dumbbell curls, this exercise helps to add both mass and peak to your biceps.

Starting Position—You will need a flat exercise bench about 2½–3 feet high for this movement. If you don't have one that high, you will have to boost the height of your existing bench by placing its legs on either thick blocks of wood or barbell plates. Grasp two moderately weighted dumbbells and lie facedown on the bench, your arms hanging directly down from your shoulders. Rotate your wrists so your palms are facing forward as you do the exercise. Be sure that you hold your upper arms motionless throughout your set.

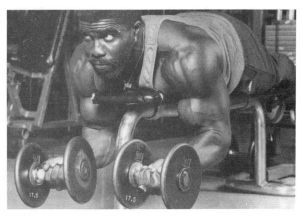

Prone Dumbbell Curl (midpoint)

Movement Performance—Use biceps strength to slowly curl the dumbbells forward and upward in semicircular arcs to your shoulders. Hold this peak-contracted position for a moment, then slowly lower the weights back along the same arcs to the starting point. Repeat.

Training Tips—Try doing your curls a bit to the sides on some of your sets.

Lying Dumbbell Curls

Emphasis—Since your biceps are fully stretched at the start of this exercise, you will find lying dumbbell curls to be a very effective way to add both mass and peak to your biceps muscles.

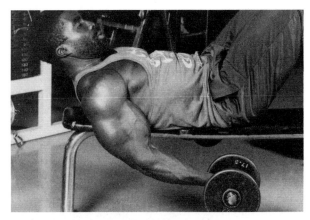

Lying Dumbbell Curl (just past bottom)

Starting Position—Again, you will need a flat exercise bench 2½–3 feet high. Grasp a pair of moderately weighted dumbbells and lie back on the exercise bench. Allow your arms to hang straight down from your shoulders. Rotate your wrists so your palms face forward throughout the movement.

Movement Performance—Use biceps strength to curl the dumbbells directly forward and upward to shoulder level. Hold this peak-contracted position for a moment, intensely tensing your biceps muscles, then lower slowly back along the same arcs to the starting point.

Training Tips—Try different curling arcs from time to time.

Dumbbell Preacher Curls

Emphasis—This is an excellent overall biceps mass builder, and it particularly adds mass to the lower biceps insertion down near the elbow.

Starting Position—Grasp two moderately weighted dumbbells and lean over a preacher bench, your arms running parallel to each other down the angled surface of the bench. The upper edge of the bench should be wedged under your armpits. Supinate your hands and slowly straighten your arms.

Movement Performance—Use biceps strength to slowly curl the dumbbells directly upward to shoulder level. Return the dumbbells slowly back along the same arcs to the starting point.

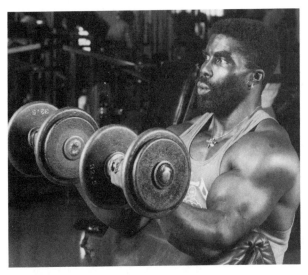

Dumbbell Preacher Curl (midpoint)

Training Tips—Be sure that you don't attempt to bounce the weights in the bottom position, because your biceps are vulnerable to injury when your arm is fully extended. Ease the weights down every repetition. It's important as you curl the weights upward and then lower them back to the starting point that the dumbbells are carried in arcs somewhat wider than the placement of your elbows. You can also do this exercise with one arm at a time, which allows you to concentrate somewhat harder on the biceps of the working arm.

One-Arm Incline Preacher Curls

Emphasis—If you don't have a preacher bench available, you can conveniently use a regular 30- or 45-degree incline bench for preacher curls. As you already know, preacher curls are

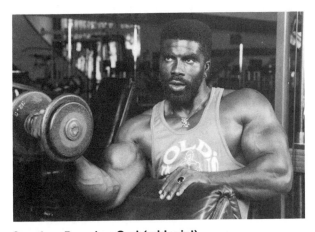

One-Arm Preacher Curl (midpoint)

good for building biceps mass, particularly down near the elbow.

Starting Position—Grasp a moderately weighted dumbbell in your left hand and run your left upper arm down the angled surface of the bench, the upper edge of the bench wedged beneath your armpit. Slowly straighten your arm.

Movement Performance—Use biceps strength to slowly curl the dumbbell from the starting position on the bench up to shoulder level. Hold this peak-contracted position for a moment, intensely tensing your biceps, then slowly lower back to the starting point. Repeat the movement. Be sure to do the same number of sets and reps with each arm.

Training Tips—Be sure to avoid bouncing the dumbbell off the surface of the bench.

Kneeling Dumbbell Curls

Emphasis—Since you can supinate your hands as you do this movement, it is excellent for building quality biceps muscle mass.

Starting Position—Place a rubber pad or folded towel on the gym floor and kneel down on it. Grasp a pair of moderately weighted dumbbells and kneel erect with your arms hanging straight down at your sides. Your palms should be facing inward toward each other. Press your upper arms against the sides of your torso and keep them motionless in this position throughout your set.

Movement Performance—Use biceps strength to curl the dumbbells directly forward and upward in semicircular arcs to shoulder level. Hold this peak-contracted position for a moment, intensely tensing your biceps, then lower back along the same arcs to the starting point. Be sure to supinate your hands as you curl the weights upward and pronate your hands as you lower the dumbbells back to the starting point.

Training Tips—You can also perform kneeling dumbbell curls alternately, or with one dumb-

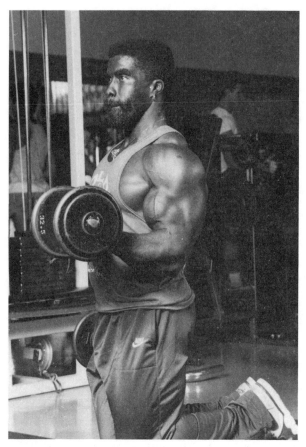

Kneeling Dumbbell Curl (alternate arms version)

bell at a time. Kneeling makes the exercise quite a bit more strict than standing dumbbell curls.

Kneeling Alternate Dumbbell Curls

Emphasis—Since you can supinate your hands as you do this movement, it is excellent for building quality biceps muscle mass. Also, doing kneeling dumbbell curls alternately makes the movement even more strict than when the dumbbells are curled upward simultaneously.

Starting Position—Place a rubber pad or folded towel on the gym floor and kneel down on it. Grasp two moderately weighted dumbbells and kneel erect with your arms hanging straight down at your sides. Your palms should be facing each other. Press your upper arms against the sides of your torso and keep them motionless in this position throughout your set.

Movement Performance—Curl the weight in your left hand up to your shoulder, then as you

begin to lower it start curling the weight in your right hand upward. Continue curling the dumbbells in seesaw fashion until you have completed the desired number of repetitions with each arm.

Training Tips—As you already know, you can curl the weights upward simultaneously if you wish, but curling them alternately makes the movement more strict.

Kneeling Hammer Curls

Emphasis—Like other variations of hammer curls, this exercise places almost equal stress on the biceps, brachialis, and forearm supinator muscles.

Starting Position—Place a rubber pad or folded towel on the gym floor and kneel down on it. Grasp two moderately weighted dumbbells and kneel erect with your arms hanging straight down at your sides. Your palms should be facing inward toward each other. Press your upper arms against the sides of your torso and keep them motionless in this position throughout your set. You should keep your palms facing each other over the exercise's complete range of motion.

Movement Performance—Use arm strength to curl the dumbbells directly forward and upward in semicircular arcs to shoulder level. Hold this peak-contracted position for a moment, intensely tensing your biceps muscles, then lower slowly back to the starting point.

Training Tips—Rather than curling the dumbbells upward simultaneously, you can curl them alternately in seesaw fashion.

Standing Cable Curls

Emphasis—This is a good exercise for the biceps. Secondary stress is placed on the brachialis and forearm flexor muscles.

Starting Position—Attach a straight bar handle at least two feet long to the end of a cable running through a floor pulley. Take a shoulder-width undergrip on the pulley handle, set

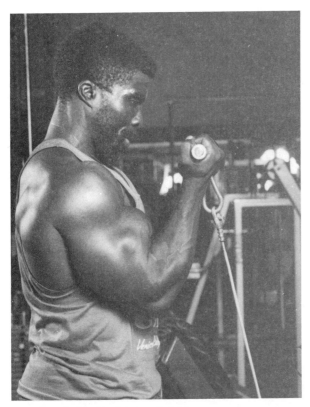

Standing Cable Curl (near finish)

Starting Position—Attach a straight bar handle at least two feet long to the end of a cable running through a floor pulley. Take a shoulder-width overgrip on the pulley handle, set your feet about shoulder width apart 1–1½ feet back from the pulley, and stand erect with your arms hanging straight down at your sides and the pulley handle resting across your upper thighs. Press your upper arms against the sides of your torso and keep them motionless in this position for your entire set. You must also avoid moving your upper body as you do the exercise.

Movement Performance—Use arm strength to curl the pulley handle in a semicircular arc from the front of your thighs up to a point beneath your chin. Hold this peak-contracted position for a moment, intensely tensing your biceps, then lower slowly back along the same arc to the starting point.

Training Tips—Experiment with various grip widths.

your feet about shoulder width apart 1–1½ feet back from the pulley, and stand erect with your arms hanging straight down at your sides and the pulley handle resting across your upper thighs. Press your upper arms against the sides of your torso and keep them motionless in this position for your entire set. You must also avoid moving your upper body as you do the exercise.

Movement Performance—Use biceps strength to curl the pulley handle in a semicircular arc from the front of your thighs up to a point beneath your chin. Hold this peak-contracted position for a moment, intensely tensing your biceps, then lower slowly back along the same arc to the starting point.

Training Tips—Try a wide variety of grip widths. You can also experiment with standing various distances away from the pulley.

Standing Cable Reverse Curls

Emphasis—Doing reverse curls with a cable places almost equal stress on the biceps, brachialis, and forearm supinator muscles.

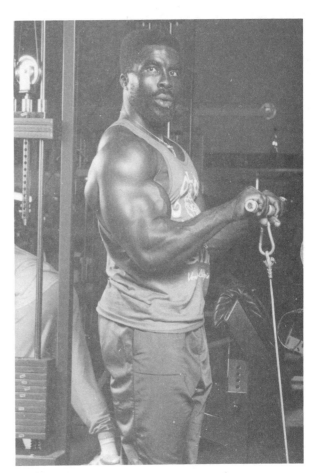

Standing Cable Reverse Curl (midpoint)

Lying Cable Curls

Emphasis—This is a very direct biceps movement, with secondary stress placed on the brachialis and forearm flexor muscles.

Starting Position—Attach a straight bar handle at least two feet long to the end of a cable running through a floor pulley. Take a shoulder-width undergrip on the pulley handle and lie on your back with your feet toward the pulley. Your arms should be straight at your sides. Pin your upper arms against the sides of your torso and hold them in this position throughout your set.

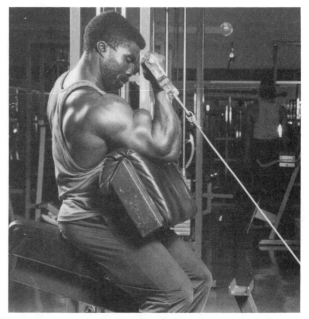

Cable Preacher Curl (finish—one-arm variation)

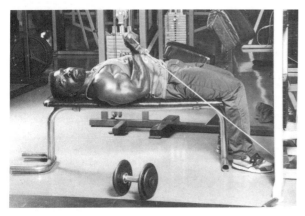

Lying Cable Curl

Movement Performance—Use biceps strength to curl the pulley handle from your thighs up to a point near your chin. Tense your biceps for a moment in this peak-contracted position, then lower slowly back to the starting point.

Training Tips—Vary the width of your grip on the pulley handle.

Cable Preacher Curls

Emphasis—This superior movement places stress on the entire biceps muscle complex, particularly the lower biceps down near the elbow. Because of the continuous tension possible when using cables, many bodybuilders find this exercise to be superior to preacher curls performed with either a barbell, two dumbbells, or a single dumbbell.

Starting Position—Attach a straight bar handle at least two feet long to the end of a cable

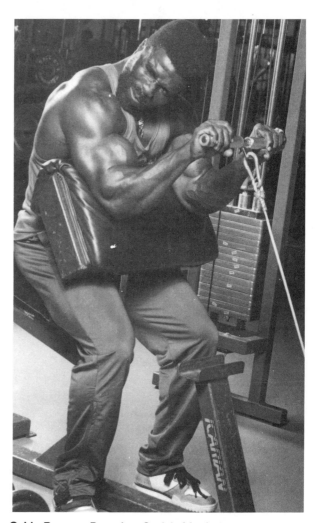

Cable Reverse Preacher Curl (midpoint)

running through a floor pulley. Take an under-grip about 3–4 inches wider than your shoulders on the pulley handle. Lean over a preacher bench and run your upper arms parallel to each other down the angled surface of the bench, your hands at the lower end toward the pulley. The upper edge of the preacher bench should be wedged beneath your armpits. Fully straighten your arms.

Movement Performance—Use biceps strength to curl the pulley handle forward and upward in a semicircular arc to a position beneath your chin. Hold this peak-contracted position for a moment, powerfully tensing your biceps muscles, then slowly lower back along the same arc to the starting point.

Training Tips—You can use a reverse grip on this movement in order to place greater stress on your brachialis and forearm supinator muscles. Regardless of the type of grip, you should also experiment with different grip widths. By attaching a loop handle to the end of the cable, you can also do this movement with one arm at a time.

Loop Handle Cable Curls

Emphasis—While this is a fairly good mass builder, you will generally do loop handle cable curls as a biceps peaker. Secondary stress is placed on the brachialis and forearm flexor muscles.

Starting Position—Attach a loop handle to the end of a cable running through a floor pulley. Grasp the handle with your left hand, stand with your feet a comfortable distance apart a foot or so back from the pulley. Press your left upper arm against the side of your torso and keep it motionless in this position throughout your set. Supinate your hand and keep it supinated throughout your set.

Movement Performance—Use biceps strength to curl the pulley handle directly forward and upward in a semicircular arc to shoulder level. Hold this peak-contracted position for a moment, powerfully tensing your biceps. Lower slowly back along the same arc to the starting

point. Be sure that you do an equal number of sets and reps with each arm.

Training Tips—You'll most often see this movement performed in alternate fashion using two pulleys and two handles in commercial gyms. Most bigger gyms have two pulleys close enough to each other to permit this movement. At home, however, you may have only one floor pulley with which you can work.

Nautilus Curls

Emphasis—The Nautilus arm machine allows you to do curls which are beneficial for building both mass and a high biceps peak. Minimum secondary stress is placed on the brachialis and forearm flexor muscles.

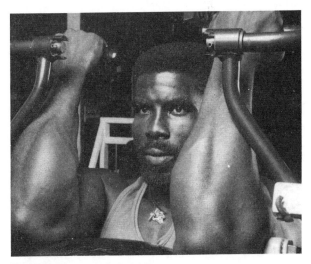

Nautilus Curl (near finish)

Starting Position—Adjust the height of the machine's seat so you can sit in the machine and extend your arms directly upward at the same angle as the padded surface of the machine. Rest your upper arms on that pad with the outer section against the vertical pad on each side. Either grasp the handles (if provided) or slip your wrists beneath the smaller pads attached to the ends of the lever arm. Fully straighten your arms.

Movement Performance—Slowly flex both arms completely, holding the peak-contracted position for a moment while powerfully tensing your biceps muscles. Lower slowly back to the starting point.

Training Tips—This movement can also be done with one arm fully flexed at all times. Start this variation by curling both arms fully. Holding your right arm completely bent, slowly straighten and then bend your left arm. Then holding your left arm completely flexed, slowly straighten and then flex your right arm. Continue alternating arms until you have completed the correct number of repetitions with each arm.

Machine Curls

Emphasis—There are many brands of curling machines on the market, most of which work similarly to the Nautilus biceps machine. Using any of these curling machines will place a very high quality of developmental stress on the working biceps muscles.

Starting Position—Sit on the machine seat and run your upper arms parallel to each other down the angled surface of the pad. The upper edge of the pad should be wedged beneath your armpits. Take a shoulder-width undergrip on the machine handle and slowly straighten your arms.

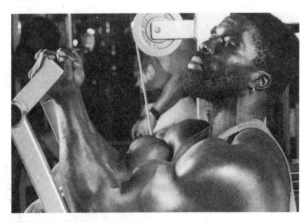

Machine Curl (midpoint)

Movement Performance—Use biceps strength to slowly curl the machine handle upward until it reaches a position directly beneath your chin. Tense your biceps fiercely in this position for a moment, return slowly to the starting point.

Training Tips—You can do reverse curls on this machine, too, as well as experiment with a variety of grip widths to see which combination works best on your biceps.

Seated Dumbbell Concentration Curls

Emphasis—This is the standard movement used by almost all top-level bodybuilders to add to the height of their biceps peak. Minor secondary stress is placed on the brachialis and forearm flexor muscles.

Starting Position—Sit at the end of a flat exercise bench with your feet set about 4–6 inches wider than your shoulders on the floor. Grasp a light dumbbell in your left hand and brace the back of your left triceps against the inside of your left knee a little away from your knee. Your free hand can either be rested on your right knee or wedged behind the triceps of your working arm. Completely straighten your arm. Your palm should be facing forward in the fully supinated position.

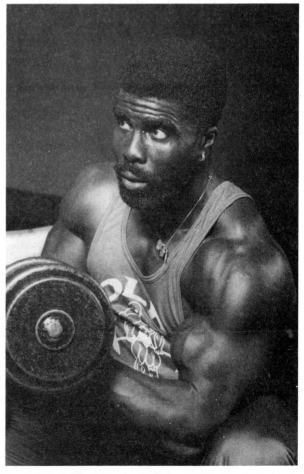

Seated Dumbbell Concentration Curl (midpoint)

Movement Performance—Use biceps strength to slowly curl the dumbbell up to your shoulder. Tense your biceps as strongly as possible in this peak-contracted position, then lower slowly back along the same arc to the starting point.

Training Tips—The real key to this movement is mustering the maximum amount of mental focus on your working biceps.

Standing Dumbbell Concentration Curls

Emphasis—An alternative to seated concentration curls, this exercise adds height to your biceps peak. Secondary stress is placed on the brachialis and forearm flexor muscles.

Starting Position—Grasp a moderately weighted dumbbell in your left hand, set your feet about shoulder width apart 2–2½ feet away from a high bench or dumbbell rack, and bend forward at the waist to rest your right hand on the bench or rack, your right arm straight throughout the movement. Your left arm

should be hanging straight down from your shoulder, with your hand supinated. You must keep the upper arm on your left side perfectly motionless throughout your set.

Movement Performance—Use biceps strength to slowly curl the dumbbell up to your shoulder. Hold this peak-contracted position for a moment while intensely tensing your biceps muscles. Lower slowly back along the same arc to the starting point.

Training Tips—You can curl the weight either directly forward, across the midline of your body, or at any angle intermediate between these two extremes.

Close-Grip Chins

Emphasis—While this movement is primarily intended to increase the width of your lats, you can also intensely stress your biceps with it as

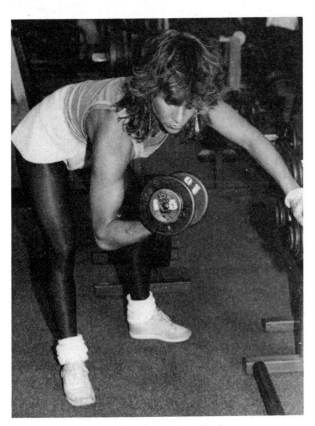

Standing Dumbbell Concentration Curl

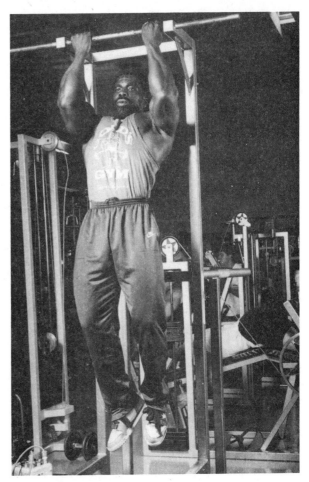

Close-Grip Chins (midpoint)

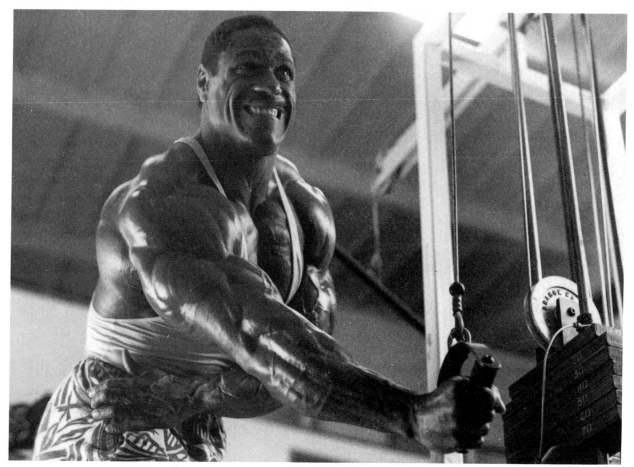

Reverse-Grip Lat Machine Pulldown

well. Secondary stress is on the brachialis, forearm flexor, trapezius, and posterior deltoid muscles.

Starting Position—Jump up and take a narrow undergrip on a chinning bar (there should be only 6–8 inches of space showing between your hands). Fully straighten your arms. You can either hold your legs relatively straight, or bend and cross them.

Movement Performance—Slowly pull yourself up to the bar by bending your arms. At the top point, your chin should be above the bar. Hold this peak-contracted position for a moment, then lower yourself back to the starting point.

Training Tips—Any width of grip from shoulder width inward until your hands are touching will bomb your biceps.

Reverse-Grip Lat Machine Pulldowns

Emphasis—As with narrow-grip chins, this movement is primarily intended to develop the lats, but very intense stress is also placed on the biceps muscles. Secondary emphasis is on the brachialis, forearm flexor, trapezius, and posterior deltoid muscles.

Starting Position—Attach a straight bar handle to the end of a cable running through an overhead pulley. Take an undergrip on the bar, your hands set 6–8 inches apart in the middle of the handle. Straighten your arms and allow your body to sink down onto the seat, at which point you should force your knees far beneath the restraint to keep yourself from rising up as you pull down on the bar handle. Alternatively, you can bend your legs and either sit or kneel directly beneath the pulley. In this case, you should have a training partner standing behind you to press down on your traps on each side of your neck to keep your body from coming up off the floor during each heavy repetition.

Movement Performance—Use lat and biceps strength to pull the bar directly downward until the backs of your hands touch the upper part of your chest. Hold this peak-contracted position for a moment, then slowly lower back to the starting point.

Training Tips—You can use a range of grip widths from about shoulder width inward until your hands are actually touching in the middle of the bar handle.

SUGGESTED BICEPS ROUTINES

Virtually everyone who has read this far in the book will be well past the beginning and intermediate stages of development and training experience. Still, there will be a few less-experienced trainees reading this chapter, so I have included a series of routines in this section which can be used by beginners, intermediates, and advanced bodybuilders. Be sure to change to the next highest routine after you have spent 4-6 weeks on the current program.

BEGINNING ROUTINE

Exercise	Sets	Reps
Standing Barbell Curls	3-4	8-12

LOW-INTERMEDIATE ROUTINE

Exercise	Sets	Reps
Seated Dumbbell Curls	3	8-12
Seated Dumbbell Concentration Curls	2	8-12

HIGH-INTERMEDIATE ROUTINE

Exercise	Sets	Reps
Wide-Grip Standing Barbell Curls	3	6-10
Incline Dumbbell Curls	2	8-12
Barbell Concentration Curls	2	8-12

LOW-ADVANCED ROUTINE

Exercise	Sets	Reps
Barbell Preacher Curls	3	8-12
Nautilus Curls	3	8-12
Standing Dumbbell Concentration Curls	2	8-12

HIGH-ADVANCED ROUTINE

Exercise	Sets	Reps
Standing Alternate Dumbbell Curls	3	8-12
Cable Preacher Curls	3	8-12
Loop Handle Cable Curls	3	8-12

OFF-SEASON, CONTEST-LEVEL ROUTINE

Exercise	Sets	Reps
Dumbbell Preacher Curls	4	8-12
Lying Dumbbell Curls	3	8-12
Prone Incline Dumbbell Curls	3	8-12

PRECONTEST CONTEST-LEVEL ROUTINE

Exercise	Sets	Reps
Standing Narrow-Grip Barbell Curls	3	10-15
Machine Curls	3	10-15
Seated Dumbbell Curls	3	10-15
Standing Dumbbell Concentration Curls	3	10-15

BICEPS ROUTINES OF THE CHAMPS

I am giving you more than 35 biceps training programs from the world's top bodybuilders as examples of how you should train this flashy body part. Feel free to modify your favorite superstar's biceps routine to meet your unique recuperative ability between workouts. Beginning bodybuilders should do no more than 4-5 total sets of biceps work; intermediates, 6-8; and advanced men, 10-12.

Lee Haney

Exercise	Sets	Reps
Standing Barbell Curls	4	8-12
Barbell Preacher Curls	3	8-12
One-Arm Cable Curls, or . . . Seated Dumbbell Concentration Curls	3	10-15

Rich Gaspari

OFF-SEASON

Exercise	Sets	Reps
Standing Barbell Curls	4	8-10
Incline Dumbbell Curls	3	8-10
Barbell Preacher Curls	3	8-10

PRECONTEST

Exercise	Sets	Reps
Standing Barbell Curls	4	10-12
Incline Dumbbell Curls	4	10-12
Barbell Preacher Curls	4	10-12
Standing Dumbbell Concentration Curls	4	10-12

Albert Beckles

Exercise	Sets	Reps
Standing Dumbbell Curls	5	10-12
Seated Dumbbell Concentration Curls	5	10-12
Standing Barbell Curls	5	10

Sergio Oliva

Exercise	Sets	Reps
Standing Barbell Curls	6	8-10
Seated Alternate Dumbbell Curls	6	8-10
Barbell Preacher Curls	6	8-10

Bertil Fox

Exercise	Sets	Reps
Standing Barbell Curls	4	8-10
Barbell Preacher Curls	4	8-10
Dumbbell Incline Curls	4	8-10
Barbell Concentration Curls	4	8-10

The exercises are performed as a giant set.

Berry de Mey

Exercise	Sets	Reps
Standing Barbell Curls	3	8-10
Barbell Preacher Curls	3	8-10
Incline Dumbbell Curls	3	8-10
Seated Dumbbell Curls	3	8-10

Josef Grolmus

Exercise	Sets	Reps
Standing Barbell Curls	4	6-8
Standing Dumbbell Curls	3	6-8
Barbell Reverse Curls	3	6-8

Mike Christian

Exercise	Sets	Reps
Standing Barbell Curls	4	10-12
Incline Dumbbell Curls	4	10-12
Nautilus Curls	4	10-12
Lying Lat Machine Curls	4	10-12
Barbell Preacher Curls	4	10-12

Scott Wilson

Exercise	Sets	Reps
Wide-Grip EZ-Bar Preacher Curls	4	6-10
Close-Grip EZ-Bar Preacher Curls	4	6-10
Standing Barbell Curls	4	6-10
Incline Dumbbell Curls	4	6-10
Seated Dumbbell Concentration Curls	4	6-10

Bob Birdsong

Exercise	Sets	Reps
Nautilus Curls	4-5	8-12
Barbell Preacher Curls	4-5	8-12
Standing Barbell Curls	4-5	8-12

Frank Zane

Exercise	Sets	Reps
Alternate Dumbbell Curls	4	8-10
Pulley Preacher Curls	4	8-10
Low-Incline Dumbbell Curls	4	8-10

Robby Robinson

Exercise	Sets	Reps
Standing Barbell Curls	3-4	8-10
Incline Dumbbell Curls	3	8-10
Standing Dumbbell Concentration Curls	2-3	10-12

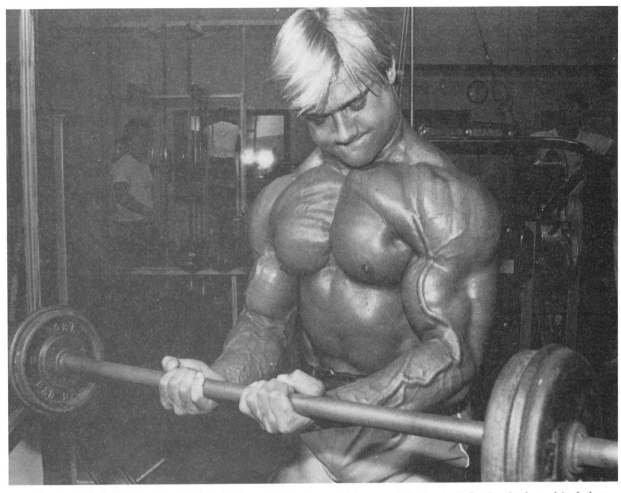

Mr. Universe Tom Platz gives it to his biceps with a set of Narrow-Grip Barbell Curls, designed to bring out the outer head of the muscle group, as is highly evident in this action photo. You can almost see the brain waves emanating toward his biceps.

Gunnar Rosbo

Exercise	Sets	Reps
Standing Barbell Curls	4-5	8-12
Seated Dumbbell Curls	4-5	8-12
Barbell Preacher Curls	4-5	8-12
Seated Dumbbell Concentration Curls	4-5	10-12

Lou Ferrigno

Exercise	Sets	Reps
Alternate Dumbbell Curls	4-5	8-10
Incline Dumbbell Curls	4-5	8-10
Close-Grip Barbell Preacher Curls	4-5	8-10
Cable Reverse Curls	4-5	8-10

Chris Dickerson

Exercise	Sets
Standing Barbell Curls	4
Incline Dumbbell Curls	4
Cable Preacher Curls	
Seated Cable Curls	

Lance Dr

Exercise
Incline Dumbbell Curls
Standing Dumbbell Co Curls
Nautilus Curls

Roy Callender

Exercise	Sets	Reps
Standing Barbell Curls	5-6	8-10
Incline Dumbbell Curls	5-6	8-10
Seated Dumbbell Concentration Curls	4-5	10-12

Dennis Tinerino

PRECONTEST ROUTINE

Exercise	Sets	Reps
Alternate Dumbbell Curls	4	10-12
Machine Curls	3-4	10-12
Wide-Grip Barbell Curls	3-4	10-12
Seated Dumbbell Concentration Curls	3-4	10-12
Cable Curls	3-4	10-12
Barbell Preacher Curls	3-4	10-12

Tom Platz

Exercise	Sets	Reps
Standing Alternate Dumbbell Curls	4-5	8-10
Standing Barbell Curls	4-5	8-10

Bronston Austin, Jr.

Exercise	Sets	Reps
Barbell Reverse Curls	6	10
Standing Barbell Curls	6	10
Seated Barbell Curls	6	10
Dumbbell Preacher Curls	6	10

Tim Belknap

Exercise	Sets	Reps
Standing Barbell Curls	3	10
Seated Dumbbell Curls	3	10
One-Arm Cable Curls	3	10

Boyer Coe

Exercise	Sets	Reps
Preacher Curls	4-5	8-10
Dumbbell Curls	4	8-10
Dumbbell Concentration	4	8-10
Cable Curls	4	8-10

Casey Viator

Exercise	Sets	Reps
Seated Dumbbell Concentration Curls	4	10-12
One-Arm Cable Curls	4	10-12
Standing Barbell Curls	4	10-12
Seated Alternate Dumbbell Curls	4	10-12

Bob Jodkiewicz

Exercise	Sets	Reps
Barbell Preacher Curls	4	10-12
Machine Curls	2	10-12
Seated Dumbbell Concentration Curls	2	10-12
One-Arm Cable Curls	2	10-12

Ed Corney

Exercise	Sets	Reps
Standing Barbell Curls	3-4	8-10
One-Arm Dumbbell Preacher Curls	3-4	8-10
Cable Concentration Curls	3-4	10-12

Larry Scott

Exercise	Sets	Reps
Incline Dumbbell Curls	3	6
Dumbbell Preacher Curls	3-4	6
Barbell Preacher Curls	3-4	6
Reverse Curls	3-4	6

Do four burns at the end of each set of every exercise.

Mike Mentzer

Exercise	Sets	Reps
Barbell Preacher Curls	2	6-8
Seated Dumbbell Concentration Curls	1-2	6-8
Alternate Dumbbell Hammer Curls	2	6-8

Mike does forced reps at the end of most sets.

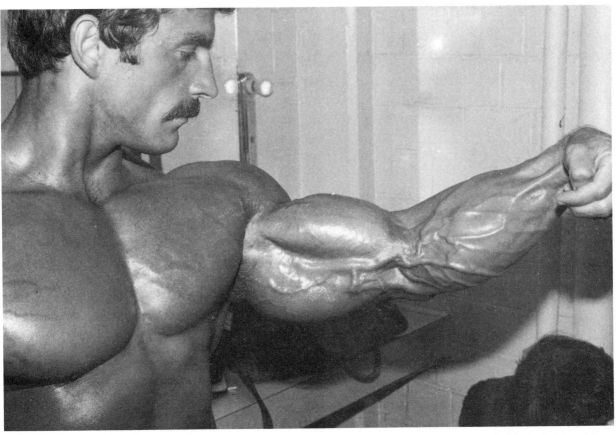

Multitalented Mike Mentzer shows what a bodybuilder's arm can look like even when held straight out to the side and tensed. Look at the fantastic tie-ins between his forearm and upper-arm muscles.

Ron Teufel

Exercise	Sets	Reps
Incline Dumbbell Curls	5	10
One-Arm Cable Curls	5	8–10
Standing Barbell Curls	4	8–10

Arnold Schwarzenegger

Exercise	Sets	Reps
Standing Barbell Curls	4	6–10
Dumbbell Curls	4	6–10
Seated Dumbbell Concentration Curls	4	6–10

Arnold often does descending sets, taking two weight drops.

Danny Padilla

Exercise	Sets	Reps
Seated Dumbbell Curls	5	6–8
Seated Dumbbell Concentration Curls	5	8–10
Incline Dumbbell Curls	4	8–10
Standing Barbell Curls, or . . . Barbell Preacher Curls	4	8–10

Lee Labrada

Exercise	Sets	Reps
Barbell Concentration Curls	2	8–10
Dumbbell Preacher Curls, or . . . Standing Alternate Dumbbell Curls	2	8–10
Alternate Dumbbell Hammer Curls	2	8–10

Greg DeFerro

Exercise	Sets	Reps
Barbell Preacher Curls	4	8–10
Seated Alternate Dumbbell Curls	2–3	8–10
Standing Pulley Curls	3	8–10

Matt Mendenhall

Exercise	Sets	Reps
Standing Barbell Curls	5	6–8
Barbell Preacher Curls	5	8
Seated Dumbbell Concentration Curls	5	8

John Terilli

Exercise	Sets	Reps
Standing Barbell Curls	4	8–12
Seated Dumbbell Curls	3	8–12
One-Arm Cable Concentration Curls	2	8–12
Standing Barbell Reverse Curls	2	8–12

Rory Leidelmeyer

Exercise	Sets	Reps
Standing Barbell Curls	4	8–10
Alternate Dumbbell Curls	4	8
Lying Pulley Curls	4	5–7
Barbell Concentration Curls	4	8

19
Building Huge,
Diamond-Shaped Calves

I have always believed that calves are the one muscle group that separates the men from the boys at high-level bodybuilding competitions. All of the really great bodybuilders have awesome calves that blend perfectly with the rest of their physiques. Some of the greatest bodybuilders with unparalleled calf development are Chris Dickerson, Mike Mentzer, Arnold Schwarzenegger, Tim Belknap, Tom Platz, and Gary Strydom.

Many bodybuilders believe that the calves are virtually impossible to build up, and therefore they completely surrender in the calf wars. They have probably trained calves hard for a few months, noticed no particular improvement in the contour of the muscle group, and given up the struggle.

Persistence is a hallmark of every champion bodybuilder in the history of the sport. They never give up in their quest to build up every muscle group, including their calves. And many a bodybuilder who previously had underdeveloped calves has ended up with calves to boast about.

One such champion is the incomparable Arnold Schwarzenegger, who came over to the United States from Europe in the late 1960s to train under me, boasting very puny calf development. But by prioritizing calf development by cutting off the legs of all his warm-up pants so he'd constantly be reminded of how weak his calves were, and using a heavy program of calf training, Arnold was able to build a pair of the greatest calves in bodybuilding history.

Lee Haney has also had to work extra hard to bring up initially puny calves. Lee has always been one of the leading exponents of the Weider Muscle Priority Training Principle, and has used that principle in bringing up his calves. He always trained them first in a workout, when he could put maximum effort into his calf program.

Haney relentlessly kept after his calves, and gradually they came up to a Herculean level which he never initially dreamed he could achieve. Week after week, he kept bombing his calves with heavy weights and absolutely pin-

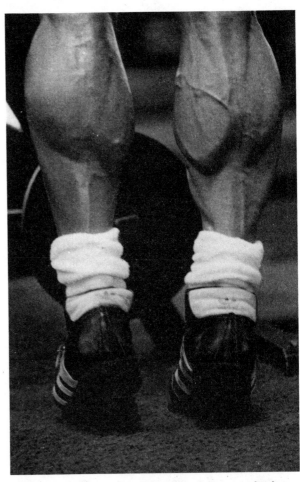

The calves of Tom Platz, IFBB Mr. Universe, who has also placed in the top three at Mr. Olympia (1981). Tom is currently pursuing an acting career.

point mental concentration on the working muscles. He also was scrupulously careful to avoid overtraining his calves. And by combining all of these factors, he was able to build huge, diamond-shaped calves, which are now the envy of most upcoming bodybuilders.

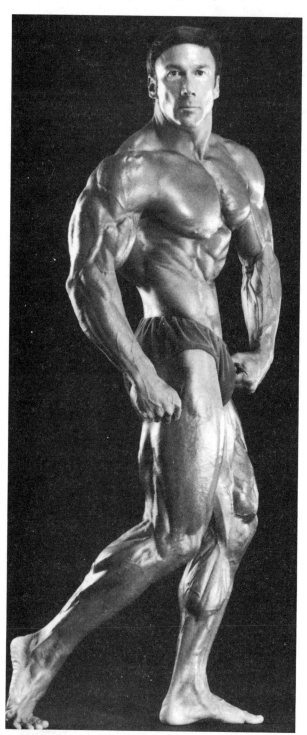

A unique side calf display from Boyer Coe, one of the all-time greats. Boyer started training at age 15 and was Teenage Mr. America by 18 years of age.

I'll try to give you all of the secrets of the champs that I have gleaned over the years of training these exceptional athletes. But rather than give you every calf-training strategy I've discovered, I'll give you only those techniques that I've consistently used with top bodybuilders who needed calf development and used my coaching to achieve it.

CALF ANATOMY AND KINESIOLOGY

There are many small muscles in the lower leg, but I'll only discuss the structure and function of the three largest muscles which contract to flex and extend your foot. The first of these muscles, a long one which runs down the shins, is called the *tibialis anticus*, which contracts to flex the toes toward the knee. In everyday practice, few bodybuilders work this muscle group directly, because it seems to come up merely through normal calf training.

On the back of your leg, there is a long, broad muscle connecting the lower part of the upper leg with the end of the heel called the *gastrocnemius*. It flexes to extend the toes when the leg is straight, as well as to flex the entire leg, such as in a leg curl, which stresses the gastrocnemius muscles as much as the biceps femoris.

Beneath the gastrocnemius is a shorter and flatter muscle called the *soleus*, which connects the upper part of your shin bone with your heel. This muscle can only be contracted completely when your gastrocnemius is not involved, as is the case when your leg is bent at a 90-degree angle. As a result, the only movement that successfully develops the soleus is heel raises on a seated calf machine.

CALF TRAINING TIPS

"If you lack width to your calves," says *Lee Haney*, "you should concentrate your efforts on seated calf raises either in a machine, or with a heavy barbell resting on your knees. This exercise adds width to your soleus, which is the widest muscle in your calf complex. Seated calf raises are also excellent for carving deep cuts in the outer sides of your calves, so it serves a dual purpose.

"You can't depend on seated calf raises to make up your entire lower leg routine, however. While they add width to your calves and cuts when the lower legs are viewed from the sides, they do little to improve the appearance of your calves when viewed from the rear. To bring up your gastrocs, which give that rear-view impressiveness, you have to do plenty of standing calf raises, donkey calf raises, one-legged calf raises, and calf presses on leg press machines."

Successful IFBB pro bodybuilder, *John Hnatyschak* enlarges on the concept of different reps for different calf exercises: "The calves are a great muscle group on which you can use the Weider Holistic Sets Training Principle. With this training technique, you will use a variety of rep schemes for a particular body part. For the soleus and gastrocnemius muscles, you can occasionally do low reps in the range of 6-10, medium repetitions in the range of 10-15, and some other sets in the higher range of 20-30 counts. Each rep range affects your calves somewhat differently, and it is the accumulation of many exercises and many repetition ranges that will ultimately develop terrific calves for your next onstage competitive experience."

Lou Ferrigno tells how he improved his once weak calves prior to winning his Mr. America and Mr. Universe titles: "When I was in my late teens, I realized I had to drastically improve my calves if I ever wanted to win any high-level bodybuilding titles. So I studied all of the hundreds of back issues of various muscle magazines I had, looking for a calf routine which might work for me.

"The calf-training program I hit upon was a three-day cycle. On the first day I did 6-8 very heavy sets—after a good warm-up, of course—of 8-10 reps on seated calf raises. The second day I did 4-5 total sets of 15-20 reps of standing calf raises on a calf machine. Then I rested one day and repeated the cycle on the fourth day. In only about a year of using this simple calf program, I was able to put 1½ inches of new muscle on my calves, and I won my Mr. America title as a result. Another year on the same type of routine, and I had won Mr. Universe and Mr. International titles. I hope my calf-building routine works as well for you as it did for me!"

Most champion bodybuilders believe that consistent stretching of the lower-leg muscles is essential if you want to build great calves. *Boyer* Coe is typical of these champs: "I made my best gains in calf muscle mass and quality when I began stretching my calves before my workout and between calf-training sets. In only a year of stretching, I was able to add more than an inch of solid muscle to my calves, a terrific increase.

"The best way to stretch calves is to face a wall while standing about 2½-3 feet from the wall. Lean forward and place your hands about shoulder width apart and at shoulder level on the wall. Straighten your legs and torso so your body makes one long line from the floor to the wall. If you can place your heels flat on the floor in this position, step back a few more inches, and attempt to again place your heels on the floor with your legs held straight. When you can barely touch the floor with your heels, you should hold this stretched position for 10-15 seconds, release for 5-10 seconds, and repeat the stretch 5-10 times.

"You can also do this with one leg at a time, bending the nonstretching leg and concentrating on stretching your calf muscle on the leg that is held straight. I personally find this a better way to stretch calves than doing it with both legs simultaneously. But whichever variation you choose, be sure to stretch consistently if you expect to get any results in calf development."

Rich Gaspari warns against overtraining the calves: "I see many inexperienced young bodybuilders do 15-20 total sets of calf training six days a week in an effort to develop their diamonds. They never seem to make any progress because they are doing too many sets too frequently, thereby preventing the calves from recovering between workouts. As a result, you become overtrained, and you don't make any progress at all from continued hard calf-bombing sessions. And in some extreme cases, you can even lose calf muscle mass and tone by overtraining.

"If you fall into this category, the best thing you can do is begin training your calves on an every-other-day system. One of the days, you can do 5-6 heavy sets of standing calf raises, and two days later you can perform a lighter series of 5-6 sets on seated calf raises. You can then continue alternating this program, never doing a particular calf routine more frequently than every fourth day. I'd suggest about 10–12 reps on the heavy movements and 15–20 reps on the lighter exercises.

"This type of program should prevent you from overtraining in the future. And as long as you consistently have 100% mental concentration on the working muscles on every repetition of each set, you will make great progress in building up your calves. And perhaps that will one day help you to win a National or World Championship like I did at only 20 years of age."

Calf training is an excellent place in which to follow the Weider Peak Contraction Training Principle. This particular principle advocates having a heavy weight on the working muscles when they are maximally contracted. Each calf movement allows you to use peak contraction. I suggest that you hold the top position of the movement for a slow count of three to add to the peak contraction effect, then slowly lower back to the starting point.

For all machine calf raises you can also use the Weider Retro-Gravity Training Principle by emphasizing the amount of weight placed on the negative (lowering) phase of each repetition. Let *Ron Love* (National Heavyweight Champion and IFBB Pro World Champion) tell you how to emphasize the negative part of each calf movement: "I can best illustrate this method by sitting you in a Universal Gym leg press machine, your legs straight and only your toes and the balls of your feet in contact with the lower set of pedals.

"When you are in position with a weight which would restrict you to about 15–20 full positive and negative reps, start out with 5–6 strict repetitions. When you have the weight pressed out as far from you as possible, bend your right leg to shift full resistance to your left calf, then slowly lower back to the fully stretched calf position. Be sure that you fight mightily to resist the downward pressure of the weight on each leg. Then push the pedals back out with both legs, bend your left leg and lower the weight while resisting only with the calf muscles on your left leg. Continue alternating legs in this manner, until you literally can't push the pedals into the finish position with both legs.

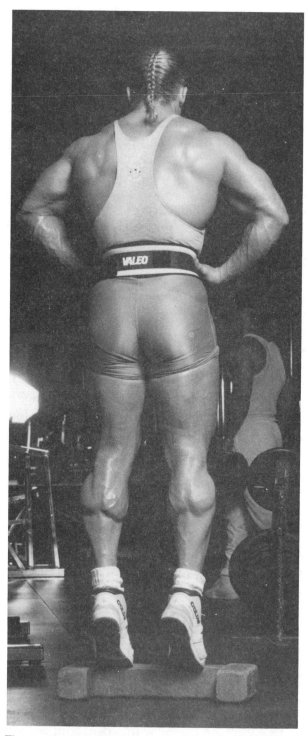

The contracted calves of Andreas Cahling (IFBB Pro Mr. International), model for most of the exercises in this chapter.

"You'll discover a new definition of growth burn in your calves when you use this technique on them. But you have to consistently fight through this pain barrier if you want to build your calves up to an international standard. This is a technique I used after turning pro, and I credit it with the improved calf development which allowed me to win my Pro World Championship."

As a final tip, I want to give you a nonresistance calf routine that will help to balloon your calves and rip them to the limit for a competition. It consists of a superset of one-legged calf raises performed with no added resistance in a stairwell where you can do 25 reps with one leg, 25 with the other, 20 for the first, and then 20 for the second set of calf muscles, all nonstop. And you should do this little superset with your toes angled outward on every set.

Now for the part of this superset that really works wonders for calf mass, shape, and muscular definition. An hour after the first superset, step into the stairwell and do another superset. Over a period of a couple of weeks, you can gradually add to the number of total supersets you perform, all with at least one hour between them. Ultimately, I'd like you to work up to 8–10 total supersets. In practice, you'll be pumping up your calves virtually all day. And I have found this routine is best used in conjunction with a normal calf workout with heavy weights. I suggest a four-day training cycle. On the first day, do the weightless superset; on the second day, do your heavy calf workout, restricting it to about 6–8 total sets with low reps and very heavy weights; on the third day, repeat the weightless supersets; and on the fourth day rest.

I've put a lot of bodybuilders on this type of routine about 6–8 weeks before a competition, and it's not unusual to see someone pump his calves up a full inch in only this short period of time, while ripping his calves to shreds. It's a real winner of a calf training program, and I hope you will give it a good trial in your own calf training philosophy.

As a concluding note on calf training, listen to *Shane DiMora:* "One trick I've learned through experience in the gym is to never do my calf workout prior to my thigh routine. If you do calves before thighs, you will find that your legs tend to vibrate so much when squatting that you simply can't get in a good leg workout. The solution to this problem is to either do calf training *after* legs, or on a separate training day. Then you shouldn't have any problems with leg vibration."

CALF EXERCISES
Standing Barbell Calf Raises

Emphasis—If you don't have a standing calf machine, but do have good balance, you can use this movement to isolate stress on the grastrocnemius muscles. Secondary emphasis is on the broad, flat soleus muscles beneath the gastrocs.

Starting Position—Power clean a moderately heavy barbell to your shoulders and push it up over your head to a position resting on your

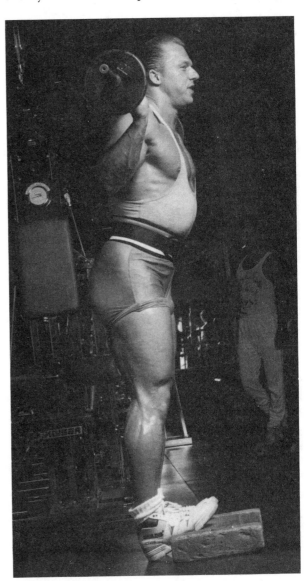

Standing Barbell Calf Raises (start)

trapezius muscles behind your neck. Balance the bar in this position by grasping the bar on each side out near the collars. Step on to a thick block of wood (4×4 inches is a good size), with only your toes and the balls of your feet in contact with the block of wood. Stand erect throughout your set. Relax your calves and allow your heels to travel as far below the level of your toes as possible, thereby prestretching your calf muscles.

Movement Performance—Use calf strength to rise up as high as possible on your toes. Hold this peak-contracted position for a moment and then lower back to the starting point.

Training Tips—Most frequently, this movement is performed with the feet about shoulder width apart and toes angled straight forward.

However, you can stress your calves somewhat differently by moving your feet either closer to each other or wider apart. You can also experiment with different toe angles such as pointed outward at 45-degree angles, or pointed inward in a pigeon-toed position. By varying foot stance width and angle, you can intensely stress your calves with at least 10–12 different variations unique from all of the rest.

Standing Machine Calf Raises

Emphasis—This is a much more secure movement for isolating stress on the gastrocnemius muscles than the free-standing barbell version just described. Minor secondary stress is also placed on the soleus muscles lying beneath the gastrocnemius muscles.

Starting Position—Stand facing a standing calf machine, bend your legs and fit your shoulders beneath the yokes attached to the weight. Next place your toes and the balls of

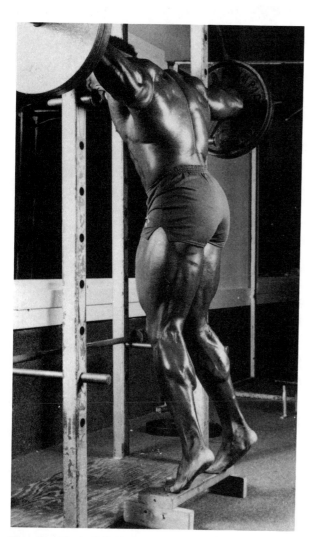

Standing Barbell Calf Raises (finish—model: Lee Haney)

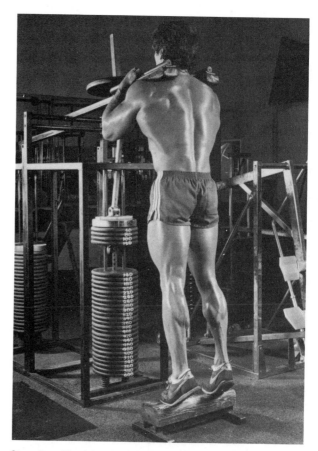

Standing Machine Calf Raises (finish—model: Frank Zane)

your feet on the calf block, your feet about shoulder width apart and toes pointed straight ahead. Stand erect and relax your calves to allow your heels to sink as far below the level of your toes as is comfortably possible, thereby prestretching your calf muscles. Keep your torso and legs positioned in one long and unbroken line throughout the movement, and lock your legs out straight for the entire set.

Movement Performance—Use calf strength only to rise up as high as possible on your toes. Hold this peak-contracted position for a slow count of two to enhance the intensity of the repetition, then slowly lower back to the starting position.

Training Tips—As with standing barbell calf raises, you can vary the width of your foot stance, plus the angle of your feet (either in, out, or straight ahead). But you can also do this movement with only one leg at a time, which automatically intensifies it. Whenever you must concentrate your mental focus on two legs or two arms, you lose some of the value of the movement.

Seated Barbell Calf Raises

Emphasis—This movement is the forerunner of the popular one performed on a seated calf machine, so you don't see it used much unless a seated calf machine is unavailable. It does a very good job of isolating stress on the soleus muscles, with minimal secondary assistance from the gastrocs.

Starting Position—Pad the middle of a heavy barbell handle by rolling a towel around it. Position a calf block about 2–2½ feet from the end of a flat exercise bench. Lift the barbell up to knee height and then sit down at the end of the bench with the barbell resting across your lower thighs down near your knees. (Alternatively, you can sit down and have a training partner position the bar across your lower thighs.) Place your toes and the balls of your feet on the calf block. Allow the weight to push your heels as far below the level of your toes as possible. There should be about 1½–2 feet of space between your heels, and your toes should be pointed directly forward.

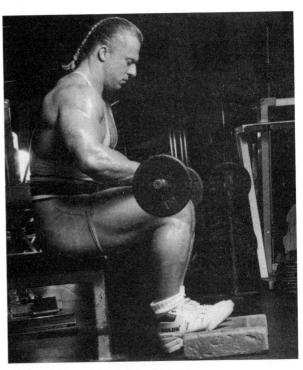

Seated Barbell Calf Raises (finish)

Movement Performance—Push down with your toes and extend your feet as completely as possible, actually rising up on your toes if possible. Hold this peak-contracted position for a moment, then slowly lower back to the starting point.

Training Tips—Due to the length of the calf block, you won't be able to use an excessively wide foot spacing, but you should nonetheless experiment with different foot placement widths, from feet nearly touching in the middle of the calf block, to as wide a stance as the block permits. You should also experiment with angling your toes inward and outward at approximate 45-degree angles in addition to pointing your toes directly forward.

Seated Machine Calf Raises

Emphasis—A more convenient and secure movement, this is directly equivalent to seated barbell calf raises. So it places isolated stress on the soleus muscles of the lower legs, with only minimal secondary assistance from the gastrocnemius muscles.

Starting Position—By pulling a pin out of the two sliding columns that attach the knee pads

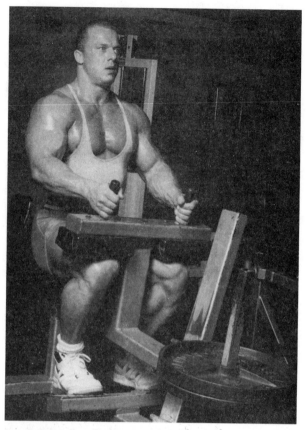

Seated Machine Calf Raises (start)

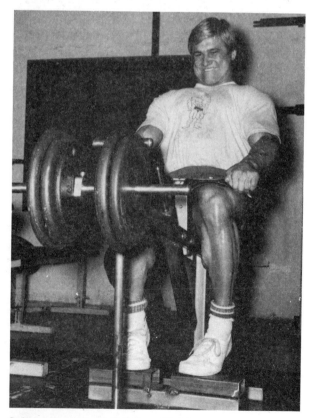

Seated Machine Calf Raises (finish—model: Tom Platz)

to the lever arm of the machine, you can adjust the relative height of the pads to match the length of your lower legs. In any case, adjust the length of the column so that you can place your feet on the foot bar, wedge the pads over your knees comfortably snug, and then push down slightly with your toes to free the weight. Sit down on the machine seat and place the toes and balls of both feet on the foot bar, your heels and the rest of your foot hanging off into space. Pull the pads to the rear and snugly over your knees. Push down with your feet and release the stop bar to free the machine for the movement. This stop bar is different from machine to machine, but usually it moves either forward or off to the side to free the lever arm. (Be sure that you relock the machine by returning the stop bar to its original position when you have finished your set, and before exiting the machine.)

Movement Performance—Allow the weight attached to the pads over your knees to force your heels as far below the level of your toes as comfortably possible. This prestretches the calf muscles. Without bouncing in the bottom of the movement, slowly push downward with your toes and rise up as high as possible on your toes, fully extending your feet. Hold this peak-contracted position for a slow count of two, then slowly lower back to the position in which your calf muscles are completely stretched.

Training Tips—Experiment with the width of your foot placement on the foot bar, as well as with your toe angle as you do the movement.

Calf Presses

Emphasis—This is an excellent way to isolate stress on your gastrocnemius muscles while minimizing assistance from the soleus muscles.

Starting Position—This exercise can be performed on a vertical, angled, or horizontal leg press machine, and there are both Nautilus and Universal Gym machines which allow a horizontal attack. I will explain the Universal Gym variation; from that, you can easily infer how to do the movement on the other types of machines. Sit down in the machine seat and adjust

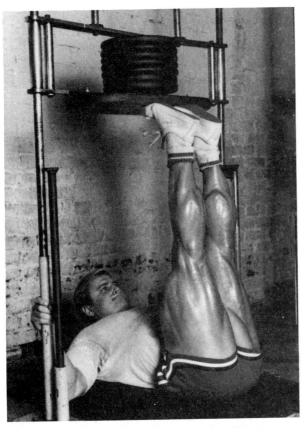

Calf Presses (vertical machine variation—finish)

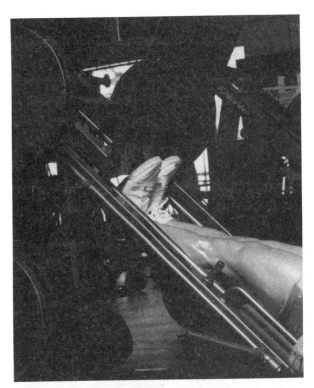

Calf Presses (angled machine variation—start)

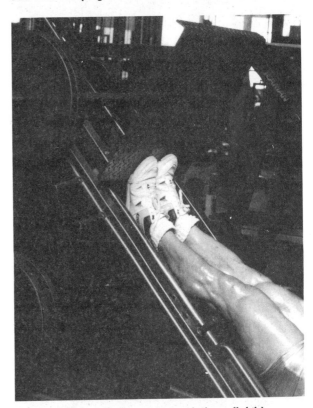

Calf Presses (angled machine variation—finish)

the seat to a position as far from the foot pedals as possible. Place your feet on the lower set of pedals (if there are two sets) and straighten your legs. When you have your legs locked out straight, slide your heels from the lower edges of the pedals, until only your toes and the balls of your feet are in contact with the pedals. Be sure to keep your legs locked out straight throughout your set. Allow the weight attached to the lever arm of the machine to force your toes as far toward your body as comfortably possible. This effectively prestretches the calf muscles.

Movement Performance—Push slowly down with your toes against the machine pedals and fully extend your feet. Hold this peak-contracted position for a slow count of two, then slowly return to the starting point without bouncing in the bottom position of the exercise.

Training Tips—Vertical and angled leg press machines allow a wide variety of foot placement widths, and all leg press machines allow you to experiment with a more narrow range of foot placement widths. You should also experiment with various toe angles as you place your feet for calf presses.

Donkey Calf Raises

Emphasis—This movement allows a better stretch in the calf muscles at the beginning of each repetition, so it is a very good isolation exercise for gastroc development. There is only a minimum of synergistic assistance from the soleus muscles.

Starting Position—Place a calf block at the side of a flat exercise bench about 2-2½ feet back from the bench. Place your toes and the balls of your feet on the block, heels about 16-20 inches apart and toes pointed directly forward. Bend forward at the waist so your torso is in a position parallel with the gym floor, and rest your hands on the bench with arms straight to maintain this position. Have a heavy training partner jump up astride your hips, as if he was riding a horse. It is essential, however, that he ride as far back as possible. Riding forward near the shoulders places minimum extra resistance on the working calf muscles. Allow the weight of your training partner to push your heels as far below the level of your toes as possible, prestretching your calf muscles.

Movement Performance—Push down with your toes and rise up as high on your toes as possible. Hold this peak-contracted position for a slow count of two, and then return slowly to the starting point without bouncing in the low position of the movement.

Training Tips—You should experiment with different foot placement widths and toe angles. If you need more resistance than your training partner can supply, he should hold a heavy barbell plate or dumbbell against your back as close to his crotch as possible. Again, it does little good if he rests the added weight against your upper back.

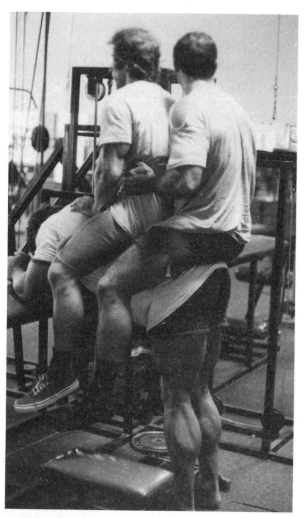

Arnold Schwarzenegger with Eddie Guiliani and Dan Howard providing extra resistance—often Arnold would have one man jump off partway through, so he could continue a set using the Weider Descending Sets Training Principle.

Nautilus Multi Machine Calf Raises

Emphasis—This equivalent of donkey calf raises is unique to the Nautilus multi machine. It places direct, high-quality stress on the gastrocnemius muscles and lesser stress on the soleus muscles.

Starting Position—Place the machine belt around your hips as low on your waist as possible. Bend your knees and attach the ring on the belt to the end of the machine lever arm. Stand up bearing the weight of the machine, and place the toes and the balls of your feet on either the upper or lower steps of the machine, your feet set about shoulder width apart and toes pointed directly forward. (I really don't feel it makes any difference on which step you place your feet.) Keep your legs straight throughout the movement. Allow the weight of the plate stack to pull your heels as far below the level of your toes as possible to prestretch your calf muscles.

Movement Performance—Push down with your toes and completely extend your feet, rising up as high as possible on your toes. Hold this peak-contracted position for a slow count of two, then slowly lower back to the starting position. Do not bounce the weights in the bottom part of the movement.

Training Tips—Experiment with the usual foot-placement width variations and toe angles. It is also possible to do this movement with one leg at a time, although you will need to drastically reduce the amount of weight you use. When doing the exercise, you can either rest your forearms on the cross members of the machine at waist height, or grasp these bars in your hands. You can also stand virtually erect as you do the movement.

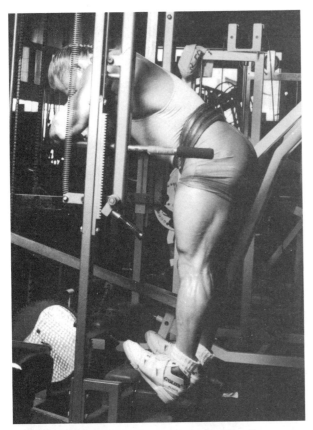

Nautilus Multi Machine Calf Raises (start)

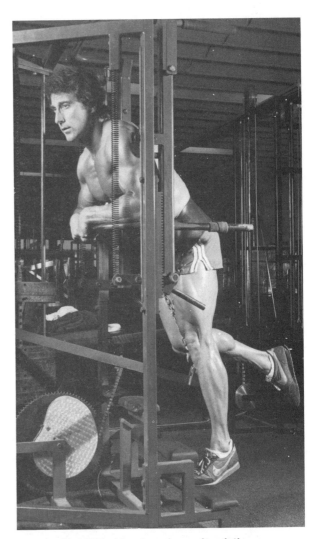

Nautilus Multi Machine (one-legged variation—midpoint)

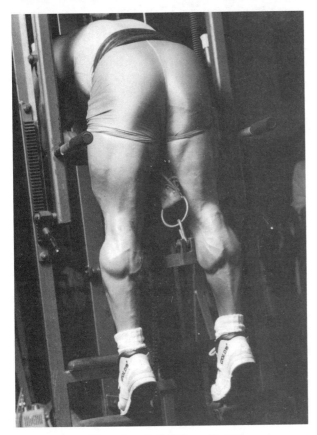

Nautilus Multi Machine Calf Raises (finish)

One-Legged Calf Raises

Emphasis—The all-time universal calf exercise is one-legged calf raises. The only piece of equipment needed for the movement is a dumbbell and either a thick block of wood or a stairwell, so everyone can do this calf exercise, regardless of how limited his equipment is. And one-legged calf raises are a very direct gastrocnemius movement which also places limited stress on the soleus muscles.

Starting Position—Hold a moderately heavy dumbbell in your right hand and stand with toes and the ball of your right foot on the calf block or stair riser. Bend your left leg at a 90-degree angle to keep it out of the movement. Balance your body in place by grasping a sturdy upright or by pressing your hand against a wall as you do the movement. Keep your right

leg straight throughout your set. Allow the weight of your body with the extra dumbbell to push your right heel as far as possible below the level of your toes.

Movement Performance—Use calf strength to rise up as high as possible on the toes of your right foot. Hold this peak-contracted position for a slow count of two, then slowly lower back to the starting point. Be sure to do an equal number of sets and reps with each leg.

Training Tips—The most common mistake when doing this exercise is inadvertently pulling up with the hand which should be balancing your body. This destroys some of the value of the movement, and is an action which should only be undertaken to provide 2–3 forced reps at the end of a normal set to failure.

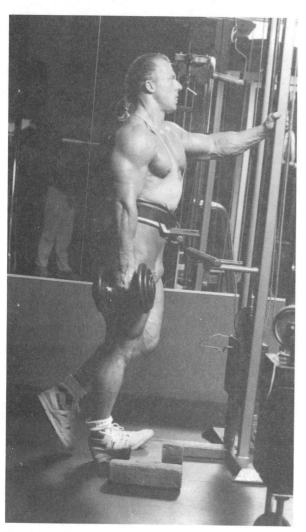

One-Legged Dumbbell Calf Raise (start)

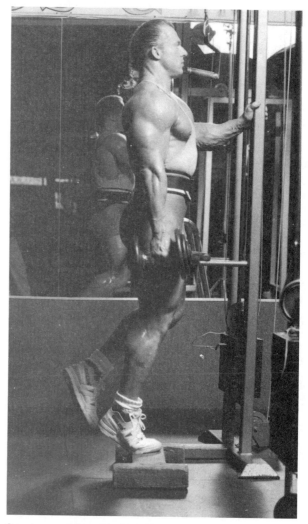

One-Legged Dumbbell Calf Raise (finish)

Hack Machine Calf Raises

Emphasis—This is an excellent, although often ignored, movement for isolating stress on the grastrocs while marginally involving the soleus muscles.

Starting Position—While this exercise can be performed on a yoke-style hack machine, it is best done on the sliding-platform hack machine. Facing the machine, reach down and grasp the handles at the sides of the lower part of the sliding part of the machine. Pull up on the handles to bring the sliding platform up high enough so you can press your chest and upper abdomen against the padded surface. Slide your feet backward until only your toes and the balls of your feet are in contact with the angled foot platform at the start of the machine. Straighten your legs and keep them straight throughout your set. Allow the weight of the machine to push your heels as far below the level of your toes as comfortably possible.

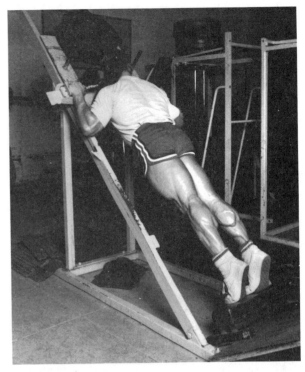

Hack Machine Calf Raises (finish)

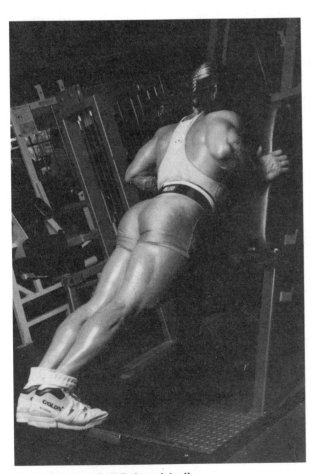

Hack Machine Calf Raises (start)

Movement Performance—Use calf strength to rise up on your toes as high as possible. Hold this peak-contracted position for a slow count of two. Then slowly lower back to the starting position without bouncing in the bottom of the movement.

Training Tips—It is also possible to do this movement on a yoke-type machine, although there will obviously be no platform against which to press your chest. All you need to do with the yoke-type machine is reverse your body position from the one you would use for hack squats (e.g., you will be facedown).

Jumping Squats

Emphasis—This dynamic movement stresses all of the leg muscles, but particularly those of the calves.

Starting Position—Place a moderately weighted barbell across your shoulders behind your neck and hold it in position by grasping the barbell handle out near the plates. Set your feet about shoulder width apart.

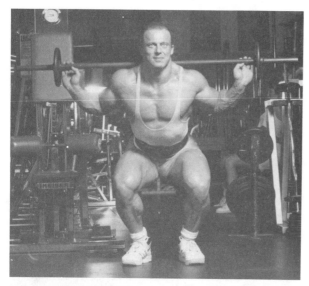

Jumping Squat (start)

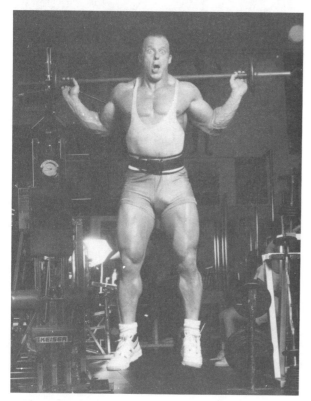

Jumping Squat (finish)

Movement Performance—Keeping your torso erect, slowly sink down into a squatting position until your thighs are parallel with the gym floor. Reverse the movement and come erect, sharply accelerating the movement and actually springing off the floor at the top of the exercise. Bend your legs to absorb the shock of landing, and begin sinking back down to start a repetition.

Training Tips—You can also do this movement while holding moderately weighted dumbbells in your hands.

Tibialis Raises

Emphasis—This is the only direct movement you have for isolating stress on the tibialis anterior muscles at the fronts of your shins.

Starting Position—Sit at the end of a flat exercise bench with your feet flat on the floor and close to each other. Have a training partner place a heavy barbell plate over your toes.

Movement Performance—Raise the barbell plate from the floor by flexing your feet upward as high as possible. Hold this peak-contracted position for a slow count of two, then lower back to the starting point.

Training Tips—If you haven't been working your tibialis anterior muscles directly, you will find that they become pumped up and reach

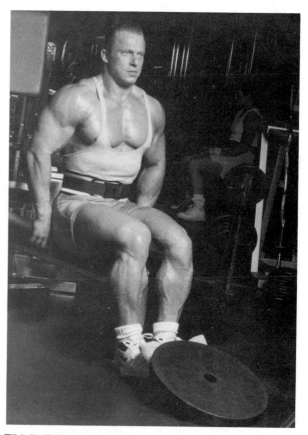

Tibialis Raise (midpoint)

muscular failure after only a few reps. But with time you can treat them like any other muscle group. You can also do this movement with one foot at a time.

SUGGESTED CALF TRAINING PROGRAMS

As with any other muscle group, you will over-train your calves if you attempt to do an Olympian-level routine without first gradually building up your recovery ability and muscle strength levels. To counteract overtraining, I have formulated four successively more-difficult calf-training schedules which you can use one after another, 6–8 weeks on each routine, until you have developed sufficient recovery ability to thrive on a more complex and extensive calf-training program, such as the calf routines of the champions at the end of this chapter.

BEGINNING-LEVEL ROUTINE

Exercise	Sets	Reps
Standing Calf Raises	2–3	15–20
Seated Calf Raises	2–3	10–15

LOW-INTERMEDIATE-LEVEL ROUTINE

Exercise	Sets	Reps
Seated Calf Raises	3	12–8*
Calf Presses	2–3	15–20
One-Legged Calf Raises	2–3	12–15

Exercises marked with an asterisk have weights and reps pyramided, the poundage increased and repetitions decreased with each succeeding set.

HIGH-INTERMEDIATE-LEVEL ROUTINE

MONDAY–THURSDAY

Exercise	Sets	Reps
Seated Calf Raises	4	12–6*
Donkey Calf Raises	2–3	15–20

TUESDAY–FRIDAY

Exercise	Sets	Reps
Standing Calf Raises	4	15–8*
Jumping Squats	2–3	10–15

ADVANCED-LEVEL ROUTINE

MONDAY–THURSDAY

Exercise	Sets	Reps
Seated Calf Raises	4	12–6*
Calf Presses	3	12–15
One-Legged Calf Raises	3	15–20

TUESDAY–FRIDAY

Exercise	Sets	Reps
Standing Calf Raises	4	15–8*
Hack Machine Calf Raises	3–4	15–20

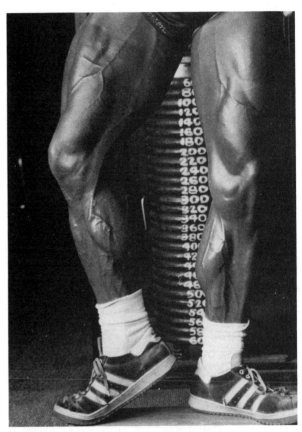

A pair of the most famous calves in bodybuilding belong to Chris Dickerson, 1982 Mr. Olympia and the IFBB all-time pro victories leader.

CALF ROUTINES OF THE CHAMPIONS

In this section I will give you personal calf routines submitted by 20 IFBB superstar bodybuilders. Rather than just adopting the calf routine of your favorite star, you should try all of the routines out in some systematic fashion and then adopt parts of the training philosophies or routines of several great bodybuilders. In this manner, you will ultimately develop the perfect individualized approach to personal calf training.

Lee Haney

DAY ONE

Exercise	Sets	Reps
Standing Calf Raises	5	10-15
Calf Presses	5	15-20
Donkey Calf Raises	5	12-15

DAY TWO

Exercise	Sets	Reps
Seated Calf Raises	6-8	10-12
One-Legged Calf Raises	5-6	15-20

Frank Zane

Exercise	Sets	Reps
Nautilus One-Legged Calf Raises	4	20
{ Seated Calf Raises	5-6	15
{ Angled Calf Presses	5-6	15

Bracketed exercises are supersetted.

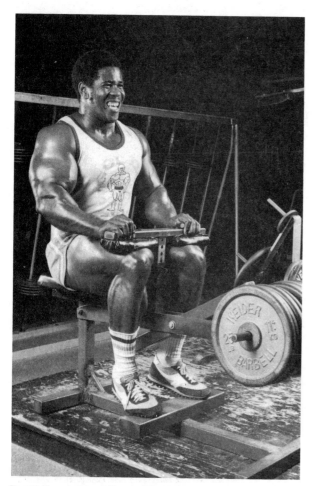

Bertil Fox, several times Mr. Universe, goes heavy on Seated Calf Raises to add width to his soleus muscles.

Rich Gaspari

DAY ONE

Exercise	Sets	Reps
Standing Calf Raises	5	10-15
Seated Calf Raises	5	8-12
Donkey Calf Raises	5	15-20

DAY TWO

Exercise	Sets	Reps
Calf Presses	4-5	15-20
One-Legged Calf Raises	4-5	15-20

Robby Robinson

DAY ONE

Exercise	Sets	Reps
Seated Calf Raises	10	8-10
Donkey Calf Raises	5	15-20

DAY TWO

Exercise	Sets	Reps
Standing Calf Raises	5	10-12
Calf Presses	5	20-25

Peter Hensel

DAY ONE

Exercise	Sets	Reps
Standing Calf Raises	5	10-15
One-Legged Calf Raises	5	15-20

DAY TWO

Exercise	Sets	Reps
Seated Calf Raises	5-6	10-12
Hack Machine Calf Raises	5-6	15-20

DAY THREE

Exercise	Sets	Reps
Angled Calf Presses	3	20-25
Vertical Calf Presses	3	20-25

Mike Mentzer

Exercise	Sets	Reps
Calf Presses (Nautilus)	2	8-12
Seated Calf Raises	2	8-12
Standing Calf Raises	1	8-12

John Hnatyschak

Exercise	Sets	Reps
Donkey Calf Raises	4	15-20
Hack Machine Calf Raises	4	15-20
Seated Calf Raises	4	10-15
Calf Presses	4	20-25

Dennis Tinerino

Exercise	Sets	Reps
Standing Calf Raises	4-5	15-20
Seated Calf Raises	4-5	15-20
Donkey Calf Raises	4-5	15-20

Tim Belknap

Exercise	Sets	Reps
{ Standing Calf Raises	5	15-20
{ Donkey Calf Raises	5	15-20

Lee Labrada

DAY ONE

Exercise	Sets	Reps
Standing Calf Raises	4	15-6*
Calf Presses	2-3	15-20

DAY TWO

Exercise	Sets	Reps
Seated Calf Raises	4	12-8*
One-Legged Calf Raises	2-3	15-20

Boyer Coe

DAY ONE

Exercise	Sets	Reps
{ Calf Presses (horizontal machine)	6	10-12
{ Standing Calf Raises	6	10-12

DAY TWO

Exercise	Sets	Reps
{ Calf Presses (angled machine)	10	10
{ Donkey Calf Raises	10	10

Chris Dickerson

Exercise	Sets	Reps
Seated Calf Raises	3-5	25-30
Standing Calf Raises	3-5	25-30
Donkey Calf Raises	3-5	25-30

Josef Grolmus

DAY ONE

Exercise	Sets	Reps
Standing Calf Raises	5-6	10-15
Seated Calf Raises	5-6	10-15

DAY TWO

Exercise	Sets	Reps
Calf Presses	3-4	15-20
Donkey Calf Raises	3-4	15-20

Ali Malla

Exercise	Sets	Reps
Seated Calf Raises	4	10
Donkey Calf Raises	5	10
Calf Presses	5	8-10

A case of problem calves solved. Dennis Tinerino had flat feet and experienced extreme difficulty in developing his calves. But through perseverance and awesome intensity, Denny brought his calves up to the level of the rest of his outstanding physique.

Mike Christian

DAY ONE

Exercise	Sets	Reps
Standing Calf Raises	6-8	10-15
Seated Calf Raises	6-8	10-15

DAY TWO

Exercise	Sets	Reps
Donkey Calf Raises	5-6	15-20
Calf Presses	5-6	15-20

Tom Platz

Exercise	Sets	Reps
Standing Calf Raises, or . . .		
Seated Calf Raises, or . . .		
Calf Presses (angled machine)	4-5	15-20
Donkey Calf Raises	2-3	15-20

Herman Hoffend

Exercise	Sets	Reps
Donkey Calf Raises	3-4	15-20
Seated Calf Raises	3-4	8-10
Standing Calf Raises	3-4	12-15

Ray Mentzer

Exercise	Sets	Reps
Standing Calf Raises	2	8-10
Seated Calf Raises	2	8-10

Steve Davis

DAY ONE

Exercise	Sets	Reps
Standing Calf Raises	10	10

DAY TWO

Exercise	Sets	Reps
Seated Calf Raises	5	20
Calf Presses	5	20

DAY THREE

Exercise	Sets	Reps
Donkey Calf Raises	5	15
Standing Calf Raises	5	15

Bertil Fox

Exercise	Sets	Reps
Standing Calf Raises	5	8-12
Calf Presses	5	8-12
Seated Calf Raises	5	8-12
Donkey Calf Raises	5	8-12

20
Championship
Chest Development

There is nothing so impressive in the sport of bodybuilding as a pair of striated, slab-like pectoral muscles resting over a deep rib box. Four-time Mr. Olympia Lee Haney is a perfect example of this terrific type of chest development. Both his side-chest and most-muscular poses display his huge and muscular pecs to perfect advantage.

Only one man, Arnold Schwarzenegger, has won more Mr. Olympia titles than Haney, and the Austrian Oak won most of his Olympias in the same dominating manner that Lee has made his trademark over the years. Undoubtedly, you will look at the smashing chest development of these two great Olympia winners and conclude that you have to beef up your chest if you're ever going to win the big titles you hanker to call your own.

It's essential that you take pains to expand your ribcage as you progressively build up your pectorals, or you'll end up with shallow, flat-looking chest development. That might have won shows back in the Dark Ages of the sport, but today's champ is fully developed in every part of his body, including a deep rib box.

Back in those Dark Ages, a bodybuilder could get along with doing almost nothing but bench presses in order to bring up his chest muscles. But the pecs became unbalanced from benches, thick around the lower and outer edges of the pectoral muscles, but correspondingly shallow in the upper and inner sections of the fan-like muscle complex.

Today's superstar has pectorals equally thick over the entire area of the muscle group, from top to bottom and from side to side. And this type of development can only be achieved by incorporating a wide variety of exercises in your chest routine, including incline work for

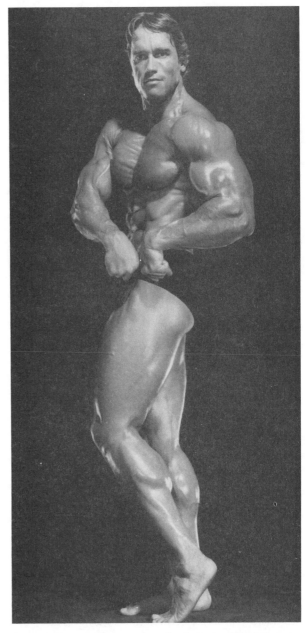

One of the most impressive chests in bodybuilding, displayed by Arnold Schwarzenegger in a contracted side-chest shot.

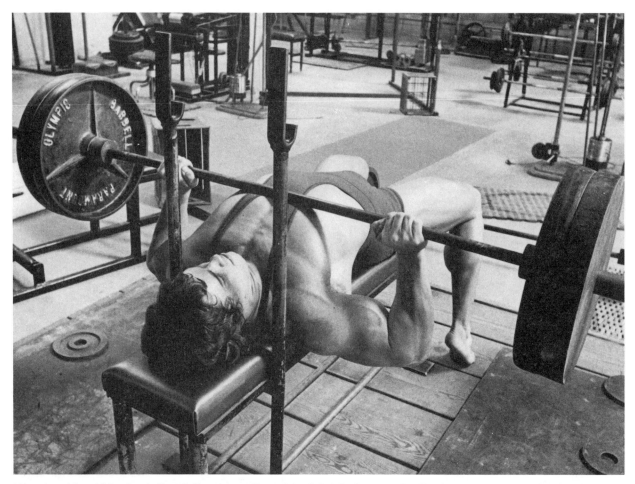

How Arnold got his chest: Bench Presses at the original Gold's Gym on Pacific Avenue in Venice, California.

the upper chest and pec-deck flyes for the inner pecs. This is obviously the type of development you should be after if you want to win plenty of bodybuilding trophies.

It is essential as you balance your pectoral development within the muscle complex that you don't fail to keep your pecs in proportion with surrounding muscle groups (e.g., delts, arms, lats, traps). It's easy to allow your pecs to lag if you fail to work them with sufficiently high training intensity. But it's equally easy to allow your chest muscles to grow too large if you decide that pectorals will be your favorite muscle group.

Great bodybuilders don't have favorite body parts, because having them invariably leads to unharmonious balance between various muscle groups. You will invariably work a favorite muscle group much harder than any other one, which will lead to overdevelopment. Don't ever allow this to happen in your own chest workouts!

ANATOMY AND KINESIOLOGY

The pectorals are large squares with rounded corners, which cover the upper part of the rib box. A large tendon attaches the pectoral muscle on each side to the humeris, or upper-arm bone. A pectoral contraction pulls via that tendon on the upper arm bone and draws it forward.

In order to demonstrate pectoral function to yourself, raise your arms out to the sides and stiffen them. Now without dropping them, move your arms to the rear as far as possible. This is the starting position of the pectoral contractile function. Then slowly contract your pecs to pull your arms directly forward and toward each other, actually contracting so completely that your arms cross each other in front of your chest. You have just demonstrated the full range of motion your arms can achieve as a result of pectoral contraction.

Through correct selection of bodybuilding

exercises, you can actually isolate stress to various portions of the pectorals. For example, presses (with barbell, dumbbells, or machine) and flyes performed on an incline bench will isolate stress on the upper pecs. The same movements done on a decline bench isolate stress on the lower and outer pectorals. And to place maximum stress on the inner pecs, you can do pec-deck flyes and narrow-grip bench presses. The accumulation of movements performed from a variety of angles will ultimately give you perfect pectoral development.

TRAINING TIPS

According to *Dr. Franco Columbu,* "The most basic exercise for pectoral development is the bench press. I think that just by using bench presses, and the closely allied incline presses and decline presses, I could have developed exceptional pectorals, perhaps almost as good as I eventually displayed when winning my Mr. Olympia titles. All of the other pectoral movements are just fluff, and other than various types of dumbbell flyes and dips are not in the same class with benches."

Many other top champs, however, believe that bench presses are just another good pec movement, and not one that's any better than the rest of the available chest exercises. But virtually all bodybuilders have used the bench press extensively in their workouts, particularly in the early years of their involvement in the activity.

I have concluded that benches are excellent for use at the beginning and intermediate stages of bodybuilding. Use bench presses to build up basic upper-body power, and particularly to strengthen the pectorals, anterior delts and triceps, which are most intensely used in this exercise. As you advance, however, you will need to use other exercises to shape and define the chest you've built.

"One of the best methods for training chest," reveals *Dennis Tinerino,* winner of both Pro and Amateur Mr. Universe titles, "is using the Weider Isolation Training Principle. While you will build good general chest muscle mass using basic exercises like benches, inclines, and dips, you simply won't bring out all of the little striations necessary in your pecs at contest time without using plenty of pectoral isolation movements. Nor will you be able to develop fullness in every part of your chest complex without using plenty of isolation exercises.

"The best way to develop an ultimate in pectoral muscle mass and detail is to combine generous amounts of both basic and isolation movements. The basic exercises will give you great overall pectoral fullness, while the isolation movements will etch in the details and give you completeness of pectoral muscle development unattainable in any other fashion."

So you will be able to choose the best basic and isolation movements for each section of your chest complex, here is a complete list of such exercises:

Pectoral Section	Basic Exercises	Isolation Exercises
Upper pecs	Barbell/Dumbbell/Machine Incline Presses	Dumbbell/Cable Incline Flyes
Lower-outer pecs	Barbell/Dumbbell/Machine Decline Presses, Parallel Bar Dips	Dumbbell/Cable Decline Flyes, Cable Crossovers
Inner pecs	Narrow-Grip Bench Presses	Pec-Deck Flyes, Cable Crossovers
Pecs (in general)	Barbell/Dumbbell/Machine Bench Presses	Dumbbell/Cable Flat-Bench Flyes

"One of my favorite new principles for developing the chest and various other muscle groups," notes *Mike Christian*, "is using the Weider Eclectic Training Principle. With this method, you will use a wide variety of chest exercises in an effort to build up optimum pectoral development.

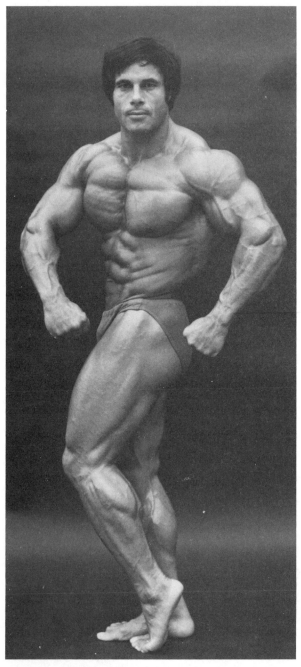

Two-time Mr. Olympia Franco Columbu was noted for the unique (and very deep) split between upper and lower pectoral masses. Phenomenally strong in all exercises, Franco has benched more than 500 pounds for reps. Now retired from competition he works as a doctor of chiropractic medicine.

"When you are using the Eclectic Principle, you should pick one basic exercise for your pectorals, say bench presses or incline presses, and do 5-6 sets of 5-8 reps, increasing the weight after every set. The rest of the routine should then be made up of 1-2 sets each of 6-8 reps choosing 5-15 different exercises for your chest muscles, choosing movements that will stress the pecs from a maximum number of angles. In time, using this principle will give you great chest development."

A sample chest routine using the Weider Eclectic Training Principle just enumerated by Mike Christian appears below:

Exercise	Sets	Reps
Incline Presses (30-degree bench)	5-6	5-8
Parallel Bar Dips (weighted)	2	6-8
Flat-Bench Cable Flyes	2	6-8
High-Incline Dumbbell Presses	2	6-8
Decline Dumbbell Flyes	2	6-8
Cross-Bench Dumbbell Pullovers	2	6-8
Dips Between Benches	2	6-8
Cable Crossovers	2	8-10

Take 1-2 minutes rest between sets of presses, and about 60 seconds rest between sets for all other exercises.

"My idea of a good chest workout is one in which I do plenty of forced reps," says *Berry de Mey*, the youngest man to ever win a Mr. Europe title. "The Weider Forced Reps Training Principle allows me to push some of my bench press and incline press sets past the point of momentary muscle failure as a result of accumulated fatigue within the working muscles.

"There are several ways in which you can push past normal failure and thereby force your muscles to grow larger and stronger at a faster rate of speed. The simplest method is cheating reps, but when you cheat up a repetition in any movement, you will invariably cheat either too much or too little. It's much easier to have exactly the amount of weight removed from the bar that allows you another repetition. You can accomplish this by having a training partner grasp the middle of the bar when you are benching and pull upward with the exact minimum amount of force necessary to allow you to complete the repetition. It should go without saying that your partner will be forced to pull

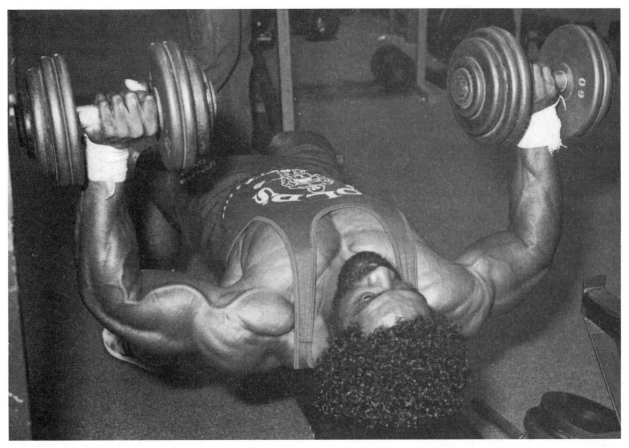

A former captain of the University of California/Berkeley gymnastics team, Charles Glass won NPC National and IFBB World Middleweight championships in 1983 in order to qualify as a competing IFBB pro bodybuilder. Although he has an engineering degree, Charles works as a personal trainer at the famous Gold's Gym in Venice, California.

up a bit more on the bar with each succeeding forced rep as a consequence of your working muscles growing progressively more fatigued. This is forced reps in action.

"The third method for pushing the working chest muscles past the point of momentary fatigue-related failure is use of the Weider Descending Sets Training Principle. Arnold Schwarzenegger called this method 'stripping.' You will find it easiest to use descending sets when you are doing bench presses on a Universal or similar exercise machine. With a training partner stationed at the weight stack, the selection pin close at hand, you begin your set by forcing out as many reps as possible with the first weight. When you fail, your training partner moves the pin up the stack to lighten the load, and you continue with the reduced poundage for 3–5 reps. In this manner, you can do several weight drops, pushing your working muscles to the absolute limit using descending sets."

National and World Middleweight Champion *Charles Glass* tells us about one of his favorite Weider Training Principles for chest development: "I find that pre-exhaustion used from time to time is a good way to bump my chest muscles back into a growth cycle whenever they have been stuck at a certain level for a few weeks. Normally, I do a lot of heavy barbell benches and inclines, which have done wonders for my chest muscles over the years, but occasionally I simply don't get the gains I need from these basic movements.

"One problem with basic chest exercises like benches is that the triceps muscles are involved in pushing the weights up and usually fail long before the pecs and delts have been exhausted to the limit with such exercises. As a result, your weaker arm muscles may be holding back your progress in developing your chest muscles.

"The best way to make your arms briefly stronger—and therefore allow you to push your pecs and delts to the limit with basic move-

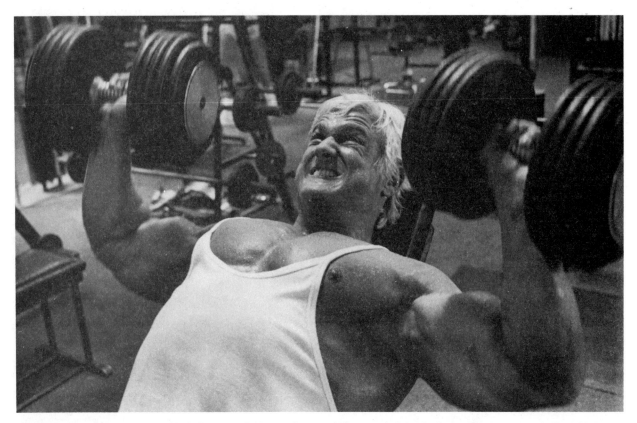

Going heavy on Incline Dumbbell Presses (he's used up to 180-pound dumbbells in the movement), Tom Platz works on his upper pecs.

ments—is to fatigue or weaken your chest muscles before stressing out your triceps. And the best way to do this is to use the Weider Pre-Exhaustion Training Principle, which consists of supersets of isolation exercises for the pectorals and basic movements in which your arms are involved in pressing the weights upward. Such pre-ex supersets allow you to train your pectorals tremendously hard, thereby pushing them to new growth."

Here are three sample pre-exhaustion supersets for your chest muscles, which you can try out in your own training philosophy:

Upper pecs =	Incline Flyes	+ Incline Presses
Lower-outer pecs =	Decline Flyes	+ Decline Presses
General pecs =	Flat-Bench Flyes	+ Bench Presses

Be sure that you rest no more than 4–5 seconds between exercises of a pre-exhaustion superset. The fatigued pectoral muscles will very quickly regain their strength and endurance when allowed to rest, up to 50% of it in no more than 10–12 seconds. Therefore, you must rest minimally between pre-exhaustion exercises in order to preserve the pre-ex effect.

RIBCAGE EXPANSION

If you are still growing, it is possible to enlarge the volume of your chest cavity. This is accomplished by supersetting movements that stimulate breathing with exercises that stretch the ribcage.

But the ribcage is all bone! You can't stretch the bones, can you? No, you can't lengthen bones, but you *can* stretch and lengthen the cartilages which attach the ribs to the sternum, or breast bone. And this, in effect is the same as lengthening the bones themselves. But once you have finished your natural growth cycle, these once-pliable cartilages begin to harden, and as an adult you won't be able to appreciably enlarge your ribcage.

The movements that you will superset are breathing squats and breathing pullovers, doing about 20–25 reps per set. Beginning bodybuilders will need only 1–2 of these supersets, intermediates about 2–3, and advanced bodybuilders no more than 4–5 total supersets.

Breathing squats are normal squats performed with exaggerated breathing between repetitions. Take a light weight, no more than

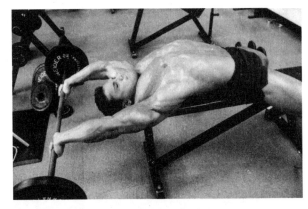

Breathing (Stiff-Arm) Pullovers (bottom)

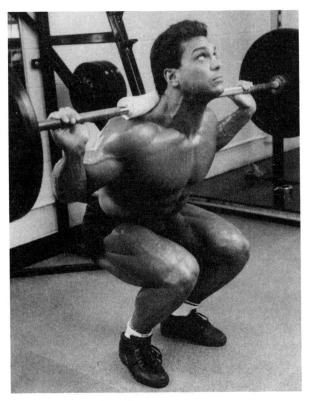

Breathing Squats (midpoint)

All chest exercises modeled by Rich Gaspari, photographed by Bill Dobbins at World Gym, Venice, California.

bodyweight, and assume the starting position for squats. Before you squat down in your first repetition, you should take three very deep breaths, making sure that you completely empty and then completely fill your lungs on each repetition. Hold the third breath and squat down, exhaling only when you are half-way erect. Repeat the breathing between each of your repetitions, taking three breaths between reps 1–10, four breaths between reps 11–20, and five breaths between reps 21–25.

You should be breathing quite heavily at the end of your set. Take advantage of this breathless state by immediately lying down on a flat exercise bench and doing a set of 20–25 reps of breathing pullovers. For this movement, you should take a shoulder-width grip on a light barbell (only 25–30 pounds will be needed) and lie back on the bench, placing your feet flat on the floor to balance your body in position during the movement. Extend your arms directly upward as for the start of a bench press rep and hold your arms stiff throughout your set.

When you have assumed the correct starting

position, simultaneously inhale very deeply and slowly lower the barbell to the rear and downward in a semicircular arc to as low a position as possible. (You will probably be able to lower the weight to a position 6–8 inches below the level of your head on the bench.) Hold the breath and slowly raise the weight back along the same arc to the starting point, exhaling only when you have reached the original starting position. Repeat the movement.

CHEST EXERCISES

On the following pages, you will find 30 basic chest movements precisely described and illustrated with action exercise photos. There are several variations on most of these movements, which in the end will give you at least 50 exercises you can incorporate into your chest routines.

Bench Presses

Emphasis—This is the most basic movement for the pectorals, and perhaps the best of all upper-body exercises. It places particular stress on the lower and outer pectorals, anterior deltoids, and triceps. Secondary stress is on the remainder of the chest muscle complex, medial deltoids, and those upper-back muscles that impart rotational movement to the scapulae.

Starting Position—Adjust the weight on a barbell resting on the uprights of a pressing bench to the correct level for a set of bench presses. Lie on your back on the bench with your shoulders 3–5 inches away from the uprights. Place your feet flat on the floor on each side of the bench to

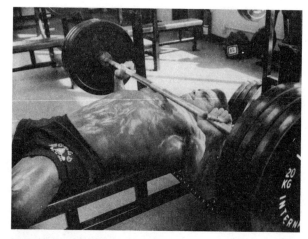

Barbell Bench Press (start)

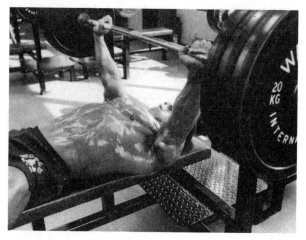

Barbell Bench Press (finish)

balance your body on the bench during your set. Reach up and take an overgrip on the barbell with your hands set 3–5 inches wider than your shoulders on each side. Straighten your arms to lift the barbell from the rack to a position at straight arms' length directly above your shoulder joints.

Movement Performance—Allowing your upper-arm bones to travel directly out to the sides, bend your arms, and slowly lower the barbell downward and slightly forward until it lightly touches the middle of your chest, a couple of inches above the lower pectoral line. Without bouncing the weight off your chest, slowly extend your arms and press the weight back up along the same arc to the starting point.

Training Tips—Avoid arching your back as you press the weight upward, because this is a

cheating movement which both removes stress from the muscles that should be receiving it, and dangerously compresses your lower spinal vertebrae. To avoid such a torso arch, you might consider raising your feet from the floor by curling your legs up over your lower torso. You can vary the width of your grip on the bar to one as wide as the length of the bar permits inward to one as narrow as having your hands touch each other in the middle of the bar. Each change of grip width stresses your chest, shoulder, and arm muscles from a different angle. On all bench presses, you must have a spotter at the head end of the bench to rescue you in case you get stuck under the weight, or have any tendency to pass out when holding your breath and exerting during a heavy rep.

Narrow-Grip Bench Presses

Emphasis—When you use a narrow grip on the barbell, stress shifts primarily to the triceps and inner pectorals, with secondary emphasis placed on the remainder of the pectoral structure, anterior deltoids, and those muscles of the upper back that impart rotational movement to the scapulae.

Starting Position—Adjust the weight of a barbell resting on the upright rack attached to the end of a pressing bench. Lie on your back on the bench with your shoulders 3–5 inches away from the uprights. Place your feet flat on the floor on each side of the bench to balance your body on the bench during your set. Reach up

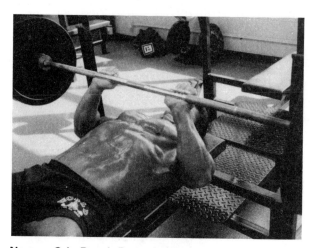

Narrow-Grip Bench Press (midpoint)

and take an overgrip on the barbell with your hands set about 6 inches apart in the middle of the bar. Straighten your arms to lift the bar off the rack to a position at straight arms' length directly above your shoulder joints.

Movement Performance—Allowing your elbows to travel out to the sides away from your torso, slowly bend your arms and lower the barbell downward and slightly forward until it lightly touches your mid-chest. Without bouncing the weight off your chest, slowly press the weight upward along the same arc until it reaches the starting point.

Training Tips—You can vary the width of the grip inward until your hands are actually touching, or outward to a point where your hands are 12–14 inches apart. You can also curl your legs up over your torso to make the movement more strict. And it is possible to do the same exercise on a Smith machine.

Barbell Incline Presses

Emphasis—When you do presses (whether with a barbell, two dumbbells or a machine) on an incline bench set at an angle ranging between about 15 degrees and as much as about 75 degrees, you shift major emphasis to the upper-pectoral muscles, anterior deltoids, and triceps. Strong secondary stress is also placed on the inner and medial pectorals, medial deltoids, and those upper-back muscles that contract to rotate the scapulae. All types of incline

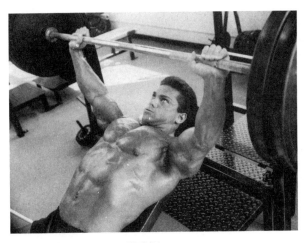

Barbell Incline Press (finish)

presses are ideal for developing pec-delt tie-ins so necessary for success in competitive bodybuilding.

Starting Position—Place a bar on the support rack attached to an incline pressing bench, and adjust the weight on the bar to the necessary level for a set of inclines. (If you don't have such a rack attached to your incline bench, you will have to clean the bar to your shoulders, recline on the bench and push it up to straight arms' length to begin the movement.) Reach up and take an overgrip on the barbell with your hands set 3–6 inches wider than your shoulders on each side. Lie back on the bench, sitting down on the seat. Straighten your arms to pull the barbell into the correct starting position at straight arms' length directly above your shoulder joints.

Movement Performance—Being sure to keep your elbows back to achieve maximum pectoral stretch in the bottom point of the movement, slowly bend your arms and lower the barbell downward until it touches lightly on your upper chest at the base of your neck. Without bouncing the bar off your chest, slowly reverse the movement and press the bar back up to straight arms' length.

Training Tips—By varying the angle of the incline bench on which you do your presses, you can shift the stress from one muscle group to another, the same as you can change stress points when varying the width of your grip. When you use a low incline angle, most of the

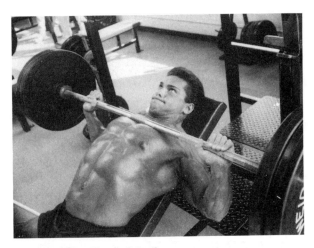

Barbell Incline Press (start)

stress is borne by the upper chest and anterior deltoid muscles, with more stress on the pectorals. But the higher you angle the pressing bench, the more stress is shifted to the anterior delts and triceps, at the expense of the upper pecs, which should be receiving maximum stress.

Barbell Decline Presses

Emphasis—When you do presses (with a barbell, two dumbbells or machine) on a decline bench, major stress is on the lower-outer pectoral muscles, anterior-medial delts, and triceps. Proportionately more stress is on the upper-back muscles than on presses on a flat or incline bench.

Starting Position—Rest a barbell on the support rack attached to one end of your decline pressing bench, and load the bar to an appropriate poundage for a set of decline presses. If

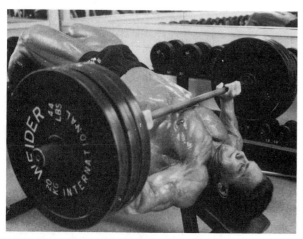

Barbell Decline Press (start)

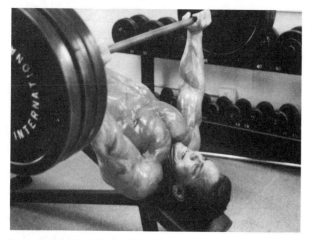

Barbell Decline Press (finish)

you don't have a rack on your decline bench, you will have to have a training partner lift the bar up to the correct starting point for a set of declines. Hook your feet under the restraint bar at the foot of the bench and lie back on the decline bench. Reach up and take an overgrip on the bar with your hands set 3–6 inches wider on each side than the width of your shoulders. When you have your grip on the bar, straighten your arms and bring the bar to straight arms' length directly above your shoulder joints.

Movement Performance—Being sure to keep your elbows back throughout the movement to achieve optimum pectoral stretch and contraction, bend your arms and slowly lower the barbell straight downward until it lightly touches your chest at the lower edge of your pectorals. Without bouncing the weight off your chest, slowly press the barbell back up along the same arc to the starting point, being sure to intensely contract your pectorals in the top position.

Training Tips—Most decline benches are set at an angle of about 25–30 degrees, which may seem a little steep to some bodybuilders. You will find that you can improvise a decline bench at an almost perfect angle if you merely set the legs of your flat bench on a thick block of wood (anything thicker than about four inches will be perfect), then doing the movement with the bench angled like this, your head at the low end. Varying the angle of the bench will stress your lower-outer pecs a bit differently, as well as varying the width of your grip on the bar. Be sure that you have a safety spotter standing at the head of the bench when you do declines, because the movement places your face and neck in a vulnerable position.

Pullovers and Presses

Emphasis—This excellent upper-body movement places intense stress on the lats, pecs, delts (all three heads of the muscle group, in fact), and triceps. In fact, it is one of the best triceps movements and finds its way into the upper-arm programs of many top bodybuilders.

Starting Position—Place a flat exercise bench in the middle of the gym floor. Reach down

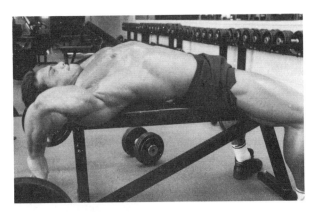

Pullover and Press (start)

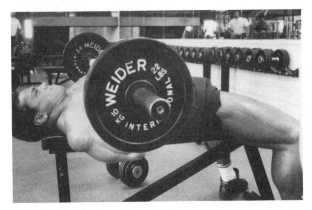

Pullover and Press (midpoint)

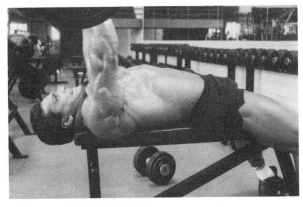

Pullover and Press (finish)

and take a narrow overgrip on the bar (your index fingers should be about 6 inches apart in the middle of the bar). Lie back on the bench with the bar resting on your chest and place your feet flat on the floor on either side of the bench to balance your body in position as you do the movement.

Movement Performance—Keeping your elbows close together and your arms bent at an approximate 90-degree angle, slowly lower the barbell in a semicircular arc past your face and downward to as low a position as comfortably

possible behind your head. Slowly reverse the movement and pull the barbell back to a position across your chest. Finally, use triceps and pectoral strength to press the barbell up to straight arms' length before lowering it back to your chest.

Training Tips—A similar movement can be done holding two fairly heavy dumbbells in your hands. With a barbell, you can vary the width of your grip from one as narrow as having your hands touch in the middle of the bar out to one set at about shoulder width.

Smith Machine Bench Presses

Emphasis—This exercise can be performed on a flat, incline, or decline bench, and as such is similar to the same exercise done with a free bar. Smith machine benches stress the entire pectoral muscle mass, incline Smith machine presses work the upper pecs, and decline Smith machine presses bomb the lower and outer sections of the pectoral complex. All three variations place intense stress on the anterior-medial delts, triceps, and those upper-back muscles that contract to rotate the sholder blade. I will describe the flat-bench version of the movement; from this description, you can easily extrapolate how the exercise is performed on an incline or decline bench.

Starting Position—Place a flat bench within a Smith machine and adjust the pins which hold the bar so it just touches your chest when you are lying on your back on the bench beneath the bar. Lie on the bench with your shoulder joints about 3–4 inches back from the bar. Place your feet flat on the floor to balance your torso on the bench as you do your presses. Reach out and take an overgrip on the bar with your hands set 3–6 inches wider than your shoulders on each side. Extend your arms to press the weight up to straight arms' length above your shoulder joints.

Movement Performance—Being sure that your upper arms travel outward at right angles with your torso, slowly bend your arms and lower the weight directly downward to lightly touch your chest. Without bouncing the weight off your chest, slowly extend your arms and press the machine slide back to the starting point at straight arms' length above your chest.

Training Tips—By varying the width of your grip on the bar you can stress your pectorals from different angles, the accumulation of which will give you incredible pectoral development. Be sure to do plenty of sets of Smith machine presses on incline and decline benches as well as on a flat bench.

Universal Bench Presses

Emphasis—This exercise can also be performed on a flat, incline, or decline bench, and as such is similar to the same exercise done with a free bar. Universal bench presses work the entire pectoral muscle mass, incline Universal presses work the upper pecs, and decline Universal presses bomb the lower and outer sections of the pectoral complex. All three variations place intense stress on the anterior-medial deltoid heads, triceps, and upper-back muscles. I will describe the incline version of the movement; from this description, you can easily extrapolate how the exercise is performed on a flat or decline bench.

Starting Position—Slide a short incline bench (one in which the seat is set very near the floor) between the angles of the bench press station of a Universal Gym machine. The bench should be positioned so your shoulder joints are directly beneath the pressing handles when you are sitting in the bench and reclining on the angled pad. Sit down and reach up to take an overgrip on the handles, your hands set in about the middle of the handles. Straighten your arms to raise the pressing handles to straight arms' length directly above your shoulders.

Movement Performance—Being sure to keep your elbows back as you do the movement, slowly bend your arms and lower the weight downward until your hands are resting at shoulder level. Without bouncing the weights in the stack, slowly press the handles upward until your arms are again straight.

Training Tips—You should experiment with a variety of grip widths (as much as the length of the handles permits) and a variety of bench angles in an effort to develop optimum pectorals.

Nautilus Bench Presses

Emphasis—This excellent machine chest movement gives you virtually the same effect as decline presses. It places intense stress on the lower-outer pectorals, anterior delts, and triceps. Strong secondary stress is on the rest of the pectoral muscle complex, medial deltoids, and those upper-back muscles which rotate the scapulae.

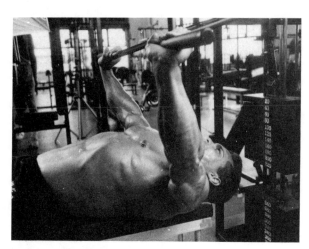

Universal Bench Press (finish)

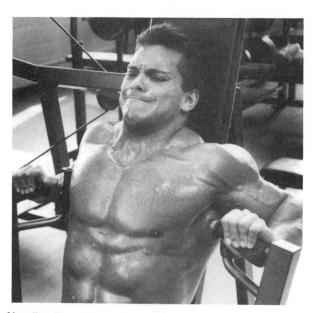

Nautilus-Type Bench Press (start)

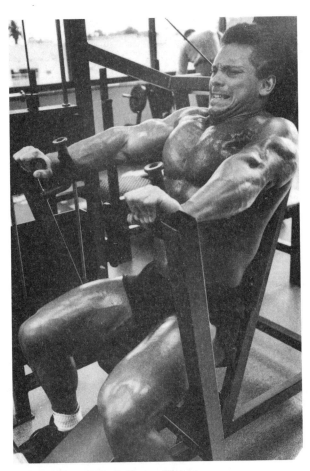

Nautilus-Type Bench Press (finish)

Starting Position—Sit down in the machine and lie back on the angled pad. (The seat can be adjusted upward or downward to suit your structure.) Buckle the seat belt across your lap. Place your feet on the large treadle in front of you, and take a grip on the handles attached to the lever arms, your palms facing inward toward each other. Push hard with both your legs and arms to bring the handles forward until your arms are locked out straight.

Movement Performance—Without pushing with your feet at any time, slowly bend your arms as completely as possible. You will find that your upper arms travel naturally into the correct pressing position. Without bouncing in the bottom position, reverse the movement and slowly press back to the starting point.

Training Tips—You can easily do negative-only reps by pushing very hard with your feet to get your arms straight, then lowering back to the starting point while strongly resisting the downward impetus of the handles.

Dumbbell Bench Presses

Emphasis—This movement affects the same muscle as normal bench presses with a barbell, except that the longer range of motion inherently possible with dumbbells actually makes dumbbell benches a somewhat more-intense movement. Dumbbell bench presses intensely stress the entire pectoral muscle complex, particularly the lower and outer sections, the anterior deltoids, and triceps. Strong secondary stress is placed on the medial delts and the upper-back muscles which contract to rotate the scapulae.

Starting Position—Grasp two heavy dumbbells, sit at the end of a flat exercise bench, and rest the weights on their ends on your knees, your feet set about shoulder width apart. To bring the weights into position for your set, keep pressing them to your knees as you roll backward on to the bench. This maneuver should bring the weights to straight arms' length directly above your shoulder joints, your wrists rotated so your hands face forward throughout the movement. (When you are finished with your set, bring your knees upward until they touch the weights, and then rock forward to bring them to the position resting on your knees. Finally, return them softly to the floor.)

Movement Performance—Being sure to keep your upper arms directly out to the sides at right angles with your torso, slowly bend your arms and lower the weights downward and a bit out to the sides to as low a position as is

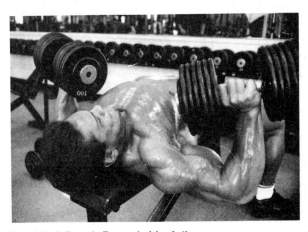

Dumbbell Bench Press (midpoint)

comfortably possible. Without bouncing the weights, slowly press the back up along the same arcs to the starting point.

Training Tips—You can also perform this exercise with your wrists rotated so your palms are facing inward toward each other throughout the movement. The real key to this exercise is lowering the weights down to as low a position beside your torso as possible, which completely stretches the pectorals before they are fully contracted at the top point of the movement.

Dumbbell Incline Presses

Emphasis—As with all variations of incline presses, the movement places intense stress on the upper pectorals, anterior deltoids, and triceps. It is the best possible movement for developing those pec–delt tie-ins so necessary in today's high-level bodybuilding competition. Strong secondary stress is placed on the rest of the pectoral complex, medial deltoids, and those upper-back muscles which contract to rotate the shoulder blades.

Starting Position—Grasp two moderately heavy dumbbells and sit back on the seat of an incline bench with the bells resting on their ends on your knees. Rock backward onto the padded surface of the bench, simultaneously bringing the weights to shoulder level. Press the weights to straight arms' length directly above your shoulders and rotate your wrists so your

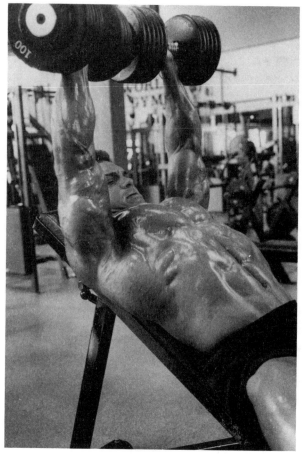

Dumbbell Incline Press (finish)

palms are facing forward throughout the movement. (Simply reverse the process used to raise the weights up to your shoulders when you are finished with your set and wish to place the weights back on the floor of the gym.)

Movement Performance—Being sure to keep your elbows back, bend your arms and slowly lower the dumbbells downward and slightly out to the sides so they are as low down on the sides of your upper torso as is comfortably possible. Slowly press the weights back up to the starting point, being sure not to bounce the weights to get them started up from the bottom point of the movement.

Training Tips—The angle of the bench can be varied to place either less or more stress on the upper pecs, the lower angle being better for the pectorals and the upper angle better for anterior deltoids. A very good bench angle for incline dumbbell presses can be achieved by merely elevating the head end of a flat exercise

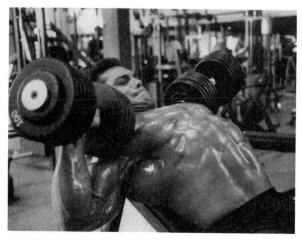

Dumbbell Incline Press (start)

bench 6–8 inches with a thick block of wood or another low exercise bench.

Dumbbell Decline Presses

Emphasis—Like all variations of decline presses, this movement places intense stress on the lower-outer pectorals, anterior-medial deltoids, and triceps. Very strong secondary stress is also placed on the upper-back muscles which impart rotational force to the scapulae.

Starting Position—Grasp two moderately heavy dumbbells and sit at the high end of a decline bench, your lower legs wedged beneath the restraint bars. Rest the dumbbells on their ends on your knees. Lie back on the angled surface of the bench, simultaneously bringing the weights to a position at straight arms' length directly above your shoulder joints. Rotate your wrists so your palms are facing forward toward your feet during the entire exercise. (If you have trouble getting the dumbbells into position for this movement, you can get a training partner to help you. The easiest method for this is for you to start with the weights lying on the gym floor at straight arms' length behind your head. If you keep your arms stiff, your training partner can easily deadlift the weights into position for your set.)

Movement Performance—Being sure to keep your elbows out to the sides as you do the movement, slowly bend your arms and lower the weights directly downward and slightly out to the sides until they are in as low a position as is

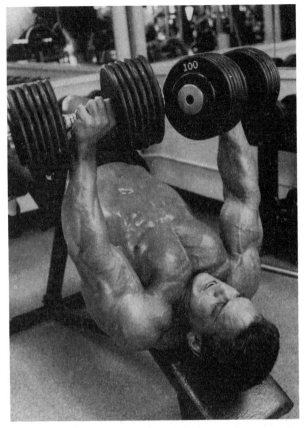

Dumbbell Decline Press (finish)

comfortably possible at the sides of your torso. Without bouncing the weights in the bottom position, slowly press the dumbbells back along the same arcs to the starting point.

Flat-Bench Flyes

Emphasis—This is considered an isolation movement for the pectorals, because it places the most intense stress on them, with only minor help from the anterior-medial deltoids, triceps, and upper-back muscles.

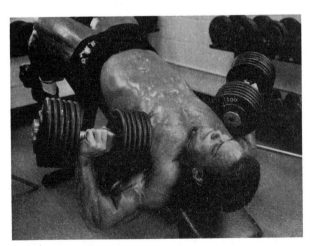

Dumbbell Decline Press (start)

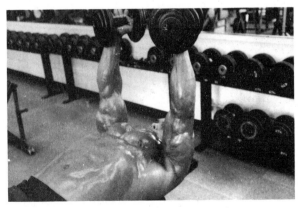

Flat-Bench Dumbbell Flyes (start/finish)

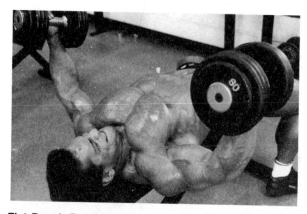

Flat-Bench Dumbbell Flyes (midpoint)

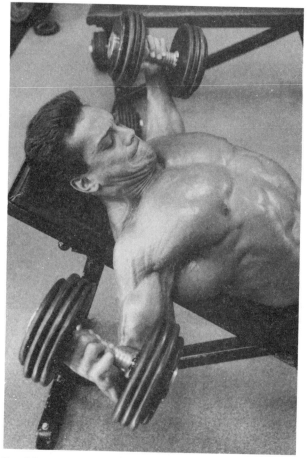

Dumbbell Incline Flyes (bottom)

Starting Position—Grasp two moderately weighted dumbbells and sit at the end of a flat exercise bench with your feet set about shoulder width apart. Raise the weights up and rest their ends on your knees. Rock backward to lie on the bench surface, simultaneously bringing the weights to a position at straight arms' length directly above your shoulder joints. Rotate your wrists so your palms are facing inward toward each other throughout the movement. Bend your arms about 10 degrees and keep them rounded like this as you raise and lower the dumbbells.

Movement Performance—Being sure that your upper-arm bones travel directly out to the sides perpendicular to your torso, allow the dumbbells to travel outward and downward in semicircular arcs until they are as far below the level of your chest as possible. Without bouncing the weights in this bottom position, slowly reverse the movement and return the dumbbells back along the same arcs to the starting point.

Training Tips—If you allow your elbows to travel forward (as they would like to travel), you will lose much of the beneficial effect of this exercise. For optimum pectoral contraction, be sure to press the weights together hard when they are touching each other directly above your chest.

Incline Dumbbell Flyes

Emphasis—As with variations of the incline press, this flye movement most intensely stresses the pec–delt tie-ins, upper pectorals, and anterior deltoids. As such, it is a very good

isolation movement for the upper pecs. Minor secondary stress is placed on the medial deltoids and triceps.

Starting Position—Grasp two moderately light dumbbells, and lie back on the incline bench, simultaneously raising the weights to straight arms' length directly above your shoulder joints. Rotate your wrists so the palms of your hands are facing each other throughout the set. Bend your arms about 10 degrees and keep them rounded like this throughout your set.

Movement Performance—Being sure to keep your elbows back as you do the movement, slowly lower the weights out to the sides and downward in semicircular arcs to as low a position as is comfortably possible. Without bouncing the weights in the low position, reverse the movement and slowly raise the dumbbells back along the same arcs to the starting point with the dumbbells pressed strongly together directly above your chest.

Training Tips—By varying the angle of the incline bench, you can intentionally shift stress to specific areas of your upper-pectoral muscles.

Decline Dumbbell Flyes

Emphasis—As with variations of decline presses, this flye movement places intense stress on the lower-outer pectorals, but decline flyes isolate most of the stress to that part of the pecs. Minor secondary stress is placed on the anterior deltoids, and proportionately less stress on the triceps.

Starting Position—Grasp two light dumbbells and sit at the end of a decline bench, the bells resting on their ends on your knees. Hook your feet under the restraint bar and lie back on the bench, simultaneously bringing the weights to a position supported at straight arms' length

directly above your shoulder joints. Rotate your wrists so your palms face each other throughout your set. Bend your arms about 10 degrees and keep them rounded like this for your whole set.

Movement Performance—Keeping your elbows back as you do the movement, slowly lower the dumbbells directly out to the sides and downward in semicircular arcs to as low a position as is comfortably attainable. Without bouncing the weights in the bottom position, use pectoral strength to raise the dumbbells back along the same arcs to the starting point, pressing the weights together in this finish position to intensely contract your pectorals.

Training Tips—Try a variety of decline bench angles in order to stress the lower-outer pecs from a variety of angles.

Stiff-Arm Dumbbell Flyes

Emphasis—Performed with stiff arms on a flat, incline, or decline bench, this exercise is very similar to bent-arm flyes. Incline stiff-arm flyes isolate stress on the upper pecs, flat-bench stiff-arm flyes stress the entire pectoral muscle complex, and decline stiff-arm flyes isolate stress on the lower and outer pecs. I will describe the flat-bench variation; from this description, you can easily extrapolate correct performance of the incline and decline versions of the same movement.

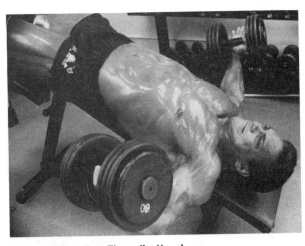

Dumbbell Decline Flyes (bottom)

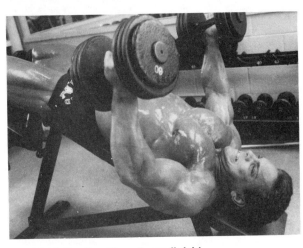

Dumbbell Decline Flyes (near finish)

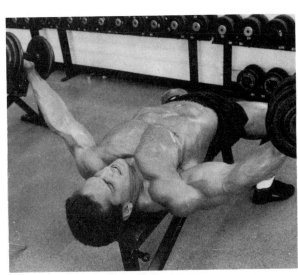

Stiff-Armed Dumbbell Flyes (flat bench—midpoint)

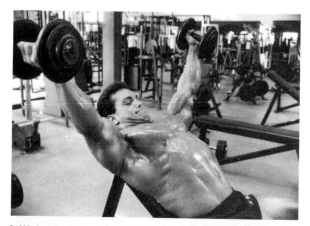

Stiff-Armed Dumbbell Flyes (incline bench—midpoint)

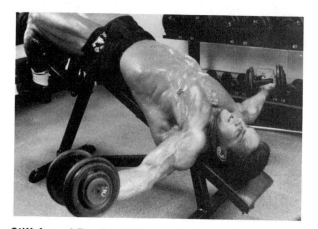

Stiff-Armed Dumbbell Flyes (decline bench—bottom)

Starting Position—Grasp two light dumbbells in your hands and lie back on a flat exercise bench with your feet flat on the floor to balance your body on the bench as you perform the movement. Extend your arms straight upward from your shoulders and rotate your wrists so your palms are facing each other throughout your set. Straighten your arms and keep them stiff throughout the movement.

Movement Performance—Being sure that your upper arms travel directly out to the sides at 90-degree angles with your torso, slowly lower the weights outward and downward in semicircular arcs to as low a position as is comfortably possible. Without bouncing the weights in the low position of the movement, use pectoral strength to raise the weights back along the same arcs to the starting point, where you should press the weights together as intensely as possible to completely contract your pectoral muscles.

Training Tips—You'll be restricted to light weights for this movement, since heavy weights will painfully stress the ligament on the inner side of each elbow. Historically, this is the reason why virtually all bodybuilders today do the exercise with the arms slightly bent throughout each repetition. Again, you can do this movement on incline and decline benches set at various angles.

Pec Deck Flyes

Emphasis—Originated about 1980, this excellent movement isolates stress on the pectoral muscles, particularly the inner and outer sections of the muscle group. Minor secondary stress is placed on the anterior and medial heads of the deltoid muscles.

Starting Position—Adjust the height of the machine seat so your upper arm bones are held parallel with the floor when you are in the correct starting position. Some of these seats can be adjusted with a pin, others by turning the seat which is attached to a large screw. Sit on the seat and press your upper back against

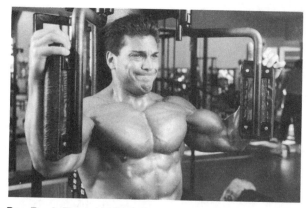

Pec-Deck Flyes (midpoint)

the vertical pad attached to the machine. Force your elbows against the padded surface of the moveable pads attached to the lever arms of the machine, your forearms running vertically up the pads, hands resting over the top edge of the pads. Allow the weight attached to the lever arms to pull your elbows (and hence the elbow ends of your upper arms) as far to the rear as possible, completely stretching the pectoral muscles.

Movement Performance—Use pectoral strength to move the pads forward and inward toward each other until the pads touch each other directly in front of your chest. Hold this peak-contracted position for a moment, then slowly return the pads to the starting position.

Training Tips—To vary the stress of this movement, you can perform it with the seat set markedly higher or lower than normal. You can also do the exercise with only one arm at a time, which serves to intensify the stress on your pectorals. Movements performed with one arm or leg at a time automatically intensifies the stress of the exercise, since you no longer split your mental focus between two working limbs.

Nautilus Flyes

Emphasis—One of two movements which can be performed on a Nautilus double-chest machine (the other is bench presses, which have already been described), this exercise isolates stress on the lower-outer and inner pectoral muscles.

Starting Position—Adjust the height of the machine seat so your upper arm bones are parallel with the gym floor when you are in the correct starting position. Sit down in the machine and recline against the angled pad. Buckle the seat belt across your lap. Force your elbows against the pads set at the ends of the lever arms of the machine, forearms running vertically and hands grasping the upper or lower set of hand grips. Allow the weight attached to the lever arms to pull your elbows as far to the rear as is comfortably possible, thereby stretching the pectoral muscles.

Movement Performance—Use pectoral strength to move the pads forward and toward each other until they touch directly in front of your chest. Hold this peak-contracted position for a moment, then slowly return the pads to the starting position.

Training Tips—If you want to do this exercise with one arm at a time, you can use your free hand to grasp the handle provided above and a

bit in front of your head. With both variations, you can vary the height of the machine seat to stress your pectorals from somewhat different angles.

Cable Flyes

Emphasis—Performed on flat, incline, or decline benches, this movement isolates stress on the entire pectoral muscle complex, but particularly on the inner and outer sections of the pectorals. Minor secondary stress is placed on the anterior deltoids. When you use cables, you will find that you can exercise your pecs with a more continuous form of tension than is possible with dumbbells. Flat-bench cable flyes work the entire pectoral mass, while incline cable flyes shift major stress to the upper pecs and decline cable flyes work primarily the lower and outer sections of the pectoral muscle complex. I will describe the incline version of this movement first; from this description, you can easily extrapolate the method of performance for flat-bench and decline variations.

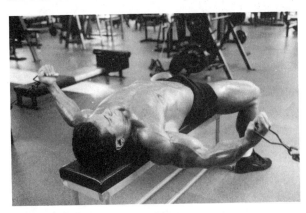

Cable Flyes (flat bench—start)

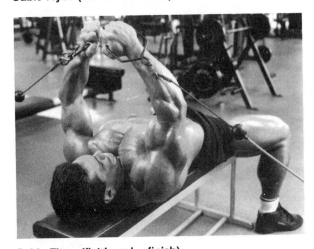

Cable Flyes (flat bench—finish)

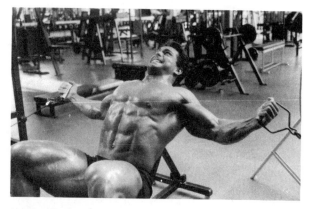

Incline Cable Flyes (start)

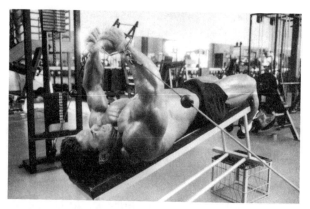

Decline Cable Flyes (finish)

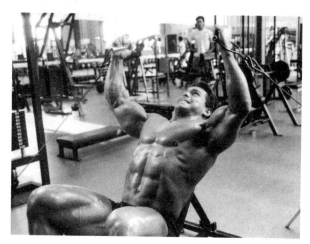

Incline Cable Flyes (finish)

Starting Position—Attach loop handles to the ends of cables running through floor pulleys. Place a 30–45-degree incline bench between the pulleys, so your shoulders are directly even with the two pulleys when you are lying back on the incline bench. Grasp the pulleys and lie back on the incline bench, bringing your hands together directly above your chest. Bend your arms about 10 degrees and keep them rounded like this throughout your set.

Movement Performance—Being sure that your upper arms travel directly out to the sides toward the pulleys, allow the weights attached to the ends of the cables to pull your hands outward and downward in semicircular arcs to as low a position below your upper chest as possible. Without bouncing your hands, use pectoral strength to raise the pulley handles back along the same arcs to the starting point. Hold this peak-contracted position for a moment, intensely contracting your pectoral muscles.

Training Tips—As already mentioned, you can do this exercise on flat and decline benches as well.

Parallel Bar Dips

Emphasis—This is an excellent upper-body movement which places intense stress on the pectorals (particularly the lower and outer sections of the muscle complex), anterior deltoids, and triceps. Strong secondary stress is placed on the medial deltoids and the muscles of the upper back which rotate the scapulae.

Starting Position—While this exercise can be performed on parallel bars which are actually parallel, it is best done on bars which angle inward at one end. The angled bars allow you to take various widths of grip, the width depending on which part of the bars you jump up and take your grip. Grasp the bars so your palms will be facing each other as you do the movement, and jump up to support yourself at straight arms' length above the bars, your torso hanging down from your shoulders. Bend your legs at 90-degree angles, cross your ankles,

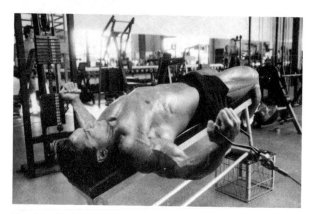

Decline Cable Flyes (start)

place your chin on your chest, and angle your torso forward, hips to the rear.

Movement Performance—Keeping your torso incline constant, slowly bend your arms and allow your body to sink as far down between the bars as possible. Without bouncing in the bottom position of the movement, slowly reverse the motion, and return to the starting point.

Training Tips—Varying the width of your grip on the bars serves to stress your pectorals from different angles. In order to keep continuous tension on your working pectorals, be sure not to lock out with your arms straight in the top position. Merely rise about three-quarters

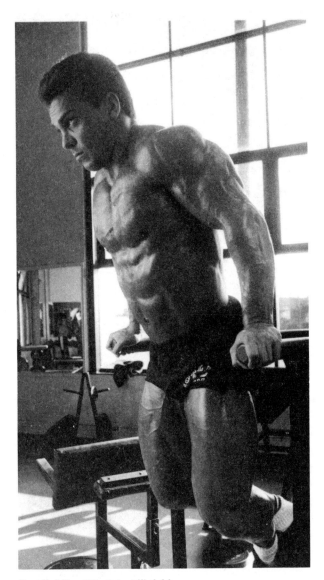

Parallel Bar Dip (start/finish)

of the way up, then immediately descend. On all variations of parallel bar dips, you can hang a dumbbell or some barbell plates around your waist with a rope or loop of nylon webbing as a means of adding resistance to the exercise.

Stiff-Arm Pullovers

Emphasis—This is the primary movement used to stretch the ribcage and expand the chest. In terms of muscular stress, the exercise emphasizes the serratus, pectoral, and latissimus dorsi muscles.

Starting Position—Take a shoulder-width overgrip on a light barbell and lie on your back on a flat exercise bench, your feet placed flat on the floor on either side of the bench to balance your body as you do the movement. Extend your arms directly upward from your shoulders, assuming the same starting position as you would for a set of bench presses. Be sure to hold your arms stiff as you do your set. (See Breathing Stiff-Arm Pullovers on page 289 for illustrations of this movement.)

Movement Performance—While slowly inhaling, lower the barbell to the rear and downward in a semicircular arc to as low a position below the bench as is possible when holding your arms straight. Exhale as you slowly return the bar back along the same arc to the starting point.

Training Tips—It can be beneficial to vary the width of your grip on the barbell, from one as wide as the length of the bar permits inward to one in which your hands are touching each other in the middle of the bar. A similar movement can be performed while holding a single dumbbell in both hands, palms against the inner sides of one set of plates, handle perpendicular to the gym floor, and thumbs encircling the handle in order to keep the dumbbell secure in your hands. You can also do the movement with a dumbbell held in each hand, which allows you much more freedom of distance between your hands as you perform the exercise.

Dumbbell Around-the-World

Emphasis—This is a great all-around chest movement, which both stretches the ribcage and develops the pectorals and serratus muscles. Strong secondary stress is also placed on the lats.

Starting Position—Grasp two light dumbbells and lie back on a flat exercise bench, your feet pressed flat on the floor to balance your body on the bench as you do the exercise. Extend your arms straight upward from your shoulders, allowing the dumbbells to touch each other with palms facing.

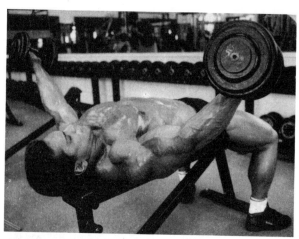

Dumbbell Around-the-Worlds (midpoint)

Movement Performance—With your arms held slightly unlocked throughout the movement, slowly lower the dumbbells in semicircular arcs out to the sides and downward to a position slightly below the level of your chest. When the weights have reached this position, begin moving them in semicircular arcs to the rear while holding them parallel to the floor. When the dumbbells touch each other behind your head (in the bottom position for stiff-arm pullovers), raise them in semicircular arcs back to the starting point, as if doing a pullover with the weights.

Training Tips—You can also do this movement in the opposite direction, that is by first lowering them to the rear as if starting a stiff-arm pullover movement.

Cross-Bench Dumbbell Pullovers

Emphasis—Again, this is a good all-around chest exercise that stretches the ribcage and builds up the pectoral, serratus, and latissimus dorsi muscles.

Starting Position—Place a moderately heavy dumbbell on end on top of a flat exercise bench, being sure to position it toward one end. Lie across the bench with only your upper back and shoulders in contact with it, your feet set about shoulder width apart to balance your body as you perform the exercise. Reach to the side and place the palms of your hands against the underside of the upper set of plates on the dumbbell, encircling the handle in order to secure the implement in your hands. Pull the weight up to a position at straight arms' length directly above your shoulder joints.

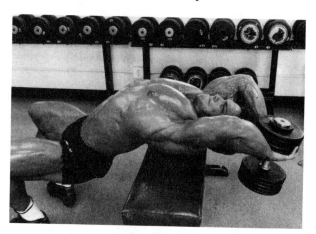

Cross-Bench Dumbbell Pullovers (bottom)

Movement Performance—Simultaneously bend your arms 10–20 degrees while lowering the dumbbell to the rear and downward in a semicircular arc to as low a position behind your head as is comfortably possible. It is best to inhale as you lower the weight and exhale as you raise it. Without bouncing in the bottom position of the movement, slowly return the dumbbell back along the same arc to the starting point.

Training Tips—You can get a much more intense stretch in the working muscles if you consciously drop your hips 3–6 inches as the weight reaches the bottom position.

Bent-Arm Pullovers

Emphasis—Purely a muscle builder rather than a movement intended for ribcage expansion, bent-arm pullovers place intense stress on the pectorals, lats, and other upper-back muscles which impart rotational movement to the scapulae.

Starting Position—Take a narrow overgrip in the middle of a fairly heavy barbell (there should be 4–6 inches of space showing between your index fingers when you have assumed the correct grip), and lie back on a flat exercise bench, pressing your feet flat on the floor on each side of the bench to balance your body in position as you do the movement. Bring the barbell up to a position resting on your chest, your arms fully bent.

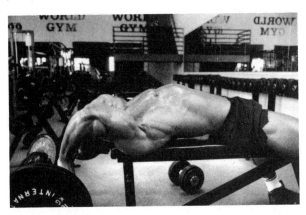

Barbell Bent-Arm Pullovers (bottom)

Movement Performance—Being absolutely certain to keep your elbows in as close to each other as possible, slowly lower the barbell past your face and down behind your head in a semicircular arc to as low a position as is comfortably possible to assume. Without bouncing the bar in the low position, pull it back along the same arc to the starting point.

Training Tips—Never allow your elbows to splay out to the sides as you do bent-arm pullovers because to do so places your shoulder joints in a weak mechanical position and they can be seriously injured. With very heavy weights, you will need to have a training partner pressing down on your knees to restrain your body on the bench.

Nautilus Pullovers

Emphasis—This exercise intensely stresses the pecs, lats, serratus, and even the upper-abdominal muscles. But unlike other pullover movements, it has little effect on chest expansion.

Starting Position—Adjust the machine seat so your shoulder joints are even with the cam pivot points when you sit down. Sit in the machine and fasten the seat belt over your lap. Push down on the T-bar-shaped treadle in front of you and bring the lever arm of the machine sufficiently forward so you can press your elbows against the pads attached to the ends of the lever arm. Grasp the handles provided. Release the treadle and allow the weight attached to the lever arm to pull your elbows upward and to the rear as far as is comfortably possible.

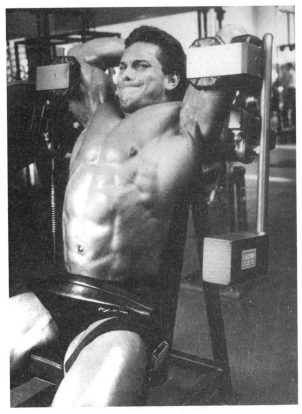

Nautilus-Type Pullovers (start)

Movement Performance—Use torso power to press your elbows against the pads and move them forward and downward in a semicircular arc until the cross member attached to the arm touches your abdomen. Hold this peak-con-

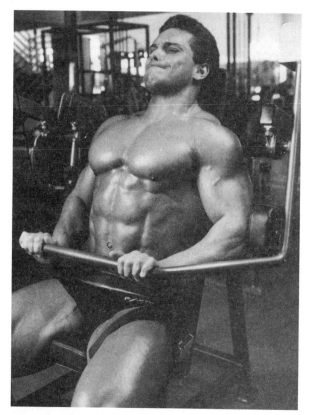

Nautilus-Type Pullovers (finish)

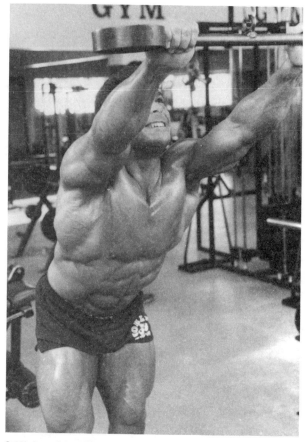

Stiff-Arm Lat Machine Pulldowns (start)

tracted position for a moment, then slowly return back along the same arc to the starting point.

Training Tips—This is a good movement on which to use the Weider Burns Training Principle. Burns consist of short, quick partial reps in the peak-contracted position of an exercise. Eight to 10 of these burns should be performed at the end of each set, using a training partner to help you pull the cross bar completely in to touch your midsection.

Stiff-Arm Pulldowns

Emphasis—As with various types of pullover movements, this exercise places the most intense stress on the pecs, serratus muscles, and lats. Secondary stress is on the remainder of the upper-back muscles which contract to rotate the shoulder blades.

Starting Position—Place your feet shoulder width apart 2½–3 feet back from an overhead pulley. Take a narrow overgrip in the middle of the lat machine bar. With your arms slightly

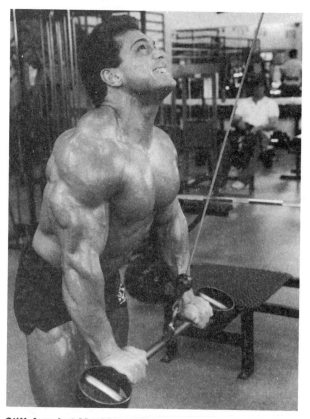

Stiff-Arm Lat Machine Pulldowns (finish)

bent, extend them toward the pulley and bend forward slightly at the waist to place stress on the working muscles. Maintain this upper-body position throughout your set.

Movement Performance—Slowly move the lat bar in a semicircular arc from the starting point forward and downward until it touches your upper thighs. Hold this peak-contracted position for a moment, then slowly return the bar back along the same arc to the starting point.

Training Tips—Vary the width of your grip on the bar. You can also use rope handles that provide you with a grip in which your hands are in a parallel position. Stiff-arm pullovers can also be done kneeling on the gym floor rather than standing.

Cable Crossovers

Emphasis—In all of its many variations, cable crossovers comprise the premier exercise for etching deep striations across the pectoral muscles. Primary stress is borne by the lower, outer, and inner pecs, plus the anterior deltoids.

Starting Position—Attach loop handles to the cables running through two overhead pulleys. Grasp the handles and stand midway between the two pulleys, your feet set about shoulder width apart. Bend a bit forward at the waist and maintain this torso angle throughout your set. Your arms should be extended upward di-

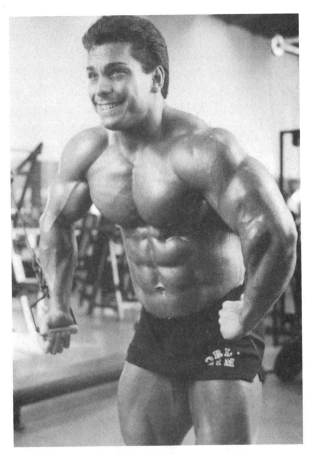

Cable Crossovers (near finish)

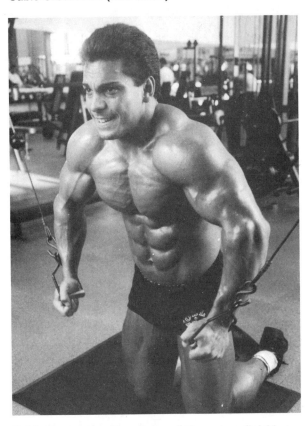

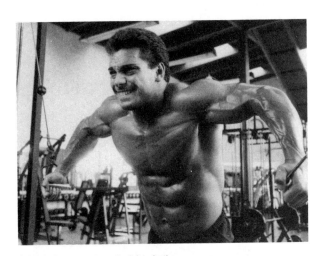

Cable Crossovers (midpoint)

Cable Crossovers (kneeling variation—near finish)

rectly toward the pulleys. Rotate your wrists so your palms are facing toward the floor throughout your set. Keep your arms slightly bent as you do the set.

Movement Performance—Use pectoral strength to move the handles out to the sides and downward in semicircular arcs until they meet about six inches in front of your hips. Hold your hands together while doing a "most muscular" pose, tensing your pecs and anterior delts, for 3–5 seconds. Slowly return the handles back along the same arcs to the starting point.

Training Tips—To make this movement more strict, you can perform it while kneeling on the floor rather than standing between the two pulleys. Crossovers can also be done with one arm at a time either while standing or kneeling on the gym floor.

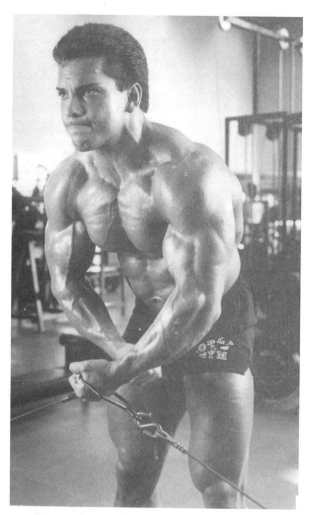

Low-Pulley Cable Crossovers (finish)

Low-Pulley Crossovers

Emphasis—Unlike the more normal crossovers performed with high pulleys, this movement is more for the upper and inner sections of the pectorals. As with normal crossovers, low-pulley crossovers are great for etching deep striations across your pectorals.

Starting Position—Attach loop handles to cables running through floor pulleys. Grasp the pulley handles and stand midway between the two pulleys, your feet set about shoulder width apart. Bend forward at the waist until your torso is inclined at about a 45-degree angle with the gym floor, and maintain this torso position throughout your set. Rotate your wrists so your palms are facing the floor, and maintain this hand orientation throughout your set.

Movement Performance—With your upper arms moving approximately perpendicular to the floor, slowly move your hands in semicircular arcs forward, downward, and toward each other until they touch. Hold this peak-contracted position for a moment, then return to the starting point.

Training Tips—You can also do this exercise either kneeling on the gym floor, or with one arm at a time while standing or kneeling.

Push-Ups Between Benches

Emphasis—A good finishing-off movement, push-ups between benches stress the entire pectoral muscle mass, along with the anterior del-

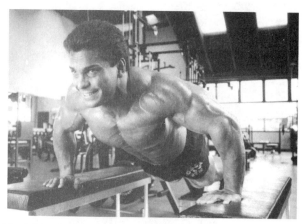

Push-Ups between Benches (midpoint)

toids, triceps, and those upper-back muscles which rotate the scapulae.

Starting Position—Position three benches so you can assume a standard push-up starting position while having your toes on one bench and each of your hands on a different bench. Keep your torso and legs rigid as you do your set.

Movement Performance—Bend your arms and lower your torso as far below the level of your hands as comfortably possible. Without bouncing in the bottom position of the movement, slowly push yourself back to the starting position.

Training Tips—If you wish to shift stress to the upper pecs, elevate your feet at least 1½–2 feet higher than your hands as you do the movement. Resistance can be applied to this exercise by having a training partner push down on your upper torso with appropriate force as you do the movement.

SUGGESTED CHEST ROUTINES

It would be foolish to pick the chest routine of a favorite bodybuilder and use it exercise-for-exercise and set-for-set in the gym. Such a routine would be of such great volume and high intensity that you would soon overtrain.

To avoid overtraining, I will give you several chest routines of lesser intensity which you can use in your own bodybuilding workouts. Each routine is followed by one of somewhat higher intensity, which can be used once you have spent 4–6 weeks on the first training program. By following the routines one after the other, you will build up sufficient recovery ability eventually to use the routines of the actual champions.

The following routine can be used by beginners three nonconsecutive days per week:

Exercise	Sets	Reps
Barbell Bench Presses	3	10–6*
Dumbbell Incline Presses	2	8–10

Pyramid weights and reps on any exercises marked with an asterisk, reducing the reps and increasing the training poundage with each succeeding set.

This routine will work well for low-intermediate bodybuilders:

Exercise	Sets	Reps
Barbell Incline Presses	4	12–6*
Dumbbell Bench Presses	3	8–10
Decline Flyes	2	8–10

And the following routine will work well for high-intermediate bodybuilders, who can use it either two or three times per week:

Exercise	Sets	Reps
Smith Machine Incline Presses	4	12–6*
Parallel Bar Dips	3	12–8*
Flat-Bench Flyes	3	8–10

Once you have reached the advanced level of bodybuilding, this routine will be typical of how you will train in an off-season building cycle:

Exercise	Sets	Reps
Dumbbell Incline Presses	5	12–5*
Bench Press to Neck	4	12–6*
Decline Barbell Presses	4	12–6*
Cross-Bench Dumbbell Pullovers	2–3	10–15

CHEST ROUTINES OF THE CHAMPS

In this section, I have included more than 30 chest routines used by various IFBB superstar bodybuilders. You can use them as models of how you should be training your chest, or once you have developed good recovery ability you can actually use the complete routines as outlined.

Lee Haney

OFF-SEASON ROUTINE

Exercise	Sets	Reps
Bench Presses	4–5	5
Incline Barbell Presses	4	5
Flat-Bench Dumbbell Flyes	3	6–8

PRECONTEST ROUTINE

Exercise	Sets	Reps
Bench Presses	5	8
Incline Barbell Presses	4	8
Flat-Bench Flyes	4	10
Cable Crossovers	2–3	10

Albert Beckles

Exercise	Sets	Reps
⎰Dumbbell Incline Presses	4	12
⎱Parallel Bar Dips	4	12
High-Incline Dumbbell Presses	4	12
Dumbbell Incline Flyes	4	12
Close-Grip Barbell Incline Presses	4	12
Incline Dumbbell Pullovers	4	12

Bracketed exercises throughout this section are supersetted.

Mike Christian

Exercise	Sets	Reps
Incline Dumbbell Presses	5	8–12
Parallel Bar Dips	5	10–15
Incline Dumbbell Flyes	5	8–12
Cable Crossovers	5	10–15
Pec Deck Flyes	4	8–12
Cross-Bench Dumbbell Pullovers	4	10–15

Rich Gaspari

Exercise	Sets	Reps
Incline Dumbbell Presses	7	8–10
Dumbbell Bench Presses	3–4	8–10
Incline Dumbbell Flyes, or . . .		
Pec Deck Flyes	3–4	8–10

For a contest, Rich adds in four sets of 10–12 reps of cable crossovers.

Bob Reis

Exercise	Sets	Reps
Bench Presses	5	15–8*
Incline Barbell Presses	3	10
Flat-Bench Dumbbell Flyes	3	20+

Robby Robinson

Exercise	Sets	Reps
Incline Dumbbell Presses	4–5	8–10
Bench Presses (to neck)	3–4	8–10
Parallel Bar Dips (weighted)	3–4	10–15
Flat-Bench Flyes, or . . .		
Cable Crossovers	3–4	8–10

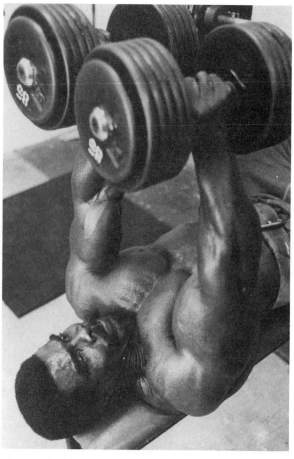

The Black Prince, Robby Robinson, starts a rep of Flat-Bench Dumbbell Flyes with a pair of 85-pounders. Robby has won a multitude of IFBB professional titles.

Danny Padilla

Exercise	Sets	Reps
Bench Presses	5	12
Flat-Bench Flyes	5	12
Incline Barbell Presses	5	12
Barbell Decline Presses	5	12
⎰Cross-Bench Dumbbell Pullovers	5	12
⎱Cable Crossovers	5	12

Greg DeFerro

Exercise	Sets	Reps
Smith Machine Incline Presses	4–5	8–10
Flat-Bench Dumbbell Flyes	4	8–10
⎰Bench Presses	3–4	8–10
⎱Cable Crossovers	3–4	8–10
Parallel Bar Dips	3–4	8–10
Cross-Bench Dumbbell Pullovers	3–4	8–10

Frank Zane

Exercise	Sets	Reps
Bench Presses	5	15-6*
Incline Dumbbell Presses	3	20-6*
Decline Dumbbell Flyes	3	8-10
Cross-Bench Dumbbell Pullovers	3	10

Lou Ferrigno

Exercise	Sets	Reps
Bench Presses	5-7	15-6*
Barbell Incline Presses	5	6-10
Barbell Decline Presses	5	6-10
Flat-Bench Dumbbell Flyes	5	10-12
{Cross-Bench Dumbbell Pullovers	3	15
{Cable Crossovers	3	10-15

As with all exercise charts in this book, exercises marked with an asterisk have reps and training poundages pyramided.

Arnold Schwarzenegger

Exercise	Sets	Reps
Bench Presses	5	6-10
Machine Incline Presses	5	6-10
Parallel Bar Dips	5	10-15
Flat-Bench Dumbbell Flyes	5	8-12
Cross-Bench Dumbbell Pullovers	5	10-15
Cable Crossovers	5	8-12

Jusup Wilkosz

ROUTINE #1

Exercise	Sets	Reps
Incline Barbell Presses	5	10-12
Narrow-Grip Bench Presses	5	10-12
Parallel Bar Dips	5	10-12
Cable Crossovers	5	10-12

ROUTINE #2

Exercise	Sets	Reps
Bench Presses	5	10-12
Barbell Incline Presses	5	10-12
Barbell Pullovers	5	10-12
Cable Crossovers	5	10-12

Roy Callender

Exercise	Sets	Reps
{Dumbbell Incline Presses	6-10	8-12
{Incline Dumbbell Flyes	6-10	8-12
{Parallel Bar Dips	6-8	8-12
{Cross-Bench Dumbbell Pullovers	6-8	8-12
Flat-Bench Dumbbell Flyes	6-8	8-12
Cable Crossovers	6-8	8-12

Pat Neve

Exercise	Sets	Reps
Bench Presses	5-6	10
Barbell Incline Presses	4-5	10
Flat-Bench Dumbbell Flyes	4-5	15-20
Parallel Bar Dips	4-5	10-15
Cross-Bench Dumbbell Pullovers	3-4	20

Tim Belknap

Exercise	Sets	Reps
Bench Presses	4	8-12
Barbell Incline Presses	3	8-10
Low-Incline Dumbbell Flyes	3	10
Parallel Bar Dips	1	15-25

Chris Dickerson

Exercise	Sets	Reps
Pec Deck Flyes	5	20-12*
Incline Dumbbell Flye-Presses	5	12-6*
Dumbbell Bench Presses	5	12-6*
Cable Crossovers	3-5	12

Dennis Tinerino

Exercise	Sets	Reps
Barbell Incline Presses	4	6-8
Smith Machine Incline Presses	4	6-8
Bench Presses	4	6-8
Parallel Bar Dips	4	8-12

Ron Teufel

Exercise	Sets	Reps
{Bench Presses	7	12-6*
{Cross-Bench Dumbbell Pullovers	7	10-12
{Machine Incline Presses	5	8
{Decline Dumbbell Presses	5	8
{Barbell Incline Presses	5	8
{Cable Crossovers	5	10

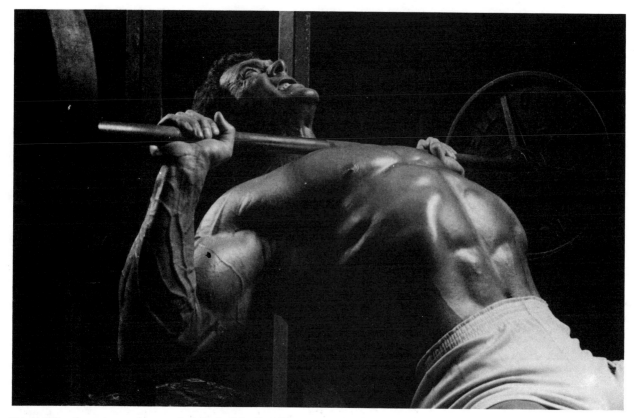

Scott Wilson warms up for a set of Barbell Incline Presses at Gold's Gym in Venice, California. Scott works as the manager of the Gold's in San Jose.

Gary Leonard

Exercise	Sets	Reps
Bench Presses	5-6	15-6*
Incline Barbell Presses	5-6	8-5*
{ Incline Dumbbell Flyes	3-4	8-10
{ Cable Crossovers	3-4	10-15

Bertil Fox

Exercise	Sets	Reps
Bench Presses	6-8	15-6*
Incline Dumbbell Presses	6-8	8-10
Flat-Bench Dumbbell Flyes	6-8	8-10
Parallel Bar Dips	6-8	8-10
Cable Crossovers	6-8	8-10

Edward Kawak

Exercise	Sets	Reps
Flat-Bench Flyes	4	12-15
Incline Barbell Presses	4	10-12
Bench Presses	6	12-4*
Cross-Bench Dumbbell Pullovers	3-4	15
Cable Crossovers	3-4	15-20

Charles Glass

Exercise	Sets	Reps
Bench Presses	4	12-15
Incline Barbell Presses	4	12-15
Cross-Bench Dumbbell Pullovers	4	12-15
Decline Dumbbell Presses	4	12-15
Pec Deck Flyes	4	12-15
Incline Dumbbell Flyes	4	12-15
Pec Crunches*	4	12-15

―――――――――――――

Pec crunches are short burns done slowly in the peak-contracted position of pec deck flyes.

John Terilli

Exercise	Sets	Reps
Dumbbell Bench Presses (warm-up)	2	20
Dumbbell Bench Presses	3-4	15-6*
Barbell Incline Presses	3	12-8*
Flat-Bench Dumbbell Flyes	3	8-12
Cross-Bench Dumbbell Pullovers	2	15
Parallel Bar Dips	1	max.

Ian Dowe

Exercise	Sets	Reps
Bench Presses	4-6	30-6*
Close-Grip Bench Presses	3	8-12
Incline Dumbbell Presses	4	8-12
{Flat-Bench Dumbbell Flyes	5	8-10
{Parallel Bar Dips	5	10-15
{Cross-Bench Dumbbell Pullovers	3	10-15
{Stiff-Arm Lat Machine Pulldowns	3	10-15

Boyer Coe

Exercise	Sets	Reps
Machine Incline Presses	3-4	8
Pec Deck Flyes	3-4	8
Vertical Machine Bench Presses	3-4	8
Incline Machine Flyes	3-4	8

Dr. Franco Columbu

Exercise	Sets	Reps
Bench Presses	7	6-8
Incline Barbell Presses	4	6-10
{Flat-Bench Dumbbell Flyes	2-3	8-12
{Parallel Bar Dips	2-3	10-15

Bob Jodkiewcz

Exercise	Sets	Reps
Bench Presses	5	8-12
Incline Barbell Presses	5	8-12
Parallel Bar Dips	5	8-12
Incline Dumbbell Flyes	5	8-12
Cable Crossovers	5	8-12

Scott Wilson

Exercise	Sets	Reps
Incline Barbell Presses	4-5	6-8
Barbell Bench Presses	4-5	6-8
Incline Dumbbell Flyes	4-5	8-10
Pec Deck Flyes	4-5	8-10

21
Fabulous Forearms!

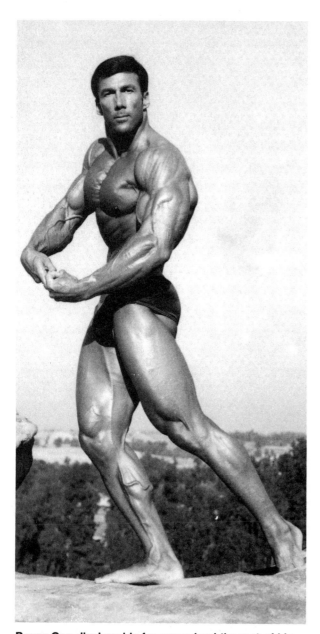

Boyer Coe displays his forearms (and the rest of his great physique) just befor heading off to Australia for the 1980 Mr. Olympia, where he placed third behind Arnold Schwarzenegger and Chris Dickerson.

Forearms—some bodybuilders have them in spades without even directly training the muscle group, while other less-fortunate men never have fantastic forearms regardless of how hard they work the body part.

For every *Mike Mentzer,* who built a pair of the sport's greatest forearms merely by "squeezing the barbell and dumbbell handles" when doing upper-body exercises, there are ten unfortunates who are forced to slave away on forearms two or three times per week for many years just to acquire a moderately good lower-arm development.

In the late 1800s and early 1900s most bodybuilders were also weightlifters, and invariably they had forearms that Popeye would envy. This development came through cleaning and snatching exceedingly heavy barbells, pinchgripping thick barbell plates, arm wrestling for fun, and fooling around with such forearm-oriented strength feats as maxed-out reverse curls and odd lifts requiring tremendous, crushing grip strength.

As the sport began to mature in the 1940s and 1950s, less emphasis was placed on lifting ability and grip strength and more on pure bodybuilding movements. And as an unfortunate consequence, an overall regression in forearm development began to take place among the best bodybuilders.

When bodybuilding experienced a terrific surge in popularity during the 1970s and 1980s, emphasis shifted to total development of every body part, including forearms. And bodybuilders who didn't have naturally good forearm development began to train hard to acquire it. Now virtually all great pro and amateur bodybuilders at the national and international level have exceptional forearms.

Perhaps you are lucky enough to have optimum genetics for fabulous forearm development, in which case you can forget reading this chapter. But if you are like most of us and have average or below-average potential for forearm mass and muscularity, you will need to digest and apply all of the detailed forearm developmental information in this chapter. So when you are beginning to make your mark nationally, no one is going to score you lower than you should place because your forearms are underpar. They'll be thick and corded with muscles from elbow to wrist!

FOREARM ANATOMY AND KINESIOLOGY

There are more different muscles in your forearms than in any other large body part. These muscles are capable of exerting crushing grip force, or the delicate manipulations of a heart surgeon. For your purposes, however, we will deal with only three general categories of forearm muscle structure and function.

The first category is the *forearm supinator* muscle complex, a large, meaty muscle out the outer-upper part of your forearm. This muscle contracts with great intensity when you do barbell reverse curls, hammer curls, and Zottman curls. And in most cases, you will only be able to develop this muscle group to the maximum extent by hard, consistent, heavy training on these three curling movements.

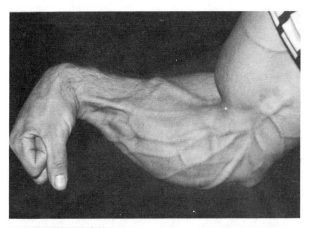

The most massive forearm on the planet belongs to Mike Mentzer, a former editor of *Muscle & Fitness* magazine. The real shocker here is that Mike claims to have seldom ever done any direct training for his forearm muscles, yet they're H-U-G-E!

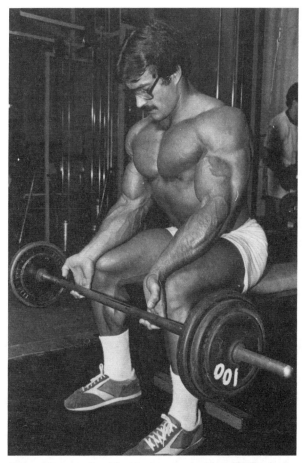

Mike wrings every bit of stress from Barbell Wrist Curls.

The second category is the *forearm flexor* muscles, which are a bundle of many small muscles on the inside of your forearm. When you have your arms down at your sides and palms facing each other, the forearm flexors act on the large group of muscles on the insides of your forearms. This group of muscles contracts to close your fist, or to flex your fist, as in barbell wrist curls.

The final general category of forearm muscles is the *forearm extensors*, or the smaller bundle of muscles on the outer sides of your forearms. These muscles contract to extend your fingers from a position in which you have made a fist. They also contract to extend your hand in relation to your forearm, as is the case in barbell reverse wrist curls.

To develop optimum forearms, you will therefore need to do three types of movements: reverse curls, wrist curls with your palms facing upward, and wrist curls with palms facing the floor. In order of total mass, the forearm flexors are potentially the largest, followed by the forearm supinator muscles and then the forearm extensors.

FOREARM TRAINING TIPS

Training forearms is a basic task with very few refinements. Therefore, there really aren't any secrets you'll need to know when building up your forearm muscles. There are a couple of tricks you *should* know, however.

Regardless of how weak your forearms might be, you won't be able to use the Weider Muscle Priority Training Principle on them. When you train forearms hard, you will have difficulty in gripping weights for other exercises later in your sessions. Your forearm muscles will be so pumped up, in fact, that you won't even be able to write notes in your training diary. Therefore, *all* serious bodybuilders save forearm work for last position in each training session. But since the muscles are relatively small in mass when compared to the leg, back, and chest muscles, you won't need much energy remaining at the end of a training session in order to bomb them with absolute intensity.

While some bodybuilders train forearms virtually every day, you *can* overtrain the muscle group. I firmly believe that you will make your best progress in adding to forearm muscle mass and contour on only 2–3 direct forearm training sessions per week, preferably with at least 48 hours of rest between forearm workouts.

Finally, you must always bear down on your forearms if you want to build them up. The muscle group *will* come up with consistently hard training, but it is very difficult to see any progress in them from month to month. So it becomes very easy to throw up your hands in disgust because you don't seem to be making any gains in forearm development, and abandon training them altogether. It doesn't take a genius to realize that this approach won't win you any Mr. Olympia titles. Therefore, you must always train consistently heavy and hard if you want to end up with fabulous forearms.

Photographed by Paula Crane at Gold's Gym, Venice, California

FOREARM EXERCISES
Barbell Reverse Curls

Emphasis—All variations of reverse curls place primary stress on the upper-outer forearm muscles, brachialis muscles, and biceps. Secondary stress is on the forearm flexors.

Starting Position—Take a shoulder-width overgrip on a moderately weighted barbell. With your feet set a comfortable distance apart, stand erect with your arms hanging down at your sides and the barbell resting across your upper thighs. Straighten your arms and press your upper arms against the sides of your ribcage until you have completed your set. You should also keep your wrists straight.

Movement Performance—Without allowing your torso to move forward or backward, slowly curl the barbell upward in a semicircular arc from your upper thighs to a point directly under your chin. Squeeze your forearm and upper-arm muscles as tightly as possible for a moment, then slowly lower the weight back along the same arc to the starting point.

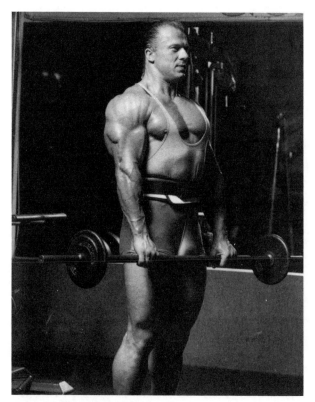

Barbell Reverse Curls (start)

ment with more narrow grip widths. While you won't be able to use as much weight with a narrower grip, you often get more out of the movement anyway.

Cable Reverse Curls

Emphasis—All variations of reverse curls place primary stress on the upper-outer forearm muscles, biceps, and brachialis muscles. Secondary stress is on the forearm flexors.

Starting Position—Attach a straight bar handle to the end of a cable running through a low pulley. Take a shoulder-width overgrip on the pulley handle, set your feet a comfortable distance apart 6-8 inches back from the pulley, and stand erect with your arms running

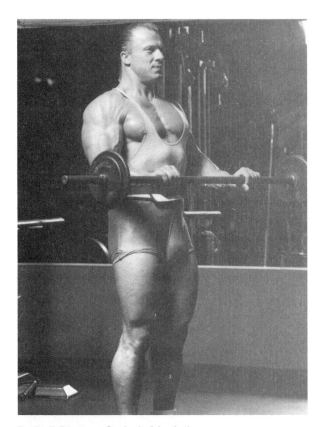

Barbell Reverse Curls (midpoint)

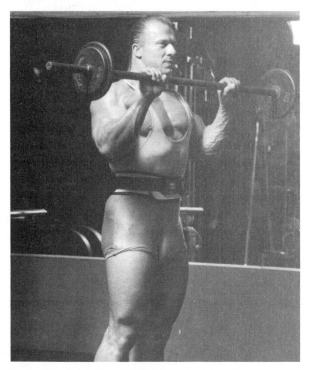

Barbell Reverse Curls (finish)

Training Tips—It is very difficult to use a grip wider than your shoulders when performing reverse curls, but you should definitely experi-

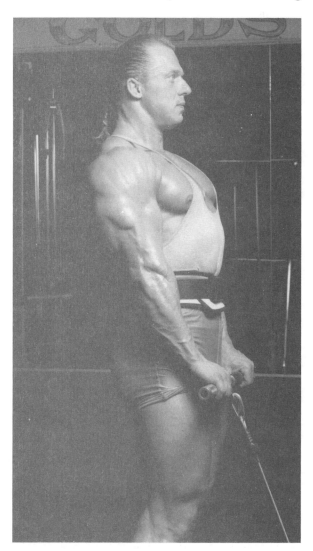

Cable Reverse Curls (start)

straight downward from your shoulders directly toward the pulley. Press your upper arms against the sides of your torso in this position, and keep them motionless like this throughout your set. Keep your wrists straight.

Movement Performance—Without allowing your torso to move forward or backward, slowly curl the pulley handle upward in a semicircular arc from the starting point to a position directly beneath your chin. Tense your upperarm and forearm muscles as tightly as possible in this position for a moment, then return the handle back along the same arc to the starting point.

Training Tips—As with barbell reverse curls, you should experiment with a variety of more narrow grip widths.

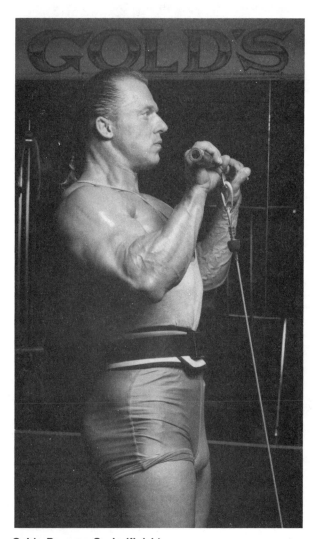

Cable Reverse Curls (finish)

Barbell Reverse Preacher Curls

Emphasis—All variations of reverse curls place primary emphasis on the upper-outer forearm muscles, biceps and brachialis muscles. Secondary stress is on the forearm flexors. But when the upper arms are braced on a preacher bench, the movement is much more strict than when performed in a standing position.

Starting Position—Take a shoulder-width overgrip on a fairly light barbell. Lean over the top of a preacher bench so the top edge of the bench is under your armpits and your upper arms are running down the angled surface of the bench parallel with each other. You can either stand or sit on the bench seat if one is provided, but be sure you keep your arm-chest juncture pressed firmly against the upper edge of the bench. Fully straighten your arms.

Movement Performance—Slowly curl the barbell upward in a semicircular arc from the starting point to a position beneath your chin. Tense your upper-arm and forearm muscles as tightly as possible in this position, then slowly lower the barbell back along the same arc to the starting point.

Training Tips—Experiment with various grip widths. Be careful at all times to never bounce the weight in the bottom position, because such a training error can tear arm muscle tendons relatively easily when the arm-flexing muscles are fully extended and in a poor mechanical position.

Cable Reverse Preacher Curls

Emphasis—All variations of reverse curls place primary emphasis on the upper-outer forearm muscles, biceps, and brachialis muscles. Secondary stress is on the forearm flexors. But when the upper arms are braced on a preacher bench, the movement is much more strict than when performed in a standing position.

Starting Position—Attach a straight bar handle to the end of a cable running through a floor pulley. Place a preacher bench about 2–3 feet back from the pulley with the angled surface of the bench toward the machine. Take a shoulder-width overgrip on the pulley handle and drape yourself over the bench so the upper edge of the bench is pressed firmly under your armpits and your upper arms are running down the angled surface of the bench parallel with each other. You can either stand or sit on the bench seat if one is provided. Fully straighten your arms.

Movement Performance—Slowly curl the pulley handle upward in a semicircular arc from the starting point to a position directly beneath your chin. Tense all of your upper-arm and forearm muscles in this position for a moment, then slowly return the handle back along the same arc to the starting point.

Training Tips—Experiment with different grip widths. Be careful at all times to never bounce the weight in the bottom position, because such a training error can tear arm muscle tendons relatively easily when the arm-flexing muscles are fully extended and in a relatively poor mechanical position.

Hammer Curls

Emphasis—Also called thumbs-up occasionally, hammer curls are excellent for developing the upper-outer sections of the forearms, biceps, and brachialis muscles.

Starting Position—Grasp a moderately heavy pair of dumbbells, set your feet about shoulder width apart, and stand erect with your arms running straight down at your sides, palms facing your legs (toward each other). Press your upper arms against the sides of your torso and keep them motionless in this position throughout your set. At all times when performing hammer curls, your palms should be facing each other.

Movement Performance—Use arm strength to curl the dumbbells forward and upward in semicircular arcs to about shoulder level. Tense all of your arm muscles tightly in the top posi-

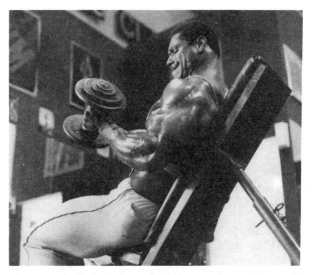

Hammer Curls (one-armed version, performed seated on an incline bench—midpoint)

Model: Mike Christian

tion, then slowly lower the weights back along the same arcs to the starting point.

Training Tips—If you have trouble with your torso wafting forward and backward during a set, you should either do the movement seated astride a flat exercise bench, or standing with your back pressed against the gym wall as you do the movement.

Zottman Curls

Emphasis—Named after the movement's originator, George Zottman, Zottman curls place intense stress on the biceps, brachialis, upper-outer forearm, and forearm flexor muscles.

Starting Position—Grasp two moderately weighted dumbbells, set your feet about shoulder-width apart on the gym floor, and stand erect with your arms running straight down at your sides, palms facing each other. Press your upper arms against the sides of your torso, and keep them motionless in this position throughout your set.

Movement Performance—With palm facing upward, slowly curl the weight in your left hand forward and upward in a semicircular arc to shoulder level. At the level of your shoulder, rotate your wrist, so your palm is facing downward as you lower the weight back to the start-

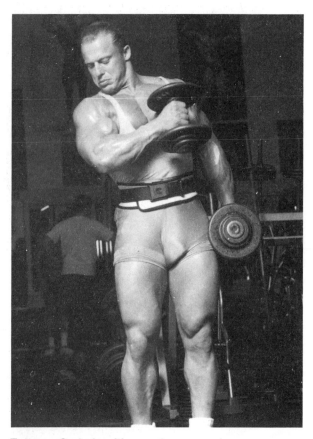

Zottman Curls (position one)

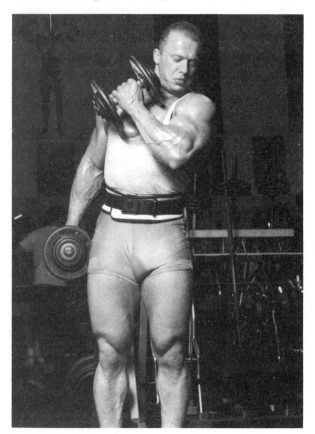

Zottman Curls (position two)

ing point at the side of your upper thigh. This is the movement for one arm. To add in the other arm, start to curl the weight in your right hand upward (palm upward) as the weight in the other one is being lowered, then rotate your hand so your right palm is facing downward toward the floor as you lower the weight back to the starting point. Continue curling the weights in seesaw fashion, being sure each palm is facing upward as the weight in that hand is being curled upward, and is facing downward as the dumbbell in that hand is being lowered.

Training Tips—You can also do this movement while seated astride a flat exercise bench, or in a standing position with your upper back pressed against the gym wall throughout your set.

Barbell Wrist Curls/Reverse Wrist Curls

Emphasis—When performed with palms facing upward, wrist curls isolate stress on the forearm flexor muscles; when performed with palms facing downward, reverse wrist curls isolate stress on the forearm extensor muscles.

Starting Position—I will describe wrist curls with palms facing upward to you, and from this description you can easily extrapolate how to perform reverse wrist curls with palms facing downward. Take a shoulder-width undergrip on a moderately weighted barbell. Sit at the end of a flat exercise bench with your feet set about shoulder width apart. Run your fore-

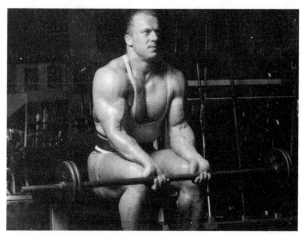

Barbell Wrist Curls (start)

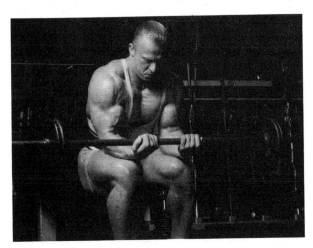

Barbell Wrist Curls (finish)

arms down over your thighs so your wrists and hands are hanging over the edge formed by your knees. Be sure that you keep your forearms pressed firmly against your thighs at all times when doing wrist curls. Allow the weight of the bar to pull your fists downward as far as possible to prestretch the forearm flexor muscles.

Movement Performance—Use forearm strength to curl the barbell upward in a semicircular arc to as high a position as possible. Hold this peak-contracted position for a moment while powerfully flexing your forearm flexors, then slowly lower the weight back along the same arc to the starting point.

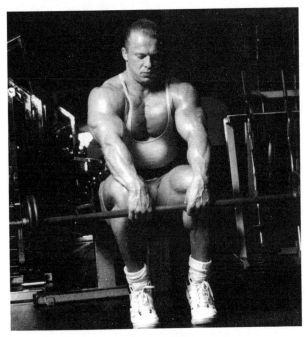

Barbell Reverse Wrist Curls (start)

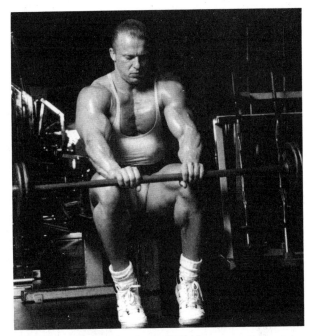

Barbell Reverse Wrist Curls (finish)

Training Tips—While most bodybuilders do wrist curls with their thumbs encircling the bar, a few top men believe that they achieve a better contraction in their forearm flexors by curling the barbell upward with their thumbs curled under the bar rather than around it. For a somewhat more secure movement, you can support your forearms over a flat exercise bench rather than running them down your thighs. And to increase the peak contraction effect on your working forearm muscles, you can support your forearms down along the 45-degree-angled surface of a preacher bench.

Dumbbell Wrist Curls/ Reverse Wrist Curls

Emphasis—When performed with palm(s) facing upward, dumbbell wrist curls isolate stress on the forearm flexor muscles. And when you might infrequently perform the movement with palm(s) facing downward, dumbbell reverse wrist curls isolate stress on the forearm extensor muscles.

Starting Position—I will describe dumbbell wrist curls performed with one arm at a time supported on a flat exercise bench. If you wish to either do dumbbell reverse wrist curls, or either dumbbell wrist curls or reverse wrist

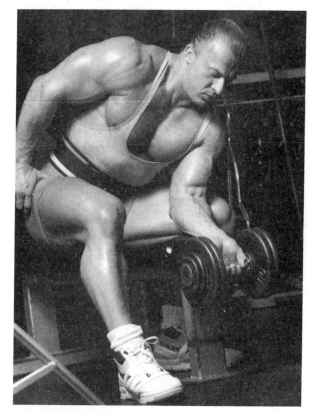

Dumbbell Wrist Curls (one-armed version—start)

And for a greater peak contraction effect when doing dumbbell wrist curls, you can support your forearm with a preacher bench rather than a flat exercise bench. You can also support the weight on your thigh if you like, although it is usually a less secure movement than one in which your forearm is supported by an exercise bench.

Cable Wrist Curls/Reverse Wrist Curls

Emphasis—When performed with palms facing upward, cable wrist curls place isolated stress on the forearm flexor muscles. And when performed with palms facing downward, cable reverse wrist curls place isolated stress on the forearm extensor muscles.

Starting Position—I will explain how to perform cable wrist curls, and from that explanation you can easily extrapolate how to do cable reverse wrist curls. Attach a straight bar handle to the end of a cable running through a floor pulley. Place a flat exercise bench or stool about

curls with forearms running down your thighs, you can easily extrapolate correct performance for the variation of the explained movement. Grasp a moderately weighted dumbbell in your right hand and run your right forearm down the surface of a flat exercise bench, wrist and hand hanging off the end of the bench (you can sit astride the bench near the middle). Your palms should be facing upward. Allow the weight to pull your fist down as far toward the floor as possible.

Movement Performance—Use forearm strength to curl the weight upward as high as possible in a semicircular arc, holding the peak-contracted position for a moment while intensely flexing your forearm muscles. Then lower slowly back along the same arc to the starting point. Without bouncing the weight in the bottom position of the exercise, be sure to perform an equal number of sets and reps with each arm.

Training Tips—You can experiment with placing your thumb both around the bar and under the bar for your dumbbell wrist curls.

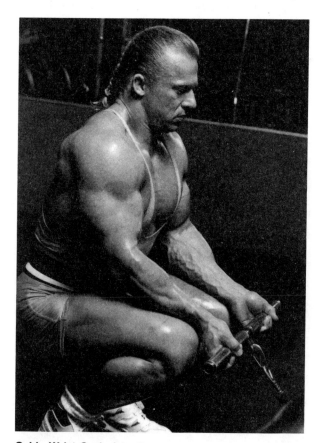

Cable Wrist Curls (start)

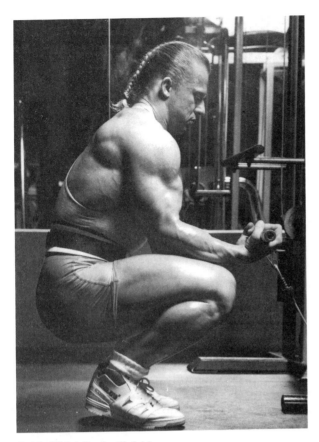

Cable Wrist Curls (finish)

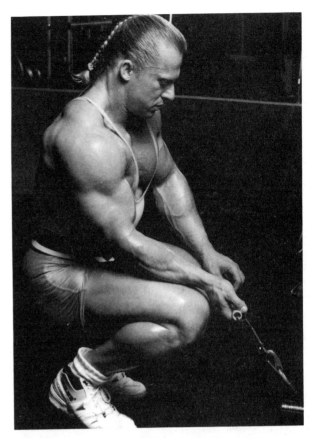

Cable Wrist Curls (one-armed variation—start)

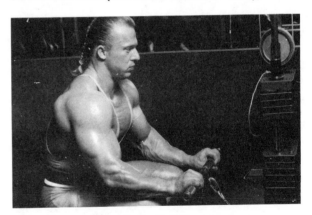

Cable Reverse Wrist Curls (finish)

1½–2 feet back from the pulley. Take a shoulder-width undergrip on the pulley handle and sit down at the edge of the exercise bench, your forearms running down the surface of your thighs, wrists and hands hanging off the edge of your knees. Allow the weight attached to the end of the cable to pull your fists downward toward the pulley as far as comfortably possible.

Movement Performance—Use forearm flexor strength to curl the pulley handle upward in a tight semicircular arc to as high a position as comfortably possible. Hold this peak-contracted position for a moment while intensely flexing your forearm muscles. Slowly return to the starting point.

Training Tips—You can also do this movement supporting your forearms by resting them across a flat exercise bench. Or to increase the peak contraction effect of the movement, you can run your forearms down the angled surface of a preacher bench.

Standing Barbell Wrist Curls

Emphasis—Since it provides an optimally intense peak contraction effect in the working muscles, this is one of the best exercises for isolating stress on the forearm flexors.

Starting Position—Place a moderately heavy barbell crossways on a high, flat exercise bench. Back up to the bench and take a shoulder-width grip on the bar with your hands set 3–4 inches wider than your shoulders on each side. Stand

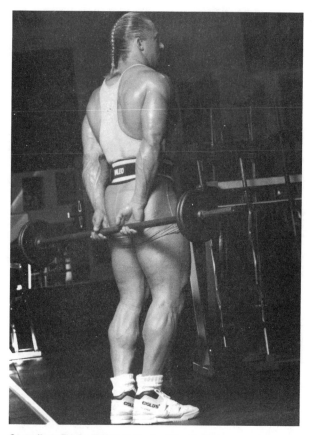

Standing Barbell Wrist Curls (start)

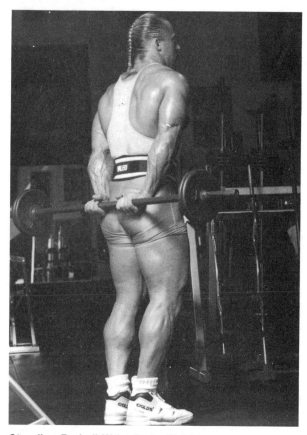

Standing Barbell Wrist Curls (finish)

erect with your arms hanging straight downward from your shoulders, the bar resting across the backs of your upper thighs.

Movement Performance—Use forearm flexor strength to curl the barbell to the rear and upward in a small semicircular arc to as high a position as possible. Hold this peak-contracted position for a moment while intensely flexing the working forearm muscles. Then slowly lower the barbell back along the same small arc to the starting point.

Training Tips—You can do a very similar movement with a pair of heavy dumbbells hanging at arms' length from your shoulders, curling them inward and upward in small semicircular arcs.

SUGGESTED FOREARM ROUTINES

Beginning bodybuilders can usually achieve sufficient forearm stimulation merely from doing barbell curls and other upper-body movements which also stress the forearm muscles. But after the first 8–10 weeks of steady training, you will need to begin doing direct forearm training as a means of further stimulating forearm muscle growth. Here are three successively more intense routines which you can follow for 6–8 weeks, 2–3 times per week, as you progress in the sport.

LEVEL "A" ROUTINE

Exercise	Sets	Reps
Barbell Reverse Curls	3	8–12
Barbell Wrist Curls	3	10–15

LEVEL "B" ROUTINE

Exercise	Sets	Reps
Barbell Preacher Reverse Curls	4	8–10
Supported Dumbbell Wrist Curls	3	10–15
Supported Barbell Reverse Wrist Curls	3	10–15

LEVEL "C" ROUTINE

Exercise	Sets	Reps
Hammer Curls	4–5	8–10
Standing Barbell Wrist Curls	4	10–15
Cable Reverse Wrist Curls	4	10–15

FOREARM ROUTINES OF THE CHAMPIONS

In this section, I have listed a dozen routines from 10 great IFBB bodybuilding stars. You should use these training programs primarily as models upon which you should base your own forearm training programs. Just be sure that you don't exceed the total number of sets of forearm work from which you can safely recover and make good gains.

Jusup Wilkosz

ALTERNATIVE "A"

Exercise	Sets	Reps
Barbell Wrist Curls	4	10–12
Barbell Reverse Curls	4	10–12

ALTERNATIVE "B"

Exercise	Sets	Reps
Zottman Curls	4	10–12
One-Arm Dumbbell Wrist Curls	4	10–12

Lee Haney

Exercise	Sets	Reps
Barbell Reverse Curls	5	6–10
Barbell Wrist Curls	5	8–12
Barbell Reverse Wrist Curls	5	8–12

Larry Scott

Exercise	Sets	Reps
Machine Reverse Curls	3–4	8
Seated Barbell Supported Wrist Curls	2–3	20
Standing Barbell Wrist Curls	2–3	20

Mike Mentzer

Exercise	Sets	Reps
Barbell Wrist Curls	2–3	10–12
Barbell Reverse Wrist Curls	2–3	10–12

Jorma Räty

Exercise	Sets	Reps
Barbell Reverse Curls	3–4	8–10
Barbell Wrist Curls	3–4	10–15
Barbell Reverse Wrist Curls	3–4	10–15

Dave Draper

Exercise	Sets	Reps
Barbell Reverse Curls	4–5	8–10
Supported Barbell Wrist Curls	4–5	10–15

Matt Mendenhall

Exercise	Sets	Reps
Barbell Reverse Curls	4	8–10
Barbell Wrist Curls	4–6	10–12
Barbell Reverse Wrist Curls	4–6	10–12

Bracketed exercises are supersetted.

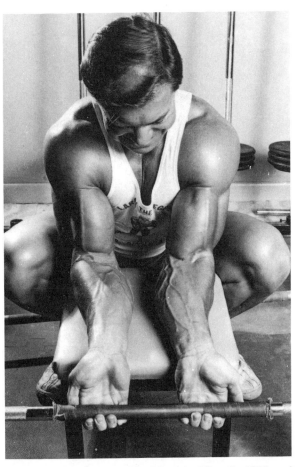

Winner of the first two Mr. Olympia titles (in 1965 and 1966), Larry Scott pumps out a set of Barbell Wrist Curls using a narrow grip and resting his forearms on a flat exercise bench for support. This photo was taken when Larry was 50 and still in great shape. He's a successful businessman in Salt Lake City, Utah.

Casey Viator

DAY 1

Exercise	Sets	Reps
Zottman Curls	5	6–10
Barbell Wrist Curls	5	15–20
Barbell Reverse Wrist Curls	5	15–20

DAY 2

Exercise	Sets	Reps
Barbell Reverse Curls	5	6–10
One-Arm Dumbbell Wrist Curls	5	15–20
Supported Barbell Reverse Wrist Curls	5	15–20

Mike Christian

Exercise	Sets	Reps
Cable Reverse Curls	4–5	8–10
Barbell Wrist Curls	4–5	10–12
Barbell Reverse Wrist Curls	4–5	10–12

Bob Birdsong

Exercise	Sets	Reps
Zottman Curls	4	8–12
Standing Barbell Wrist Curls	4	12–15
Supported Barbell Reverse Wrist Curls	4	12–15

22
Building a
Column of Neck Muscle

A lot of champions talk about how a body-builder actually wears his sport. His body is so highly developed that the average person *knows* a man is a bodybuilder. And no part of the human body is more visible year-round than the neck.

The champs also joke about "pencil necks," or guys who don't train and as a result have puny, weak-appearing bodies. Even if you don't train your neck muscles directly, however, you will never be accused of being a pencil neck. The neck muscles of a bodybuilder expand in mass merely as a side effect of hard training for the upper torso muscles. Almost all of us therefore have thick necks, somewhat like marble columns of muscle.

NECK ANATOMY AND KINESIOLOGY

There are many muscles in your neck, and they contract to accomplish two basic functions—rotation of the head in relation to your torso, and flexion of your head in relation to your torso. Neck flexion takes place in four main directions—forward, to either side, and to the rear—as well as a myriad of subdirections between these four main poles.

The two prominent neck muscles you need to know about are the main muscle at each side of the front of your neck, called the *sternocleido mastoid* muscle, and the back of your neck, the *trapezius* (an upper-back muscle) inserts at the upper point nearly at the base of your skull. Each muscle contracts to provide head flexion, and the sternocleido mastoid also assists in head rotation.

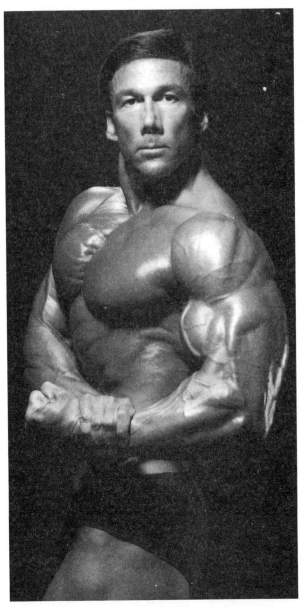

In this classic side-chest shot, Boyer Coe also shows how his neck has developed as an indirect result of balanced, heavy-duty training.

NECK TRAINING TIPS

Most of the bodybuilders with truly outstanding neck development were wrestlers and/or football players prior to moving into the Iron Game. Both of these sports place a premium on strong neck development, and wrestlers and football players spend time nearly every training session doing direct exercises for their necks.

While you may learn that your neck needs a few weeks or months of direct training to bring it up to the desired level, you must be careful to avoid overdeveloping your neck. An overly thick neck can actually detract from the illusion of shoulder width that is so important to a top bodybuilder's symmetry. Work your neck, but don't overdo it.

NECK EXERCISES

There are only a few direct neck exercises available for your use. In this section I'll illustrate and fully describe each of them.

Wrestler's Bridges

Emphasis—Performed faceup, this movement stresses the neck flexor muscles at the back of your neck. Performed facedown, it strengthens and develops the neck flexor muscles at the front and sides of your neck.

Starting Position—You should do this movement on an exercise pad, which will provide a cushion for your head. Alternatively, you can do it with a towel, folded over several times, for your head pad. Lie on your back on the gym floor with the back of your head resting on the pad. Pull your feet up toward your buttocks until you can place them flat on the floor about where your knees were resting. Arch upward as high as possible, as illustrated.

Movement Performance—Slowly rock toward the rear, rolling your head along the floor pad, until your forehead is almost touching the floor. Rock the other direction as far as you can as well. Continue to rock forward and backward until your neck muscles have become fully fatigued (normally about 6-8 repetitions).

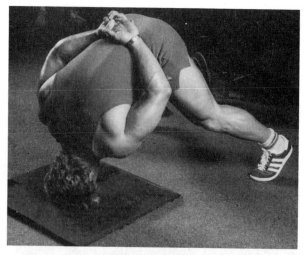

Wrestler's Bridges

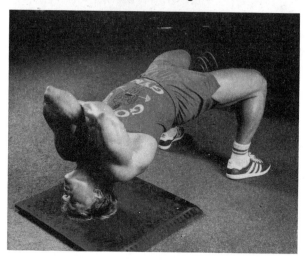

Training Tips—You can also do this movement facedown, starting with your forehead against the floor pad. On the faceup version of wrestler's bridges, you can add resistance to the movement by holding a loose barbell plate or light dumbbell across your upper abdomen.

Partner Hand Pressure Neck Movement

Emphasis—When you are resisting your partner as he is pressing straight downward, you are developing the neck flexors at the back of your neck. When you are resisting his pressure directly to either side, you are developing the flexors at the side of your neck.

Starting Position—Kneel on the floor of the gym on your hands and knees. Move your head

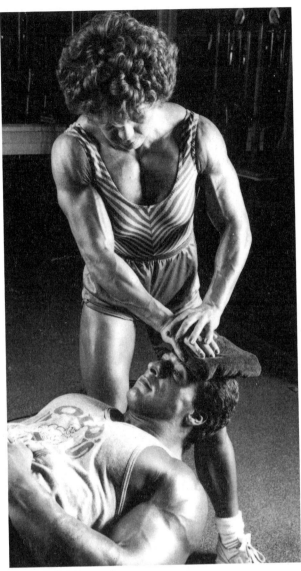

Partner Hand Pressure Neck Movements

holds on to the opposite upper arm for additional leverage.

Neck Strap Movement

Emphasis—If you can find a good neck strap in a sporting goods store, you can use it to develop all of your neck muscles.

Starting Position—Slip the harness over your head and sit at the end of a flat exercise bench with your hands placed on your knees to support your torso at a slight forward angle. With a weight on the end of the chain or rope, slowly move your head forward until your chin is resting on your chest.

Movement Performance—Slowly move your head directly to the rear as far as possible. Pause a second, then return to the starting point.

Training Tips—You can also do this movement with the chain/rope hanging down your back and your torso inclined somewhat to the rear. Or you can lean to the left or right and move your head in that direction.

Safety Tip—With very heavy weights, you can pad the head harness by slipping a thick towel over your head before you slide on the apparatus.

Nautilus Four-Way Neck Machine Movement

Emphasis—Depending on which direction you move your head against resistance, you can develop the flexor muscles at the back, front, or either side of your neck. And you can use much greater resistance on this movement that any other neck exercise you might care to utilize.

Starting Position—Adjust the height of the seat so your head rests against the pads on the movement arm without having to stretch or hunch over excessively. Face toward the lever arm and bend forward to place the back of your head against the pads. Grasp the handles provided to steady your body in the machine as you do the movement.

forward until your chin is on your chest. Your partner places his hands on the back of your head to add resistance to the movement by pressing down with appropriate force.

Movement Performance—Slowly rotate your head upward and to the rear as far as possible. When your partner increases resistance, try to stop the movement of your head back to the starting point. Repeat until your neck muscles have become fully fatigued.

Training Tips—You can also do this movement side-to-side while your partner pushes against the side of your head with one hand and

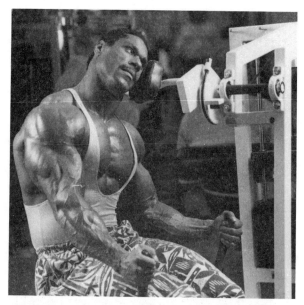

Nautilus Four-Way Neck Machine Movement (side)

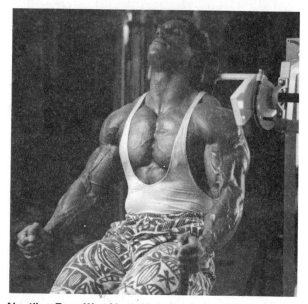

Nautilus Four-Way Neck Machine Movement (rear)

Movement Performance—Use neck strength to move your head in a semicircular arc as far to the rear as possible. Hold this position for a moment, then return to the starting point.

Training Tips—You can also do the movement facing away from the lever arm to stress the front neck flexors, or with either side facing the arm.

Upright Rows

Emphasis—Upright rows strengthen and develop the trapezius muscles of the upper back,

as well as the deltoids, biceps, brachialis, and forearm flexor muscles.

Starting Position—Set your feet about shoulder width apart on the gym floor. Bend over and take a narrow overgrip in the middle of a barbell handle (there should be about 4–6 inches of space showing between your index fingers when you have assumed the correct grip). Stand erect. Extend your arms directly downward from your shoulders until they are straight. In the correct starting position, the barbell handle in your fists should be resting across your upper thighs.

Movement Performance—Keeping the weight close to your body and your elbows well above the level of your hands at all times, slowly pull the barbell directly up to a position where the backs of your hands are touching the underside of your chin. Rotate your shoulders back at this point and press your shoulder blades together, holding the top position for a slow count of two. Slowly lower the weight back along the same arc to the starting point.

Training Tips—You can also do this movement with a straight bar handle attached to the end of a cable running through a floor pulley, or with two moderately weighted dumbbells. Whatever the apparatus used, you must consciously resist torso swing forward and backward as you do the exercise.

SUGGESTED NECK ROUTINE

The type of routine you can perform 2–3 days per week for your neck depends on which exercise apparatus you have available. Try this one:

Exercise	Sets	Reps
Barbell Upright Rows, or . . .		
Cable Upright Rows, or . . .		
Dumbbell Upright Rows	3–4	8–10
Wrestler's Bridges, or . . .		
Neck Strap (four ways), or . . .		
Partner Neck Presses (four ways),		
or . . .		
Nautilus Four-Way Neck		
Movement	2–3	max.

Be sure that you do any of the last four exercises for the suggested sets and reps in each available direction.

23
Training
Thighs and Hips

It is absolutely essential for you to do plenty of heavy squats in your thigh workouts in order to develop the lower body to its maximum potential, and such heavy work is rather fatiguing and painful. As a result, it takes terrific dedication and training drive to build the thigh and hip girdle muscles to a championship level. Only the best bodybuilders are able to develop huge columns of ripped-to-shreds muscle in their legs, plus full, rounded buttock development.

There is a school of thought—largely discredited in recent years—that the hip and buttock muscles should not be fully exercised. This theory was championed by Vince Gironda, a famous gym owner in California. And to discourage performing squat exercises, which he feels will overdevelop the buttocks, Gironda does not have a squat rack in his gym. His charges are expected to develop fully their quads and hamstrings with hacks, leg extensions, and other leg exercises.

Can you imagine Sergio Oliva, Arnold Schwarzenegger, or Lee Haney without their fully developed buttocks? Certainly not! The obvious power in these men's physiques would be largely dissipated if they didn't have this superior development of a body part Vince Gironda shuns. As a result, I am a firm promoter of the full squat as one of bodybuilding's greatest exercises.

Styles have changed dramatically over the years in terms of quadriceps and hamstring development. During the 1940s and early 1950s, it was sufficiently advanced to merely have huge thighs, even though there was little detail to the muscular development. No real effort was devoted to proportional balance and symmetry within the muscle group. Steve Reeves hap-

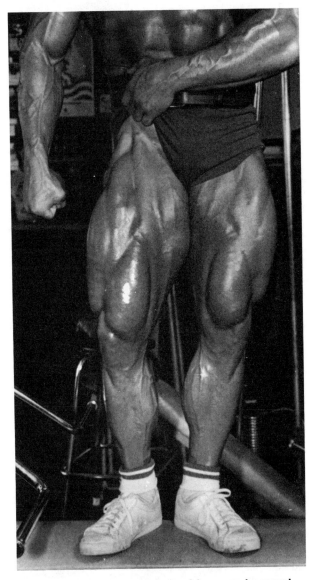

The standard against which quadriceps and general leg development is currently—and perhaps will always be—measured is the awesome development of Tom Platz, IFBB Mr. Universe. These massive, highly muscular legs were capable of doing 10 rock-bottom squats with 600 pounds before Tom turned his talents to acting.

pened to have full development and muscularity *par excellence* in the late 1940s and early 1950s, but that was more a matter of his natural genetics than anything calculated. Most of the other men of his era just had big, hammy thighs.

For about 15 years, beginning in the middle

1950s, thigh mass was tempered with attention to developing the lower aspects of the quadriceps, as well as the inner quadriceps and outer quad sweep. The result was a new type of proportional leg development—still lacking some of the sharp muscularity in vogue today—that superceded the older, carrot-shaped thighs of bodybuilders up to about 1955. One top bodybuilder who characterized this style of leg development was Bill Pearl (Mr. America, Mr. USA, and winner of four NABBA Mr. Universe titles).

Toward the end of the 1970s, bodybuilders like Arnold Schwarzenegger and Frank Zane, both winners of many Mr. Olympia titles, began to take thigh development into the stratosphere, adding the ultimate in deep cuts and even cross striations in the quads, as well as deep vertical rips along the length of the biceps femoris muscles at the backs of the thighs and along the sides of the thighs. After building optimum muscle mass and proportion, this was the only direction the great IFBB stars could take thigh development.

As everyone who has picked up a bodybuilding magazine or seen a bodybuilding competition will know, the ultimate in thigh development is currently embodied in the legs of Tom Platz, IFBB Mr. Universe. His thighs are hugely developed from top to bottom, with the ultimate degree of muscle mass in both quads and hamstrings. And when he is in top shape for a Mr. Olympia competition, Tom is so ripped up that you can almost hide a dime in the cross striations in his quads!

ANATOMY AND KINESIOLOGY

More than 200 muscles make up the lower body—the vast majority of them in the thighs, hips, and buttocks. It would be impossible to deal with every one of these often-small muscles, so I will restrict my discussion of leg and buttock development to the main muscle groups and functions of each one.

The thigh muscles are among the largest in the human body, and the main muscles are the *quadriceps* and *hamstrings* groups. The quads consist of four moderately large muscles that contract to straighten the leg completely from a fully or partially bent position. The primary

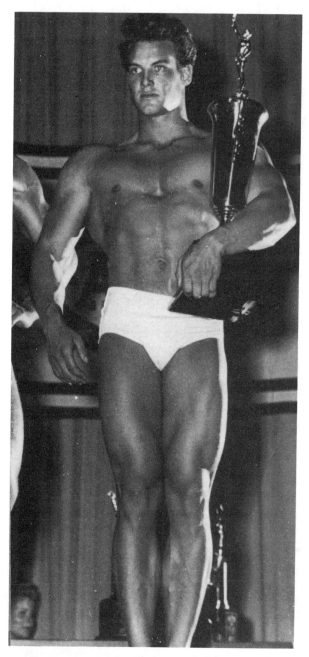

Taken on the occasion of his victory at the '47 Mr. America competition in Chicago, Steve Reeves displayed the type of leg development that led the world in the 1940s and early 1950s. We've come a long way, Baby!

muscle group at the back of the thigh is the *biceps femoris*, which is often called the leg biceps. The biceps femoris muscle complex contracts to bend the leg fully from a straight or partially bent position.

The primary muscle group of the buttocks is the *gluteus maximus*, which are called the glutes when you talk about both sides of the body. The gluteus maximus contracts to help straighten the line of legs and torso from a position in which the body is completely or partially flexed at the waist.

The leg adductors, primarily the *sartorius* muscles, help to pull your legs together toward each other from a position in which they are partially or completely spread apart. The sartorius muscle, incidentally, is the longest single muscle group in the human body. In contrast, the leg abductors, primarily the *gluteus minimus* at the sides of the hips, help you to spread your legs apart.

Up until the last few years, most bodybuilders used only squats (of various types), leg presses, leg extensions, lunges, and leg curls (of various types) to completely develop the thigh and hip muscles. But there are now many more exercises available that work many of the quadriceps muscles in relative isolation from the rest of the thigh muscles. There are now even a variety of machines with which you can work the leg adductors and abductors. Use of all of these new pieces of bodybuilding equipment on which you can train your leg muscles—plus many new training techniques and routines promoting maximum muscular definition—has resulted in the space-age development now displayed on the top amateur and professional bodybuilders.

TRAINING TIPS

Ed Kawak feels that the biggest key to ripping up the quadriceps is use of the Weider Iso-Tension Training Principle. Ed says, "Often bodybuilders can't bring out the deep cuts—let alone the myriad of striations along and across the various quadriceps muscles—because they don't have good control over posing their legs. As long as your body fat percentage is as low as it should be for a competition, you should be able to display ripped-up quads and hamstrings.

"The Iso-Tension Principle consists of many 'rep' flexes of each muscle group, holding the limbs in different positions. Simply flex the muscle group on which you are using iso-tension as completely as possible for 6–8 seconds, then relax for 8–10 seconds to partially rest the working muscle. When you are in a peaking cycle, you should work on iso-tension virtually

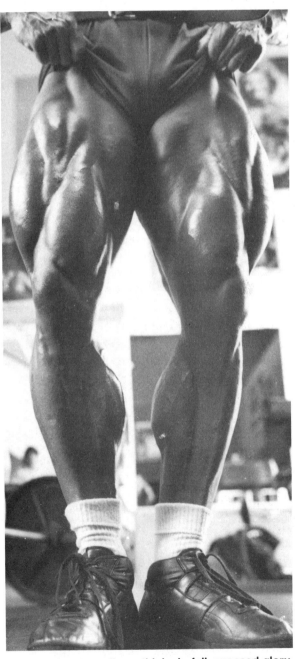

Tom Platz's extraordinary thighs in full, exposed glory.

every day, working up to 40–50 'rep' flexes on each body part.

"I believe that it is best to do iso-tension work in front of a mirror, usually at a time separated from your actual workout. But you will no doubt see many top bodybuilders doing these little muscle flicks in front of the mirror between sets of an actual workout."

"One of the keys to my own success in ripping up my thighs has been use of the Weider Peak Contraction and Slow, Continuous Tension Training Principles during precontest phases," says *Robby Robinson* (Mr. America, Mr. World, Mr. Universe). "Peak contraction consists of having a heavy weight on the working muscles when they are fully contracted. I feel that it also consists of holding the weight in this position for a few seconds to increase the peak contraction effect of the movement before returning to the starting point.

"As good as the squat is for developing all of the leg muscles, it does not provide a peak contraction effect to the leg and buttock muscles. As you can discern for yourself, you are actually supporting the bar on a continuous column of bone when you are standing erect with the barbell.

"On the other hand, leg curls and leg extensions allow you to keep contracting your quads and hamstrings when you have reached the finish point of either movement. This is why top bodybuilders do a lot more leg extensions close to a competition than during an off-season cycle.

"Continuous tension involves moving the weight very slowly over the full range of motion of an exercise while powerfully contracting the quads and hamstrings as you do the exercise. This way you can develop stronger and stronger contractions in your working muscles, which eventually leads to more muscle detail."

IS THE SQUAT A GOOD LEG EXERCISE?

In powerlifting terms, Dr. Squat, *Fred Hatfield*, is the greatest squatter ever to don a lifting belt. He has set world squat records in five weight classes and has officially squatted with more than 1,000 pounds in both the 242- and 275-

pound weight classes. And unbeknownst to most bodybuilders, Fred was a very respectable bodybuilder before turning to full-time powerlifting.

Dr. Squat says, "Squats are indeed important, even though a rare bodybuilder here and there can get along without doing them. Mohamed Makkawy doesn't do squats in his leg workouts, for example, and his legs are quite good. However, when you compare them with the legs of Tom Platz, who has done thousands of tons of squats over the years, you have to believe that there's really something valuable about squats. You certainly couldn't get Tom's thigh development without doing squat workouts. So I do think that squats are indispensable, despite the attitude of many other so-called experts.

"Here's why: squats allow the bodybuilder to maximize the intensity he places on his thighs. You get perfect isolation doing leg extensions and leg curls but you can't develop mass with these exercises. While extensions and leg curls give you fine cuts and muscle definition, you can't load up the kind of poundage your quads need for actual growth. You need muscle mass before you can carve in the striations with isolation exercises.

"Squats are great for the quads, providing that you do them properly. For a bodybuilder, I think the correct style would be to go down with the torso perpendicular to the floor. Let the knees extend out over the feet as far as possible. If you don't have ankle flexibility, place a block of wood under your heels. I suggest a shoulder-width-or-less stance. The toes should be pointed either straight forward or slightly outward. Your knees should go out *directly over your feet*, regardless of the angle of foot placement.

"The bar should remain high on the back. Make the movement hard on yourself, so you can get the most out of the intensity of squats. I'm dead set against wearing a belt or knee wraps. When you start hitting extremely heavy weights, I'd recommend a belt, but not until then. You want your muscle tissue to bear the intensity of the movement, not the supports of leather and fabric."

Dr. Squat doesn't feel there's any point in changing foot stance from one set to another. "There's a common tendon of insertion for three of the four quads. You can get a better stretch of the medial head, however, with a slightly wider stance when you squat. It's prestretched in this position, although I'm not entirely convinced that the prestretch offers sufficient stress to add to the differential development. Still, I don't believe in much of this because of the noncontiguous innervation problem.

"I've been doing squats longer than most men and I've never noticed any great change in thigh shape over the years, regardless of the type of squats I do. I do, however, believe that you have to do both isolation and intensity exercise to achieve maximum thigh development. If you have too much of one or the other, you won't get optimum results."

Fred gave his recommendations for how a bodybuilder should approach his squat workout: "When your objective is to do heavy squats in the range of 5–8 reps, you'll be able to handle 85%–95% of your max. This depends on your level of muscular endurance. If the objective is to do 5–8 repetitions, your major goal should be to increase strength, which then allows you to achieve better overload over the long term. Every bodybuilder's training cycle should have a period in which strength improvement is a primary objective. With increased strength, size will come.

"After an initial warm-up of three—at most four—lighter sets, you should be at your maximum poundage level. Just for the sake of argument, let's say that it's 85% of your maximum for eight reps. You do your eight reps with 85% and you can either stay there for a couple more sets, perhaps only seven the second set and six reps the third. But if your endurance is good, you might even be able to get to 90% for five reps. Then drop down in your weight for sets of eight, perhaps with slightly descending weights.

"Bodybuilders must also avoid getting carried away with doing ego-building single reps in the squat. For bodybuilders, I think five would be the lowest productive number of repetitions in a set. I can't think of a single instance where triples would be valuable, since they are only to prepare the nervous system for maximum efforts. And, of course, you have a much greater chance of getting injured when you do very heavy singles in your squat workouts."

A SUCCESS STORY

Hundreds of thousands of young bodybuilders fail to squat heavily, ending up with deficient leg development. Even hulking *Lou Ferrigno* suffered from this problem. But he was able to correct it. Here's how: "By the age of 18, I had been bodybuilding for a couple of years, and my upper body had become fairly massive. But my leg development, particularly my thighs, had not kept pace. I had made the classic mis-

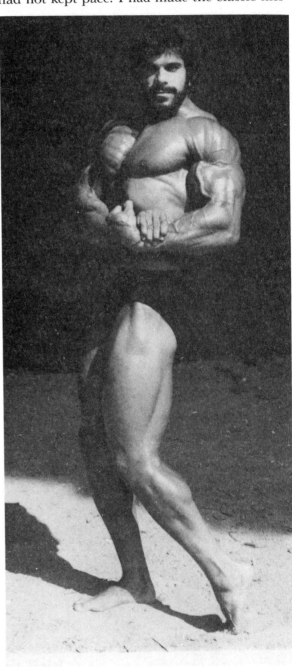

Had it not been for his television career, Lou Ferrigno feels confident he would have added a Mr. Olympia title to his vast collection of trophies.

take of training to build a showy upper body while neglecting my leg development.

"I realized that if I was to succeed as a bodybuilder, I'd need to bring my legs into balance with my upper body. I also knew it would be tough sledding to accomplish this transformation, because my upper body had exploded in growth. For example, my arms had increased from 17 to 20 inches in just a year and a half.

"During the summer and fall when I was 18, I embarked on a specialized program of heavy leg training. I worked my calves hard, and I squatted until I was blue in the face. As a result, my legs grew tremendously. Within a year they were perfectly proportioned to the rest of my body, and both my thighs and calves were ripped to shreds.

"Bodybuilding history has shown how effective my thigh specialization workouts actually were. Within three years I had won Teenage Mr. America, Mr. America, Mr. International, and Mr. Universe, plus I placed second to Arnold Schwarzenegger in the Mr. Olympia competition. Had I not chosen to forego my competitive bodybuilding career to become television's 'Incredible Hulk,' I'm confident I could have won the Mr. Olympia title while still in my middle 20s."

In order to bring up his legs, Lou used one of the Weider Training Principles most relevant to specialized training of a weak body part, the Weider Muscle Priority Training Principle. With this principle, you train the weak body part first in your routine when you have optimum mental and physical energies to devote to all-out high-intensity bombing and blitzing. In extreme cases, you can use the Muscle Priority Principle by working a single large muscle group by itself one day with specialized effort, then come back the next day and train the remainder of your body.

Lou's thigh development lagged far behind his upper body, so he decided to priority train his legs twice per week, then split up the balance of his body for four other weekly workouts, two for each remaining half. Here is an example of how Lou Ferrigno split up his routine to give priority to his lagging thighs and calves: on Mondays and Thursdays he trained his thighs; on Tuesdays and Fridays, his chest, back, calves, and abs; and on Wednesdays and Saturdays, his shoulders, arms, and forearms.

Note how Lou would do only an all-out, thigh-bombing session on the one workout day. And he did two very heavy calf sessions each week separate from the thigh-training session. If your own legs are weak, you can use Lou's suggestions for bringing them up to the level of the rest of your body parts.

Platz's Thigh-Building Secrets

Without a doubt, Tom Platz possesses the most superior thigh development in the history of bodybuilding: "But you probably wouldn't believe how thin my thighs were when I first started working them," he confesses. "Like so many beginning bodybuilders, I got carried away with training my showy arm, chest, back, and shoulder muscles, totally neglecting my legs. It's a common beginner's mistake.

"I finally got into leg training because there were a lot of powerlifters in the gym where I trained in Detroit at the time. If I didn't squat hard, they wouldn't let me walk out of the gym. And when I squatted hard, I'd have trouble walking out of the gym anyway, so I was getting hit coming and going.

"They really made me work. I made progress quickly as a result, which got everyone going on my case even harder. I very quickly worked up to 10–12 sets of squats, using a light weight and working up to the heaviest possible set of five reps one workout day and one rep the next. I also began doing hack squats. Early on, I found that fatigue from doing leg extensions tended to keep my squat poundages down. Eventually, I started to throw in a few sets of leg curls at the end of my routine.

"From day one, I had good leg workouts, and in fact I have never really had a bad one. Today I can do one set of squats and my thighs blow up like balloons. This is because I am immediately able to make a strong link between my mind and my thighs, a requisite for good workouts for any muscle group. It took 3–4 years to develop this ability for my arm workouts, but from the first training session I could feel the link with my legs.

"The heavy work in thigh training has always been enjoyable to me. It reminds me of football practice when I was in high school. I leave the gym with the inner satisfaction that I've given 100%. I like the feeling of handling enormous poundages, hearing the deep rattle of five or six 45-pound plates on each end of the bar as I squat.

"In competition, I lifted 600 pounds in the squat at 198 pounds body weight. For reps I've done 28 with 405 pounds and 52 with 350. Prior to the 1977 Mr. American competition, I was also doing 10 straight minutes of squatting with 225 pounds, which must have been over 100 reps every workout!"

Tom believes the squat will put muscle on anyone's thighs. "However," he says, "the amazing thing to me is that most bodybuilders don't squat correctly. It's a very basic exercise, but usually the feet are too far apart, the squat depth is too shallow, and they lean too far forward.

"To begin with, I place the bar high on my traps, holding it about halfway between the plates and my shoulders in order to balance it correctly for my set. My feet are set slightly more narrow than shoulder width, toes pointed slightly outward. (I'm experimenting with putting my heels close together, which has had an excellent effect on my thigh shape, but let's get the basics down cold, first.) I keep my head up when squatting, which keeps my back straight and upright.

"I take a deep breath and sink slowly all of the way down, allowing my knees to travel directly out over my toes. I don't bounce in the bottom position because it would probably cause an injury, and I keep my back and torso muscles tensed throughout the movement. Then I come back up to the starting position, being careful not to lean forward.

"After a good set of squats, I'm breathless and have difficulty walking. There's an overwhelming desire to sit down, but I fight it. Instead, I walk around the gym to recover more quickly for the next set."

THIG, HIP, AND BUTTOCK EXERCISES
Squats

Emphasis—This is the most basic of all leg exercises, and possibly the single best bodybuilding movement in existence. The heavy work involved in squatting can actually turn your metabolism anabolic, allowing you to gain muscle mass in your upper body as well as in your legs. When you do squats, primary stress is placed on the quadriceps, buttocks, and lower-back muscles. Significant secondary stress is also placed on the middle- and upper-back muscles, hamstrings, abdominals, and other upper-body muscle groups.

Starting Position—Place a barbell on a squat rack and load it up with a sufficient poundage for a heavy set of squats. Duck under the bar and position it across your shoulders with your trapezius muscles contracted to act as padding.

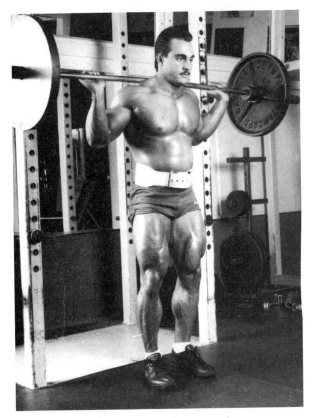

Squat (start)

Photographs taken by Greg Aiken at Gold's Gym, Venice, California.   Model: Shane DiMora

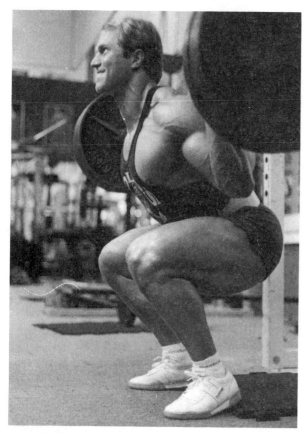

Squat (finish—at parallel-thighs position)

Model: Gary Strydom

The bar should be at about the level of your shoulders, and you can pad it with a towel if you feel that it is cutting into your spine too sharply. Grasp the bar out near the plates on each side to balance it in position. Set your feet about shoulder width apart and straighten your legs to lift the bar from the rack. Step one pace back from the rack, keeping your feet about shoulder width apart, your toes angled slightly outward. Your spinal erectors, abdominals, and upper-back muscles should be tensed throughout your set. Focus your eyes on a point at eye level on the wall in front of you in an effort to keep your torso upright as you do your squats. Your spine should be either straight or slightly arched throughout your set.

Movement Performance—Keeping your torso upright, slowly bend your legs and sink down into a full squatting position, your knees traveling forward and out over your toes as you sink downward. Without bouncing in the bottom position, slowly reverse the movement and return to the upright starting position.

Training Tips—You should wear a weightlifting belt tightly cinched around your waist when doing heavy squats. And if your knees have been injured in the past, it is also a good idea to wear neoprene rubber and/or fabric wraps around your knees to protect them from further injury. If your ankles are inflexible, you won't be able to do full squats with your feet flat on the floor. In such a case, you should squat with your heels resting on a 2 × 4-inch block of wood or on two thick barbell plates.

Partial Squats

Notes—There are several types of partial squats that you can use to stress your quads and buttocks with somewhat heavier weights than is possible when doing full squats. You can do quarter squats (squatting down only a quarter of the way toward a full squat), half squats, three-quarter squats, and parallel squats (sinking downward until your thighs are parallel with the floor, as in the type of squat powerlifters do in competition). You can also do bench squats by straddling a flat exercise bench and squatting down until your buttocks lightly touch the bench before returning to the starting point. On all forms of squats—and particularly when doing partial squats—you should have a spotter standing behind you, or two

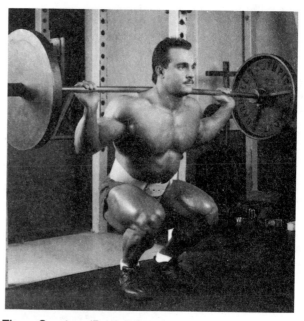

Three-Quarters (Partial) Squat

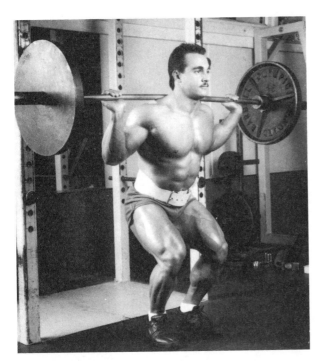

Half (Partial) Squat

Jumping Squats

Emphasis—When you do jumping squats, you work the same muscles as normal squats, plus the gastrocnemius muscles of your lower legs.

Starting Position—Place a light barbell on a squat rack, step under it, and lift it off the rack. Step back and assume the correct starting position for a squat, except that you cannot elevate your heels when doing jumping squats.

Movement Performance—Keeping your torso as upright as possible, slowly sink down into a full squatting position. Without bouncing in the bottom position (which will sooner or later injure your knees), reverse the movement and begin to slowly come erect. As you reach the halfway point back up to the erect starting position, accelerate your upward momentum and actually spring into the air as high as

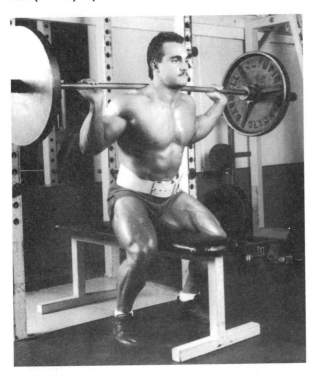

Bench Squat

spotters at each end of the bar to rescue you in case you fail to complete a repetition or get the bar a bit out of the correct groove when doing squats. When you have a single spotter to help you come erect with a difficult rep, he can hug the middle of your torso from behind to pull you erect.

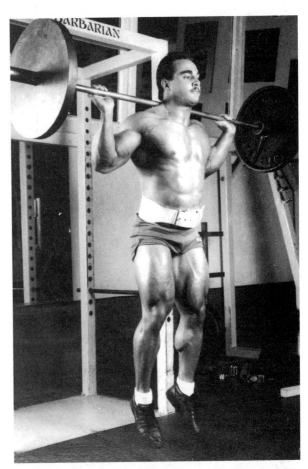

Jumping Squat (finish). Do not use as heavy a weight as depicted here until you've had practice with lighter weights.

possible. Bend your legs slightly to absorb the shock of landing back on the floor.

Training Tips—For more of a calf-building effect, you can do your jumping squats sinking only about halfway downward before springing out of the squatting stance. Jumping squats are one of the best movements for athletes who require quickness and power for participation in their sport.

Dumbbell Squats

Emphasis—As with normal full barbell squats, this movement places intense stress on the quadriceps, buttocks, and upper-back muscles. While there is intense stress on the forearm flexors, there is proportionately less stress on the lower-back muscles when you do the movement holding a pair of heavy dumbbells in your hands.

Starting Position—Stand between a pair of heavy dumbbells and reach down to grasp them. Stand erect with your arms hanging

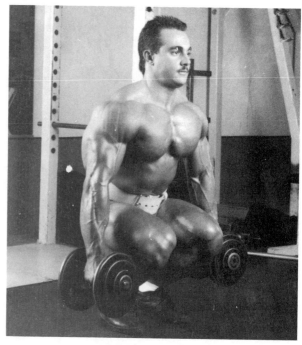

Dumbbell Squats (finish)

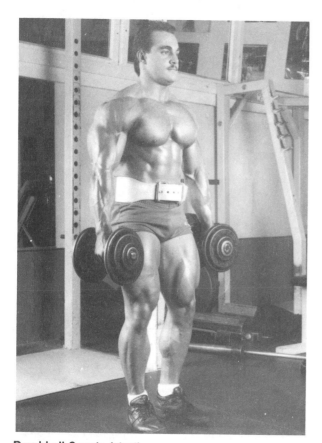

Dumbbell Squats (start)

down at your sides and your wrists rotated so your palms are facing inward, toward your legs. Position your feet about shoulder width apart, your toes angled slightly outward. (You can elevate your heels if you feel that your ankles are too inflexible to allow a comfortable full squat.) Focus your eyes on a point at eye level on the wall in front of you, and tense both your back and abdominal muscles in an effort to keep your torso upright as you do this movement.

Movement Performance—Keeping your torso erect, slowly sink down into a full squatting position. Without bouncing in the bottom position, reverse the movement and slowly straighten your legs until you are again standing erect.

Training Tips—You can also do jumping squats with two dumbbells rather than a barbell. And you can hold the dumbbells behind your buttocks, which makes this movement similar to a barbell hack squat.

Jefferson Squats

Emphasis—The "Jefferson lift" was a way of proving basic body strength back in the early days of bodybuilding. Today it can be an excellent leg exercise that places primary stress on the quads and glutes without undue stress on the lower back. Secondary emphasis is on the traps, delts, and forearm flexors.

Starting Position—Stand straddling a heavy barbell with your feet set about shoulder width apart and toes angled slightly outward. Bend your legs sufficiently so you can grasp the bar with your hands set about shoulder width apart, both hands facing inward toward the midline of your body. Keeping your arms straight throughout the movement, slowly stand erect.

Movement Performance—Slowly bend your legs as fully as possible (downward until the weight again lightly touches the floor) and then return to the starting point.

Training Tips—If you want a longer range of motion of this exercise, you can do it while standing on a thick block of wood or a barbell plate.

Front Squats

Emphasis—Front squats place primary emphasis on the quadriceps (particularly down close to the knee), buttocks, and the lower- and upper-back muscles. Secondary stress is on the hamstrings and abdominals.

Starting Position—Place a moderately heavy barbell on a squat rack. (You will be able to front squat with only about 60% of the weight you can use for back squats.) Step up to the bar and position it across your deltoids at the base of your neck. With your upper arms held parallel with the floor, cross your arms over the weight. As long as you keep your elbows up as you do this movement, the bar will be sure at your shoulders. Lift the bar off the rack, step back a few feet, and set your feet about shoulder width apart, toes angled slightly outward. Tense all of your back and midsection muscles and keep them tensed throughout your set. Focus your eyes high on the wall in front of you in order to keep your head up and back straight as you do front squats.

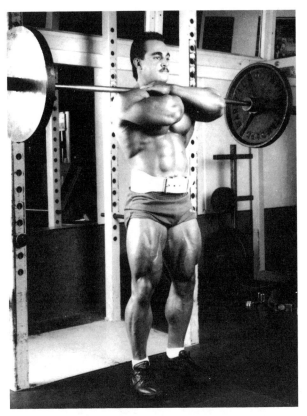

Front Squat (start—note: arms crossed and elbows held high throughout movement to keep bar comfortably in position)

Movement Performance—Keeping your torso upright, slowly sink down into a full squatting position. Without bouncing in the bottom position of the movement, reverse directions and slowly straighten your legs to return to the starting point.

Training Tips—If you find it difficult to hold the weight at your shoulders with your arms crossed, you can hold it with your hands gripping the handle slightly outside of your shoulders, as you would when doing standing barbell presses. As long as you keep your elbows up when doing front squats, this variation of grip on the bar will work well for you. Regardless of the grip used, you will probably need to wear a weightlifting belt as you do front squats.

Barbell Hack Squats

Emphasis—With the advent of various types of hack machines over the past decade, barbell hack squats have lost favor. Still, there are a few bodybuilders who still do them, including su-

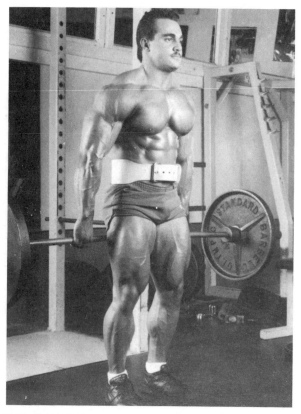

Barbell Hack Squat (start)

Training Tips—The more you lean back as you do barbell hack squats, the more you can isolate stress on the lower quadriceps.

Machine Hack Squats

Emphasis—If you have carrot-shaped thighs, this is the best movement for correcting the condition. Hack squats performed on a machine place intense stress on the quadriceps muscles, particularly the lower and outer sections of the muscle complex.

Yoke-Type Machine Starting Position—Position your shoulders beneath the yokes attached to the machine. Place your feet close together on the foot platform, toes angled outward at approximate 45-degree angles. Straighten your legs to bear the weight of the machine. Rotate the stop bars up near your shoulders to release the carriage slide.

Platform-Type Machine Starting Position—Bend your legs enough so you can rest your back against the padded surface of the carriage

per-massive Bertil Fox. Barbell hacks place intense stress on the quadriceps while involving the lower back and buttocks proportionately less intensely. The movement places primary stress on the lower and outer sections of the quadriceps muscle complex.

Starting Position—Step up to a barbell lying on the gym floor and turn your back toward the bar. With your feet set about shoulder width apart, reach down and take an overgrip on the bar with your hands set slightly wider than your shoulders on each side. Stand erect with the weight resting at straight arms' length behind your upper thighs. Keep the bar pressed against your buttocks in this position and your torso erect as you do your set.

Movement Performance—Slowly bend your legs and sink down as deeply as possible in a squatting position. Without bouncing in the bottom position, reverse the movement and return to the starting point by straightening your legs.

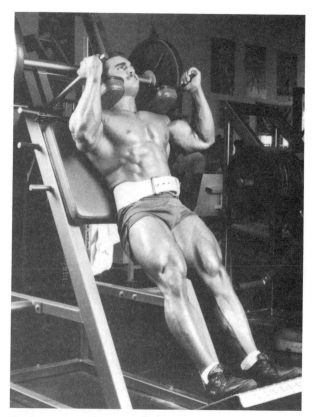

Machine Hack Squat (start)

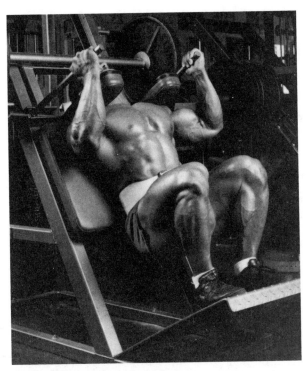

Machine Hack Squat (finish)

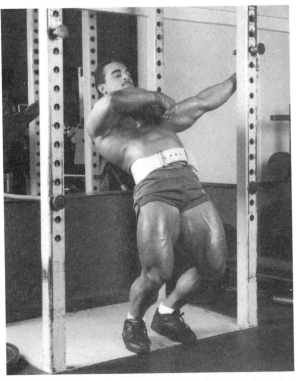

Sissy Squats (midpoint—note how loose barbell plate is held on chest for added resistance, while free hand grasps upright for balance)

slide and rest your feet close together on the foot platform, toes angled outward at approximate 45-degree angles. Grasp the handles down near your hips on each side. Straighten your legs to bear the weight of the machine.

Movement Performance—Keeping your feet flat on the platform of each machine, slowly bend your legs as completely as possible. Without bouncing in the bottom position, reverse the movement and return to the starting point.

Training Tips—Tom Platz does a very effective quadriceps movement on this type of machine. It is very much like a sissy squat. It starts in the standard position and continues that way until you reach the bottom position of the movement. But as Tom does it, the hips are shifted forward and the knees thrust as far forward as possible while rising up on the toes to finish the repetition. On all types of machine hack squats, you can experiment with different widths of foot placement and various toe angles.

Sissy Squats

Emphasis—Sissy squats isolate stress on the quadriceps muscles at the front of each thigh.

This is the premier movement for etching deep cuts between and across the quads when peaking for a competition.

Starting Position—While you can do this movement while holding on to a single sturdy upright with one hand, it is best learned while standing between the dipping bars in your gym. Place your feet 8–10 inches apart, your toes pointed directly forward. Reach up and grasp the bars with your hands in order to balance your body as you do the movement. Avoid pulling up with your hands, however.

Movement Performance—Inclining your torso backward, slowly bend your legs while thrusting your knees as far forward as possible during the movement. You will find that you need to go up on your toes in order to completely bend your legs in the bottom position of the movement. As you bend your legs, you should progressively increase the backward lean of your torso, until it is only a bit above a position parallel to the floor when you reach the bottom point of the movement. Reverse the movement to return to the starting point.

Training Tips—For a really great quadriceps superset, try doing leg presses followed immediately by sissy squats. If you find that you need to add weight to your sissies, you should hold a barbell plate of appropriate weight against your chest with your free hand as you execute the movement.

Leg Presses

Emphasis—All variations of leg presses place intense stress on the quadriceps and buttocks, lesser stress on the hamstrings.

Vertical Machine Starting Point—Adjust the angled pad beneath the machine so you can lie on it with your hips at the upper end of the pad and your hips directly below the movement carriage. Set your feet about shoulder width apart on the foot plate, toes angled slightly outward. Place your hands on the stop bars at the sides of the machine. Straighten your legs and rotate the stop bars to free the carriage for your set.

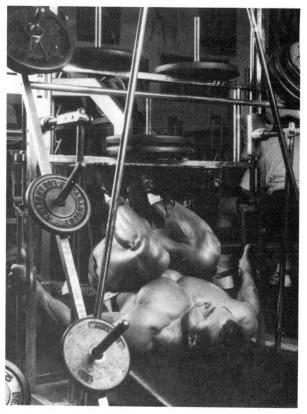

Vertical Leg Press (finish)

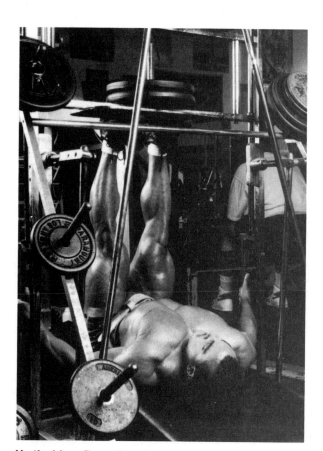

Vertical Leg Press (start)

Angled Machine Starting Position—Sit in the machine with your buttocks in the corner where the back and seat pads meet. Lie back against the angled back pad. Place your feet about shoulder width apart on the foot plate attached to the carriage, toes angled slightly outward. Straighten your legs and rotate the stop bars at the sides of your hips to release the carriage for your set.

Nautilus Machine Starting Position—Adjust the seatback forward far enough so your legs are almost completely bent in the bottom position of the movement. This adjustment can be made with an adjustment handle at the right side of the seat. Sit down and fasten the seat belt around your waist. Set your feet in the middle of the pedals in front of yourself, toes angled slightly outward, and grasp the handles at the sides of the seat to steady your body in position as you do the movement. Extend your legs until they are completely straight.

Universal Gym Machine Starting Position—Adjust the seatback forward far enough so your legs are almost completely bent in the bottom

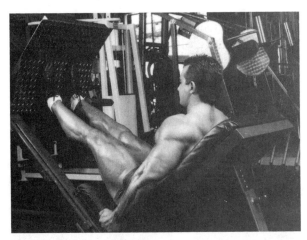

Angled Leg Press (start)

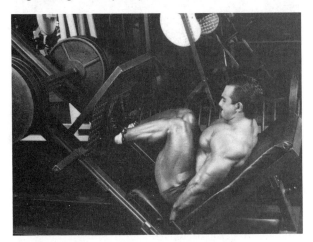

Angled Leg Press (finish)

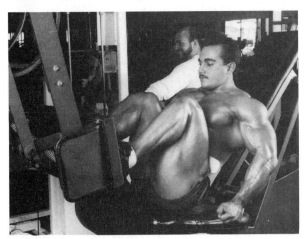

Nautilus Leg Press (midpoint)

Movement Performance—Slowly bend your legs as completely as possible while being sure that your knees travel out to the sides of your chest. Without bouncing in the bottom position of the movement, reverse direction and press the weight out until your legs are again straight.

Training Tips—On Universal leg presses, you can also use the upper set of pedals when using very heavy weights. However, you will get a better quality of movement when you stick to using the bottom pedals of the leg press machine.

Barbell Lunges

Emphasis—As you undoubtedly know, you alternate forward legs when doing lunges. On the front leg, stress is on the buttocks and quadriceps down near the knee; back-leg emphasis is on stretching the upper quadriceps and hip flexors. Most of the top guys use this movement to bring out muscle separation in the upper quads and hip flexors.

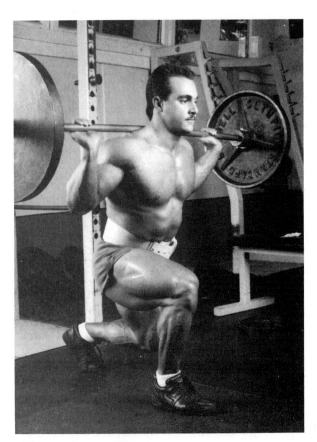

Barbell Lunges (midpoint)

position of the movement. This adjustment can be made with a pin at the front end of the seat. Sit down and grasp the handles at the sides of the seat to restrain your body as you do the movement. Set your feet in the middle of the lower set of pedals, toes angled slightly outward. Extend your legs until they are straight.

Starting Position—Lift a light barbell up to a position across your shoulders behind your neck, balancing it there by grasping the barbell bar out near the plates on each side. Stand erect with your feet about 8-10 inches apart, toes pointed directly forward.

Movement Performance—Step forward 2-2½ feet with your left foot. Then while keeping your right leg relatively straight, bend your left leg as fully as possible. In the bottom position, your right knee should be 2-4 inches above the floor, and your left knee should be 3-5 inches in front of your left ankle. Forcefully straighten your left leg to push yourself back to the starting position with your feet on the same plane 8-10 inches apart. Do the next rep with your right foot forward.

Training Tips—For a different effect, try lunging forward with your front foot up on a thick block of wood rather than merely set on the floor. When doing such a variation, you simply step onto the block with your forward foot each repetition. You'll find that this variation puts more stress on the buttock muscle and upper-hamstring muscle of your forward leg.

Dumbbell Lunges

Emphasis—As with barbell lunges, the front leg has stress on the buttocks and quadriceps down near the knee, while the rear leg feels stress as a stretch of the upper thigh and hip flexor muscles.

Starting Position—Grasp two moderately heavy dumbbells and stand erect with the weights hanging at straight arms' length at your sides. Your feet should be set about 8-10 inches apart, your toes angled straight forward.

Movement Performance—Step directly forward 2-2½ feet with your left foot. Then while keeping your right leg relatively straight, bend your left leg as fully as possible. In the bottom position, your right knee should be 2-4 inches above the floor, and your left knee should be 3-5 inches in front of your left ankle. Forcefully straighten your left leg to push yourself back to

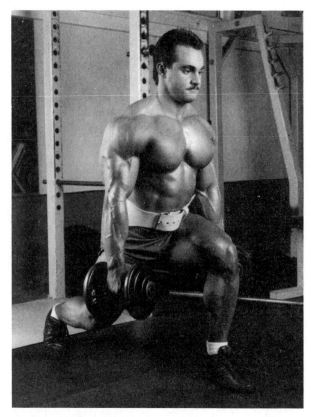

Dumbbell Lunges (midpoint)

the starting position with your feet on the same plane 8-10 inches apart. Do the next rep with your right foot forward.

Training Tips—As with barbell lunges, you can step onto a thick block of wood with your forward foot on each repetition. You'll find that this variation puts more stress on the buttock muscle and upper-hamstring muscle of your forward leg.

Leg Extensions

Emphasis—This is the best quadriceps isolation movement, and it is used by most bodybuilders primarily to rip up the front thigh muscles. The entire quadriceps muscle mass is stressed in isolation from the rest of the body.

Starting Position—There is a wide variety of leg extension machines, but the movement performance is almost identical on each apparatus. Sit in the machine with the backs of your knees against the edge of the padded surface of the machine toward the lever arm. Slip your

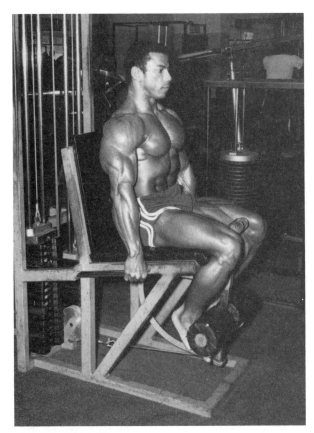

Leg Extension (start)

Model: Chris Dickerson

in a semicircular arc to a position in which your legs are straight. Hold this peak-contracted position for a moment before slowly returning your feet back along the same arc to the starting point.

Training Tips—Normally, you will do leg extensions with your toes pointing directly forward, but for a different quadriceps effect, you can angle your toes either inward or outward at approximately 45-degree angles. You can also perform leg extensions with one leg at a time, which automatically increases training intensity on your quadriceps.

Lying Leg Curls

Emphasis—Variations of leg curls, this one included, allow you to isolate stress on the biceps femoris muscles at the back of your thighs.

toes and insteps under the lower set of roller pads (if there are two sets). With your legs bent at a 90-degree angle or greater, grasp the handles provided beside your hips or the edges of the padded surface to brace your body in position for the movement.

Movement Performance—Use quadriceps strength to move your feet forward and upward

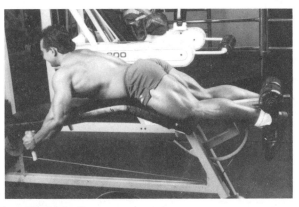

Leg Curl (start)

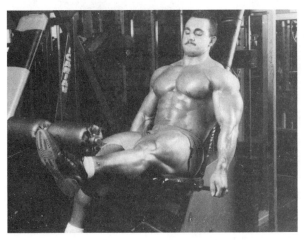

Leg Extension (finish—one-legged variation)

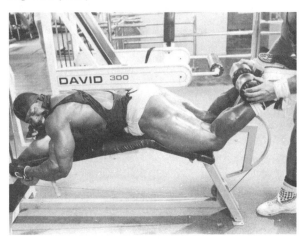

Leg Curl (midpoint)

Model: Mike Christian

Starting Position—Many gym equipment companies sell leg curl machines, but performance is very similar on each type of apparatus. Lie facedown on the padded surface of the machine, your knees at the edge of the pad toward the machine lever arm. Hook your heels under the upper set of roller pads (if there are two sets) and straighten your legs. Grasp either the handles provided on each side of the head end of the pad, or the edges of the pad itself to steady your torso in position on the machine as you do the movement. As you perform your lying leg curls, be sure that you don't allow your hips to come up off the surface of the machine.

Movement Performance—Use leg biceps strength to curl your feet upward in a semicircular arc until your legs are as fully bent as possible. Hold this peak-contracted position for a moment, then lower back to the starting point.

Training Tips—Normally, you will do leg curls with your toes pointing directly forward, but for a different hamstrings effect, you can angle your toes either inward or outward at a 45-degree angle. You can also perform leg curls with one leg at a time, which automatically increases training intensity. For a unique peak-contraction effect in your hamstrings, try doing the entire movement with your shoulders held up off the padded surface of the machine. You can best accomplish this by resting the weight of your upper body on your elbows.

Seated Leg Curls

Emphasis—The machine which allows this movement is relatively new, but it still effectively isolates stress on the hamstrings. Compared to lying leg curls, which seem to work the lower section of the biceps femoris muscle complex, seated leg curls tend to place the greatest amount of stress on the upper quads, where they attach to a point beneath the buttocks.

Starting Position—The roller pad on the level arm can be adjusted forward or backward on the lever arm so it matches the length of your legs. Sit in the machine and rest your heels over the roller pad, your legs straight. By pulling out a pin and resetting it, you can pull the leg restraint down to press against your upper thighs. You can occupy your hands by grasping the thigh restraint pad.

Movement Performance—Moving only your lower legs, contract your leg biceps muscles to move the roller pad downward in a semicircular arc to a position in which your legs are as fully bent as possible. Hold this peak-contracted position for a moment, then allow the roller pad to return back along the same arc to the starting point with your legs straight.

Training Tips—The exercise can be done with one leg at a time. Or you can vary the angle of your feet to stress different sections of your biceps femoris muscles.

Standing Leg Curls

Emphasis—This is also a relatively new movement, although one which has been rescued

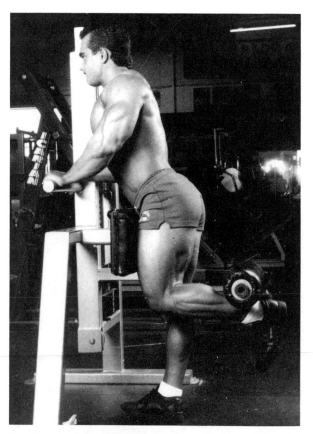

Standing Leg Curl (finish)

from the darker days of the sport when it was done with an iron boot attached to the foot. Using one leg at a time, you can isolate stress to the biceps femoris muscle of each leg.

Starting Position—Stand facing toward the machine and hook your right heel under the roller pad. Your right knee should be pressed against the restraint pad in front of it. Straighten your leg and grasp the machine to restrain your upper body as you do the movement.

Movement Performance—Use leg biceps strength to curl the roller pad up to a position in which your leg is as fully bent as possible. Hold this peak-contracted position for a moment, then return to the starting point.

Training Tips—Try angling your toes differently to allow various effects on your hamstrings.

Nautilus Hip And Back Machine

Emphasis—This machine movement places intense stress on the buttocks and erector spinae, secondary stress on the upper hamstrings.

Starting Position—Lie on your back on the padded surface of the machine, your hips toward the lever arms. Grasp the handles at the sides of your hips, curl your legs up over your chest (being sure that your lower legs go over the roller pads), and use your hands to pull against the handle and move your hips as far forward as possible in the direction your hips are facing. This should compress your knees against your chest. The backs of your knees should be against the roller pads. Once you have achieved this position, fasten the lap belt over your hips to restrain your torso in position as you do the movement. Arch your back and keep it arched as you do your entire set. Finally, push down with your knees and straighten your legs, so your legs are relatively straight and parallel with the floor.

Movement Performance—Keeping your right leg motionless, allow the weight of the machine to pull your right knee upward and toward

your chest in a semicircular arc. When your left knee has lightly touched your chest, push down with your left leg to return to the starting position. Repeat the movement with your right leg moving and left leg held stationary.

Training Tips—You will probably find this movement best for rounding your buttocks, so if you don't have a hip and back machine available, you need not worry. You can still build rounded glutes doing full squats with a barbell.

Cable Back Kick

Emphasis—This unique cable movement primarily stresses the buttocks and upper hamstrings, with secondary emphasis on the spinal erectors.

Starting Position—Attach an ankle cuff to the end of a cable running through a floor pulley. Fasten the cuff around your right ankle. You should stand on a block of wood (which allows

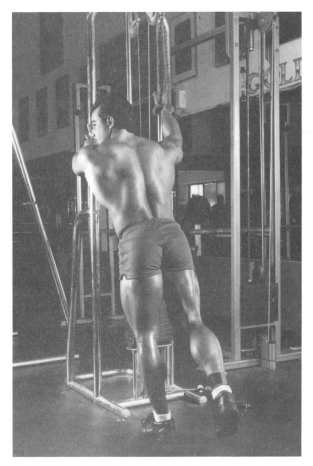

Cable Kick Back (finish)

you to swing your leg freely without your foot bumping on the floor) about 2½-3 feet back from the pulley, facing the machine weight stack. Grasp a sturdy upright or two to restrain your upper body as you do your back kicks. Hold both legs relatively straight as you do the movement. Allow the weight at the end of the cable to pull your right foot forward as far toward the pulley as comfortably possible.

Movement Performance—Use buttocks strength to move your foot in a semicircular arc from the starting point to the rear and upward as high as comfortably possible. Hold this peak-contracted position for a moment, then slowly return your foot back along the same arc to the starting point. Be sure to do the same number of sets and reps for each leg.

Training Tips—This exercise can be used to specialize on buttocks development, or to finish off your leg and hip development for a competition.

Cable Front Kick

Emphasis—This interesting cable movement places direct stress on the upper quadriceps and hip flexors. Strong secondary stress is on the rectus abdominis muscle complex, particularly the lower section of that muscle wall.

Starting Position—Attach an ankle cuff to the end of a cable running through a floor pulley. Fasten the cuff around your right ankle. You should stand on a block of wood (which allows you to swing your leg freely without your foot bumping on the floor) about 2½-3 feet back from the pulley, facing away from the weight stack. Grasp a sturdy upright or two to restrain your upper body as you do the movement. Allow the weight at the end of the cable to pull your right foot to the rear as far toward the pulley as comfortably possible. Hold both legs relatively straight as you do your set.

Movement Performance—Use quadriceps and hip flexor strength to move your foot forward and upward in a semicircular arc from the starting point to as high a position in front of your body as possible. Hold this peak-con-

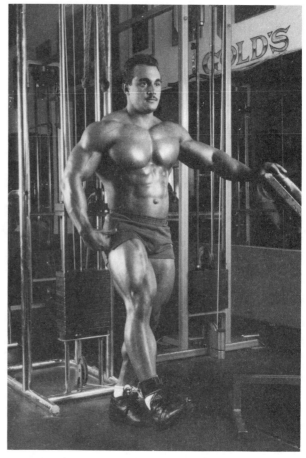

Cable Front Kick (finish)

tracted position for a moment, then lower your leg back along the same arc to the starting point. Be sure to do the same number of sets and reps for each leg.

Training Tips—As with cable front kicks, this is primarily a movement to finish off your leg and hip flexor development for a competition. In point of fact, it is a favorite exercise of Gary Strydom (National Champion) for precisely this purpose.

Cable Adduction

Emphasis—Another unique movement, cable adductions intensely stress the adductor muscles of the legs and hips, most prominently the sartorius.

Starting Position—Attach an ankle cuff to the end of a cable running through a floor pulley and fasten the cuff around your right ankle. You should stand on a block of wood (which allows you to swing your leg freely without your foot bumping on the floor) about 2½–3 feet back from the pulley, your right side facing the weight stack. (To do your left leg, position your left side to face the stack.) Grasp a sturdy upright or two to restrain your upper body as you do the movement. Allow the weight at the end of the cable to pull your right leg away from the midline of your body and as far toward the pulley as comfortably possible. Hold both legs relatively straight as you do your set.

Movement Performance—Pull your right leg toward and then across the midline of your body as far as you can. Hold this peak-contracted position for a moment, then return your leg to the starting position. Be sure to do an equal number of sets and reps with each leg.

Training Tips—This movement is primarily performed by women bodybuilders, but it's one which should be done by more men. It results in very impressive inner thigh development.

Cable Abductions

Emphasis—The final unique cable movement in your leg training arsenal, cable abductions intensely stress the abductor muscles of the thighs and hips.

Starting Position—Attach an ankle cuff to the end of a cable running through a floor pulley, then fasten the cuff around your right ankle. You should stand on a block of wood (which allows you to swing your leg freely without your foot bumping into the floor) about 2½–3 feet back from the pulley, your left side facing the weight stack. (To do your left leg reps, position your right side toward the stack.) Grasp a sturdy upright or two to restrain your upper body as you do the movement. Allow the weight at the end of the cable to pull your right leg across the front of your body and as far toward the pulley as comfortably possible. Hold both legs relatively straight as you do your set.

Movement Performance—Pull your right leg across your body and out to the side to as high a position as comfortably possible. Hold this

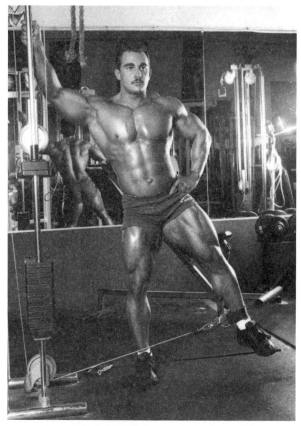

Cable Abduction (finish)

peak-contracted position for a moment, then return your leg to the starting position. Be certain to perform an equal number of sets and reps with each leg.

Training Tips—As with cable adductions, this movement has long been known as a women's exercise, but it's an excellent one for male bodybuilders as well.

Nautilus Adductions/Abductions

Emphasis—Depending on the direction toward which you exert against the weight, you work either the adductor or abductor muscles of the legs and hips.

Starting Position—A lever at the side of the machine allows you to select whether you wish to do adductions or abductions. There are also two movable pads attached to the leg restraints which must be shifted for either adduction or abduction. Sit in the seat and run your legs out the lever arms of the machine. Fasten the seat

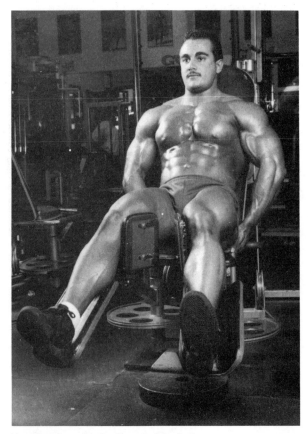

Nautilus Leg Abduction (midpoint)

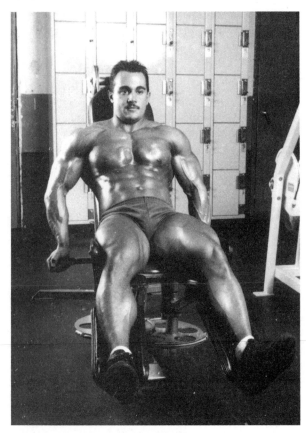

Nautilus Leg Abduction (midpoint)

belt across your lap and grasp the handles at the sides of your seat.

Movement Performance—Depending on how you have set the machine, you can either force your legs together from a spread position (adductions), or force them apart from a position where they start out together (abductions). Be sure to move the lever arms over an exaggerated range of motion, and resist the weight as you lower it slowly back to the starting point on each repetition.

Training Tips—Up until 1984 or 1985, there probably weren't 20 bodybuilders who used this movement with any regularity. But now there are so many bodybuilders including it in their leg routines that it is difficult to count them.

SUGGESTED LEG ROUTINES

If you attempted to perform one of the routines of the champs with which I conclude this chapter without first building up a champion's energy reserves and recovery ability, you would undoubtedly overtrain or injure yourself. Therefore, I have included several beginning- and intermediate-level routines which you can perform in an effort to build up your energy reserves and recovery ability. By using each routine for 6–8 weeks, you can gradually build yourself up to the point where you can profit from the routines of the champions themselves. (Note: Exercises marked with an asterisk are pyramided, the weight increased and repetitions decreased with each succeeding set.)

BEGINNING-LEVEL ROUTINE

Exercise	Sets	Reps
Squats	4	12–6*
Lying Leg Curls	2–3	8–12

INTERMEDIATE-LEVEL ROUTINE

Exercise	Sets	Reps
Angled Leg Presses	5	12–5*
Leg Extensions	3	8–12
Seated Leg Curls	3–4	8–12

LOW-ADVANCED-LEVEL ROUTINE

Exercise	Sets	Reps
Leg Extensions	3-4	8-12
Squats	5	12-5*
Standing Leg Curls	3	8-12
Stiff-Legged Deadlifts	2-3	10-15

LEG ROUTINES OF THE CHAMPIONS

In this concluding section to my Master Blaster leg and hip training chapter, I will give you more than 20 thigh routines of the top IFBB bodybuilders. Be sure that you use them primarily as examples of how you should organize your own leg workouts, since your object at this point should be to boil down the routines and training methods of all of the champions into a formula which works for your own unique physique.

Tom Platz

Exercise	Sets	Reps
Squats	8-10	20-5*
Hack Squats	5	10-15
Leg Extensions	5-8	10-15
Lying Leg Curls	6-10	10-15

Lee Haney

Exercise	Sets	Reps
Squats	4-6	6-8
Leg Extensions	3-4	8-10
Lying Leg Curls	4-5	8-10
Lunges (precontest only)	3	12-15

Jusup Wilkosz

Exercise	Sets	Reps
{ Leg Extensions	4-6	15-8*
{ Squats	4-6	15-8*
{ Lunges	4-6	15-8*
{ Hack Squats	4-6	15-8*
Lying Leg Curls	5	20-10*

Bertil Fox

Exercise	Sets	Reps
Squats	6	15-8*
{ Barbell Hack Squats	5	8-10
{ Leg Extensions	5	8-10
Lying Leg Curls	5	15-8*

Mike Mentzer

Exercise	Sets	Reps
Nautilus Leg Extensions	2	6-8
Vertical Leg Presses	1-2	8-10
Squats	1	8-10
Nautilus Leg Curls	2	6-8

Many sets are extended by forced reps.

Chris Dickerson

Exercise	Sets	Reps
Angled Leg Presses	6-8	8-10
Squats	4-5	8-10
Leg Extensions	5-6	8-10
Lying Leg Curls	7-8	8-10

This is an off-season workout.

Dennis Tinerino

Exercise	Sets	Reps
Leg Extensions	4-5	6-8
Squats	5	6-8
	2	10-12
Hack Squats	4	6-8
Lying Leg Curls	5	6-8
Lunges (precontest only)	4	20

Mohamed Makkawy

Exercise	Sets	Reps
Leg Extensions	5	10
Lying Leg Curls	5	10
Hack Squats	5	10

Exercises enclosed by brackets are supersetted.

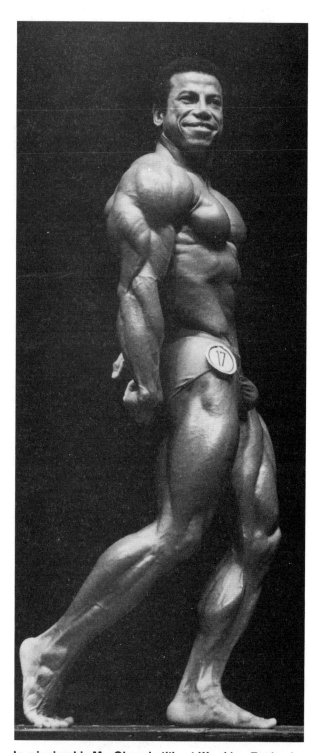

In winning his Mr. Olympia title at Wembley, England, in 1982, Chris Dickerson showed excellent overall development, particularly in his quads. Note the outstanding inner- and outer-quad cuts in this impressive side triceps shot taken in the middle of his free-posing program.

Gary Strydom

Exercise	Sets	Reps
Squats	4–5	8–10
Leg Extensions	3–4	8–10
Cable Front Kicks*	3–4	10–15
Lying Leg Curls	4–5	8–10
Stiff-Legged Deadlifts	4–5	10–15

Precontest only.

Tom Terwilliger

Exercise	Sets	Reps
Lying Leg Curls	8	15–8*
Stiff-Legged Deadlifts	4	10–12
Leg Extensions	5	15–8*
Squats	6	15–6*
Angled Leg Presses	5	12–8*

Rich Gaspari

Exercise	Sets	Reps
Leg Extensions	7	8–10
Angled Leg Presses	4–5	12–15
{Hack Squats	4	8–10
{Leg Extensions	4	8–10
Lunges	4	8–10
Lying Leg Curls	9–10	8–12

Christer Ericsson

Exercise	Sets	Reps
Squats	6	10–6*
Angled Leg Presses	4	10–6*
Leg Extensions	4–5	8–10
Lying Leg Curls	5–6	8–10

Frank Zane

Exercise	Sets	Reps
Leg Extensions	5–6	20–8*
Leg Curls	5–6	20–8*
Squats, or . . .	4–5	12–8*
Nautilus Lunges	4–5	10

Lee Labrada

Exercise	Sets	Reps
Leg Extensions (warm-up)	1-2	20-30
Leg Extensions	2-3	12-15
Angled Leg Presses	2-3	10
Squats	2	15-20
Lying Leg Curls	4-5	10-15
Stiff-Legged Deadlifts	2-3	10-12
Hamstrings Stretches (for three minutes)	—	—

Lou Ferrigno

Exercise	Sets	Reps
Front Squats	5-6	10-15
Hack Squats	4-5	10-15
Leg Extensions	4-5	10-15
Lying Leg Curls	5-6	10-15
Lunges	3-4	10-15

Berry de Mey

Exercise	Sets	Reps
Squats	3-4	15-20
Vertical Leg Presses	3-4	10-15
Hack Squats	3-4	10-15
Leg Extensions	3-4	10-15
Lying Leg Curls	3-4	10-15
Standing Leg Curls	3-4	10-15

Ali Malla

Exercise	Sets	Reps
Squats	4-5	10-15
Hack Squats	4	10
Angled Leg Presses	3	8-10
Leg Extensions	3-4	8-10
Lying Leg Curls	6-8	10
Standing Leg Curls	4	8

Bob Paris

Exercise	Sets	Reps
Leg Extensions	6	30
Angled Leg Presses	6	25
Hack Squats	6	15-20
Lunges	6	30
Squats	6	15
Standing Leg Curls	6	15-20

24
Sculpting
Stupendous Shoulders

One of the surest marks of a rugged male physique is broad shoulders. Combine a wide shoulder structure with mellon-sized deltoids, flaring lats, and a small waist–hip structure,

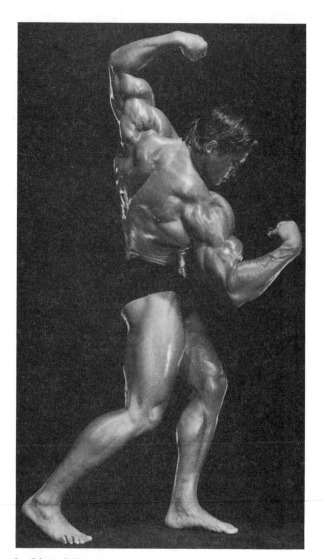

In this twisting three-quarters back shot, Arnold Schwarzenegger displays the type of shoulder development which won him thirteen world titles in all, seven of them Mr. Olympia victories.

and you have the type of symmetry that wins bodybuilding competitions.

Obviously, it is impossible to broaden the bone structure of your shoulder girdle. But you can dramatically increase the mass and quality of your shoulder muscles. When you add enough muscle mass to the medial heads (the side aspects) of your deltoids, you can add several inches to the width of your shoulders.

To my mind, the first great bodybuilder who displayed broad shoulders tapering down to a very narrow midsection was Steve Reeves. Reeves had won the Mr. Pacific Coast competition prior to entering and winning the 1947 Mr. America show, but he was still a relative unknown in national bodybuilding. But when he arrived in Chicago for the competition, his physique caused quite a stir. He won the show on a tie-breaker over Eric Pederson by virtue of his terrifically wide shoulders, flaring lats, and exceptionally narrow waist and hips.

Over the past 20 years or so, no bodybuilder who has won American national competitions has done so with weak deltoids. It seems as though everyone has developed his deltoids to the maximum, building balanced thickness from front to back and the ultimate degree of muscularity. No one with mediocre deltoid development will probably ever win a big show because the delts are such a key muscle group.

Why are the deltoids so important to a competitive bodybuilder? Simply put, the delts are visible from every angle when posing, and weak deltoids can be seen from every angle as well. You can sometimes hide weak calves or arms, but never weak deltoids. So the deltoids both add to shoulder width and improve virtually every pose in your contest program.

The deltoids are the one muscle group that requires three types of movement for complete

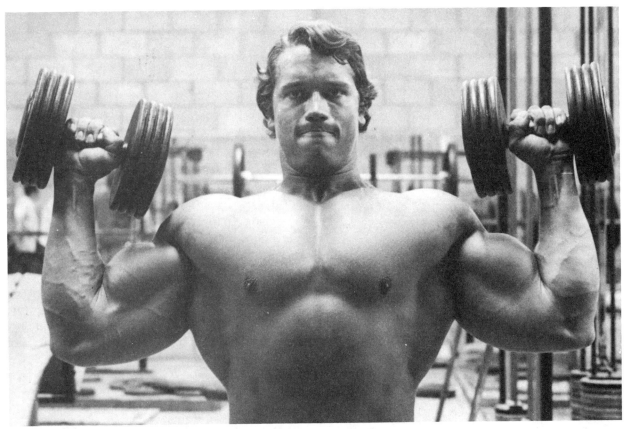

Seated Dumbbell Presses formed the basis of many a Schwarzenegger deltoid routine. He commonly worked up to dumbbells weighing more than 100 pounds in each hand.

development: pressing, pulling, and leverage exercises. You will seldom find a top bodybuilder who doesn't use at least two types of movement for shoulders, and a majority of them will use all three.

You will probably find that it takes several years to develop quality deltoids, somewhat more time than is required for other body parts to be brought up to a high standard. But if you put in the time and always train deltoids with 100% intensity, ultimately you will have very good shoulder development.

ANATOMY AND KINESIOLOGY

The primary shoulder muscle group is the deltoid, which contracts to move the upper arm bone in a variety of directions. The deltoid is segmented into three lobes, called heads. The anterior head is the front lobe; the medial head, the middle lobe; and the posterior head, the rear lobe. And each head of the deltoid is contracted harder than the others in order to move the upper arm bone in three different directions.

Let's assume that you are standing erect with your arms down at your sides. Holding your right arm straight, slowly raise it directly forward, a movement which isolates stress on the anterior deltoid head. When you raise your arm directly out to the side, the medial head takes up the job. And when you raise it to the rear, the medial head is contracted.

While there are a few exercises that isolate stress on a single deltoid head, most movements involve two or three deltoid heads acting in concert. Exercises that work two or more heads of the deltoids, as well as some other muscle group along with the delts, are called basic movements. And exercises that isolate stress on only one head of the muscle group are called isolation movements.

There are several other small muscle groups involved in the shoulder structure, called collectively the rotator cuff. These muscles are so small that they can be easily injured. To avoid injuring the rotator cuff muscles when doing heavy benches or standing presses, be sure to do a thorough warm-up prior to pumping the really heavy iron.

TRAINING TIPS

According to *Dennis Tinerino*, who has tremendous deltoid development, "It is essential during the first two or three years to stick to basic movements like overhead presses and upright rows. This basic work gives you a good foundation of deltoid muscle mass, which you can later refine using isolation movements during a peaking cycle.

"If you'd like a good routine, I would suggest 4–5 sets each—between six and eight reps per set—of standing barbell presses, seated dumbbell presses, and barbell or cable upright rows. Do the movements slowly and under strict control. And don't be afraid of doing 2–3 forced reps on a couple sets of each exercise.

"Get in a thorough warm-up prior to your first movement, then build up the weight each succeeding set. Your final set of each exercise should be done with the heaviest weight you can use on that movement."

"One of my deltoid training secrets," says *Tom Terwilliger* (National Light-Heavyweight Champion), "is pre-exhausting the muscle group prior to doing my pressing exercises. I find that I get much more building stimulus

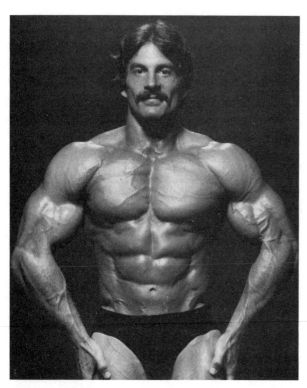

The broad shoulders of Mike Mentzer are set off by his rounded deltoids. Mike is one of the best writers in the sport, working currently for *Flex* magazine.

from the overhead presses if I've already done my side laterals. This is the exact opposite of what most top bodybuilders do, because they generally perform their pressing exercises first and then work down to the lighter leverage and dumbbell movements toward the end of their deltoid workouts. But if you give my theory a trial, I'm sure you will find that it works best if you do the presses after all of the laterals."

The incredible 6'7" IFBB World Champion, *Ralf Möller*, also is an advocate of working shoulders using the Weider Pre-Exhaustion Training Principle: "When you are working shoulders hard with overhead pressing movements, you will discover that your comparatively weaker triceps muscles will fatigue and cause you to fail on a rep quite a bit before your larger and stronger deltoids would become completely fatigued and cause you to fail the repetition. The way around this problem and hence, the way to push your delts much harder than usual using presses, is to utilize the pre-exhaustion technique.

"To pre-exhaust the deltoids, you should first do an isolation exercise, such as dumbbell side laterals, pushing the set to the point of failure. This fatigues the deltoids, making them briefly weaker than the triceps. So when you superset the laterals with seated presses behind the neck, you can really make your anterior and medial deltoids scream for mercy. You will literally push your deltoids twice as hard with a pre-ex superset than is possible doing straight sets for the muscle complex.

"It's vitally important that you take the briefest possible rest interval between exercises of a pre-ex superset. The longer you rest between the movements, the more quickly your delts recover from the pre-exhaustion isolation movement, thereby destroying the pre-ex effect. Rest only 3–4 seconds between the exercises, just enough to drop the dumbbells and pick up the barbell."

Big Ralf contributed the following deltoid pre-exhaustion supersets:

- Dumbbell Side Laterals + Standing Barbell Presses
- Barbell Front Raises + Seated Dumbbell Presses
- Dumbbell Side Laterals + Seated Barbell Presses

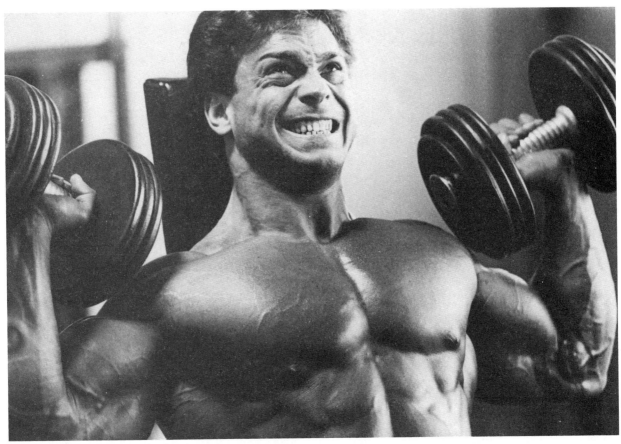

Always working hard, Rich Gaspari always works hard on his delts. Here he's doing Dumbbell Presses seated with his back braced against a high incline bench to support his back as he bombs anterior delts.

And if you wish to use the Pre-Exhaustion Principle for rear deltoids, you can superset dumbbell bent laterals with barbell bent rows, also for several sets of 8-10 reps each.

Flashy *Rich Gaspari* believes that there is an almost direct correlation between deltoid muscle mass and density and the amount of weight that can be pressed overhead for a minimum of 5-6 repetitions per set. He notes, "I have done 6-8 reps of seated presses behind the neck with 315 pounds. And that is one of the main reasons why my deltoids are so thick, hard, and striated onstage at a Mr. Olympia competition." Wise words from a champion who has placed as high as second in the Mr. Olympia event.

DELTOID EXERCISES

Standing Barbell Presses

Emphasis—This is the most basic deltoid exercise. It intensely stresses the anterior deltoids and places significant secondary emphasis on the medial delts as well. Standing presses also intensely stress the triceps and place secondary stress on the upper pectorals and those upper-back muscles which impart rotational movement to the scapulae.

Starting Position—Take an overgrip on a moderately heavy barbell resting on the gym floor, your hands set 3-4 inches wider than your shoulders on each side. Set your feet about shoulder width apart, dip your hips, and clean the barbell to your shoulders. Start the movement with your elbows directly beneath the bar, and keep them under the bar throughout your set. Stand erect and don't bend backward as you do the movement.

Movement Performance—Use deltoid and arm strength to press the barbell directly upward, close to your face, until it is at straight arms' length directly above your shoulder joints. Return the barbell back along the same arc to the starting point.

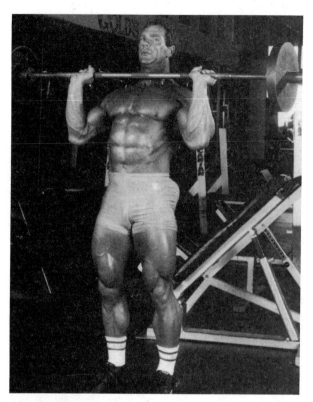

Standing Barbell Presses (start)

Exercises photographed at Gold's Gym by Paula
Crane   Exercise model: Scott Wilson

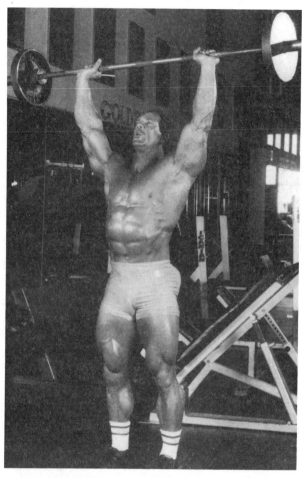

Standing Barbell Presses (finish)

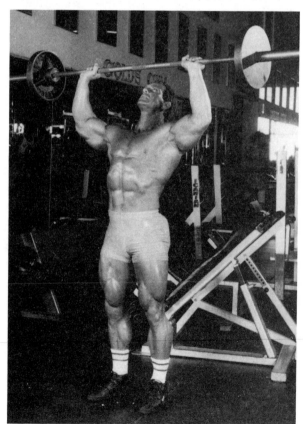

Standing Barbell Presses (midpoint)

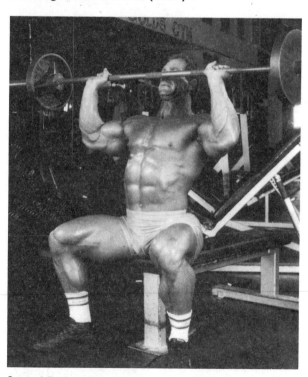

**Seated Barbell Front Presses (a variation of Standing
Barbell Presses)**

Training Tips—If you have difficulty in keeping your torso erect (i.e., you bend backward at the waist to help cheat up the bar), you should do seated barbell presses in which you sit astride a flat exercise bench as you do your overhead presses. In any case, you should wear a lifting belt when doing all overhead pressing exercises as a means of protecting your lower back and abdomen from injury. To stress your deltoids from slightly different angles, you should experiment with different widths of grip, from one in which your hands are shoulder width apart, out to one as wide as the length of the barbell handle allows.

Presses Behind Neck

Emphasis—This movement places somewhat more direct stress on the anterior and medial deltoids than front presses. It also places surprisingly more stress on the posterior heads of

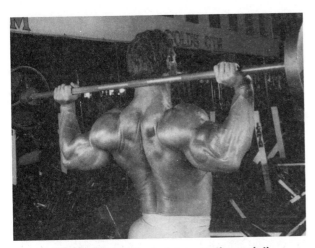

Presses Behind Neck (just above starting point)

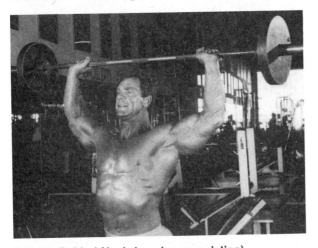

Presses Behind Neck (nearing completion)

the deltoids as well. Significant secondary stress is on the triceps muscles, and tertiary stress on the trapezius and other upper-back muscles.

Starting Position—While it can be performed standing, this movement is most frequently done while sitting astride a flat exercise bench. Take an overgrip on the barbell handle with your hands set 3–5 inches wider than your shoulders on each side. Clean it to your shoulders, push it over your head to rest across your trapezius muscles behind your neck, and sit down on the bench. Start the movement with your elbows directly beneath the bar and keep them under the bar for your entire set.

Movement Performance—Use shoulder and arm strength to press the barbell directly upward until it is locked out at straight arms' length directly above your shoulder joints. Lower it slowly back to your traps, and start another repetition.

Training Tips—For the sake of variety, you might like to do some of your overhead presses alternating one rep from the front of your neck with one from the back of it. Varying the width of your grip on the bar allows you to stress the deltoids from somewhat different angles. When I do presses behind the neck, I personally like to set the bar on the rack of a bench-pressing bench and sit down on the bench a couple of feet back from the rack. This way I can take my grip on the bar, dip my head under it, and then sit erect to start my set. Then at the end of the set, I merely bend forward a bit and place the barbell back on the bench rack.

Smith Machine Presses

Emphasis—All types of overhead presses on a Smith machine intensely stress the anterior and medial heads of the deltoid complex. Lesser stress is placed on the triceps, and even less on the upper-back muscles.

Starting Position—You can do either front presses or presses behind the neck on this convenient machine. Set the bar at shoulder level and load it up with the correct number of plates to set the weight for your set. Sit directly beneath it and take an overgrip on the bar with

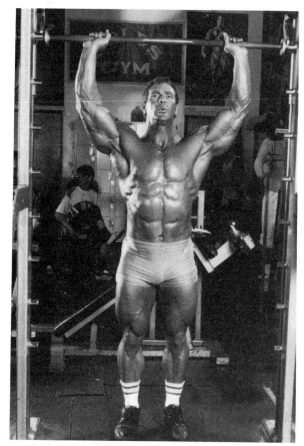

Smith Machine Presses (this can also be performed in a seated position, either in front of or behind the neck)

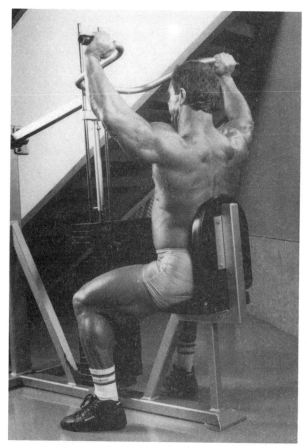

Seated Machine Press (for both Nautilus shoulder press and Universal machine shoulder press—midpoint)

your hands set 3-5 inches wider apart than your shoulders on each side. Either start with the bar on your upper chest in front of your neck, or resting across your traps behind your neck. Rotate your elbows beneath the bar and keep them under the bar for your entire set.

Movement Performance—Use deltoid and triceps strength to press the bar directly upward until it is locked out at straight arms' length directly above your shoulder joints. Pause briefly and then lower it back to shoulder level.

Training Tips—If you aren't too tall, you can also do this movement standing, but the seated version is used by the majority of top bodybuilders. Try varying the width of your grip on the bar from time to time.

Universal Shoulder Presses

Emphasis—As with all overhead pressing exercises, this movement places intense stress on

the anterior-medial deltoids and triceps. Secondary emphasis is on the upper pectorals and those upper-back muscles.

Starting Position—Place the stool which comes with a Universal Gym machine directly beneath the handles of the overhead pressing station of the apparatus. Sit on the stool facing the weight stack and take an overgrip on the pressing handles with your hands set 3-5 inches wider than your shoulders on each side. Sit erect and keep your elbows directly beneath the bar throughout your set.

Movement Performance—Use shoulder and arm strength to press the handles directly upward until your arms are locked out straight. Lower slowly back to the starting point.

Training Tips—When you do this exercise facing toward the weight stack, it corresponds with front barbell presses. Facing away from the machine, the movement is very similar to barbell presses behind the neck. As with all overhead barbell and machine presses, you should experiment with a variety of grip widths in as much as the length of the handles attached to the machine's lever arm allow.

Nautilus Shoulder Presses

Emphasis—As with all types of overhead presses, this exercise places the most intense stress on the anterior-medial deltoids and triceps, with secondary stress on those upper-back muscles which impart rotational force to the shoulder blades. In general, Nautilus machines are engineered to provide a somewhat more intense form on the working muscles than do free-weight equivalents of the same movement. On the down side, Nautilus provides very little variety, with only 2–3 movements for most body parts, including shoulders.

Starting Position—Adjust the height of the seat to place your shoulder joints at the level of the pressing handles when you sit in it. Sit in the seat, fasten the lap belt over your hips, and cross your ankles beneath the seat. Grasp the pressing handles with your palms facing each other.

Movement Performance—Use deltoid and triceps strength to press the handles upward until your arms are locked straight. Lower slowly back to the starting point.

Training Tips—On machine movements, you can use a very effective form of negative reps. On the Nautilus pressing machine, you can do this by pushing the handles upward with both arms, then lower it with only one arm, powerfully resisting the downward force provided by the machine. Be sure to alternate arms on the lowering phase of each repetition, so you fatigue each side of your body equally.

Dumbbell Presses

Emphasis—Dumbbell presses give you an overhead movement in which your hands are not restricted to a set distance apart. The movement places the most intense stress on the anterior-medial deltoids and triceps, with secondary emphasis on the upper pectorals and upper-back muscles.

Starting Position—Grasp two moderately weighted dumbbells, set your feet about shoulder width apart, and clean the dumbbells to your shoulders. Rotate your hands so your palms are facing directly forward as you do your set. Stand as erectly as possible. Be sure you keep your elbows under your hands throughout each rep.

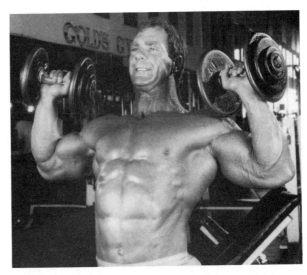

Dumbbell Presses (standing position—can also be performed seated—start)

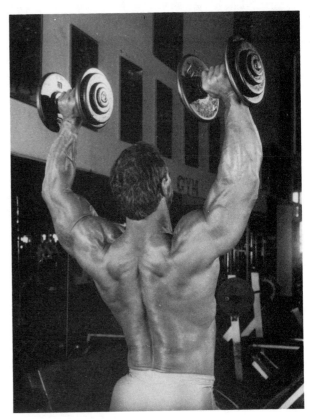

Dumbbell Presses (very near finish)

Movement Performance—Press the weights directly upward, then in toward each other near the top of the movement, so they touch directly over your head when your arms are locked out straight. Lower slowly back along the same arcs to the starting point.

Training Tips—There are many variants of dumbbell presses, each of which can be performed either standing or in a seated position. You can, for example, perform the exercise with your wrists rotated so your palms are facing each other throughout your set. You can also do dumbbell presses alternately, pushing the dumbbell in your right hand upward as the one in your left hand descends, continuing in seesaw fashion.

"Arnold" Presses

Emphasis—Whether or not Arnold Schwarzenegger actually originated this exercise is problematical, but he did popularize it through articles in various bodybuilding magazines. This variation of dumbbell presses allows you to move the weights over a greater range of motion than is possible with normal dumbbell presses. Therefore, it places a higher quality of stress on the anterior-medial deltoids and triceps. Secondary emphasis is on the upper pectorals and upper-back muscles.

Starting Position—Most frequently, top bodybuilders will do this exercise seated on a flat

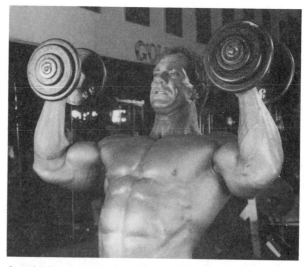

Arnold Presses (midpoint)

exercise bench, or on a bench with a vertical back support. Grasp two moderately heavy dumbbells, clean them to your shoulders, and sit down on the bench. In the starting position, your hands should be fully supinated, so your palms are facing toward your body, as in the finish position of a dumbbell curling movement.

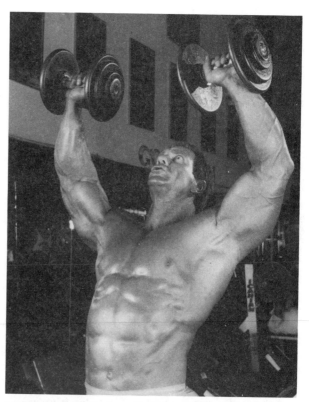

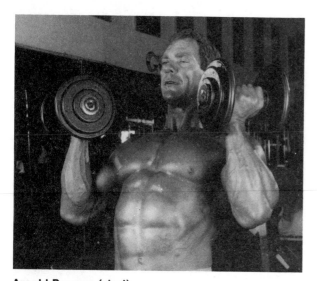

Arnold Presses (start)

Arnold Presses (finish—rotation of dumbbells during movement and lack of a lockout at the top)

Movement Performance—Slowly press the dumbbells directly upward, simultaneously rotating your hands so your palms face forward during the last part of the movement. You can either press the weights up all of the way, until they touch each other directly above your head, or you can keep continuous tension on your pressing muscles by terminating the upward part of the movement about three-quarters of the way up. Lower slowly back along the same arcs to the starting point, rotating your hands 180-degrees in the opposite direction.

Training Tips—You can also do this exercise with one arm at a time, standing erect and holding on to a sturdy upright with your free hand in order to brace your torso in an erect position.

One-Arm Dumbbell Presses

Emphasis—This exercise also stresses the anterior-medial deltoids and triceps, with secondary stress on the upper chest and back muscles. Generally speaking, one-armed movements place a higher quality of stress on the working muscles because you are no longer forced to concentrate with a split mental focus on each arm.

Starting Position—Grasp a moderately heavy dumbbell in your right hand, stand with your feet a bit wider than your shoulders, and grasp

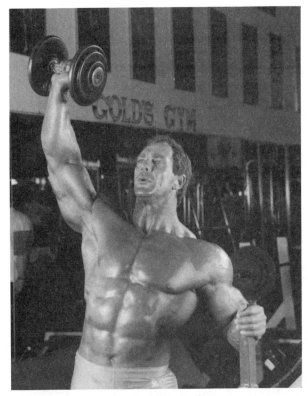

One-Arm Dumbbell Press (finish)

a sturdy upright with your free hand to steady your torso in an upright position as you do your set. Clean the dumbbell to your shoulder, and rotate your wrist so your palm is facing forward throughout your set.

Movement Performance—Use arm and shoulder strength to press the dumbbell directly upward until your arm is locked out straight and the dumbbell is supported directly above your shoulder joint. Lower slowly back to the start. Be sure to switch arms so you do an equal number of sets and reps with each arm.

Training Tips—You can also do this movement with your wrist rotated so your palm is facing in toward the midline of your body as you do the exercise.

Barbell Upright Rows

Emphasis—This is the best movement for developing delt-trap tie-ins. It directly stresses the trapezius and other upper-back muscles, as well as the anterior and medial heads of the deltoids. Secondary stress is on the biceps, brachialis, and forearm flexor muscles.

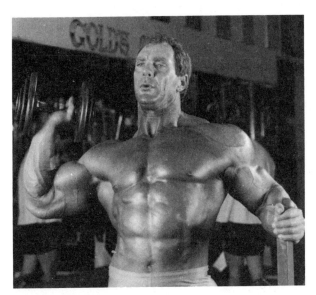

One-Arm Dumbbell Press (start—note hold on solid upright to brace body)

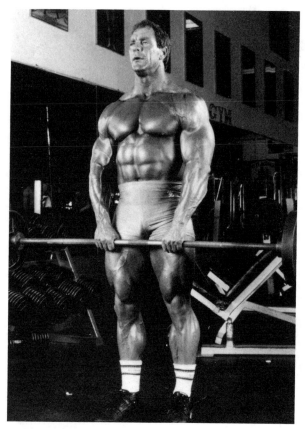

Barbell Upright Rows (start)

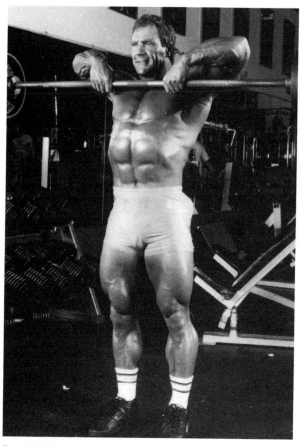

Barbell Upright Rows (finish)

Starting Position—Take a narrow overgrip in the middle of a barbell handle. There should be 4-6 inches of space showing between your index fingers when you have the correct grip on the bar. Set your feet about shoulder width apart, and stand erect with your arms straight down at your sides, the barbell resting in your hands across your upper thighs. Keep your torso upright and as motionless as possible as you do your set.

Movement Performance—Moving only your arms, slowly pull the barbell directly upward close to your body until the backs of your fists touch the underside of your chin. It is important as you do this movement, both upward and downward, that you keep your elbows well above the level of your hands gripping the barbell. At the top point of the movement, you should rotate your shoulders to the rear and press your shoulder blades together briefly before slowly lowering back along the same arc to the starting position.

Training Tips—If you wish to shift stress away from your trapezius muscles and onto your

medial delts, you should do this exercise with your hands set about shoulder width apart on the bar. You won't be able to pull the weight any higher than about the lower edge of your pecs, but even this short a range of motion will intensely stress your medial delts and add to the apparent width of your shoulders.

Cable Upright Rows

Emphasis—The cable equivalent to barbell upright rows, this excellent exercise places intense stress on the anterior-medial deltoids and triceps, with secondary stress on the biceps, brachialis, and forearm flexors.

Starting Position—Attach a bar handle to the end of a cable running through a floor pulley. Take a narrow overgrip on the handle, about 4-6 inches of space showing between your index fingers. Set your feet a comfortable distance apart a foot or so back from the pulley and stand erect with your arms hanging straight down from your shoulders, the bar handle resting in your hands across your upper thighs.

Movement Performance—Keeping your upper body motionless and your elbows above the level of your hands throughout your set, slowly pull the handle directly upward close to your torso until the backs of your hands slightly contact the underside of your chin. In the top position, you should emphasize the elbows-up position, rotate your shoulders to the rear, and press your shoulder blades together for a moment. Lower slowly back along the same path to the starting point.

Training Tips—You can experiment with different widths of bar grip. On all types of upright rows, it is vitally important that you lower the weight slowly back from the top position, rather than just allowing the bar or handle to drop. Dropping the weight robs you of about 50% of the value you should receive from a set of upright rows. When using a cable apparatus, you will find that you can profitably do your upright rows while seated at the end of a flat exercise bench, as well as in the normal standing position.

Dumbbell Upright Rows

Emphasis—As with all variations of upright rows, this dumbbell movement stresses the delts and traps most intensely, with secondary emphasis placed on the biceps, brachialis, and forearm flexor muscles.

Starting Position—Grasp two moderately heavy dumbbells, set your feet a comfortable distance apart, and stand erect with your arms hanging directly downward from your shoulders, the dumbbells resting on your upper thighs. Keep your palms facing the rear throughout your set, and try to keep your upper body motionless, save for the movement of your arms.

Movement Performance—Keeping your elbows well above the level of your hands throughout the movement, slowly pull the dumbbells directly upward close to your torso until they are at shoulder level. Lower slowly back to the starting point.

Training Tips—When you use dumbbells, you can pull the weights upward along a myriad of

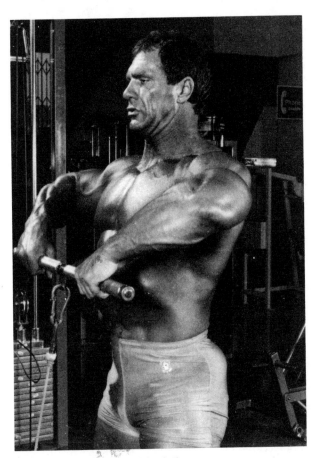

Cable Upright Rows (midpoint)

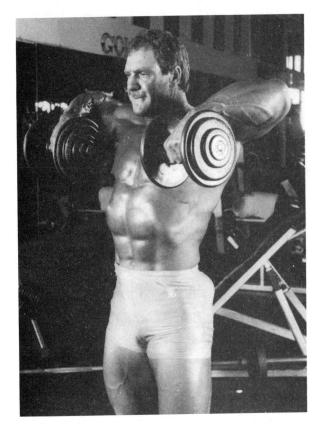

Dumbbell Upright Rows (finish)

arcs, either close together or out wide apart. Each new arc stresses your working muscles from a new angle, and the accumulation of many such upward arcs will give you the maximum degree of shoulder girdle development.

Standing Dumbbell Side Laterals

Emphasis—This movement effectively isolates stress almost exclusively on the medial heads of the deltoids, with very little assistance from the anterior delts and trapezius muscles.

Starting Position—Grasp two light dumbbells, set your feet about shoulder width apart. Stand erect with your arms hanging down at your sides. With your palms facing each other, press the dumbbells together 4-6 inches in front of your hips. Bend your arms 10-15 degrees, and keep them rounded like this throughout the movement. Bend slightly forward at the waist and maintain this torso inclination throughout your set.

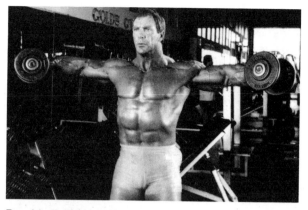

Dumbbell Side Laterals (finish)

Movement Performance—Being sure to keep your palms facing toward the floor, use deltoid strength to raise the dumbbells in semicircular arcs out to the sides and slightly forward until they reach shoulder level. In the top position, you can most effectively isolate stress on the

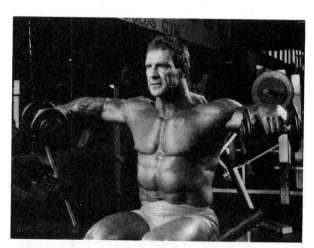

Seated Dumbbell Side Laterals (variation of Standing Side Laterals—finish)

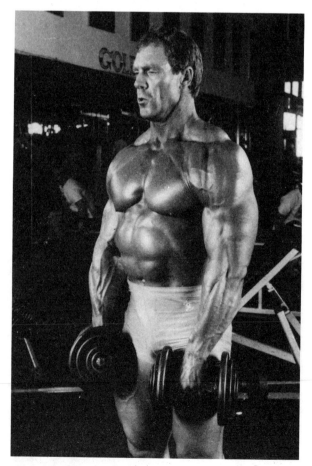

Dumbbell Side Laterals (start)

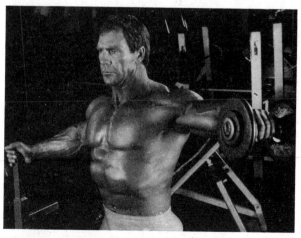

One-Arm Dumbbell Side Lateral (variation of Standing or Seated Side Laterals—finish)

medial delts, and you can rotate your hands forward a bit, so the front edge of the dumbbell on each side is a little below the level of the back end. Slowly lower the weights back along the same arc to the starting point.

Training Tips—Never allow your palms to face forward when attempting to isolate stress on the medial deltoids, because such a movement places the most intense stress on the anterior heads of the muscle complex. You can also do dumbbell side laterals either in a seated position, or with one arm at a time standing, your free hand grasping a sturdy upright to brace your torso in an erect position as you do the exercise.

Cable Side Laterals

Emphasis—This one-arm movement allows you to place very intense stress on your medial deltoids, since it permits a more powerful contraction of the working muscles than is possible doing side laterals with both arms simultaneously.

Starting Position—Attach a loop handle to the end of a cable running through a floor pulley.

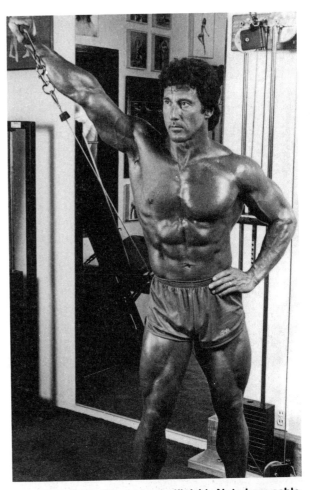

One-Arm Cable Side Laterals (finish). Note how cable runs behind body; more commonly, the movement is performed with the cable running across the front of the body   Model: Frank Zane

Grasp the handle in your right hand and turn your body so the cable runs diagonally across the front of your body. Your feet should be set somewhat wider than shoulder width, your left foot 1–1½ feet away from the pulley. Bend your right arm slightly and keep it rounded throughout the movement. Rest your left hand on your left hip throughout the set. Allow the weight on the other end of the cable to pull your right hand as far as is comfortably possible across the midline of your body.

Movement Performance—Use right-shoulder deltoid strength to move the pulley handle slightly forward and out to the side in a semicircular arc up to shoulder level. Be sure your palm is facing the floor throughout the movement. Lower slowly back along the same arc to the starting point. Be sure to do an equal number of sets and reps with each arm.

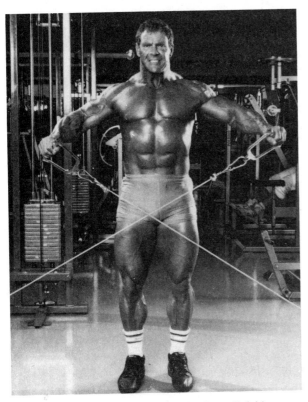

Cable Side Laterals (two-armed version—finish)

Training Tips—For a slightly different effect on your deltoids, you can also do this exercise with the cable running behind your body rather than in front of it. You can also stress your delts differently by using the arm facing toward the pulley to raise the handle in a semi-circular arc out to the side and upward.

Nautilus Side Laterals

Emphasis—This is a good way of isolating stress on your medial deltoids, with a minimum assist from your anterior delts and trapezius muscles.

Starting Position—Adjust the height of the seat so when you are sitting on it your shoulders are at the same level as the pivot points of the cams to which the lever arms are attached. Sit on the seat, fasten the lap belt, and cross your ankles beneath the seat. Slip your wrists against the inner edges of the two smaller pads, grasping the handles provided.

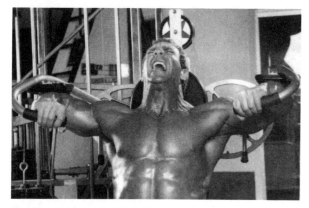

Nautilus Side Laterals (finish)

Movement Performance—Use medial deltoid strength to raise the pads outward and upward in semicircular arcs to a point a bit above shoulder level. Hold this peak-contracted position for a moment before slowly lowering back to the starting point.

Training Tips—You can do this movement with one arm at a time if you like. You will also see a lot of good bodybuilders doing the movement standing in front of the machine facing toward the seatback, which is also a very effective medial deltoid movement.

Palms-Up Dumbbell Side Laterals

Emphasis—By rotating your wrists so your palms are facing upward as you do the exercise, you shift the most intense focus to your anterior deltoids, with only minor assistance from your medial delts and trapezius muscles.

Starting Position—Grasp two moderately weighted dumbbells, set your feet a comfortable distance apart, and stand erect with your arms down at your sides. Rotate your wrists so your palms will be facing upward throughout the movement. Bend your arms slightly and keep them bent like this throughout your set.

Movement Performance—Use anterior deltoid strength to raise the dumbbells directly out to the sides and upward in semicircular arcs to shoulder level. Lower slowly back along the same arcs to the starting point.

Training Tips—You can also do this exercise with your palms facing directly forward throughout your set. Regardless of which hand orientation you use, be sure to raise the dumbbells directly out to the sides rather than somewhat forward on other variations of side laterals.

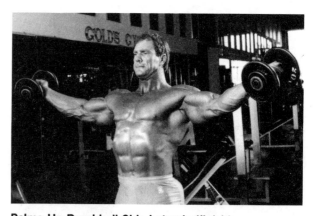

Palms-Up Dumbbell Side Laterals (finish)

Front Barbell Raises

Emphasis—If you want to isolate stress on the anterior deltoids without involving the triceps muscles, as is the case with overhead pressing movements, you should use one of the various types of front raises. Minor secondary stress is placed on the medial deltoids when you do this exercise.

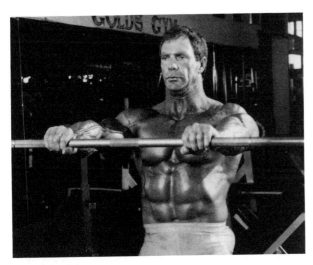

Front Barbell Raises (finish)

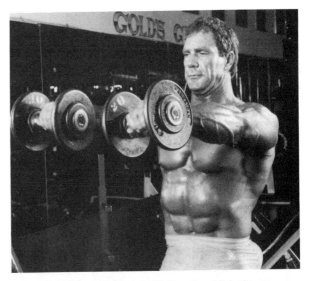

Front Dumbbell Raises (variation in which they are raised simultaneously—finish)

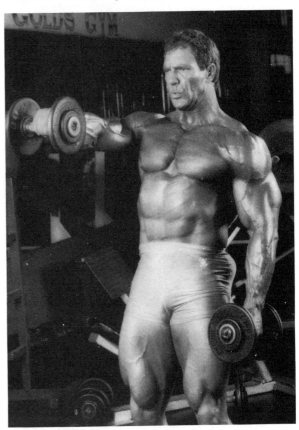

Dumbbell Alternate Front Raises (position 1)

Starting Position—Take an overgrip about shoulder width apart on a moderately weighted barbell. Set your feet a comfortable distance apart and stand erect with your arms hanging straight down at your sides, the barbell resting across your upper thighs. Keep your arms straight and torso as motionless as possible as you do your set.

Movement Performance—Use front delt strength to raise the barbell forward and upward in a semicircular arc to shoulder level. Lower back along the same arc to the start.

Training Tips—You can vary the width of your grip on the bar. As a change of pace, you can also raise the barbell all of the way upward until it is at straight arms' length directly above your shoulders in the top position.

Front Dumbbell Raises

Emphasis—The different dumbbell variations of front raises isolate stress on the anterior deltoids, with only a little emphasis on the medial delts.

Starting Position—Grasp two fairly light dumbbells, set your feet a comfortable distance apart, and stand erect. The dumbbells should be resting across your upper thighs in the starting position. Keep your arms straight and torso as motionless as possible throughout your set.

Movement Performance—Raise the dumbbell in your right hand forward and upward in a semicircular arc until it reaches shoulder level. As you begin to lower the weight in your right hand, begin to raise the dumbbell in your left hand.

Training Tips—You can also raise the dumbbells together rather than alternately, and on either variation you can raise them all of the

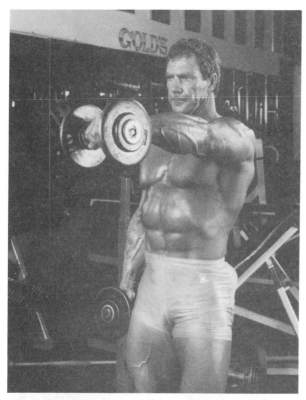

Dumbbell Alternate Front Raises (position 2)

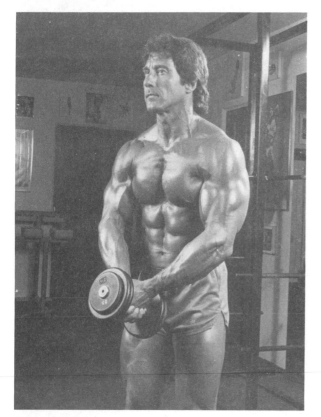

Dumbbell Front Raises (variation in which one dumbbell is raised while held in both hands—start)

Model: Frank Zane

way up to straight arms' length above your shoulders. Another dumbbell variation is performed holding a single dumbbell in both hands, your fists grasping the handle overlapping each other.

Cable Front Raises

Emphasis—As is the case with barbell and dumbbell variations of front raises, this movement isolates stress on the anterior deltoids without involving the triceps muscles, as is the case with overhead pressing exercises. Minor secondary stress is placed on the medial deltoids when you do this movement.

Starting Position—Attach a straight bar handle to the end of a cable running through a floor pulley (most types of handles used on lat machines will work well for this movement). Take a shoulder-width overgrip on the handle, set your feet about shoulder width apart (about 1½–2 feet back from the pulley), with the front

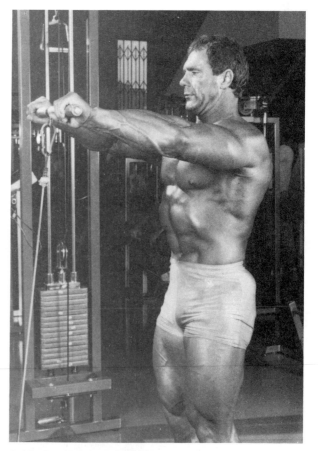

Cable Front Raises (finish)

of your body toward the pulley. Straighten your arms and allow them to hang straight down toward the pulley. Keep your arms straight throughout your set, and avoid any extraneous body movement as you do this exercise.

Movement Performance—Use deltoid strength to move the pulley handle in a semicircular arc forward and upward from the starting position to a point a bit above shoulder level directly in front of your face. Hold this peak-contracted position for a moment, then lower slowly back along the same arc to the starting point.

Training Tips—You can also raise the pulley handle up to the point at which your arms are extended straight upward from your shoulders. A somewhat narrower or wider grip can be used on the pulley handle to stress the anterior delts from different angles. If you stand facing away from the weight stack with the pulley almost directly between your feet and the cable running between your legs, you can do a similar movement which also stresses the anterior deltoids from a slightly different angle.

Incline Front Raises

Emphasis—Another variation of front raises, this movement also isolates stress on the anterior deltoids with minor secondary stress placed on the medial deltoids. But since it is done lying facedown on a bench, it is impossible to cheat up the barbell or dumbbells with extraneous body motion.

Starting Position—Take a shoulder-width overgrip on a light barbell and lie facedown on a 30–45-degree incline bench. Straighten your arms and allow them to hang directly downward from your shoulders. Keep your arms straight throughout the movement.

Movement Performance—Use deltoid strength to move the barbell forward and upward in a semicircular arc from the starting point to a position slightly above eye level. (If you can't raise the weight at least this high, you should reduce the poundage on the bar.) Hold this peak-contracted position for a moment, then lower slowly back to the starting point.

Training Tips—You can vary the width of your grip on the bar to stress your shoulder muscles from a variety of angles. You can also effectively stress your anterior deltoids using dumbbells for this movement, raising them either together or alternately.

Prone Front Raises

Emphasis—Another variation of front raises, this exercise intensely stresses the anterior deltoids and places minor secondary stress on the medial deltoids. As with incline front raises, this movement is very strict since your body is braced on the exercise bench.

Starting Position—Take a shoulder-width overgrip on a light barbell and lie facedown on a flat exercise bench, with your head hanging off one end of it. The bench must be high enough so the weight is clear of the floor when your arms are held straight and hanging straight down toward the floor, so you might have to place blocks of wood or thick barbell plates under the legs of the bench. Hold your arms straight throughout the movement.

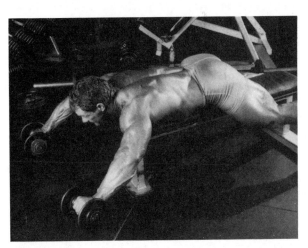

Prone Dumbbell Side Laterals

Movement Performance—Use deltoid strength to move the barbell slowly forward and upward in a semicircular arc to a point slightly above eye level. (If you cannot raise the barbell thigh high, you should reduce the poundage on the bar.) Hold the peak-contracted position for a moment, then lower the weight slowly back to the starting point.

Training Tips—You will find this movement difficult to perform with a very heavy weight, because it works your anterior deltoids with direct resistance through a range of motion it rarely experiences. You can vary the width of your grip on the bar, or use two dumbbells for the exercise, raising them either together or alternately.

Bent-Over Front Raises

Emphasis—This exercise is very much like prone front raises, except that you won't have the bench to brace your body and will consequently cheat a little on the movement no matter how hard you attempt to keep the movement strict. The exercise stresses the anterior deltoids quite intensely, and the medial delts less intensely.

Starting Position—Take a shoulder-width overgrip on a light barbell, set your feet a comfortable distance apart, and bend forward at the waist until your torso is parallel to the floor as you do the movement. Your legs and arms should be held straight throughout your set. At the start of the movement, the weight should be hanging straight down from your shoulders. If the barbell plates do not clear the floor in this starting position, you should stand on a thick block of wood as you do the exercise.

Movement Performance—Use deltoid strength to move the barbell forward and upward in a semicircular arc from the starting point to a

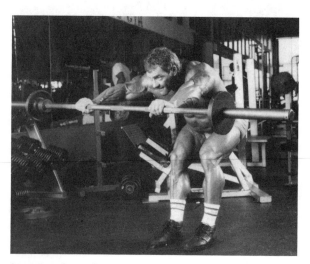

Standing Bent-Over Front Barbell Raises

position slightly above eye level. (If you cannot raise the weight at least this high without cheating, you should reduce the poundage on the bar.) Hold this peak-contracted position for a moment, then lower slowly back along the same arc to the starting point.

Training Tips—You should occasionally vary the width of your grip on the bar in order to stress your anterior delts from different angles, which will lead to more complete shoulder development. The exercise can also be performed holding two light dumbbells and raising them either simultaneously or alternately.

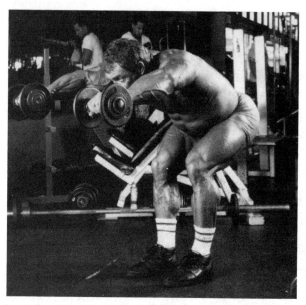

Bent-Over Dumbbell Front Raises

Prone Incline Side Laterals

Emphasis—This movement was a favorite of Larry Scott, the first Mr. Olympia winner, and for good reason. It is one of the most direct movements you can possibly perform for your medial deltoids, as well as for the medial-posterior deltoid tie-ins.

Starting Position—Grasp two moderately weighted dumbbells and lie facedown on a 30–45-degree incline bench. The dumbbells should be hanging straight down from your shoulders, with your palms facing each other throughout the exercise. Some bodybuilders like to do this exercise with their arms held straight, but I think it is best to bend them about 10 degrees and hold them rounded like this throughout your set.

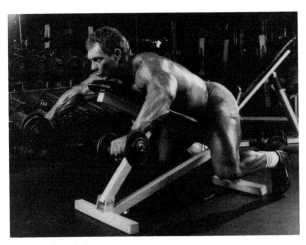

Prone Dumbbell Side Laterals

Movement Performance—Use deltoid strength to raise the dumbbells directly out to the sides and upward in semicircular arcs until they are slightly above the level of your shoulder joints. In the top position of the movement, you can make the exercise more intense by rotating your wrists so the front set of plates on each dumbbell is a bit below the level of the back set of plates. Hold this peak-contracted position for a moment, then lower slowly back along the same arcs to the starting point.

Training Tips—It's a good idea to periodically change the angle of the incline bench, as well as to experiment with raising the weights a bit forward of a position directly out to the sides. Each of these slight variations will stress your deltoid muscles from different angles, building them up to the point where they are as round and thick as cannon balls.

Side Incline Laterals

Emphasis—A favorite deltoid exercise of seven-time Mr. Olympia Arnold Schwarzenegger, side incline laterals work the medial deltoids from a unique angle, adding width to your shoulders. The movement almost perfectly isolates stress on the side delts.

Starting Position—Grasp a light dumbbell in your left hand and lie on your right side on an incline bench set at about a 30-degree angle. Alternatively, you can do the exercise lying on an inclined sit-up board set somewhere between 15–30 degrees. The dumbbell should be touching the bench directly in front of your

hips at the start, and your arm should be bent at about a 10-degree angle and held rounded throughout your set.

Movement Performance—Use deltoid strength to raise the weight upward in a semicircular arc slightly in front of your hips until you feel stress coming off your medial deltoid head. This will be at an angle of about 60 degrees with the floor. Slowly lower the dumbbell back along the same arc to the starting point. Be sure to do an equal number of sets and reps with each arm.

Training Tips—You will probably have to spread your legs and brace your feet against the floor in order to keep your body motionless on the bench. You should also try doing the exercise from time to time starting from a point behind your hips and raising the weight upward along that plane.

Floor Side Laterals

Emphasis—This is a unique movement which only has become popular in recent years. It places isolated stress on the medial and posterior heads of the deltoid muscles.

Starting Position—Grasp a light dumbbell in your left hand and lie on your right side on the floor, spreading your legs and splaying your feet on the floor to brace your body in this position as you do your set. With your arm held rounded throughout your set, start the movement with your palm facing the floor and the dumbbell lightly touching the floor just in front of your hip.

Movement Performance—Use deltoid strength to raise the dumbbell out to the side and upward in a semicircular arc from the starting point to a position wherein your arm is at about a 60-degree angle with the floor, or that point at which you begin to feel stress coming off your deltoid muscles. Lower the weight back to the starting position. Be sure to do an equal number of sets and reps with each arm.

Training Tips—You can also do the same movement starting the upward thrust of the dumbbell from a position behind your hip rather than from in front of it.

Standing Dumbbell Bent Laterals

Emphasis—This is the most basic movement for isolating stress on the posterior heads of your deltoids. There is minor stress placed on the medial heads of the deltoids and the trapezius and other upper-back muscles.

Starting Position—Grasp two moderately weighted dumbbells, set your feet about shoulder width apart, and bend forward at the waist to hold your torso parallel with the floor throughout your set. You will probably find it best to keep your legs slightly bent as you do the movement. Your arms should be hanging straight down from your shoulders, your palms facing each other throughout the movement. Bend your arms about 10 degrees and keep them rounded like this throughout the movement. Press the dumbbells together beneath your chest.

Movement Performance—Use posterior deltoid strength to raise the dumbbells in semicircular arcs directly out to the sides and upward until they are slightly above shoulder level. Hold this peak-contracted position for a moment, then slowly lower the weights back along the same arcs to the starting point.

Training Tips—The most common mistake inexperienced bodybuilders (and even some veterans) make when doing bent laterals is to raise the dumbbells to the rear of a plane running directly out to the sides, a movement which removes stress from the medial delts and transfers it to the triceps muscles. You must always raise the weights directly out to the sides, if not somewhat forward of this position.

Seated Bent Laterals

Emphasis—Another shoulder favorite of Arnold Schwarzenegger, seated bent laterals stress the posterior deltoids more intensely than any other part of the body, and put secondary emphasis on the medial delts, trapezius, and other upper-back muscles.

Starting Position—Grasp two moderately weighted dumbbells and sit at the end of a flat exercise bench with your feet touching each other and your lower legs pressed together throughout the movement. Bend forward and rest your chest on your thighs, allowing your arms to hang straight down from your shoulders, your palms facing each other throughout the movement. Bend your arms about 10 degrees and keep them rounded like this throughout your set.

Movement Performance—Keeping your chest on your thighs throughout the movement, use deltoid strength to raise the dumbbells directly out to the sides and upward in semicircular arcs until the weights are slightly above the level of your shoulders. Hold this peak-contracted position for a moment, then lower slowly back along the same arc to the starting point.

Training Tips—Even among highly experienced bodybuilders, the most common mistake when performing seated bent laterals is allowing the torso to come up off the thighs. As such, this isn't much of a problem as long as you don't rise too high. The higher your torso inclines from a position parallel with the floor, the more the exercise becomes similar to prone incline laterals, which can more beneficially be performed with your body braced on the bench to prevent cheating. Be sure not to raise the weights to the rear.

One-Arm Dumbbell Bent Laterals

Emphasis—As with normal two-armed bent laterals, this exercise intensely stresses the posterior deltoid head of each shoulder cap, with lesser emphasis on the medial deltoids, traps, and other upper-back muscles. But whenever you do an exercise with only one arm or leg, you automatically place a more intense stress on the working muscles.

Starting Position—Grasp a moderately weighted dumbbell in your left hand, set your feet about shoulder width apart, and bend forward at the waist, your left arm hanging straight down from your shoulder and your right hand grasping a piece of exercise apparatus to brace your torso parallel to the floor throughout the movement. Turn your wrist so your palm is facing in toward the midline of your body as you perform your set. Bend your left arm about 10 degrees and keep it rounded like this as you do the movement.

Movement Performance—Use posterior deltoid strength to raise the dumbbell directly out to the side and upward in a semicircular arc to a position slightly above the level of your shoulder. Hold this peak-contracted position for a moment before slowly lowering it back along the same arc to the starting point. Be sure to do an equal number of sets and reps with each arm.

Training Tips—As with other forms of bent laterals, be sure that you don't raise the weights to the rear of a plane straight out from your shoulder joint.

Cable Bent Laterals

Emphasis—This movement also places primary emphasis on the posterior deltoids and secondary stress on the medial delts, traps, and other upper-back muscles. Most bodybuilders find that they can achieve a much more benefi-

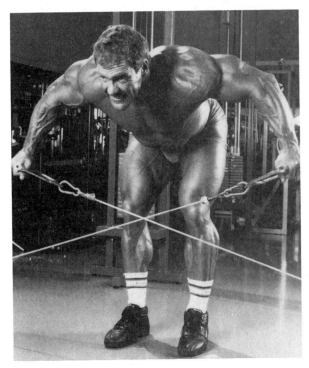

Cable Bent Laterals

cial form of continuous tension for their rear delts when they use cables for this exercise.

Starting Position—Attach loop handles to the ends of two cables running through floor pulleys about 8–10 feet apart. Reach across your body with your left arm to grasp the handle to your right, cross your arms, and reach across your body with your right arm to grasp the handle to the left. Set your feet about shoulder width apart and bend forward at the waist until your torso is parallel with the floor, a position you must maintain throughout the movement. Cross your arms as fully as possible.

Movement Performance—With the cables crossing each other directly beneath your torso, use posterior deltoid strength to raise the pulley handles directly out to the sides and upward in semicircular arcs until your hands are slightly above the level of your shoulders. Hold this peak-contracted position for a moment, then slowly lower the pulley handles back along the same arcs to the starting point of the exercise.

Training Tips—A very beneficial exercise for the medial-posterior deltoid tie-ins can be performed with the same pulley set-up while lying facedown on a 30-45-degree incline bench. Just be sure that the cables cross each other beneath the bench.

One-Arm Cable Bent Laterals

Emphasis—This is another way to place emphasis on your posterior delts, as well as lesser stress on the medial deltoids and upper-back muscles. When performed with one arm at a time, the movement is much more intense than when done with both arms simultaneously.

Starting Position—Attach a loop handle to the end of a cable running through a floor pulley and grasp the handle with your left hand. Set your feet about shoulder width apart, your right side toward the pulley, and bend forward until your torso is parallel to the gym floor, a position which must be maintained throughout the movement. Allow the weight on the cable to pull your left hand as far as possible across the midline of your body and toward the pulley.

Bend your arm about 10 degrees and keep it rounded like this throughout your set.

Movement Performance—Use posterior delt power to raise the pulley handle directly out to the side and upward in a semicircular arc until your hand is slightly above the level of your shoulder. Hold this peak-contracted position for a moment, then slowly lower the pulley handle back along the same arc to the starting point. Be sure to do the same number of sets and reps with each arm.

Training Tips—Your palm should always be facing the floor during this movement. Be sure that you don't allow yourself to ruin the effect of the exercise by raising the pulley handle toward the rear.

Prone Laterals

Emphasis—This is another excellent exercise for the posterior deltoids. Secondary stress is borne by the medial delts, traps, and other upper-back muscles. But since the movement is performed with your body braced on a bench, it is more strict than dumbbell bent laterals performed in a standing position.

Starting Position—Grasp two moderately weighted dumbbells and lie facedown on a high, flat exercise bench. (If the dumbbells are not clear of the floor in the starting position of the movement, you should raise the height of the bench a few inches by placing the legs on blocks of wood or thick barbell plates.) Allow your arms to hang straight down from your shoulders and rotate your wrists so your palms are facing inward at the start of the exercise. Bend your arms about 10 degrees and keep them rounded like this throughout your set.

Movement Performance—Use posterior deltoid strength to raise the dumbbells directly out to the sides and upward in a semicircular arc until they are slightly above the level of your shoulders. Hold this peak-contracted position for a moment, then slowly lower the weights back along the same arcs to the starting point.

Training Tips—You can also do this exercise with loop handles attached to two floor pul-

leys, the cables crossing each other beneath the bench as you raise your hands out to the sides.

Pec Deck Rear Delt Laterals

Emphasis—This is one of the few machine movements that can be used to stress the posterior deltoids, with lesser emphasis on the medial delts, trapezius, and other upper-back muscles.

Starting Position—Sit in a pec deck machine facing toward its vertical padded back support. Force your arms between the vertical pads attached to the lever arms of the apparatus, so the pads rest against the back of your upper arms. It makes little difference whether you keep your arms straight or not, so you will probably feel most comfortable keeping them slightly bent as you do the movement.

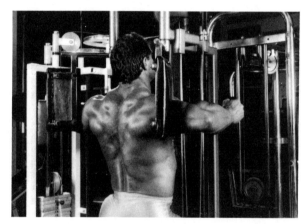

Pec-Deck Rear Delt Laterals

Movement Performance—Use rear delt strength to force your elbows to the rear in semicircular arcs as far back as comfortably possible. Hold this peak-contracted movement, then slowly return to the starting point.

Training Tips—This exercise can also be performed on a Nautilus rowing torso machine. With either variation, it can be performed with one arm at a time, which provides a more intense stress to the posterior heads of the deltoids. On each movement, you will most commonly do the exercise with your palms toward the floor, but it can also be performed with palms facing directly forward.

SUGGESTED DELTOID ROUTINES

If you are not an Olympia-level bodybuilder, you would undoubtedly overtrain and interrupt your progress if you tried the full deltoid routines of various champions with which I conclude this chapter. It is necessary to train for months, even years, with progressively more-involved routines in order to build up your recovery ability, before attempting the champions' shoulder routines.

If you are a beginner with less than 2–3 months of steady training under your belt, you can probably make your best gains from this routine performed three nonconsecutive days each week:

Exercise	Sets	Reps
Standing Barbell Presses	2–3	12–8*
Barbell Upright Rows	2–3	12–8*

On any exercise marked with an asterisk throughout this and the next section, you should pyramid your sets, increasing the weight and lowering the reps with each succeeding set.

A low-intermediate bodybuilder will make good progress with this training program, performed either two or three days per week:

Exercise	Sets	Reps
Seated Presses Behind Neck	3–4	12–6*
Dumbbell Side Laterals	2–3	8–10
Dumbbell Bent Laterals	3	8–10

If you are a high-intermediate bodybuilder, I recommend this workout:

Exercise	Sets	Reps
Seated Smith Machine Front Presses	3–4	12–5*
Nautilus Side Laterals	3	8–10
Seated Bent Laterals	3	8–10
Cable Upright Rows	2–3	12–8*

Continuing with our intensity progression, you can use this shoulder-training routine when you become an advanced bodybuilder:

Exercise	Sets	Reps
One-Arm Dumbbell Side Laterals	3–4	8–10
Seated Smith Machine Presses Behind Neck	4–5	12–5*
Cable Bent Laterals	3–4	8–10
Standing Barbell Presses	3–4	8–10

The foregoing deltoid program is very similar to what you might be doing in the off-season for the rest of your bodybuilding career. The primary allowance at the contest level of bodybuilding is only to double up on movements for whichever part of your shoulder-muscle complex is most weak. And this is just another instance of using the Weider Muscle Priority Training Principle to balance the development of a contest-level bodybuilder.

DELTOID ROUTINES OF THE CHAMPIONS

In this concluding section of my discussion of delt development, I am listing more than 30 shoulder routines of various IFBB superstar bodybuilders. You can use them either as something upon which you can model your own workout programs, or exactly as they are written and used by the champs themselves.

Frank Zane

Exercise	Sets	Reps
Universal Front Presses	5	15–6*
Dumbbell Upright Rows	5	15–8*
One-Arm Dumbbell Side Laterals	4–5	8–12
Dumbbell Bent Laterals	4–5	8–12

Weights and reps are pyramided on exercises marked with an asterisk anywhere in this section.

Albert Beckles

Exercise	Sets	Reps
Seated Dumbbell Presses	4	10
{ Dumbbell Side Laterals	4	12
{ Smith Machine Seated Front Presses	4	12
{ Barbell Upright Rows	4	12
{ One-Arm Cable Side Laterals	4	12
Barbell Incline Front Raises	4	12
Dumbbell Bent Laterals	4	12
Barbell Shrugs	4	12

Exercises enclosed by brackets are supersetted.

Lou Ferrigno

Exercise	Sets	Reps
Smith Machine Front Presses	4	8-10
One-Arm Cable Side Laterals	4	8-10
Cable Bent Laterals	4	8-10
Pulley Upright Rows	4	8-10

This is one of Lou's off-season shoulder routines.

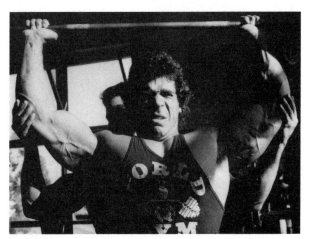

One way Lou Ferrigno got his delts: Seated Presses Behind the Neck with forced reps from a training partner, who cups his elbows to help pull up against the weight when the going gets tough!

Charles Glass

OFF-SEASON ROUTINE

Exercise	Sets	Reps
Seated Presses Behind Neck	3-4	10-6*
Dumbbell Side Laterals	4	10
Machine Shrugs	4	10
Barbell Upright Rows	4	10
Dumbbell Bent Laterals	4	10
Seated Machine Front Presses	4	10
Dumbbell Alternate Front Raises	4	10

PRECONTEST ROUTINE

Exercise	Sets	Reps
Seated Presses Behind Neck	4	15-20
Dumbbell Side Laterals	4	15-20
Machine Shrugs (Universal)	4	15-20
Barbell Upright Rows	4	15-20
Dumbbell Bent Laterals	4	15-20
Seated Machine Front Presses	4	15-20
Dumbbell Alternate Front Raises	4	15-20

Bob Paris

DAY 1

Exercise	Sets	Reps
Dumbbell Side Laterals	4	8-10*
Seated Barbell Front Presses	4	12-15
Barbell Upright Rows	4	8-10
Dumbbell Bent Laterals	4	8-12

DAY 2

Exercise	Sets	Reps
Dumbbell Side Laterals	3	12-15
Universal Seated Front Presses	3	12-20
Barbell Upright Rows	3	12-20
Prone Incline Dumbbell Laterals	3	12-20

The sets listed for the exercise marked with an asterisk are followed by a descending set with four weight drops, 8-12 reps with each weight. The program listed for Day 2 is often giant setted, or done with no rest between movements until all four exercises have been completed, then followed by a rest interval between giant sets of 2-3 minutes.

Lee Haney

Exercise	Sets	Reps
Seated Presses Behind Neck	4	10-5*
Front Barbell Raises	4	10-6*
Dumbbell Side Laterals	3	8-10
Dumbbell Bent Laterals	3	8-10
Dumbbell Shrugs	3	10-15

Mike Christian

Exercise	Sets	Reps
Barbell Upright Rows	4-5	10-12
Machine Side Laterals	4-5	10-12
Smith Machine Seated Presses Behind Neck	4-5	10
Smith Machine Seated Front Presses	4-5	10
Dumbbell Bent Laterals	4-5	10-12

Frank Richard

Exercise	Sets	Reps
Seated Bent Laterals	3	18-8
Cable Bent Laterals	3	18-8
Dumbbell Side Laterals	3	18-8
Smith Machine Seated Presses Behind Neck	3	18-8
Seated Dumbbell Presses	3	18-8
Cable Upright Rows	3	18-8
Dumbbell Shrugs	3	18-8

On each exercise, Frank decreases the number of reps and increases the weight used for the movement.

Boyer Coe

Exercise	Sets	Reps
One-Arm Cable Side Laterals	2	10
Prone Incline Laterals	2	10
Seated Front Machine Presses	4	8
Dumbbell Shrugs	2	15
Barbell Shrugs	4	10

Jacques Neuville

Exercise	Sets	Reps
Seated Presses Behind Neck	5	10-12
Seated Dumbbell Bent Laterals	5	10-12
One-Arm Cable Side Laterals	5	10-12
Barbell Upright Rows	5	10-12

Lee Labrada

Exercise	Sets	Reps
Dumbbell Side Laterals	3	10
Seated Presses Behind Neck	3	10
Seated Dumbbell Bent Laterals	3	10

Mohamed Makkawy

Exercise	Sets	Reps
Seated Presses Behind Neck	2-3	12-15
Seated Barbell Front Presses	2-3	12-15
{ Alternate Dumbbell Presses	2-3	12-15
{ Seated Dumbbell Bent Laterals	2-3	12-15

Tom Platz

DAY ONE

(WITH CHEST ROUTINE)

Exercise	Sets	Reps
Barbell Upright Rows	5-8	15-6*
Barbell Seated Front Presses	5-8	15-6*
One-Arm Dumbbell Side Laterals	5-8	15-6*
One-Arm Cable Side Laterals	5-8	15-6*

DAY TWO

(WITH BACK ROUTINE)

Exercise	Sets	Reps
Smith Machine Presses Behind Neck	5-8	15-6*
Dumbbell Bent Laterals	5-8	15-6*

Andreas

Exercise
Seated Presses Behind Neck
Dumbbell Side Laterals
Seated Dumbbell Bent Laterals
Barbell Front Raises
One-Arm Cable Side Laterals

Ron Teufel

Exercise	Sets
Nautilus Rear Delt Laterals	4
Seated Presses Behind Neck	4
Standing Dumbbell Presses	4
Dumbbell Side Laterals	4
Dumbbell Shrugs	4
Seated Dumbbell Bent Laterals	3

Dennis Tinerino

Exercise	Sets	Reps
Machine Seated Front Presses	6	6-8
Rotating Dumbbell Shrugs	4	10-15
Standing Dumbbell Presses	4	6-8
One-Arm Cable Side Laterals	5	8-10
Standing Dumbbell Bent Laterals	5	8-10

Larry Scott

Exercise	Sets	Reps
{ Standing Dumbbell Presses	4-5	6
{ Prone Incline Dumbbell Laterals	4-5	6-8
{ Cable Bent Laterals	4-5	6-8
One-Arm Dumbbell Side Laterals	5	8

Exercises enclosed by bracket are supersetted. After a warm-up, Larry starts with his heaviest poundage in each movement, then steps the weight down every time he comes back to the same exercise.

Casey Viator

Exercise	Sets	Reps
Dumbbell Side Laterals	4-5	10-15
Seated Dumbbell Bent Laterals	4-5	10-15
Seated Presses Behind Neck	6-8	15-5*
Nautilus Side Laterals	4-5	10-15
Nautilus Rear Delt Raises	4-5	10-15
Seated Smith Machine Front Presses	5-6	10-15

Bill Grant

Exercise	Sets	Reps
Dumbbell Side Laterals	5	8–10
~chine Front Presses	5	8–10
ll Upright Rows	5	8–10
~mbbell Bent Laterals	5	8–10

Ray Mentzer

Exercise	Sets	Reps
Nautilus Side Laterals	2	6–8
Barbell Front Presses	2	6–8
Nautilus Rear Delt Raises	2	6–8

The first two exercises are done with forced reps and negatives.

Dr. Franco Columbu

Exercise	Sets	Reps
Seated Dumbbell Side Laterals	4	10
Dumbbell Bent Laterals	6	10
Seated Presses Behind Neck	4	8
Dumbbell Alternate Front Raises	3	8
One-Arm Pulley Side Laterals	3	10

Cahling

Sets	Reps
2–3	8–12
2–3	8–12
2–3	8–12
2–3	8–12
1–2	8–12

Reps		Reps
8–10		
8–10	4	8–10
8–10	3–4	8–10
8–10	3–4	8–10
10		

Baldwin

	Sets	Reps
~d Neck	5	6–10
~aterals	5	8–10
~ Rows	5	8–10
~resses	3	6–10
Front Raises	3	8–10

381

25
Titanic Triceps Training

During the early years of the sport of body-building—back in the 1920s, 1930s, and 1940s—virtually all bodybuilders were also weightlifters. They did the three Olympic lifts (military presses, snatches, and cleans and jerks) as the bulk of their routines, then specialized on muscles like the pectorals and biceps which weren't directly stressed by the Olympic three toward the end of each workout.

Since these men were doing plenty of military presses and pressing assistance exercises like presses behind neck, seated dumbbell presses, and high-incline presses, they almost invariably had terrific triceps development. All overhead pressing movements place primary emphasis on the anterior heads of the deltoids, but intense secondary stress is on triceps throughout the full range of motion of each pressing exercise. So, it stands to reason that such bodybuilders had exceptional triceps development, even though they performed no direct isolation exercises for the muscle group.

Today's bodybuilders do plenty of isolation exercises in their triceps workouts, but much of their development in this muscle group still comes from pressing exercises, whether they acknowledge the fact or not. Whenever you do bench presses, inclines, declines, or dips for pectorals, you are also stressing your triceps. And whenever you do any type of overhead presses for deltoids, you are placing intense stress on your triceps muscles as well. Thus, the potential for overtraining is high when it comes to training triceps, because these arm muscles come into play in so many chest and shoulder exercises. And to aggravate the problem, they are also relatively small muscles that are even more easily overtrained than larger body parts like chest or lats.

You'll read a lot of articles about upper-arm training, stories written by top champs. Most of them will tell you that because the triceps muscles are about 40% larger than the biceps, they should receive about 40% more sets than you use to train biceps. If your triceps weren't involved in so many exercises for other body parts, I'd go along with that notion. But in most cases,

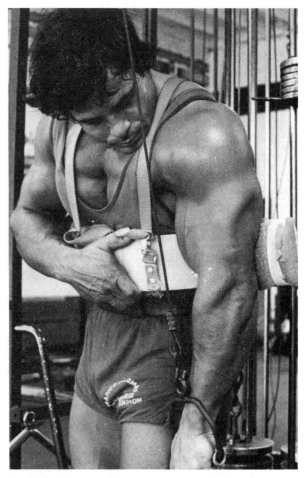

Two-time Mr. Olympia, Dr. Franco Columbu, carves out a horseshoe-shaped triceps on one arm doing Pushdowns using a Weider Arm Blaster unit.

training triceps with so many extra sets would inevitably lead to an overtrained condition.

How many sets of triceps work should you be doing in your workouts? At the beginning level of bodybuilding training, you will probably make great gains on only 3–5 total sets of triceps work. With between 3–6 months of steady training, you can probably increase this total to 5–7 sets. And even as an advanced bodybuilder, you will probably need to do no more than 8–10 total sets during an off-season cycle, and no more than 10–12 when peaking for a competition.

If you stick to the foregoing guidelines for total sets and also train very intensely, you will make great gains in triceps muscle mass and quality. Within a few years, you will probably have a set of titanic triceps the envy of everyone in the gym where you train.

TRICEPS ANATOMY AND KINESIOLOGY

I'm a big believer in studying the structure (anatomy) and function (kinesiology) of each muscle group prior to commencing a program of specialized training for that body part. In the case of triceps, the anatomy and kinesiology is very simple.

The triceps is a three-headed muscle complex that originates from insertion points at your shoulder and inserts via a large, band-like tendon over the elbow to one of the forearm bones. The primary function of the triceps muscles is to straighten your arm from a fully or partially bent position. Secondarily, your triceps contract to pull your upper arm bone forward and downward in a semicircular arc from a position in which it is extended straight upward from your shoulder to one in which it is straight down at your side. This second triceps function is covered only by pullover movements, found in the pullover and press described later in this chapter.

TRICEPS TRAINING TIPS

Throughout this book I have been stressing the importance of doing predominantly basic exercises in the off-season and primarily isolation movements during a contest peaking phase. However, there are very few basic exercises for

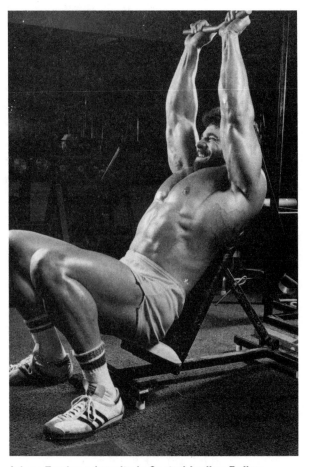

A Lou Ferrigno favorite is Seated Incline Pulley Triceps Extensions. He can usually be seen bombing away at the World Gym in Venice, Calif., when not off working on a film or television role.

triceps, so this advice more or less goes out the window when you are working triceps.

For the record, the basic movements for triceps are narrow-grip bench presses, pullovers and presses, triceps parallel bar dips, and reverse-grip bench presses. You can focus much of your triceps workout around these exercises during the off-season, then switch to almost all isolation movements—the rest of the triceps exercises described and illustrated in this chapter—when you enter a peaking cycle.

Rich Gaspari talks about supersets and triceps training: "Normally, you will compound a biceps exercise with a triceps movement when supersetting arms, but it *is* possible to do supersets just for triceps. A good pair of exercises which you can compound for triceps are pulley pushdowns and long cable triceps extensions using a high pulley. Do 6–8 reps of each movement, and you'll find you are really extending your triceps muscles to the limit!"

Mike Christian discusses his concept of the Weider Slow, Continuous Tension Training Principle in triceps training: "I normally use continuous tension on triceps when I'm in the final 6–8 weeks prior to a show, or during the classic peaking phase. And during that period, I use continuous tension on every set I perform for my triceps muscles.

"I guess it boils down really to *feeling* the exercise over its full range of motion, rather than allowing any kind of momentum to enter the movement and spoil its effect. To feel the movement optimally in the working triceps, you have to contract the antagonistic muscle group, which in this case is the biceps, and keep it contracted all of the way up and down in each triceps exercise. I also go to great lengths to build a great deal of tension into my working triceps as well.

"When you're stressing triceps correctly using continuous tension, you could almost get away with forgetting to use a weight. But adding in the resistance you use for each exercise really makes the muscles work hard. And that's what brings out the really deep striations across my triceps at contest time."

"The Weider Peak Contraction Training Principle is also important when you train triceps," says *Gary Strydom.* "If you have read much about exercise physiology, you know the muscle cells either contract completely or do not contract at all. This is called 'the all-or-nothing' model of muscle contraction. So, it should be obvious that the maximum possible number of muscle cells is contracted only when the muscles are fully flexed, or fully shortened. In the case of triceps, this occurs only when your arm is held straight and your triceps muscles are completely tensed.

"For peak contraction, you place a heavy weight on the working muscles when they are in the fully shortened state. But with most triceps exercises, there is no resistance at all on the muscles you are trying to work when they are in the fully contracted position. The only ways in which you can put weight on your triceps when they are completely shortened is to do either dumbbell kickbacks and/or triceps extensions on a machine which has a rotary cam such that there is heavy pressure on the working triceps muscles throughout the full range of motion of each repetition."

I'm always amazed when I see bodybuilders training upper arm muscle groups such as triceps *before* they bomb torso muscle groups which involve the arm muscles when doing basic exercises. If this is a little unclear, you won't want to program your triceps movements into your overall routine until *after* you have finished training both pectorals and deltoids. And the reason for this is readily apparent when you think about relative muscle size.

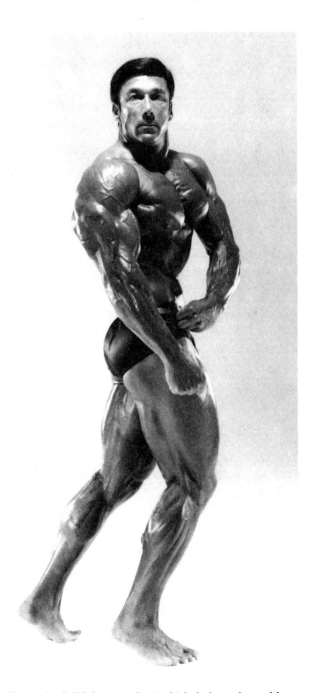

If you don't think a good set of tris help make a side-chest shot, look at this one from Boyer Coe!

"When you are doing bench presses for pectorals or standing barbell presses for deltoids," points out *Michael Ashley* (IFBB World Light-Heavyweight Champion and a leading professional bodybuilder), "you are also contracting your triceps quite powerfully as you do each repetition. But your triceps are markedly smaller than either the pectorals or deltoids. As a result, they are weaker than either of the torso muscle groups, and when you are doing a basic movement like benches or standing presses, the triceps actually fatigue completely and give out somewhat before the pecs or delts would otherwise cause you to miss a repetition.

"By choosing to use the Weider Pre-Exhaustion Training Principle for chest or shoulders, you can effectively weaken your torso muscle groups to the point where your triceps are temporarily so strong that you can push the pecs or delts to the absolute limit. But if you weaken your triceps first—as would happen if you trained arms before torso—you would make a bad situation much worse, in that you would never be able to push your chest and shoulder muscles hard enough to develop them to the limit. In effect, you would go around with great arms and no chest or shoulder development."

TRICEPS EXERCISES

In this section, I have illustrated and completely described more than 25 fundamental triceps exercises. And if you add in variations on these basic movements, you will have more than 50 triceps exercises which you can program into your workouts to build incredible triceps.

Narrow-Grip Bench Presses

Emphasis—As with normal medium-grip benches, narrow-grip bench presses place intense stress on the pectorals, anterior-medial deltoids, and triceps. But as you move your grip in toward the middle of the bar, you place

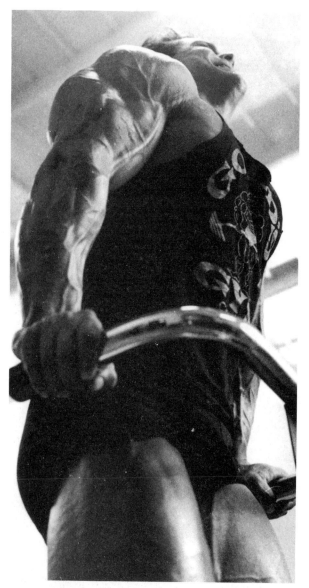

If you haven't seen Rich Gaspari work out (doing Triceps Dips in this case), you haven't seen pure bodybuilding intensity in action.

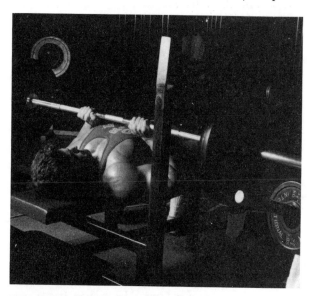

Narrow-Grip Bench Press (start)

Photos taken by Paula Crane at World Gym, Venice, California.   Model: Bob Paris

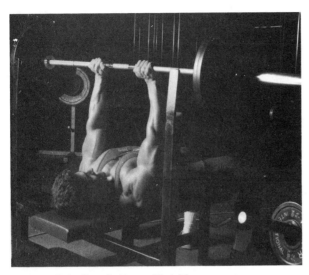

Narrow-Grip Bench Press (finish)

proportionately less stress on your pectorals and deltoids, and more on your triceps. Narrow-grip benches stress primarily the inner pecs rather than outer pectorals, as is the case with medium- and wide-grip benches.

Starting Position—Place a moderately heavy barbell on the support racks of a pressing bench and lie on your back on the bench with your shoulders 4-6 inches from the uprights. Your feet should be placed flat on the floor on either side of the bench to steady your body in position as you do the movement. Take a narrow overgrip in the middle of the bar, your index fingers 5-8 inches apart. With the assistance of your training partner, lift the weight from the rack to a position supported at straight arms' length directly above your upper chest.

Movement Performance—Being sure that your upper arms travel almost directly out to the sides in a crucifix position, slowly bend your arms and lower the bar downward and slightly forward until it lightly touches your lower chest. Without bouncing the bar, slowly push it back to the starting point.

Training Tips—This fine movement can also be performed on both incline and decline benches set at a relatively flat angle. Try occasionally varying the width of your grip on the bar to see how stress shifts to different parts of your pectorals, deltoids, and triceps.

Pullover-and-Presses

Emphasis—This is the most fundamental of all triceps exercises, as well as one of the best, particularly for the long inner head of your triceps. There is also considerable stress on the lats, pecs, and serratus muscles.

Starting Position—Lie on your back on a flat exercise bench, your head at one end and your feet pressed flat on the floor on each side of the bench to balance yourself as you do the movement. Have your training partner lift a moderately heavy barbell up to a position at straight arms' length above your upper chest. Have him bear all of the weight until you have taken a narrow overgrip in the middle of the bar, 5-8 inches between your index fingers.

Movement Performance—Slowly lower the bar down to your chest, as in the descent portion of the previous exercise. When the bar reaches

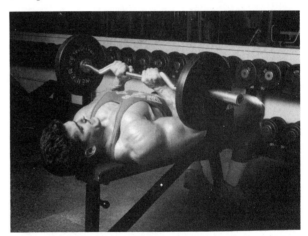

Pullover-and-Press (start)

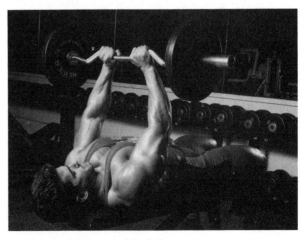

Pullover-and-Press (midpoint)

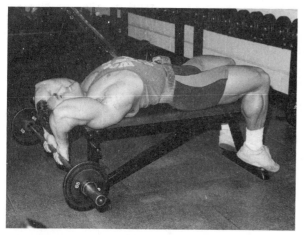

Pullover-and-Press (finish)

your chest, pull your elbows toward the mid-line of your body and then slowly lower it past your face in a semicircular arc to as low a position behind your head as comfortably possible. Without bouncing the weight in this bottom position, slowly reverse the movement and pull the weight back along the same arc to your chest. Finally straighten your arms, as in the second phase of narrow-grip bench presses.

Training Tips—If you fail to keep your elbows as close together as possible during the pullover part of this movement (i.e., you allow them to splay out to the sides), you place your shoulder joints in a weak mechanical position in which they might be easily injured.

Reverse-Grip Bench Presses

Emphasis—This movement stresses the same muscle groups as normal bench presses—pectorals, anterior delts, and triceps—but places considerably more stress on the triceps muscles.

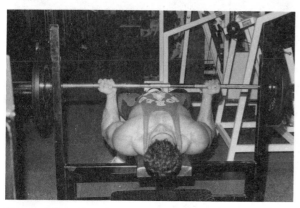

Reverse-Grip Bench Press (midpoint)

Starting Position—Place a moderately heavy barbell on the support rack of a pressing bench. Lie on your back on the bench, your head about 4-6 inches from the supports and your feet pressed flat on the floor to balance your body on the bench as you perform the movement. Take a shoulder-width undergrip on the bar, and have your training partner help you to lift the weight from the rack to a position supported at straight arms' length above your upper chest.

Movement Performance—Being certain that your elbows are kept close to the sides of your torso, slowly lower the barbell downward to lightly touch the middle of your chest. Avoid bouncing the bar off your chest as you reverse the movement and press the barbell back up to the starting point.

Training Tips—You will eventually be able to use substantial poundages on this movement, but take your time and learn how to do it correctly before you start piling on the plates. You should experiment with a variety of grip widths.

Triceps Parallel Bar Dips

Emphasis—This is usually thought of as a pectoral exercise, and when performed with the torso inclined forward it places very intense stress on the lower-outer pecs, anterior deltoids, and triceps. But when performed with the torso erect, this is one of the best triceps movements. It places correspondingly more stress on the triceps and less on pectorals.

Starting Position—Jump up to a supported position on the parallel bars, your palms facing inward, arms straight, legs bent, and ankles crossed. Be sure to keep your torso perfectly erect throughout the movement.

Movement Performance—Slowly bend your arms and lower yourself as far down between the bars as possible. Without bouncing in the bottom position, slowly straighten your arms and push yourself back to the starting point.

Training Tips—If you have parallel bars that angle inward at one end, you can experi-

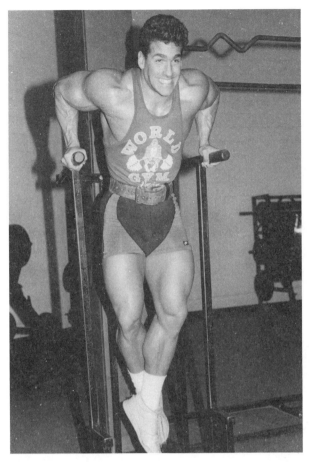

Triceps Parallel Bar Dips (midpoint)

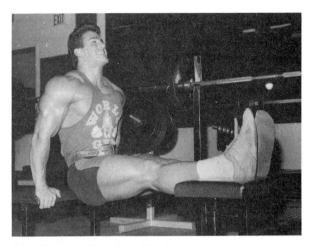

Dips Between Benches (start)

Movement Performance—Slowly bend your arms as completely as possible and lower your butt as far below the level of the two benches as possible. Slowly straighten your arms and return to the starting point.

Training Tips—To add resistance to this exercise, you can have your training partner either press downward on your shoulders, or place a dumbbell in your lap.

Lying Barbell Triceps Extensions

Emphasis—One of the most fundamental of all triceps movements, lying triceps extensions isolate stress on the triceps muscles, particularly on the medial and outer heads.

Starting Position—Take a narrow overgrip in the middle of the handle of a moderately weighted barbell. Lie on your back on a flat

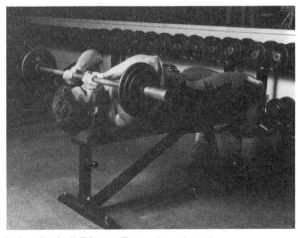

Lying Barbell Triceps Extensions (start)

ment with different widths of grip on the bars. When you become strong enough to use extra weight on this movement, you can hang a light dumbbell between your legs by looping a length of rope or nylon webbing around your waist and suspending the dumbbell in the bottom part of the loop.

Dips Between Benches

Emphasis—This is a good triceps movement, particularly for the short outer head of the muscle complex. Minimal assistance is provided by the lower-outer pectorals and anterior deltoids.

Starting Position—Place two flat exercise benches parallel to each other and 2–2½ feet apart. Place your hands close together on the bench behind yourself, fingers pointed toward your feet. Place your heels on the other bench. Assume a torso-leg angle of about 90-degrees and maintain this angle throughout your set. Straighten your arms fully.

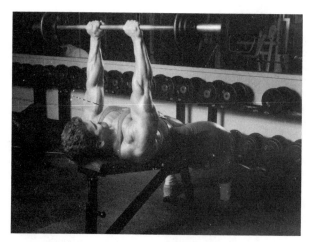

Lying Barbell Triceps Extensions (finish)

exercise bench with your feet set flat on the floor on either side of the bench to balance your body as you do the movement. Extend your arms directly upward from your shoulders. Be sure your arms are straight at the beginning of the movement.

Movement Performance—Keeping your upper arms motionless throughout your set, slowly bend your arms and allow the barbell to travel to the rear and downward in a semicircular arc until it lightly touches your forehead. Use triceps strength to reverse direction and move the barbell back along the same arc to the starting point.

Training Tips—You can vary the grip width from one as narrow as hands touching in the middle of the bar, out to one as wide as about shoulder width. You can also use an undergrip on the bar, shifting the width of your grip width from narrow to one of about medium width.

Standing Barbell Triceps Extensions

Emphasis—This is another fundamental triceps exercise. It particularly stresses the inner and medial heads of the triceps muscle complex.

Starting Position—Take a narrow overgrip in the middle of the handle of a moderately weighted barbell. Set your feet about shoulder width apart and stand erect, extending your arms straight up from your shoulders.

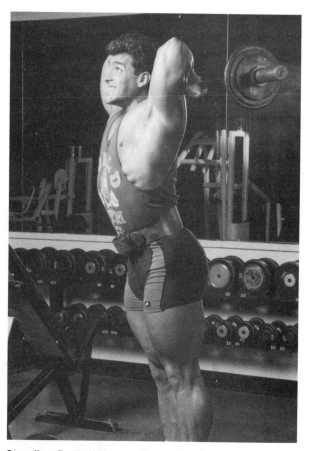

Standing Barbell Triceps Extensions (start)

Movement Performance—Keeping your upper arms motionless, slowly bend your arms and lower the barbell to the rear and downward in a semicircular arc until your arms are completely bent. Without bouncing the weight in the bottom position, use triceps strength to move it back along the same arc to the starting point.

Training Tips—As with lying triceps extensions, you can vary the width of your grip on the bar or use an undergrip when you do the movement. All grip variations can also be used when performing the exercise seated at the end of a flat exercise bench. Doing seated barbell triceps extensions isolates your legs from the movement and makes it somewhat more strict than the standing variation.

Incline/Decline Barbell Triceps Extensions

Emphasis—The basic triceps extension movement can also be performed while lying on incline or decline benches. The incline variation isolates stress on the triceps, particularly on the inner and medial heads of the muscle complex. Decline triceps extensions stress the triceps muscle complex, particularly the medial and outer heads.

Starting Position—I will describe the movement performed on an incline bench; from that description, you will have no trouble also learning how to do the version performed on a decline bench. Take a narrow overgrip in the middle of the handle of a moderately weighted barbell (there should be about 4–6 inches of space showing between your index fingers when you have the correct grip). Lie back on the incline bench, sitting on the bench seat if it has one. Extend your arms directly upward from your shoulders.

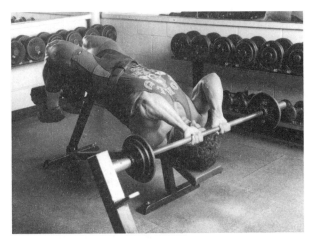

Decline Barbell Triceps Extensions (start)

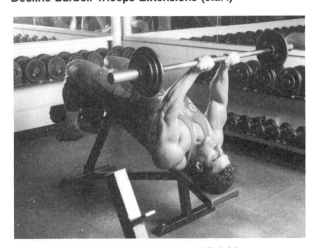

Decline Barbell Triceps Extensions (finish)

Movement Performance—Keeping your upper arms motionless, slowly bend your arms and lower the barbell to the rear and downward in a

semicircular arc until the barbell handle touches your forehead (or a position on the bench behind your head). Without bouncing the bar in the bottom position, use triceps strength to move the barbell back along the same arc to the starting point.

Training Tips—Experiment with an undergrip, as well as with a variety of grip widths on the bar.

Kneeling Barbell Triceps Extensions

Emphasis—Very similar to both standing and seated barbell triceps extensions, this movement stresses the entire triceps muscle complex, but particularly the inner and medial heads of the muscle group.

Starting Position—Kneel down on the gym floor facing a moderately weighted barbell lying on the floor. Take a narrow overgrip in the middle of the barbell handle (there should be

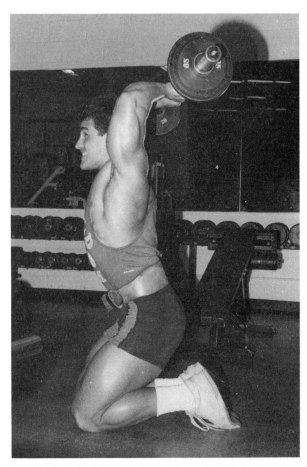

Kneeling Barbell Triceps Extensions (midpoint)

4–6 inches of space showing between your index fingers when you have taken the correct width of grip). Kneeling erect, pull the barbell to your chest and push it to straight arms' length directly above your shoulder joints.

Movement Performance—Keeping your upper arms motionless throughout your set, slowly bend your arms and allow the barbell to move to the rear and downward in a semicircular arc until your arms are completely bent. Use triceps to reverse the direction of movement and return the barbell back along the same arc to the starting point.

Training Tips—Experiment with both an undergrip on the barbell handle and with various grip widths.

One-Arm Dumbbell Triceps Extensions

Emphasis—This basic triceps movement stresses the entire triceps muscle complex, particularly the inner and medial heads of the muscle group.

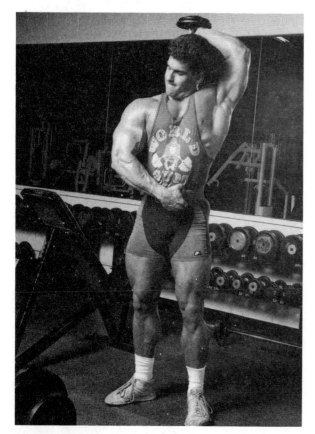

One-Arm Dumbbell Triceps Extensions (midpoint—can also be performed seated)

Starting Position—Grasp a moderately weighted dumbbell in your left hand. Place your feet a comfortable distance apart and stand erect. Extend your left arm directly upward from your shoulder joint, your palm facing toward the front. You can reach behind your head and grasp your left upper arm with your right hand to brace it in position as you do the movement.

Movement Performance—Being sure to keep your left upper arm motionless throughout your set, slowly bend your left arm and lower the dumbbell to the rear and somewhat across the midline of your body, describing a semicircular arc with the weight. Terminate the movement when your arm is as fully bent as possible, then use triceps strength to return the dumbbell back along the same arc to the starting point. Be sure to do an equal number of sets and reps with each arm.

Training Tips—This movement can also be performed while either sitting at one end of a flat exercise bench or kneeling on the gym floor, as well as while lying on an incline, flat, or decline bench. Each of these variations are somewhat more strict than the standing version of the exercise. Regardless of the body position you employ, you can experiment with lowering the dumbbell to the rear along various arcs, either directly to the rear or more across the midline of your body.

Two-Dumbbell Triceps Extensions

Emphasis—This movement can be performed while standing, seated, or kneeling, as well as lying on incline, flat, and decline benches. All variations stress the entire triceps muscle complex. Standing, kneeling, and incline variations place more stress on the inner and medial heads of the muscle group, while lying and decline variations place more stress on the medial and outer heads of the muscle group.

Starting Position—I will describe the variation performed lying on your back on a flat exercise bench; from this exercise description, you can easily learn the movement as performed while standing, kneeling, or lying on incline and decline benches. Grasp two moderately weighted dumbbells and lie back on a flat

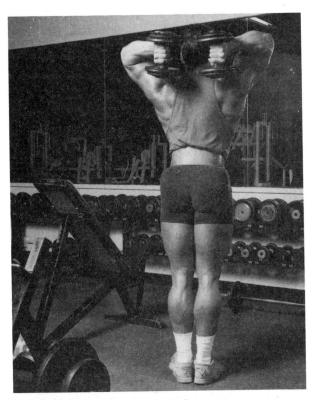

Two-Dumbbell Triceps Extensions (start)

exercise bench, your feet placed flat on the floor on either side of the bench to balance your body on the bench as you do your set. Extend your arms straight up from your shoulders, your palms facing each other.

Movement Performance—Keeping your upper arms motionless throughout your set, slowly lower the dumbbells directly to the rear (toward your head) in semicircular arcs until your arms are as fully bent as possible. Use triceps strength to return the dumbbells back along the same arcs to the starting point.

Training Tips—In addition to experimenting with various body positions on this exercise, you can also rotate your wrists so your hands are pronated as you perform your sets. Each body position and hand orientation places somewhat different stresses on the working triceps muscles.

One-Dumbbell Triceps Extensions

Emphasis—As with one-arm dumbbell triceps extensions of various types, this movement stresses the entire triceps muscle complex, but particularly the inner and medial heads of the muscle group.

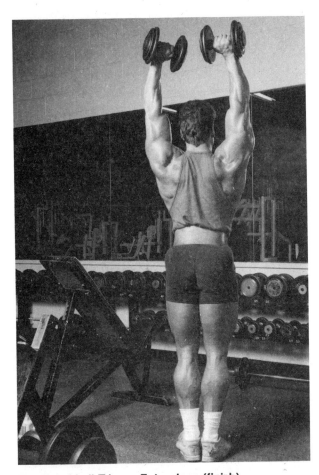

Two-Dumbbell Triceps Extensions (finish)

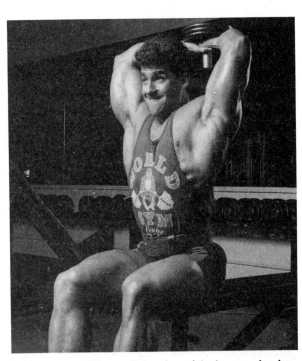

One-Dumbbell Triceps Extensions (start—can also be done standing)

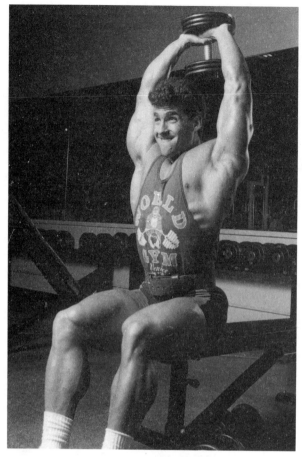

One-Dumbbell Triceps Extensions (finish)

Starting Position—Take a grip on a moderately weighted dumbbell so when the handle is hanging straight down (perpendicular to the gym floor), your palms are resting flat against the underside of the upper set of plates. Encircle the dumbbell handle with your thumbs to keep the weight from slipping from your hands as you do the movement. Set your feet about shoulder width apart, and stand erect. Pull the dumbbell upward until it is at straight arms' length directly above your head. Press your upper arms against the sides of your head and keep them motionless.

Movement Performance—Lower the weight to the rear in a semicircular arc until your arms are fully bent. Use triceps strength to return the weight back along the same arc to the starting point.

Training Tips—In order to make this movement more strict, you can do it while either sitting at the end of a flat exercise bench, or on the gym floor with your back braced against the end of the bench.

Pulley Pushdowns

Emphasis—This fundamental triceps movement places intense stress on the entire triceps, but particularly on the medial and outer heads of the muscle group.

Starting Position—While you can do pushdowns with a long, straight lat machine bar, it is best performed with a short bar angled downward at both ends, a handle which was specifically developed for this exercise. Attach the bar handle to the end of a cable running through an overhead pulley. Take an overgrip on the handle, your index fingers no more than 3–5 inches apart in the middle of the handle. Set your feet about shoulder width apart, 10–12 inches back from the handle. Bend your arms fully and press your upper arms against the sides of your torso, where they must rest throughout your set. In this position, the bar will be just below your chin. Lean slightly forward at the waist and maintain this torso position throughout your set.

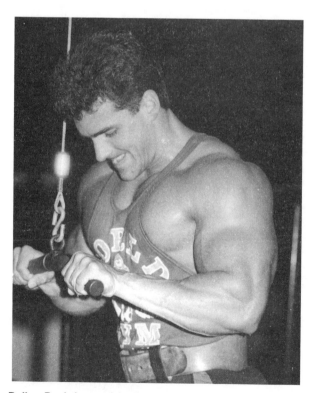

Pulley Pushdowns (start)

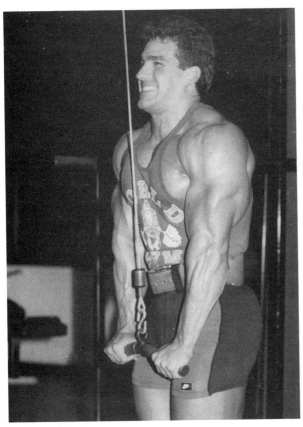

Pulley Pushdowns (finish)

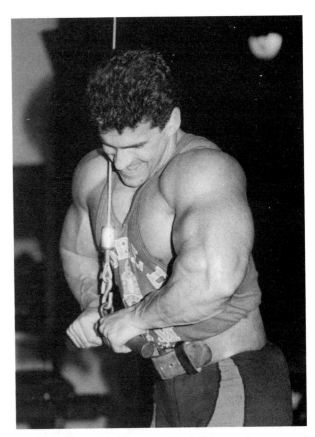

Power Pulley Pushdowns (midpoint)

Movement Performance—Moving only your forearms, slowly straighten your arms. Hold the straight-armed position for a moment, intensely tensing your triceps muscles. Slowly return the pulley handle back along the same arc to the starting point.

Training Tips—A very good variation of this movement can be performed with a rope handle which allows you to assume a parallel-hands grip as you do the movement. If you don't have a rope handle like this, you can loop a towel over the normal pulley handle and grasp the ends of the handle with a parallel-hands grip. You can also do this exercise with an undergrip on the handle. You should also experiment with a variety of grip widths on the pulley handle.

Power Pushdowns

Emphasis—Pioneered by Larry Scott, power pushdowns intensely stress the entire triceps muscle complex, particularly the outer heads of the muscles.

Starting Position—Attach the angled, short bar handle to the end of a cable running through an overhead pulley. Take an overgrip on the handle, your index fingers no more than 3–5 inches apart in the middle of the handle. Set your feet about shoulder width apart, 10–12 inches back from the pulley handle. Pull the handle forward and downward until it is at straight arms' length directly below your shoulders. You should lean forward at the waist and maintain this torso lean throughout your set. The cable can be running upward at either side of your head.

Movement Performance—Allowing your elbows to flare out to the sides, slowly bend your arms as completely as possible, the handle reaching a position at about mid-chest level. Without cheating with torso movement, slowly press the pulley handle back to the starting point.

Training Tips—Experiment with a variety of grip widths, out to one as wide as shoulder width.

Reverse Pulley Pushdowns

Emphasis—A favorite exercise of ageless Albert Beckles, this movement places intense stress on the triceps muscle complex, particularly the medial and outer heads of the muscle group.

Starting Position—Attach a short, straight bar handle to the end of a cable running through an overhead pulley. Set your feet about shoulder width apart, 10–12 inches from the pulley, with your back toward the pulley. Have a training partner pull the bar handle down so you can assume a narrow overgrip in the middle of the handle (there should be 3–5 inches of space showing between your index fingers when you have the correct grip), the handle behind your buttocks. Straighten your arms completely. Keep your torso erect as you perform your set.

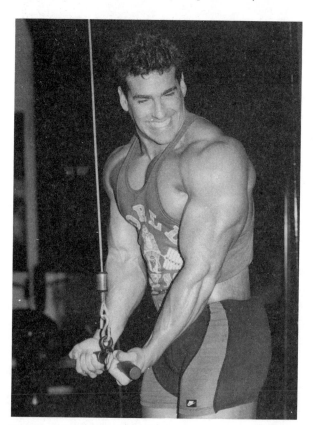

Reverse-Grip Pulley Pushdowns (near finish)

Movement Performance—Being sure to keep the handle in close to your back and allowing your elbows to move out to the sides, slowly bend your arms as completely as possible. Use triceps strength to push the pulley handle back to the starting position.

Training Tips—Experiment with a variety of grip widths, from one as narrow as hands touching out to as wide as shoulder width.

One-Arm Pulley Pushdowns

Emphasis—As with normal pulley pushdowns, the one-armed variation stresses the entire triceps muscle complex, particularly the medial and outer heads of the muscle group. However, you will find that when you no longer must split your mental focus between two arms, you will add more mental and physical intensity to each set you perform.

Starting Position—Attach a loop handle to the end of a cable running through an overhead pulley. Set your feet about shoulder width apart, 10–12 inches back from the pulley. Grasp the pulley handle in your left hand, bend your left arm fully, and press your left upper arm against the side of your torso, where it must remain throughout your set. Rotate your wrist so your palm is facing forward throughout your set. Bend slightly forward at the waist and maintain this torso lean throughout your set. You can place your free hand on your hip.

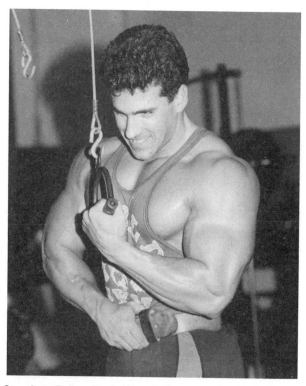

One-Arm Pulley Pushdown (palm-up variation—start)

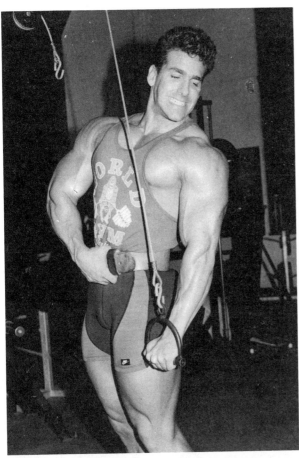

One-Arm Pulley Pushdown (palm-down variation—finish)

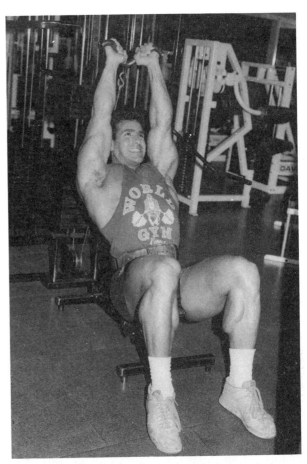

Incline Cable Triceps Extension (finish)

Movement Performance—Moving only your forearm, slowly straighten your left arm. Hold this straight-armed position for a moment while intensely flexing your triceps muscles. Return the pulley handle slowly back along the same arc to the starting point. Be sure to complete the same number of sets and reps for each arm.

Training Tips—You can also do this exercise with your wrist rotated so your palm is facing inward toward the midline of your body as you perform the movement.

Incline Cable Triceps Extensions

Emphasis—This movement is excellent for stressing the entire triceps muscle complex, particularly the inner head.

Starting Position—Attach a short bar handle (preferably the type that angles downward at each end) to the end of a cable running through

a floor pulley. Place a short incline bench (one on which your butt is very close to the floor when you are lying back on it) about 1½–2 feet from the pulley, the head end of the bench pointed directly toward the pulley. Take a narrow overgrip on the pulley handle and sit down on the bench, your back pressed flat against the angled surface of the bench. Pull the weighted end of the pulley cable upward so your arms are locked out straight and angled directly upward, perpendicular to the gym floor.

Movement Performance—Being sure to keep your upper arms motionless, bend your elbows and allow the pulley handle to descend in a semicircular arc toward the rear. When your arms are fully bent, use triceps strength to move the pulley handle back along the same arc to the starting point.

Training Tips—With a little ingenuity, you can also do this movement while lying on flat or decline benches.

Nautilus Triceps Extensions

Emphasis—This excellent machine movement places intense stress on the entire triceps muscle complex, particularly the inner and medial heads.

Starting Position—Adjust the height of the machine seat so your upper arms lie flat on the large angled pad when extending straight forward and up from your shoulders. Sit down on the seat, and press the sides of your wrists (palms facing each other) against the pads attached to the ends of the lever arms. Bend your arms fully and rest your upper arms in the corners formed by the large angled pad and the smaller vertical pads attached to the edges of the larger pad.

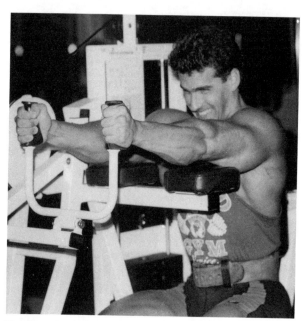

Nautilus-Type Triceps Extensions (finish)

Movement Performance—Use triceps strength to slowly straighten your arms. Hold this straight-armed position for a moment intensely flexing your triceps muscles. Slowly bend your arms and return to the starting point.

Training Tips—You can conveniently vary this movement to an alternate-arms version by first straightening both arms. Then while holding your right arm straight, you can fully bend and then straighten your left arm; then while holding your left arm straight, you can fully bend and then straighten your right arm.

High-Pulley, Long-Cable Triceps Extensions

Emphasis—This is one of the premier movements for stressing the long inner heads of the triceps muscles. It also stresses the medial head triceps very intensely and the outer triceps head somewhat less intensely.

Starting Position—Attach a short-angled bar handle to the end of a cable running through an overhead pulley. Take an overgrip on the handle, your index fingers 3–5 inches apart in its middle. Facing away from the weight stack, bend your arms fully with the cable running to one side of your head or the other, and walk 3–4 feet away from where the handle would normally hang. Split your legs fore and aft for maximum body stability as you do the movement. Bend forward at the waist so your torso is only slightly above a position parallel with the gym floor. When your arms are fully bent in this position, the handle should be approximately at the base of your neck.

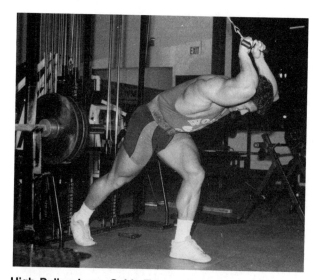

High-Pulley, Long-Cable Triceps Extension (start)

Movement Performance—Keeping your upper arms motionless, use triceps strength to move the handle forward and downward in a semicircular arc to a position in which your arms are straight. Hold this straight-armed position for a moment while powerfully tensing your triceps muscles. Slowly return the pulley handle back to the starting position at the base of your trap neck where it runs into your upper trapezius muscles.

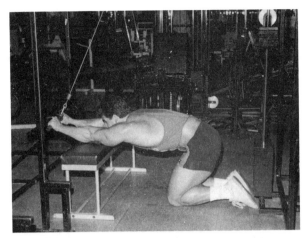

Kneeling High-Pulley, Long-Cable Triceps Extensions (finish)

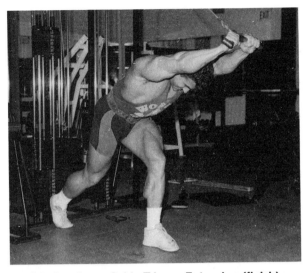

High-Pulley, Long-Cable Triceps Extension (finish)

Training Tips—With the bar handle you can experiment with a variety of grip widths, or even with an undergrip on the handle. You will find that a very intense form of this movement can be performed with a rope handle which allows a parallel-hands grip. A tremendous superset which intensely stresses all three heads of the triceps muscle complex consists of pulley pushdowns and high-pulley, long-cable triceps extensions.

Kneeling High-Pulley, Long-Cable Triceps Extensions

Emphasis—Another favorite arm exercise of two-time Mr. Olympia Larry Scott, this movement places intense stress on the entire triceps muscle complex, particularly on the inner and medial heads of the muscle group.

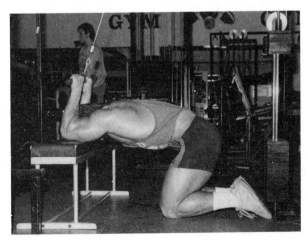

Kneeling High-Pulley, Long-Cable Triceps Extensions (start)

Starting Position—Place two flat exercise benches end to end (with the ends about 16–18 inches apart), 3–4 feet from where a short bar handle hangs from the end of a cable running through an overhead pulley. Take a narrow overgrip on the handle, 3–5 inches of space showing between your index fingers on the bar. Face away from the weight stack, then kneel down on the gym floor, leaning forward to rest your elbows on the ends of the two benches. Bend your arms fully, which will bring the pulley handle to a position at the base of your neck, where it runs into your traps.

Movement Performance—With your elbows braced on the benches so you cannot move your upper arms, slowly straighten your arms fully, holding the straight-armed position for a moment while intensely tensing your triceps muscles. Return the pulley handle back along the same semicircular arc to the starting point.

Training Tips—Try a variety of grip widths on the pulley handle, as well as an undergrip. You also can use the rope handle which permits a parallel-hands grip when you do the movement.

One-Arm High-Pulley, Long-Cable Triceps Extensions

Emphasis—As with the normal two-armed version of this movement, it stresses the entire triceps muscle complex, particularly the inner and medial heads of the muscle group.

Starting Position—Attach a loop handle to the end of a cable running through an overhead pulley. Grasp the handle in your left hand. Face away from the weight stack and step forward 3-4 feet, setting your feet fore and aft to balance yourself in position for the movement. Extend your left arm straight forward from your shoulder and position your torso slightly above parallel with the floor. Grasp your left elbow with your right hand to steady your left upper arm in a set position for your triceps extensions.

Movement Performance—With your palm facing forward throughout your set, slowly bend your left arm as fully as comfortably possible. Use triceps strength to return the pulley handle back along the same arc to the starting point. Be sure to do equal sets and reps for each arm.

Training Tips—This movement can also be performed with your hand fully supinated, or in a position where your palm faces the midline of your body throughout the set.

Barbell Triceps Kickbacks

Emphasis—This is a very intense triceps movement which particularly stresses the long inner head of the triceps muscles.

Starting Position—Take a shoulder-width overgrip on the handle of a moderately heavy barbell. Lie on your back on a flat exercise bench with your feet set flat on the floor on either side of the bench to brace your body in position for the exercise. The barbell should be resting in the middle of your chest, your arms fully bent.

Movement Performance—Slowly push the barbell directly to the rear, parallel with the gym floor, until your arms are fully straight. Hold this peak-contracted position for a moment while intensely flexing your triceps muscles. Slowly return the barbell back along the same path parallel with the gym floor to the starting point.

Training Tips—If you either deviate from the prescribed barbell movement arc, or are unable to straighten your arms, the weight is too heavy and should be reduced for your next set. You can experiment with a variety of grip widths from one as narrow as hands touching in the middle of the barbell handle outward to one in which your hands are set on the bar about shoulder width apart.

Dumbbell Triceps Kickbacks

Emphasis—All types of triceps kickback movements place a superior type of peak-contracted muscle stress on the triceps. Particular stress is placed on the inner and medial heads of the triceps muscle complex.

Starting Position—Grasp a light dumbbell in your left hand. Stand with your right side toward a flat exercise bench and bend over until your torso is parallel with the gym floor. Place

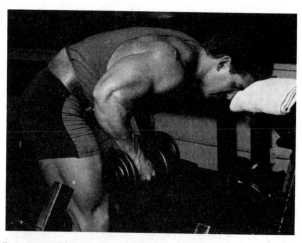

Dumbbell Triceps Kickbacks (two-dumbbell variation—start—note head braced on padded surface to steady body)

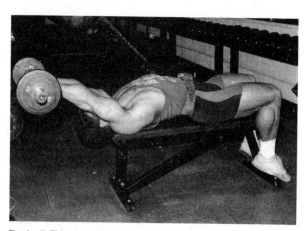

Barbell Triceps Kickback (finish)

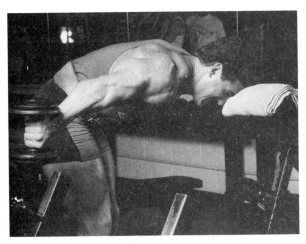

Dumbbell Triceps Kickback (finish)

your right hand on the exercise bench to brace your torso in position for your set. Press your left upper arm against the side of your torso so it is held parallel with the gym floor, and keep it in this position throughout your set. Bend your left arm at a 90-degree angle, so your forearm is perpendicular to the gym floor in the correct starting position. Rotate your wrist so your palm is facing the midline of your body throughout your set.

Movement Performance—Use triceps muscle strength to slowly straighten your left arm. Hold the straight-armed, peak-contracted position for a moment while intensely flexing your triceps muscles, then slowly return to the starting point. Be sure that you do an equal number of sets and reps with each arm.

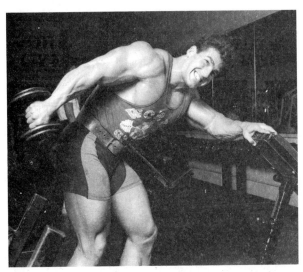

Dumbbell Triceps Kickback (one-dumbbell variation—finish)

Training Tips—You can also do this movement with your wrist rotated so your palm is facing either directly to the rear or forward as you do the exercise. You can perform dumbbell kickbacks while holding two dumbbells in your hands, bending forward until your torso is held parallel with the floor and extending your arms either simultaneously or alternatively, one weight going upward as the other descends.

Prone Incline Dumbbell Kickbacks

Emphasis—As with other variations of triceps kickbacks, this movement places a superior type of peak-contracted stress on the triceps muscle complex. Particular stress is placed on the inner and medial heads of the triceps.

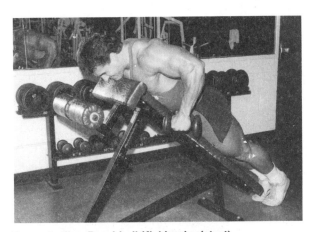

Prone Incline Dumbbell Kickbacks (start)

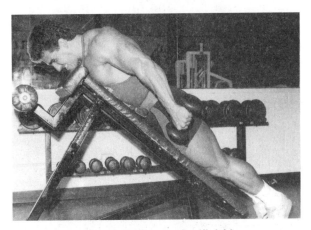

Prone Incline Dumbbell Kickbacks (finish)

Starting Position—Grasp two light dumbbells and lie facedown on an incline bench. With your palms facing each other throughout the movement, press your upper arms against the sides of your torso in a position as close to parallel with the floor as possible. Bend your arms at 90-degree angles.

Movement Performance—Moving only your forearms, slowly straighten your arms. Hold this straight-armed, peak-contracted position for a moment while intensely flexing your triceps muscles, then slowly return the weights back along the same arcs to the starting point.

Training Tips—You can also perform this movement with your palms facing either directly forward or directly to the rear as you do the exercise.

One-Arm Cable Triceps Kickbacks

Emphasis—As with dumbbell kickbacks, this movement places an intense form of peak-contracted stress on your triceps muscles, particularly on the inner and medial heads of the muscle complex.

Starting Position—Attach a loop handle to the end of a cable running through a floor pulley. Grasp the handle with your left hand, face toward the pulley, and set your feet about shoulder width apart, 3–4 feet back from the pulley. Bend forward at the waist and brace your right hand on your knee to maintain your torso in a position parallel with the floor. Bend your left arm fully and press your left upper arm against the side of your torso, holding it parallel with the floor and motionless throughout your set. Pronate your hand fully (i.e., turn

your wrist so your palm is facing toward the rear throughout your set).

Movement Performance—Use triceps strength to slowly straighten your left arm, moving the pulley handle in a semicircular arc from the starting position to one in which your arm is held straight and parallel with the floor. Hold this peak-contracted position for a moment, intensely contracting your triceps muscles, then slowly return the pulley handle back along the same arc to the starting point.

Training Tips—You can also do this movement with your palm facing the midline of your body, or with your hand fully supinated (i.e., with the palm of your hand facing forward throughout the movement).

SUGGESTED TRICEPS ROUTINES

As I have stressed many times throughout this book, one of the biggest mistakes most bodybuilders make is overtraining, or doing excessive numbers of total sets for a particular body part. If you attempted to use one of the champions' triceps routines at the end of this chapter without having at least a year of hard, steady training behind you, you would undoubtedly overtrain. Before you can use the routine of one of your favorite champions, you must pay your dues in the gym, gradually building up your recovery ability, until you are at the point where you can actually profit from such a highly intense training program.

Therefore, I am giving you four progressively more intense triceps training programs that you can use along the route toward a high-level physique of your own. You can use each of these routines for 6–8 weeks before moving on to the next one listed.

BEGINNING-LEVEL ROUTINE

Exercise	Sets	Reps
Close-Grip Bench Presses	3	12–6*
Pulley Pushdowns	2	8–12

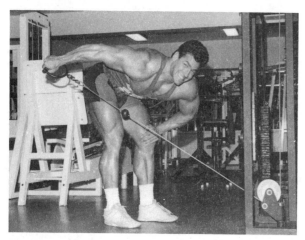

One-Arm Cable Triceps Kickbacks (finish)

Throughout this section and the next, exercises marked with an asterisk should have weights and repetitions pyramided, the poundage increased and reps decreased with each succeeding set.

LOW-INTERMEDIATE-LEVEL ROUTINE

Exercise	Sets	Reps
Triceps Parallel Bar Dips	3-4	12-6*
Incline Barbell Triceps Extensions	2-3	8-12

HIGH-INTERMEDIATE-LEVEL ROUTINE

Exercise	Sets	Reps
Single Dumbbell Seated Triceps Extensions	4	8-12
Decline Barbell Triceps Extensions	3	8-12
Pulley Pushdowns	2-3	8-12

ADVANCED-LEVEL ROUTINE

Exercise	Sets	Reps
Pullover-and-Presses	4	12-6*
Lying Barbell Triceps Extensions	4	8-12
Dumbbell Kickbacks	4	8-12

TRICEPS ROUTINES OF THE CHAMPIONS

In this concluding section, I present more than 25 triceps routines of the top champions of the sport. Rather than merely adopting the training program of a favorite champion set for set and rep for rep, you should use these training schedules as examples on which to base your own triceps-training programs. Take a little from the routine of each champion, adapt it to your own use, and ultimately you will profit maximally from formulating a triceps routine that perfectly suits your own unique bodybuilding needs.

Sergio Oliva

Exercise	Sets	Reps
Seated Barbell Triceps Extensions	6	10-15
One-Arm Dumbbell Triceps Extensions	6	10-15
Pulley Pushdowns	6	10-15

Roy Callender

Exercise	Sets	Reps
Pullover-and-Presses	6-8	8-10
Incline Pulley Triceps Extensions	5-6	8-10
Lying Dumbbell Triceps Extensions	5-6	8-10
High-Pulley, Long-Cable Triceps Extensions	4-5	10-12

Larry Scott

Exercise	Sets	Reps
Lying Triceps Extensions	4-6	6
High-Pulley, Long-Cable Triceps Extensions	4-6	6
Kneeling High-Pulley, Long-Cable Triceps Extensions	4-6	6

Bracketed exercises are supersetted. At least 4-6 burns are performed at the end of every set of this program.

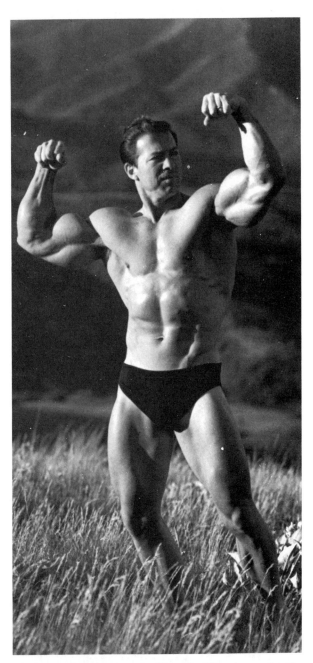

Winner of the first two Mr. Olympia titles, Larry Scott shows how a massively developed pair of triceps help to add to upper-arm mass.

Bertil Fox

Exercise	Sets	Reps
Pulley Pushdowns	4	8-10
Reverse Pulley Pushdowns	4	8-10
Lying Triceps Extensions (EZ-curl bar)	4	8-10
Parallel Bar Dips	4	8-12

Rod Koontz

Exercise	Sets	Reps
Pulley Pushdowns	4	8-12
Cable Triceps Extensions	4	6-8
Seated Single-Dumbbell Triceps Extensions	4-6	8-10

Casey Viator

Exercise	Sets	Reps
Lying Triceps Extensions (EZ-curl bar)	4	10-12
One-Arm Dumbbell Triceps Extensions	4	10-12
One-Arm Dumbbell Kickbacks	4	10-12
Seated Barbell Triceps Extensions	4	10-12

Lou Ferrigno

PRECONTEST

Exercise	Sets	Reps
Lying Triceps Extensions (EZ-curl bar)	4-5	10-12
Pulley Pushdowns	4-5	10-12
Incline Pulley Triceps Extensions	4-5	10-12
Seated Barbell Triceps Extensions	4-5	10-12
Triceps Parallel Bar Dips	4-5	10-12

OFF-SEASON

Exercise	Sets	Reps
Lying Triceps Extensions (EZ-curl bar)	5	8-12
Seated Single-Dumbbell Triceps Extensions	5	8-12
Pulley Pushdowns	5	8-12

Tim Belknap

Exercise	Sets	Reps
Close-Grip Bench Presses	3	10-12
Decline Barbell Triceps Extensions	3	10-12

Robby Robinson

Exercise	Sets	Reps
Seated Barbell Triceps Extensions	4	8-10
Lying Triceps Extensions (EZ-curl bar)	4	8-10
Pulley Pushdowns (angled handle)	4	8-10

Josef Grolmus

Exercise	Sets	Reps
Triceps Parallel Bar Dips	5	15-6*
Standing Single-Dumbbell Triceps Extensions	4	8-10
Lying Reverse-Grip Barbell Triceps Extensions	4	8-10
Barbell Kickbacks	4	10-12

Boyer Coe

Exercise	Sets	Reps
Pulley Pushdowns	3-4	8-10
Lying Triceps Extensions (EZ-curl bar)	3-4	8-10
One-Arm Dumbbell Triceps Extensions	3-4	8-10
One-Arm Dumbbell Triceps Kickbacks	3-4	8-10

Chris Dickerson

Exercise	Sets	Reps
Pulley Pushdowns	4	8
Seated Barbell Triceps Extensions	4	8
Standing High-Pulley, Long-Cable Triceps Extensions	4	10
Kneeling Pulley Pushdowns	2-3	10

John Hnatyschak

Exercise	Sets	Reps
Close-Grip Bench Presses	4-5	12-6*
Pulley Pushdowns	4	8-10
Seated One-Arm Dumbbell Triceps Extensions	3	8-10

Scott Wilson

Exercise	Sets	Reps
Lying Barbell Triceps Extensions	5	6-10
Close-Grip Bench Presses	5	6-10
Pulley Pushdowns	5	8-12

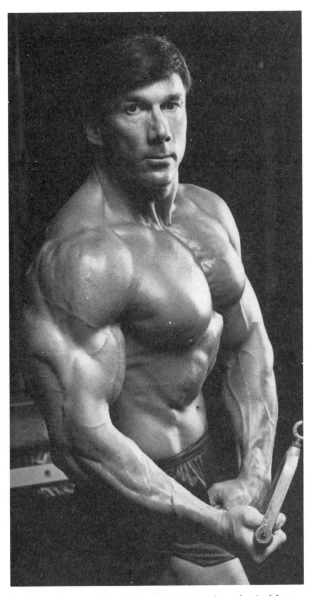

One-Arm Pulley Pushdowns with hand supinated is a favorite Boyer Coe triceps movement.

Rory Leidelmeyer

Exercise	Sets	Reps
Kneeling High-Pulley, Long-Cable Triceps Extensions	3	10
Standing High-Pulley, Long-Cable Triceps Extensions	3	10
Reverse-Grip Pulley Pushdowns	3	10
Dumbbell Kickbacks	3	12

Ron Love

Exercise	Sets	Reps
Pulley Pushdowns	4	8-10
Lying Barbell Triceps Extensions	4	8-10
Standing High-Pulley, Long-Cable Triceps Extensions	4	8-10
Dumbbell Kickbacks	4	8-10

John Terilli

Exercise	Sets	Reps
Lying Barbell Triceps Extensions	4	8-12
Pulley Pushdowns	3	8-12
One-Arm Dumbbell Triceps Extensions	2	8-12
Triceps Parallel Bar Dips	2	8-12

Chuck Williams

Exercise	Sets	Reps
Close-Grip Bench Presses	6	8-10
Seated Barbell Triceps Extensions	6	10-12
Pulley Pushdowns	5	10-12
Dumbbell Kickbacks	5	10-12

Matt Mendenhall

Exercise	Sets	Reps
Lying Barbell Triceps Extensions	5	8
Pulley Pushdowns	5	8
One-Arm Dumbbell Triceps Extensions	5	8

Albert Beckles

Exercise	Sets	Reps
Close-Grip Bench Presses	5	12
Reverse Triceps Pushdowns	5	15
Pulley Pushdowns	5	15
Incline Barbell Triceps Extensions	5	15

Mike Mentzer

Exercise	Sets	Reps
Pulley Pushdowns	1-2	6-8
Triceps Parallel Bar Dips	1-2	6-8
Lying Barbell Triceps Extensions	1-2	6-8
Nautilus Triceps Extensions	1-2	6-8

Ed Kawak

Exercise	Sets	Reps
Lying Barbell Triceps Extensions	4	10-15
Close-Grip Bench Presses	4	12
Pulley Pushdowns	4	12-15

Ali Malla

Exercise	Sets	Reps
Pulley Pushdowns	4	8–10
Standing High-Pulley, Long-Cable Triceps Extensions	4	8–10
Standing Rarbell Triceps Extensions	4	8–10
Triceps Parallel Bar Dips	4	8–10

Jusup Wilkosz

Exercise	Sets	Reps
Pulley Pushdowns	5	10–12
Triceps Parallel Bar Dips (weighted)	5	10–12
One-Arm Dumbbell Triceps Extensions	5	10–12
One-Arm Pulley Pushdowns	5	10–12

Jorma Raty

Exercise	Sets	Reps
Lying Barbell Triceps Extensions	3–4	8–10
One-Arm Dumbbell Triceps Extensions	3	8–10
Pulley Pushdowns	3	8–10

Gunnar Rosbo

Exercise	Sets	Reps
Pulley Pushdowns	4–5	8–12
Seated Single-Dumbbell Triceps Extensions	4–5	8–12
One-Arm Cable Kickbacks	4–5	10–12

PART V
THE COMPETITIVE
CYCLE

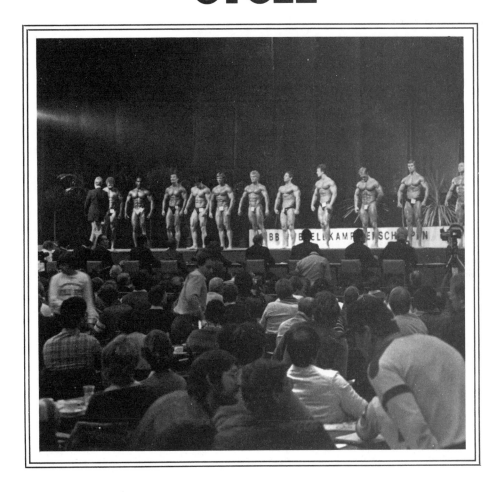

26
Training for a
Bodybuilding Competition

It would be difficult to write instructions about what you might encounter at each competition you enter. So, I suggest that you go to several shows, observe what takes place at both the prejudging and evening show, and take written notes for future reference.

Bodybuilding competitions are conducted on a wide spectrum of ability levels. You will take these competitions step by step as high as your genetic potential and hard training allow. As *Lee Haney* puts it, "I always thought of it being like climbing a mountain. I personally took it one step at a time, until I became Mr. Olympia. Don't even think about those higher steps up the mountain until you come to them. Always go one step at a time."

Let me tell you about the various levels of competition. The National Physique Committee, Inc. (NPC) conducts competitions on the local or city level, state, regional (encompassing two or more states), and national levels. They conduct novice contests up to the regional level (novice competitions are open only to bodybuilders who have never won a previous title). Teenage, past-40, collegiate, and military competitions are conducted up through the national level. Men's, women's, and mixed pairs' competitions are held at all levels.

Bodybuilders must qualify for national-level competitions by winning or placing high in lower-level shows. For city, state, and regional competitions, you usually need to live within the area covered by the contest title. For age-group shows, you will need proof of age (birth certificate).

Internationally, various continental and world championships are conducted for men, women, and pairs. Age-group competitions are also usually held on these same levels. All of these shows are sanctioned and conducted by

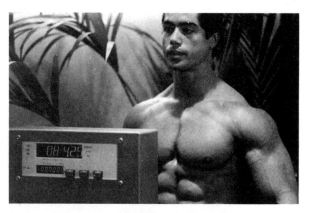

The crucial weigh-in at amateur World Championships: Moses Maldonado (USA) is easily under his 90-kilogram limit.

the International Federation of Bodybuilders (IFBB). The IFBB also conducts professional competitions internationally for men, women, and pairs.

I believe you should start out in a low-level novice or teenage show, then gradually work upward as your physique matures. Novice shows are a good place for most bodybuilders to start.

Announcements of upcoming contests are made in Coming Events sections in *Flex* and other bodybuilding magazines, as well as via bulletin boards at gyms in the area where the show will be held. Write or call for information on ticket availability, and purchase your tickets for both the prejudging and night shows as early as possible so you get seats close to the stage. It's a good idea to sit close enough to the judges at least one time so you can hear their various commands to the contestants.

HOW A COMPETITION IS JUDGED

As you will discover in my chapter on posing, there are three main rounds of posing, plus a

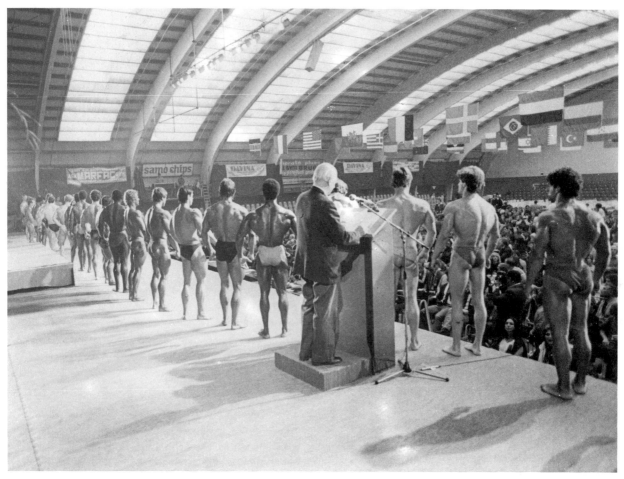

A typical prejudging scene.

final posedown for the top five athletes after the first three rounds have been conducted and scored. The first three rounds are scored at the prejudging show, and only the posedown is scored at the evening show.

The first posing round consists of seven mandatory poses, which each athlete does first individually and then in small groups for comparisons to be made. The mandatory poses are: front double biceps, front lat spread, side chest, back double biceps, back lat spread, side triceps, and a front abdominal and leg isolation.

In Round One your entire physical package will be judged in standard stances every contestant must assume. The judges will be looking for balanced proportions among various body parts, a good degree of muscle mass, sharp muscularity, and general body symmetry. In as much as you must learn to hit each compulsory pose so it shows your physique to its best advantage, your posing ability will be evaluated as well. And while it is not judged directly, personal appearance is also noted.

Since only one final prejudging score will be given after all three rounds, the judges will be making notes on each bodybuilder after the round. These notes will be used to determine your final placing, which will reflect the composite of how you looked in all three rounds.

In the second round of posing, you must stand semi-relaxed with your feet together and arms more or less down at your sides. You will be viewed from the front, left side, back, and right side in this type of stance. As in Round One you will be judged by yourself, as well as in small groups for comparison with other competitors.

All of the qualities judged in Round One are also evaluated in Round Two. But primary emphasis is on evaluation of general body symmetry and muscle tone.

In the third round of judging each bodybuilder is allowed to individually present his physique in a unique free-posing routine to his own choice of music. In Rounds One and Two you must do standard poses in which your weak points cannot be hidden. But in Round Three you can display your strong points while camouflaging your weak areas.

All of the qualities judged in Rounds One and Two are also evaluated in Round Three. But primary emphasis is on your posing ability, specifically on how effectively you show off your physique with a powerful and athletically graceful posing routine.

Based on the data they collected in all three rounds of posing conducted at the prejudging, each judge will rank you numerically somewhere between first and last place. Either five, seven, or nine judges will rank you this way, the number of judges depending on the level of competition (international and pro shows have nine, the others either five or seven). To discourage overt favoritism among the judges, the highest and lowest scores (two highest and two lowest when nine judges are used) are eliminated and the remaining place numbers are added up. The leader is the one with the lowest total.

Once the five top men have been determined, they enter the posedown at the evening show. A couple extra points can be gained in the posedown, which can be a crucial factor if two or three competitors are very close in the standings.

Learn From Watching, First

What should you be looking for? First of all, you should objectively compare your own level of development with men in the competition. This will give you an idea of whether you are ready to enter a show at that competitive level. And if you aren't ready, you'll know how much you still need to improve.

Be alert to what commands the judges give to the contestants, and how the group onstage responds to them. You'll always see some dumbo who turns left when everyone else is rotating a quarter turn to the right. Take note of how aggressively each potential champion conducts himself onstage at the prejudging, because you hope to be in his place someday.

To gradually work up your own personalized free-posing routine, you need to take special note of which transitional movements between individual poses look the best, the most creative. You should also take note of unique

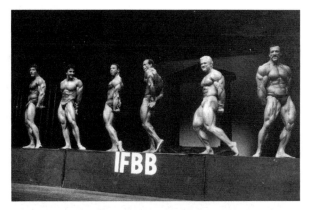

Group Compulsory Side Triceps poses (L–R: Frank Zane, Samir Bannout, Chris Dickerson, Albert Beckles, Tom Platz, and Casey Viator)

poses. All of this data will help you to choreograph your own unique routine. And all of the other data will help you conduct yourself optimally onstage at a prejudging.

GUEST POSERS

Not everyone is fortunate enough to attend every Mr. Olympia show, or even a National Championship. Hundreds of thousands of bodybuilders live in small towns or medium-sized cities. But these aspiring athletes can get a taste of what it takes to get to the top whenever a local promoter hires a guest poser for one of his shows.

One way professional bodybuilders financially support themselves is by giving guest posing exhibitions and conducting training seminars. Most of the time, a guest poser comes into an area and does one or two seminars before and/or after his or her exhibition. These are held at local gyms, and the price to attend one is nominal. It's a good idea to attend seminars to see what the champs are like as well as to get all of your nagging training and nutrition questions answered by an expert.

It's extremely difficult for most bodybuilders to stay in top shape year-round, so unless the guest poser is very close to a competition he probably will be in only 80%–90% of peak condition. But even a bit out of shape, a guest poser will still display those qualities which made him a champion: huge muscle mass, great proportional balance, classic symmetry, serious posing skill, and the charisma of a born stage performer. Take a good close look, because that'll be you one day soon!

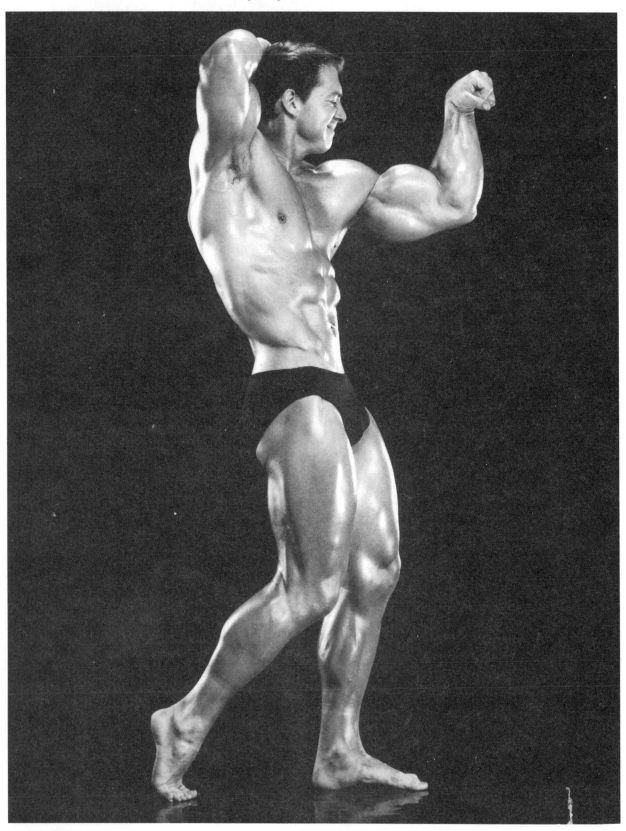

Larry Scott, 1965–66

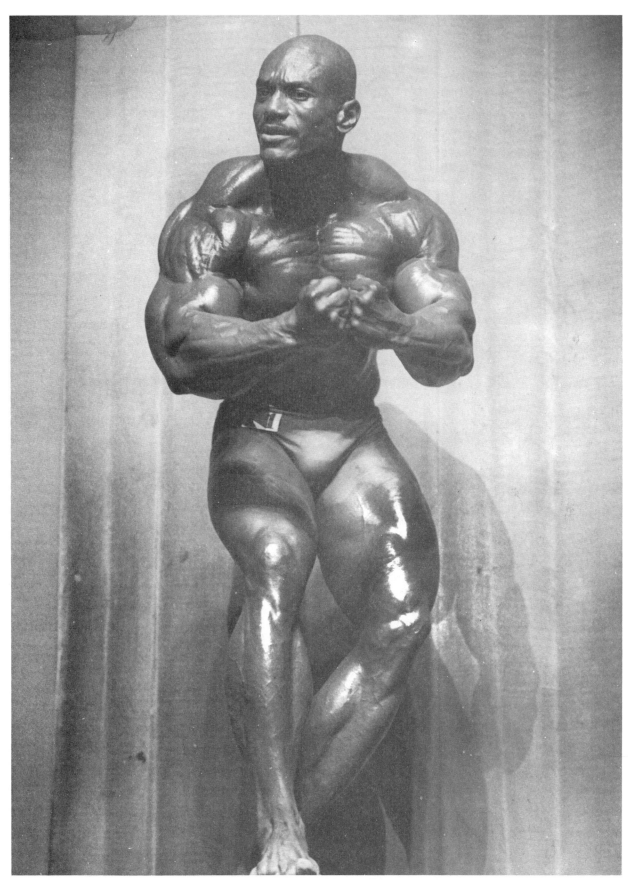

Sergio Oliva, 1967–69

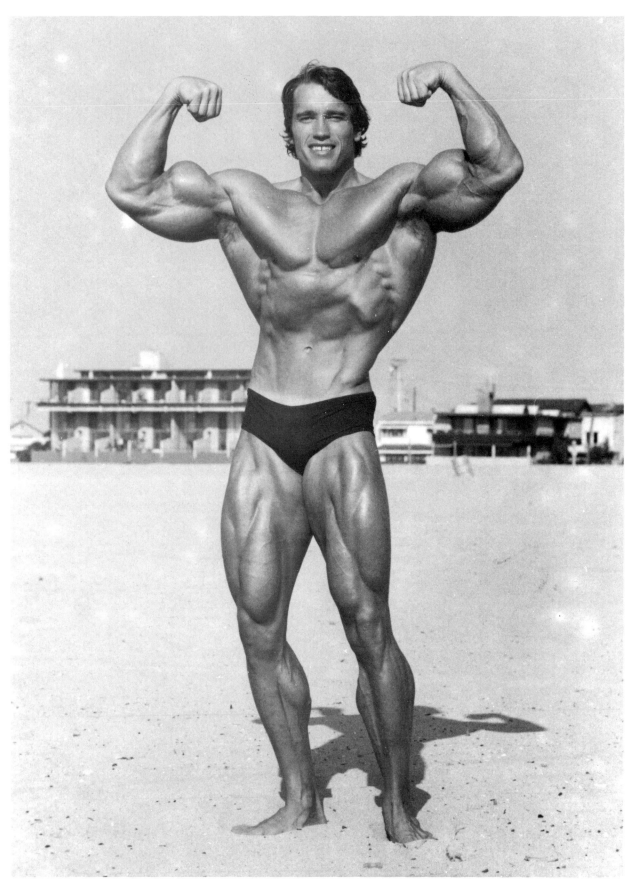

Arnold Schwarzenegger, 1970–75, 1980

414

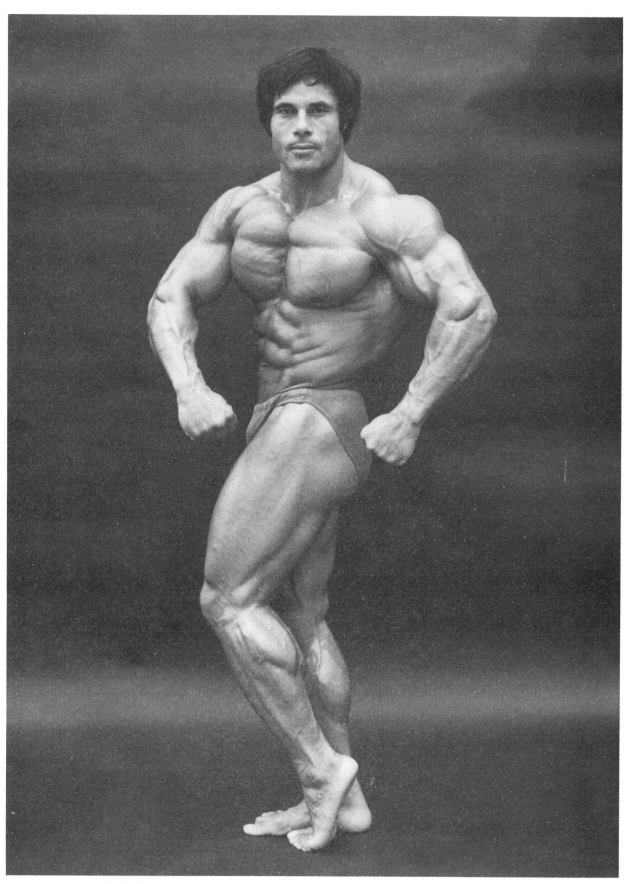

Franco Columbu, 1976, 1981

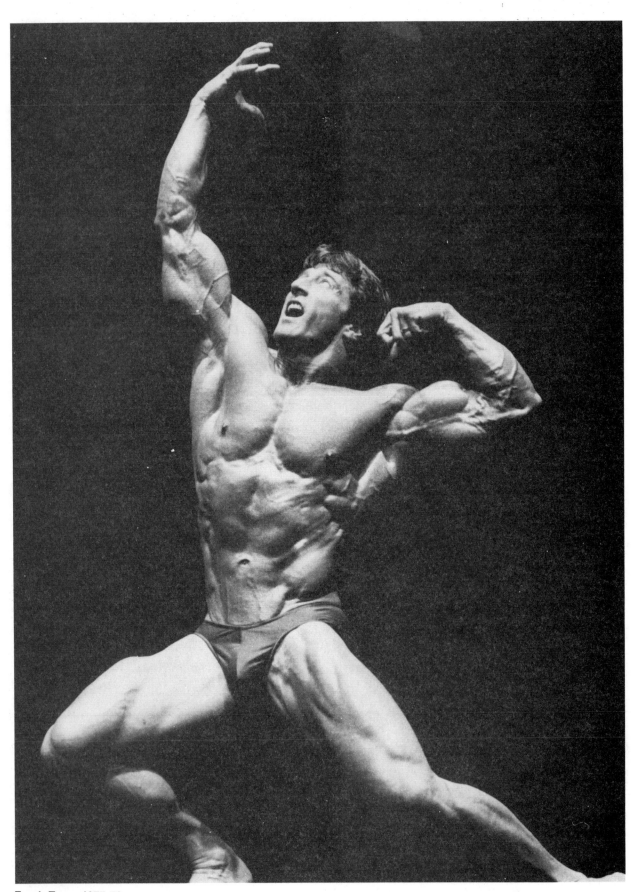

Frank Zane, 1977-79

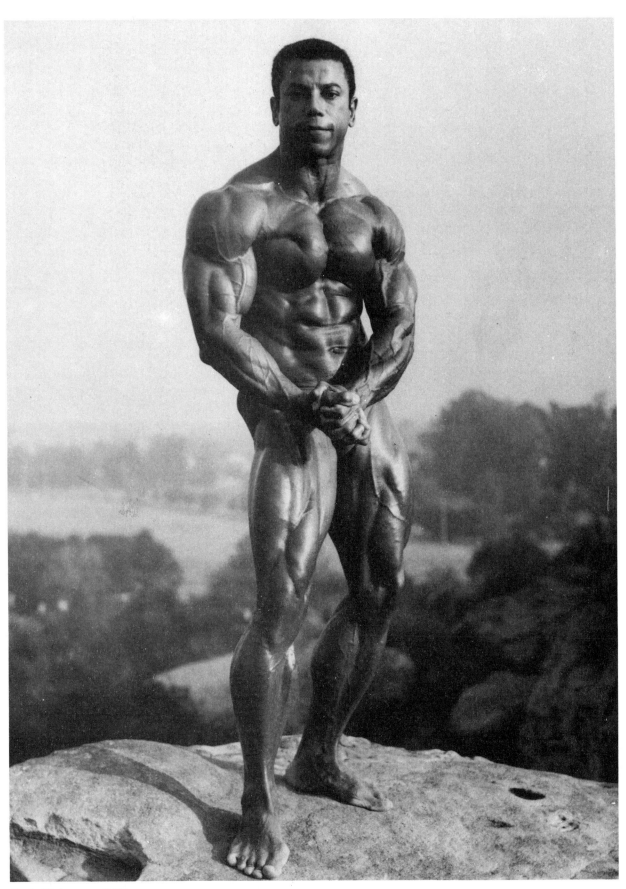

Chris Dickerson, 1982

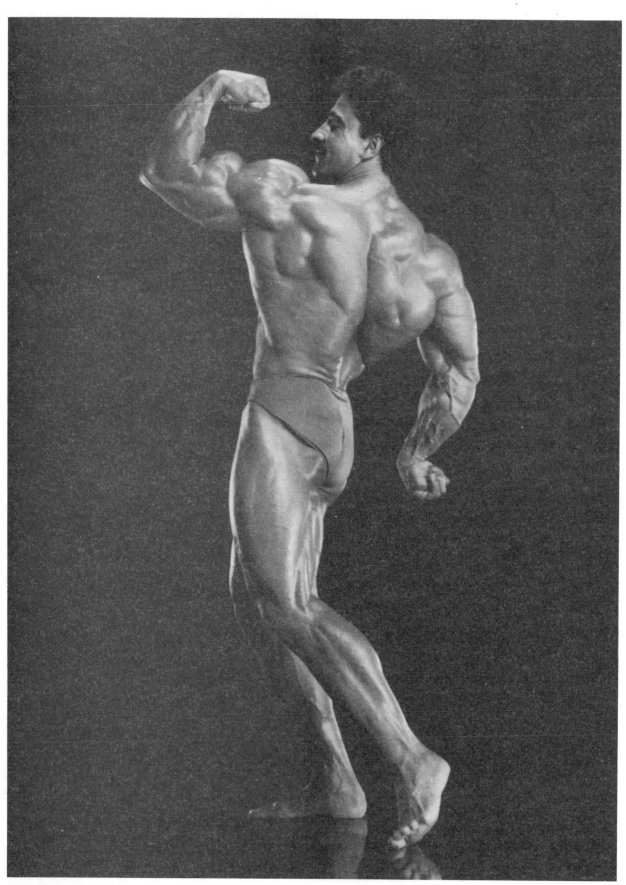

Samir Bannout, 1983

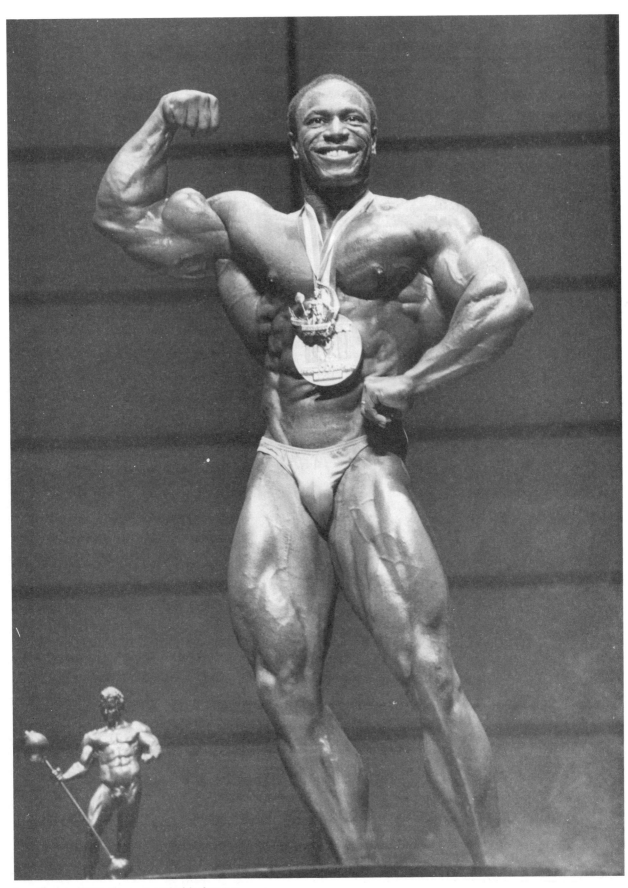

Lee Haney, 1984–88, and probably forever

THE FULL TRAINING CYCLE

No athlete can possibly train at peak intensity—nor diet super strictly—for more than 6–8 weeks at a time. Therefore, champion bodybuilders alternate off-season cycles of less intense training and relaxed diet with precompetition cycles featuring high-intensity workouts and strict dieting.

In the figure below, you will see a graph of training and dietary intensity for a one-year period in which two competitive peaks are reached. This graph shows a sine wave pattern of training and dietary intensity, which is characteristic of the cycle training philosophy used by most top bodybuilders.

The Weider Cycle Training Principle is a relatively new concept in bodybuilding, although it has been used for decades in other sports. Bodybuilders used to burn out by the dozens because they always trained at peak intensity, often while carefully monitoring their diets. Even today, you'll sometimes see this type of shooting star, a man who willfully puts it all together in terms of training and dietary intensity, usually with the assistance of heavy anabolic drug use, for a year or more to quickly reach a competitive peak, only to flame out with an injury and drop out of the sport.

Bodybuilding burnout is normally a mental state. A man has disciplined himself so rigorously and for such an extended period that he can no longer force himself to train so intensely, nor to strictly control his diet. Almost as frequently, intense training loads lead to career-ending injuries. But all of this can be avoided by intelligently following a cycle-training approach to bodybuilding.

Cycle training helps you to avoid injuries and burnout. Through cycle training, you can prolong your competitive bodybuilding career as long as you like, perhaps even as long as Frank Zane, the three-time Mr. Olympia, who competed internationally for more than 20 years.

It's a bit surprising that bodybuilders didn't take to the cycle-training system sooner, because it's been in use in such sports as track and field for more than 30 years. It didn't take middle-distance runners long to understand that they couldn't run all-out miles every day year-round. And they discovered that they could make faster progress by doing volumes of over-distance work in the off-season, followed by

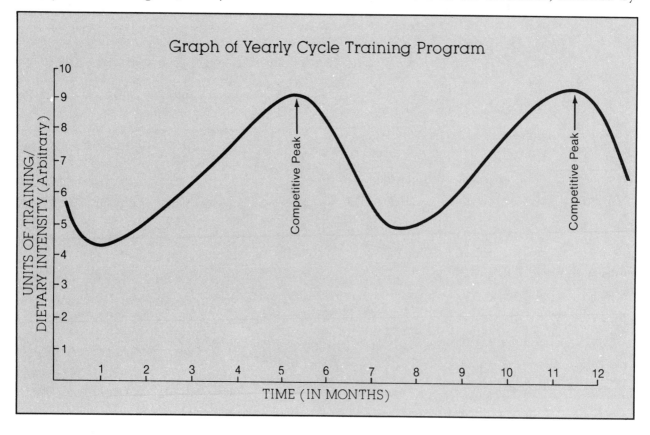

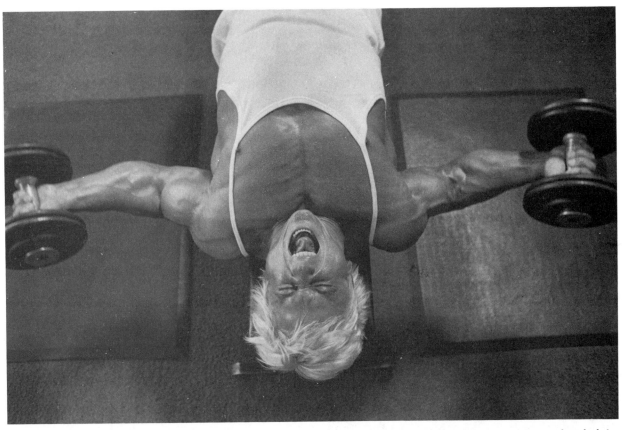

A serious hardcore trainer, Tom Platz blasts out a set of Flat-Bench Dumbbell Flyes. Tom was once so deeply into a set of this movement that he ruptured a biceps tendon without even noticing it!

very intense, shorter-distance speed training during the competitive season. Cycle training in track pushed Dr. Roger Bannister under four minutes in the mile run, and ultimately lowered the world mile record into the 3:47 range. It will push the record even lower.

In bodybuilding, we do heavy, low-rep training primarily on basic exercises during an off-season cycle, then follow this up with more intense, perhaps somewhat lighter (in terms of weight), training during a precontest cycle. And we have the added complication of alternating periods of relaxed dieting in the off-season with more intense cycles of caloric deprivation just prior to a major competition.

OFF-SEASON TRAINING

There are two similar, although slightly divergent, approaches to off-season training. One philosophy is to train primarily on heavy basic exercises year-round, with reps only slightly lower in the off-season than prior to a competition. The bodybuilder always pushes well past the failure point with forced reps, negatives, and burns. The only real difference between off-season and precontest training is that he can't maintain peak training intensity for the entire off-season preparatory cycle as he does during his precompetitive phase. Instead, he alternates periods of peak intensity with mini-cycles of lesser intensity, making sure that each peak in the intensity cycle is a bit higher than the last.

Many other champion bodybuilders—probably the majority of them—follow almost a powerlifter's approach to their workouts during the off-season, training with relatively low reps (as few as 5–6 per set) primarily on basic movements and with maximum poundages. This approach is intended to build greater overall muscle mass, although I personally don't feel that it works as well in developing or maintaining quality muscle tissue and aerobic capacity.

Aerobic training has become quite important to competitive bodybuilders, particularly during a precontest phase. Then, many bodybuilders engage in 2–3 hours of steady-state aerobics prior to a competition. During an off-season cycle, however, you should keep your aerobics threshold low (perhaps doing only one hour per week of aerobic training merely to

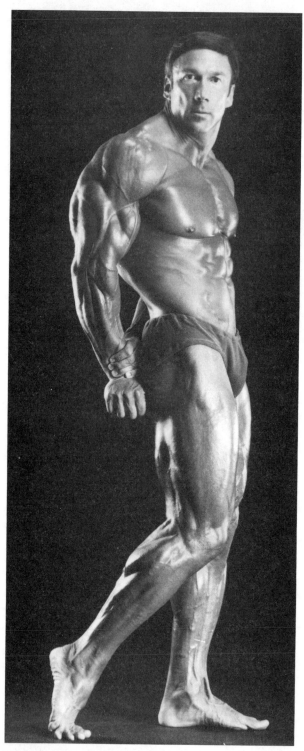

Big arm discussions often start and stop with Boyer Coe, who won more than 20 national and international titles over the years. Split biceps, peaked bis, and sweeping tris—Boyer had it all!

maintain a minimum level of conditioning), so you can receive a greater response from your aerobic workouts once you kick heavier aerobic training back into your program.

Regardless of your approach to off-season training, you *must* have two goals during this cycle: improve general muscle mass and improve a weak muscle group or two. It's virtually impossible to bring up a lagging body part during a precontest cycle, so you must do so in the off-season using the Weider Muscle Priority Training Principle and plenty of heavy, high-intensity workouts.

It's very difficult to gain muscle mass during a precontest cycle. Therefore, you will be in a prolonged off-season phase until you reach the point where you decide to enter your first competition and therefore initiate a specific peaking cycle. Your initial off-season training cycle, then, can last two, three, or more years.

Once you have entered your first bodybuilding championship, your off-season phases will become somewhat shorter, but I still feel that they should be a minimum of 3–4 months in length. With a shorter off-season cycle, you simply won't have sufficient time to improve your overall muscle mass.

Unfortunately, many young bodybuilders become so excited about entering and winning bodybuilding shows that they enter competitions virtually every weekend for several months at a time. These trophy hunters are making a big mistake, because they simply don't allow themselves sufficient time to grow, to improve their general muscle mass.

"At my level, more than one competition per year is folly," says Tom Platz. "Frequent competition would hold back my bodybuilding progress too much. Therefore, I compete only once each year, and I don't think it would be counterproductive to compete once every two years. I personally need an occasional competition to keep motivated to train at peak intensity, but I can certainly hold myself together mentally to train two years for a major show, as long as I keep firmly in mind the fact that it allows me to pack on much more muscle mass than if I entered shows every 4–6 months."

For most young bodybuilders, I believe that two competitions per year—equally spaced—is best because it allows sufficient off-season training time to make good gains, yet keeps you highly motivated to train as hard as possible. Competing every six months gives you approximately four good months to build muscle and two more months to diet and train down to reach optimum condition.

OFF-SEASON DIET

You should have three dietary objectives in the off-season:

1. Maintain a healthful, balanced diet
2. Consume sufficient protein to allow for maximum muscle growth
3. Take in enough calories to fuel all-out, high-intensity workouts and promote muscular body weight gains

With only minor individual variation, these should also be your own off-season nutritional objectives.

I've seen numerous bodybuilders—even Olympians—allow themselves to gain 40-50 pounds of body fat in the off-season, mistakenly believing that this process helps them to build additional muscle mass. However, bulking up like this does little, if anything, to add muscle mass to your physique, even though the heavier poundages that improved tissue leverage allow you to lift would *seem* to indicate that you are building muscle. And getting too heavy in the off-season makes it exceedingly difficult to reach sharp, competitive condition at the conclusion of a precontest phase.

Bodybuilders over 200 pounds competitive body weight should go no higher than 10-15 pounds over optimum condition. For smaller bodybuilders, 8-10 pounds above contest weight would be the most reasonable upper limit during an off-season cycle.

"Since I've discovered that I have difficulty gaining solid weight during an off-season phase on a low-fat regimen," reveals Platz, "I will consume plenty of whole milk, milk products, and red meat in the off-season. Eating this amount of fat also makes it much easier for me to get cut up for each competition, since my body retains those enzymes that allow it to digest, mobilize, and metabolize body fat."

"You will probably have difficulty believing me, but I've always had great trouble in gaining muscular body weight. Therefore, I can regularly consume 5,000-6,000 calories per day in

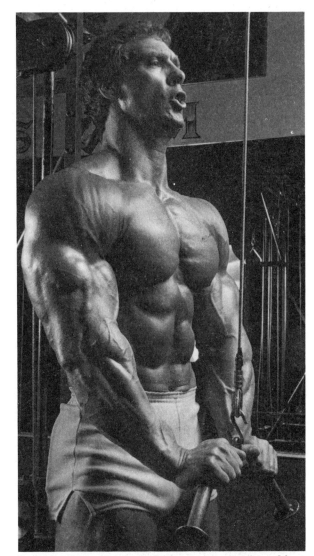

Mr. Delts himself, Scott Wilson, showing how his shoulder muscles are highly prominent even when doing a simple triceps movement like Pulley Pushdowns.

the off-season without getting particularly fat. I do gain a little weight, but a nice percentage of it is new muscle mass. Smaller bodybuilders and those with low BMRs will probably profit from keeping their caloric intake in the range of 3,500-4,000 calories a day in the off-season."

The type, amount, and timing of protein intake is particularly important. Be careful to consume complete proteins primarily from animal sources (milk, eggs, meat, fish, and poultry) in small-enough quantities to allow for complete digestion. You should even take digestive enzymes with each meal to allow you more efficient digestion of protein and other nutrients. And by eating five or six times per day during an off-season, weight-gaining cycle, you will be able to force more protein into your blood stream, where it can later be used to build new muscle tissue. This approach to eating also prevents fats from building up because of more-efficient digestion and utilization of food.

You should place emphasis on the type and amount of your carbohydrate consumption in the off-season as well, because carbohydrates give you the energy to train all-out with maximum weights. For short-term energy needs, you should consume simple carbohydrates (fruit and fruit juices), and for long-term energy needs you should eat complex carbohydrates (grains, seeds, nuts, vegetables, and whole-grain breads and pasta). During an off-season cycle, I don't think it excessive to consume 500 or more grams of carbohydrates each day.

You should purposely keep your intake of vitamins, minerals, and trace elements lower than precontest levels in the off-season, so you'll get a bigger boost from taking them during a peaking cycle. You might need as little as one or two multipacks of supplements per day, with meals.

PRECONTEST TRAINING

The main objective of a precontest training cycle is to strip away all superfluous body fat and reveal your hard-earned muscles in bold relief. Secondarily, a peaking cycle will actually harden up the muscles.

"By necessity, a precontest cycle is a time of total involvement and energy depletion," says Platz. "I find a peaking cycle to involve 10–12 hour days of training, mental conditioning, posing practice, aerobics, and other miscellaneous preparations. And the hard, long-lasting training, when even posing becomes physically exhausting, depletes your energy stores. It has to do so in order for you to strip away body fat that nature intended you have even in near-starvation situations. Correctly applied, a precontest cycle can leave you constantly fatigued.

"My own bodybuilding training varies little from one cycle to the next, except that the mental drive generated by an upcoming Mr. Olympia competition can push me to train significantly harder within each set. The mental intensity during a peaking cycle becomes absolutely awesome.

"I do much more aerobic training prior to a competition than in the off-season because aerobics automatically burns body fat for energy. And all of the posing practice that I put in further exhausts my energy reserves, gradually making my physique appear harder. Posing practice also gives me more complete control of my tensed muscles, which adds to the illusion that I am growing harder. Combined with the strict low-calorie diet that I follow during a peaking phase, this type of training approach effectively strips all surface fat from over my muscles and even from between and within my muscles."

Other bodybuilders follow a much more complicated peaking procedure. I've outlined how they diet and train in both off-season and precontest cycles in a handy chart below. In that chart, you can see that they train much more frequently, rest less between sets, do higher reps, and engage in continuous-tension and peak-contraction exercises.

"I personally do none of those things," reveals Platz, "but that doesn't mean that your body will respond exactly the way mine does. You should experiment over a period of time with all of these techniques, using your own instinctive training ability, to determine what actually works best for your body. In all likelihood, only some of my peaking philosophy will work well for you, while parts of other champions' philosophies will also find their way into your own peaking philosophy. You won't know until you actually try each variable out."

OFF-SEASON AND PRECONTEST TRAINING AND DIET
OFF-SEASON CYCLE

Training
- Primarily basic exercises.
- Low reps (3–6).
- Low sets (8–10 per body part).
- Train to failure, plus forced reps, negatives, and burns.
- Each major body part worked twice a week.
- Rest 60–90 seconds between sets.
- Low levels of aerobic training.
- Little or no posing practice.

Diet
- High protein intake.
- High carbohydrate intake.
- High fat intake.
- Low supplements intake.
- Five to six meals per day.

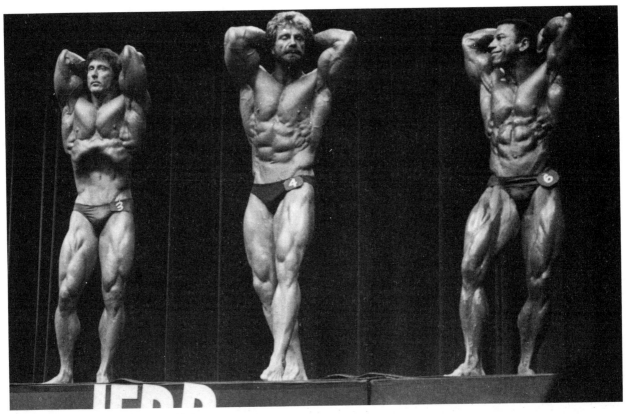

Frank Zane, Jusup Wilkosz, and Chris Dickerson.

PRECONTEST CYCLE

Training
- Primarily isolation exercises.
- High reps (10–15).
- High sets (18–20 per body part).
- Seldom train to failure, but use peak contraction, continuous tension, and iso-tension.
- Each body part worked three times per week.
- Rest 30–40 seconds between sets.
- High levels of aerobic training.
- At least one hour per day of posing practice.

Diet
- Moderate protein intake.
- Moderate carbohydrate intake.
- Lowest possible fat intake.
- Moderately high supplements intake.
- Three meals per day.

PRECONTEST DIET

"Although I have used a low-carbohydrate diet several times in the past," notes *Mike Christian*, "I now diet for competitions exclusively while using a low-fat/low-calorie diet. You will need to experiment with both low-carb and low-cal diets, then use your instinctive training ability to judge which diet works best for you. I'm sure you'll find that a low-carbohydrate diet makes it difficult for you to maintain maximum muscle mass while getting ripped up for a show.

"In general terms, my precontest diet is relatively low in calories (half or less the number of calories I consume during an off-season cycle), moderate in protein intake, relatively high in complex carbohydrate consumption, as low as humanly possible in fat intake, and relatively high in supplements consumption. Also, I reduce the number of meals from five or six down to three per day.

"At the same time I train much differently from cycle to cycle, my dietary approach is greatly modified from my off-season to my precontest phase. Virtually all champion bodybuilders follow the same yearly nutritional approach, and many more follow a low-fat/low-calorie diet than the traditional low-carbohydrate approach to precontest dieting. I'm much more sure that I can tell you how dietary factors will affect your physique than various approaches to training. Biochemistry, the study of human nutrition, is a relatively exact science in comparison to bodybuilding training."

TRANSITIONAL PHASES

Moving abruptly between off-season and pre-contest training and dietary cycles would be a great shock to your system, so it's necessary to insert transitional phases between major cycles. Transitional phases in training should last 1–3 weeks, while similar phases for dietary practices can last up to 4–5 weeks.

Traditionally, bodybuilders take a one-week to one-month layoff from training following a competitive peak. While this layoff gives your mind and body time to recuperate and allows minor injuries incurred in all-out peak training to heal, an abrupt move from hard training to total rest can be physically hard on your body. Try it, and you'll notice that you soon become restless and jumpy.

I'm far more in favor of an "active layoff" in which you practice other sports and physical activities. I suggest staying away from the gym during a post-peak layoff, but I'm very much in favor of riding your bike, playing tennis, or engaging in other physically demanding activities. And within a week or two, you will find yourself craving the feel of heavy iron, and you'll head back into the gym to build up to another, distant peak.

Can you imagine how mentally and physically difficult it would be for you to shift from eating 5,500 calories one day to consuming only 2,500 the next? You could probably maintain such a severely tightened diet for three or four days, but you'd be so weak and irritable that you'd probably end up on a junk food binge. It's a far more sensible and workable plan to lower daily caloric consumption by 200–300 calories each succeeding week, a process that allows the body to grow gradually more accustomed to caloric deprivation.

You're probably wondering how long before a show you should initiate a peaking cycle. This is a highly individual matter that depends on how far out of shape you have allowed yourself to become in the off-season (and particularly how fat you have grown), how quickly your body responds to various external stimuli, and your degree of dedication to the peaking process.

In the final analysis, you must learn to time a peak through trial and error, and use your training instinct. Very few bodybuilders peak exactly on the money the first time out of the chute. It takes several competitions and many experiments to get the process right, so don't expect to master peak timing overnight.

27
Posing, Grooming, and Publicity

Over the years, the IFBB has developed a judging system that evaluates all of the qualities that a potential bodybuilding champion must have. In the previous chapter, I described how the judges score each posing round. Now I intend to go into detail, with suggestions from stars I've coached, on what you need to do to excel in each posing round of a bodybuilding competition. I also will discuss the importance of good grooming and let the superstars provide you with their tips on the subject. Finally, I will provide you with suggestions on how to promote yourself so you can afford to continue bodybuilding and become a superstar in your own right.

ROUND ONE: COMPULSORY POSES

In this section, I will teach you how to perform the seven compulsory poses: front double biceps, front lat spread, side chest (from your choice of side), back double biceps, back lat spread, side triceps (again from your choice of side), and front abdominal and thigh isolation. The object of this round is to reveal the general level of development in standardized poses which must be duplicated by every competitor.

FRONT DOUBLE BICEPS

"As you begin to develop visible muscles," says *Tom Platz*, "it is probably natural for you to start practicing various poses that you see depicted in bodybuilding magazines. And it's equally likely that many of the first poses that you will work on are those seven compulsory poses from Round One.

"I feel that it's essential that you have an outstanding front double biceps pose in your repertoire because it is the first pose that the judges will see you perform. Communications researchers—most notably the late Marshall McLuhan—have concluded that first impressions are vital; if someone is impressed with you from the start, it will be more likely that he

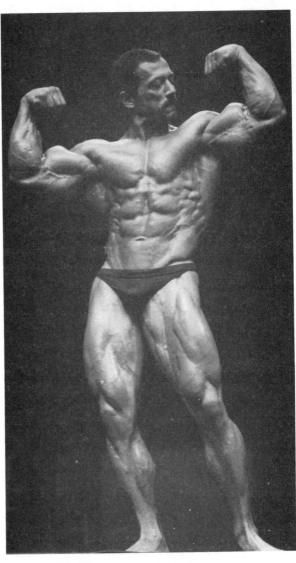

Front Double Biceps (Casey Viator)

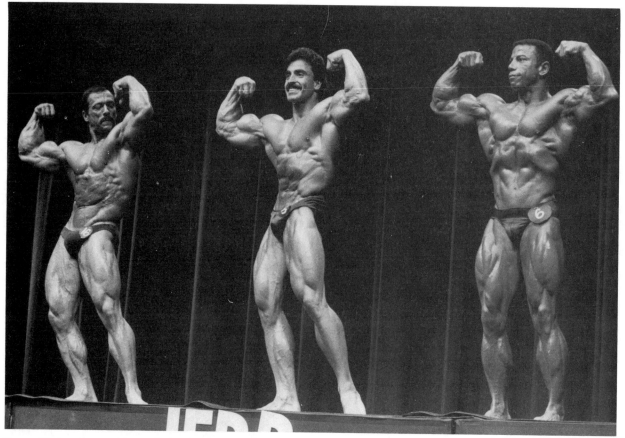

Casey Viator, Samir Bannout, and Chris Dickerson.

will remain impressed by you. Therefore, you *must* get your front double biceps shot together.

"You can do the pose either with a stomach vacuum, or with your abdominals crunched down. Some bodybuilders even do both types of double biceps poses in the same round of judging. With a vacuum, you will have more sweep to your lats and will present an image of slightly greater overall upper body mass. You lose this V-tapered look to your torso when you crunch down on your abs, but you also gain greater impressiveness through showing off your midsection.

"It's really a toss-up in terms of the value of each pose variation, so you should probably use the version that you can perform most impressively. Or, as mentioned, you can begin the pose in a vacuum position, then exhale and crunch down on your abdominals before moving on to the lat spread pose. Tony Pearson does it this way, and I'm constantly impressed with the way he is able to show off his physique with both poses.

"The degree of bend and hand supination

that you use in your arms as you do a front double biceps shot depends largely on how well-developed your biceps and triceps have become and how evenly balanced your arm shape happens to be. Very few bodybuilders have the same shape to each arm, and you'll often see some of the better men holding each arm a little differently in order to make them both appear equal in shape and mass.

"If you have a terrific biceps peak, you'll be better off bending your arms past a 90-degree angle and only half supinating your wrists. But if your biceps are not highly peaked, you may get a lot more out of holding them bent at right angles and completely supinating your wrists. Either way, I think it's more impressive to hold your elbows a bit upward and forward, so your upper-arm bones are above a line parallel with the floor.

"Leg position in all front poses depends on how well you have trained your thighs and calves. You'll get a better line to your body in a double biceps shot if you can point the toes of one foot slightly outward and bend that leg a few degrees, then extend the other leg a foot or so directly out to the side. However, you'll need highly developed thighs and calves in order to get away with this types of leg stance.

"The best leg stance for front double biceps and lat spread poses, should you not have highly developed legs, is to put your best leg's foot about four inches in front of the other, your toes on that foot pointed directly forward. And your back foot should be angled somewhat outward. Bend your legs slightly, or you won't be able to achieve maximum separation in your quads when you flex them."

FRONT LAT SPREAD

Either leg position can be used when you perform your front lat spread pose, but the best one is usually the stance with one foot behind the other. "Placing your hands correctly is the first step to bringing out your lats," notes *Joe Bucci* (Mr. World). With your palms toward the floor, place your thumbs behind your waist and your fists against your sides. This should place each

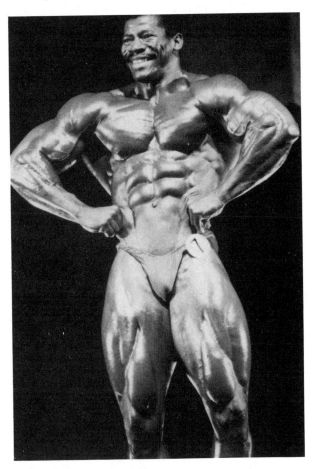

Ron Love's Front Lat Spread

arm in about a 90-degree bend at the elbow.

"Hold your shoulders down, a somewhat difficult task for most novice bodybuilders, since there is a natural tendency to shrug the shoulders when first working on a lat spread. Raising the shoulders both spoils the lines of the pose and prevents you from spreading your lats fully.

"When you press against the sides of your waist with your fists, attempt to spread your shoulder blades *and* lats outward. At first this will be difficult, because you won't have very good shoulder and scapula flexibility. But if you work at the pose—and perhaps do some shoulder flexibility movements, such as dislocates with a towel or broom stick—you'll gradually be able to spread your lats more and more completely.

"As you draw your lats outward, make sure that every muscle is flexed, from head to toe. Your lats should be spread, your quads completely flexed, your abs flattened and tensed, and your pectorals flexed and striated to the limit. When you have all of this down—and you can still smile—you've put together a perfect front lat spread pose."

SIDE POSE: CHEST

Platz advises, "Both side poses in Round One should be performed with your best side, even though your best side for a chest shot may be different from your best side for the triceps pose. Actually, doing each of these poses from a different side tips the judges off that you have balanced development on both sides of your body, but you'll see even the top Olympians performing both side shots from the same direction."

I always like to start teaching bodybuilders each pose from the ground up. There are three basic leg stances you can use on side shots, so think in terms of both the side chest and side triceps shots when I describe each of the three possible leg positions for side poses.

In the most popular leg stance, your back leg (the one away from the judges and audience) is held relatively straight, perhaps with only a few degrees of bend. The toe of the front leg is placed on the floor about 4–6 inches toward the judges from the toes of the back foot. Extend

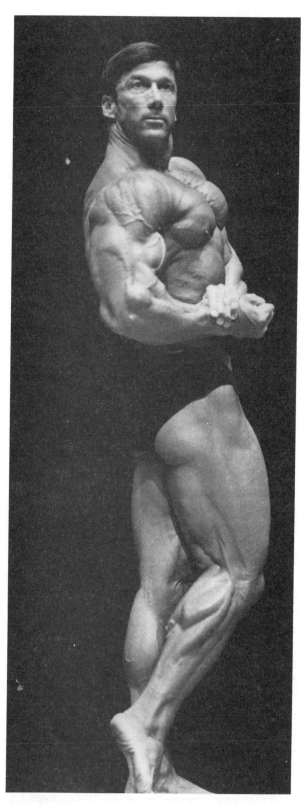

Without the kind of proper leg biceps development displayed here by Boyer Coe in one of his Mr. Olympia appearances a bodybuilder will lack width to his legs when seen from the side. Note how deeply Boyer's leg biceps are split vertically into two halves from top to bottom.

the toes of your front foot, bending your front leg about 30 degrees. Flex all of the muscles of both legs, but particularly the muscles on the outside of your front leg. You can increase the impressiveness of your legs in this stance by pulling the knee of your front leg away from the judges, across the midline of your body, pressing it against your rear leg to bring out the hamstrings of the front leg.

The next optional leg stance looks somewhat like you have been caught halfway through a step forward. The leg away from the judges is bent slightly and extended a little forward of the torso. The leg toward the judges is extended to the rear, so there is about 24–30 inches of space between the two feet. The back leg is bent about 20 degrees, and all of the leg muscles are tensed as completely as possible.

In the final side leg stance, you reverse your leg positions, so the leg away from the judges is to the rear and the other leg set forward. In this stance, you can rise up on the toes of the foot away from the audience and flex the calf of that leg maximally as you flex all of your leg muscles.

Regardless of which of the three leg stances you choose to do, the way you arrange your upper body will be pretty much the same with every bodybuilder who tries to do a side chest shot. I'll tell you how to do it from the right side; if you choose to do it left-handed, you can simply reverse my directions.

Bend your right arm about 90 degrees, with the right hand held palm up. Grasp the wrist of your right arm with your left hand, palm down. With your forearms held approximately parallel with the floor, pull your hands in against your upper abdomen, pressing your right arm against the side of your torso to flatten out your right upper arm and make it appear more impressively massive. Let out your breath about halfway and suck in your stomach while throwing out your chest.

The foregoing directions will give you a pretty good side chest shot, but you can improve it by manipulating your arms, chest, and shoulder muscles. By pulling one way with your right deltoid muscles and the other way with your pecs, you can striate both muscle groups. You should be particularly conscious of tensing and striating your left pectoral. Pressing down with your left hand while pulling up with your right will bring out your biceps and brachialis muscles on your right arm.

If necessary, you can hide weak forearm development simply by turning the palm of your right hand toward the floor, and hit the rest of the pose as described.

BACK POSES

"Turning to the two compulsory back poses," *Tom Platz* continues, "let's talk first about foot and calf position. In the back double biceps shot during Round One, you must extend one leg or the other to the rear and flex the calf of that leg. Then during the back lat spread shot, most novice bodybuilders maintain this same leg position. Better athletes tend to extend their other leg to the rear to show that they have equal calf development on both sides. I've

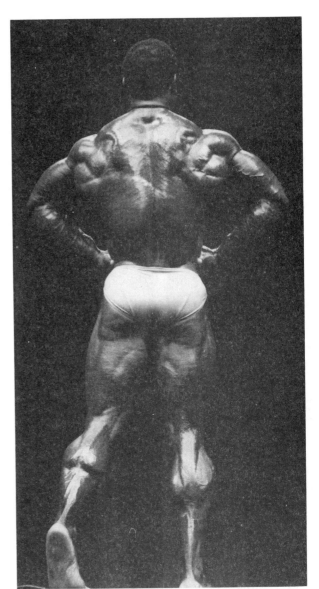

Back Lat Spread (Johnny Fuller)

coached other bodybuilders to do their lat spread poses with feet flat on the floor in a position in which, with some practice, they can bring out some incredible calf striations. This is, indeed, the leg position I use for my own back lat spread shot.

"To learn the flat-footed calf pose, start by rocking a bit forward so your weight is primarily on the balls of your feet. Then work on gripping the floor with your toes while attempting to flex your calves. At first, you probably won't be able to get any striations to show, but within a couple of hours of periodic practice you'll begin to see them peeking out. Eventually, you can put as many striations in your calves in this position as you can in your pectorals in many poses."

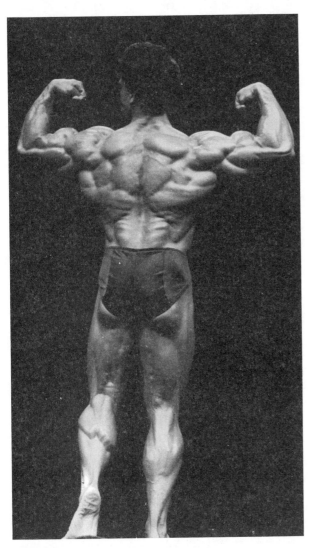

Back Double Biceps (Samir Bannout)

I've coached a great many top bodybuilders over the years on how to correctly assume a back double biceps pose. It's a little like a front double biceps shot, but with some crucial differences. The first of these is that you have to make sure your calves and hamstrings are tensed completely, since they make half of the pose. Untensed, your legs will look ridiculous if you've done the upper body correctly.

Rather than pulling your elbows forward, you should pull them toward the rear and rotate your hands rearward while keeping your elbows forward of your hands. Round your spine slightly and spread your shoulder blades as you tense your back muscles. Finally, tense your abdominal muscles to bring out your lower back and turn your head to one side or the other, a movement which adds impressive contours to your trapezius muscles.

"The back lat spread is very much like the front variation of the pose," says Platz, "except that you will round your torso forward and pull your elbows ahead of the midline of your torso as you do the pose. It's also very effective to start this pose by first pressing your shoulder blades together. This movement makes the width of your lat spread even more dramatic than it would be if you merely hit the shot with no preamble. And if your lower lats are well-developed, you'll bring out some terrific striations in them when you press your shoulder blades together like this prior to hitting your full back lat spread pose."

SIDE POSE: TRICEPS

Again, I'll describe how to do the side triceps shot from the right side. And you can reverse the instructions if you want to do it left-handed. Position your legs similarly to one of the three ways described for the side chest pose.

After choosing your leg stance, extend your right arm straight down from your shoulder. Reach across your back with your left arm and grasp your right wrist with your left hand, your left palm toward the rear. This will give you a securely braced position from which you can pull or push with your right arm to bring out your shoulder and chest musculature. This will require some experimentation, but you'll get the hang of it rather quickly if you spend some time in front of your mirror.

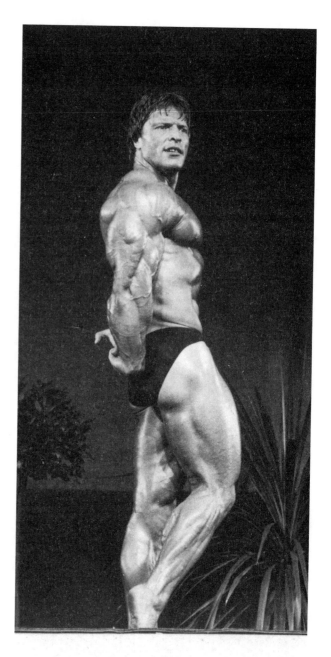

Side Triceps (Gunnar Rosbo)

You'll also need to experiment with a straight-armed position to display your right triceps, as well as with various rotations of your right arm in perspective with your shoulder. You might end up actually rotating your arm in your shoulder socket in the middle of your triceps shot, so the judges and audience can see your upper-arm development from two or more angles, all of which might be very complimentary. Either way, you should press your right upper arm against the side of your torso—the same as you did in the side chest pose—to flatten out your upper arm and make it appear even more impressive than it actually is.

Once you're in the right position, exhale halfway and crunch down on your abdominals. I taught Robby Robinson a method for bringing out the intercostals in this position, and he has elicited cheers with it. All you need to do is raise your right hip a couple of inches while crunching down on your intercostals, and you'll be able to bring them out fairly prominently the first time. With practice, the intercostals will appear like thick ropes of muscle.

As with all other poses, be sure that your legs and all of the muscles of your upper body are totally tensed in your side triceps pose. One of the biggest mistakes novice bodybuilders make is failing to keep all muscles fully flexed. You gotta keep it all going at once.

ABDOMINALS AND THIGH POSE

Again, *Tom Platz* tells you how to do the final compulsory pose: "Start by setting your feet so one foot is about 12 inches in front of the other. Your back foot should be positioned with your toes angled somewhat outward, and the toes of your front foot should be pointed straight ahead. Bend your forward leg slightly and tense your quads to bring out thigh muscularity, simultaneously flexing and spreading your calves.

"Practice bending your leg to various angles as you flex your thigh muscles, because each new degree of bend produces a different look to your leg. One gives you plenty of sartorius and little front thigh muscle, while another gives you all front thigh and very little sartorius. Pick the one that looks best, or switch between the two leg stances in the middle of the pose.

"Next, place your hands behind your neck or head, interlacing your fingers so they won't slip away. Be certain to flex your biceps while in this position, because failing to do so will detract considerably from how your upper body appears in this pose. Being sure to stand up as straight as possible, exhale and tense your abdominals. As long as you're concentrating on your rectus abdominis, intercostals, and serratus muscles when you flex your abs, this will give you an excellent conclusion to your compulsory round of poses."

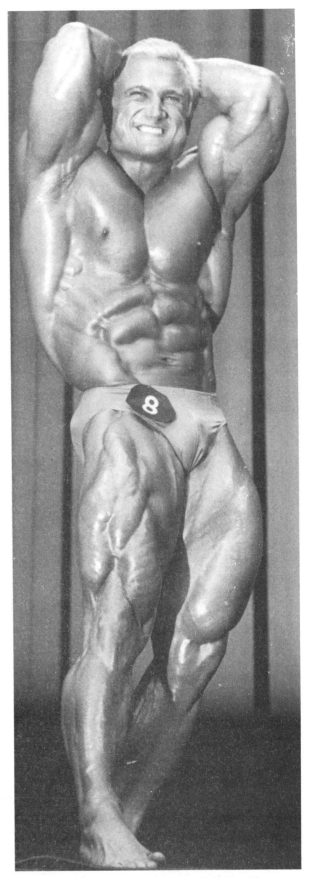

Front Ab-and-Thigh (Tom Platz)

ROUND TWO: RELAXED POSES

"The object of the Round Two poses in the IFBB system," says *Joe Bucci*, "is to bring out all of your muscularity while standing with your heels together and arms down at your sides. In this position, you are required to dis-

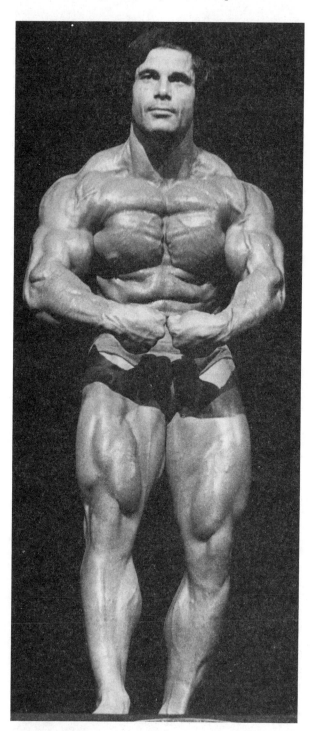

Dr. Franco Columbu, two-time IFBB Mr. Olympia, displays awesome pec-delt tie-ins and muscularity as he wins one of his major international titles.

play your body from the front, left side, back, and right side. You're supposed to stand 're-laxed,' but you'll never see any bodybuilders in Round Two actually standing relaxed. At a minimum, he will have his quads and abdomi-nals flexed nearly to the limit, and every other muscle group will probably be at least 50% tensed.

"How much you flex in the Round Two poses depends entirely on what the judges allow, so you have to take this round as it comes each time, adjusting according to what you see ev-eryone else getting away with in the lighter weight classes. Just observe everything closely, and you won't have a problem with bringing out your entire physique in these facing stances.

"There are a lot of little variations of arm, leg, and torso position that will reveal your body optimally in each of the four facing stances. These variations are highly individual, and they'll even change from one year to the next as your physique gradually fills out and matures. And the only way you can discover which positions show you off best is to spend a lot of time in front of the mirror learning how to adjust each pose for maximum effect.

"It's essential as you work on your poses to have a mirror set up on one wall with rather flat light over it. Another smaller mirror should be set up so you can look into it and see pre-cisely what your back looks like when you pose it either semirelaxed, or fully flexed in a wide variety of poses.

"The flat light will reveal your physique quite objectively. You'll have trouble telling yourself you're really in shape when the light is hot enough to reveal every ridge of body fat around your waistline. *Always* be perfectly ob-jective when you're looking at your various poses. You'll only end up a chronic loser if you lie to yourself."

Group Comparisons From Semi-Relaxed Symmetry Round

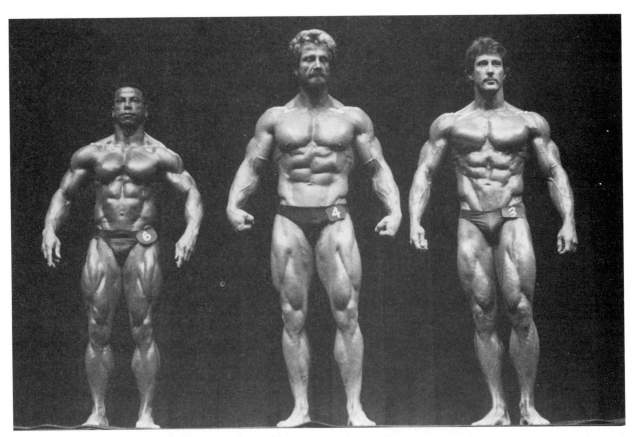

Front (L-R): Chris Dickerson, Jusup Wilkosz, and Frank Zane.

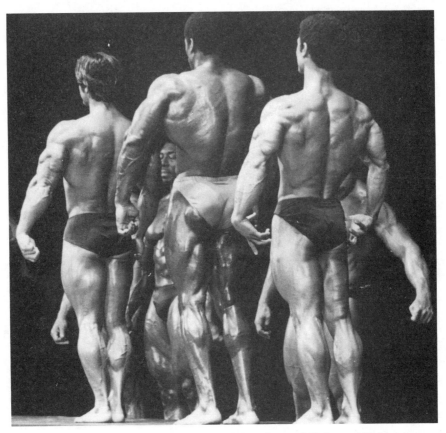

Left Side (L-R): Danny Padilla, Roy Callender, and Mohamed Makkawy.

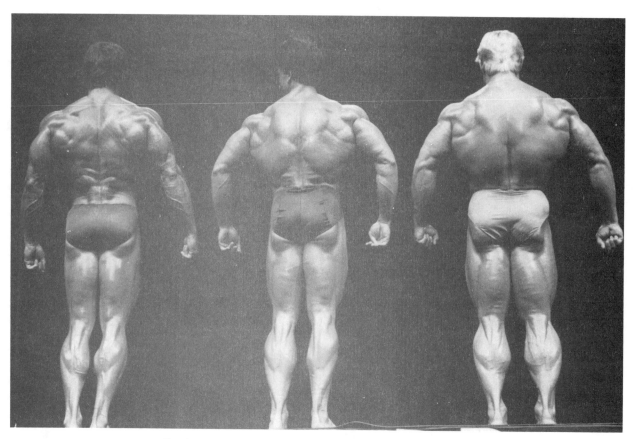

Back (L-R): Frank Zane, Samir Bannout, and Tom Platz.

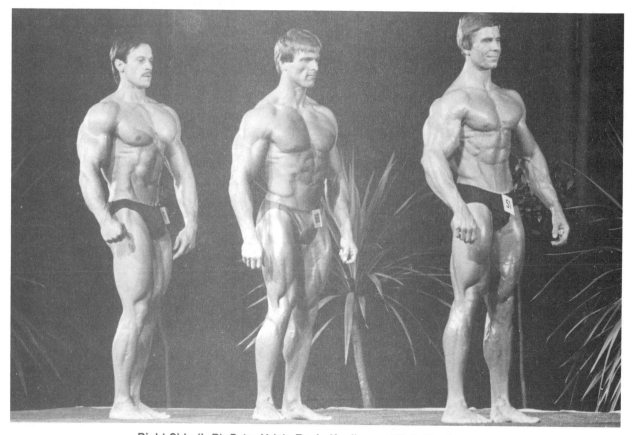

Right Side (L-R): Peter Urick, Erwin Knoller, and Dale Ruplinger.

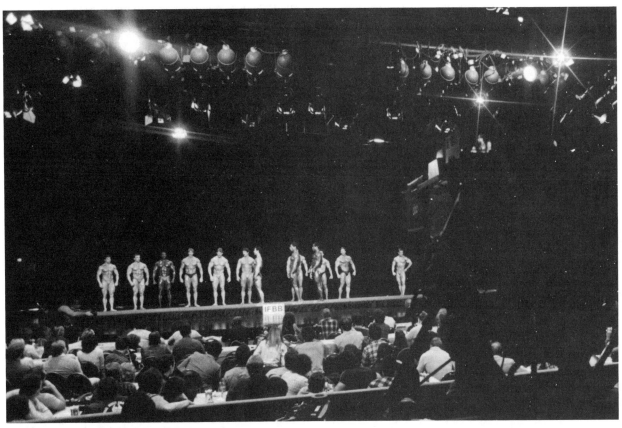

Long View: Comparison of three athletes in symmetry round, as pulled out of lineup.

ROUND THREE: FREE-POSING

"In Round Three of the IFBB Judging System, you will present your uniquely individual free-posing routine to your own choice of music," continues Platz. "The first two rounds of posing will reveal your development in the same poses as every other bodybuilder, but in Round Three you are at liberty to choose shots that highlight your strong points and camouflage the weaker areas of your physique.

"For some bodybuilders, the free-posing round becomes almost like a dance display, while for others it is merely a chance to get out there and sock it to 'em with heavy, super-muscular shots. The style of posing you choose will ultimately depend largely on your personality and on how completely you have developed your physique.

"Before you being working on your own free-posing routine, however, I strongly encourage you to attend as many competitions as possible, concentrating on how each athlete makes transitions between poses. And if you are unable for some reason to attend an actual high-level bodybuilding show, you can purchase videos of

most of the top men going through their posing routines. Such study is worth the time and money to see what is possible. And don't underestimate the inspiration great posing routines can provide.

"It's not excessive to spend at least one hour per day practicing your posing, particularly not the last 4–6 weeks prior to a competition. About half of this time should be devoted to practicing Round One and Round Two poses, while the remainder of your practice time should be devoted to Round Three and the posedown.

"One big mistake made by many novice bodybuilders is spending all of the practice time on perfecting a flashy free-posing routine. Free-posing accounts for less than half of your total score, so it makes good sense to practice the first two posing/judging rounds nearly as hard as your free-posing program.

"Your first free-posing routine will probably be based heavily on the compulsory poses of Round One, although I personally feel that it's foolish for an experienced bodybuilder to repeat mandatory poses in his free-posing program. If you do the same poses, change them

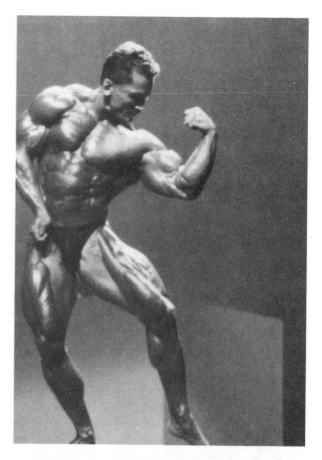

Depicted here in the middle of his free-posing routine at the 1988 IFBB Mr. Olympia show in Los Angeles, Lee Labrada has gained a reputation as one of the best onstage showmen in bodybuilding. Note particularly how he turns mundane poses into works of art, simply with a small shift of his feet, hips, arms, or some other part of his body. The shots are arranged in sequence and make up about one-fourth of his entire routine.

Photos by Bill Dobbins and Robert Reiff

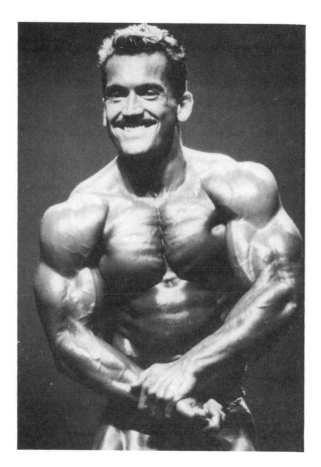

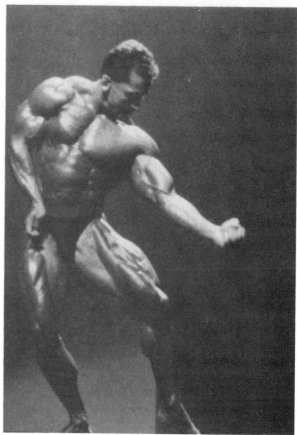

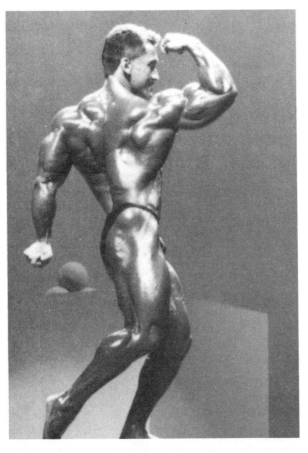

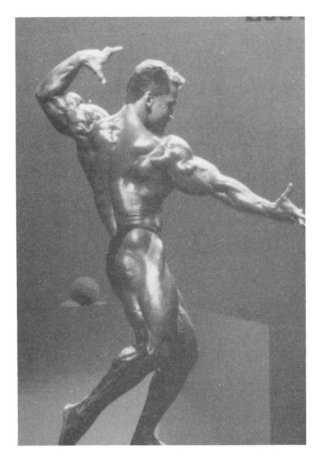

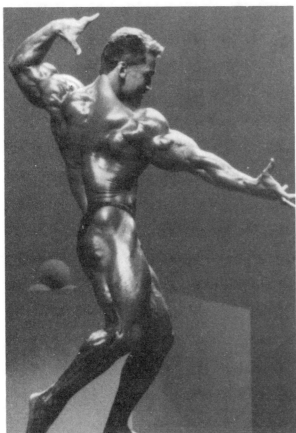

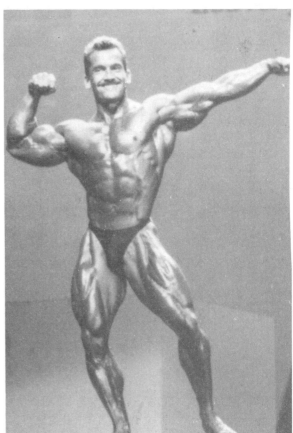

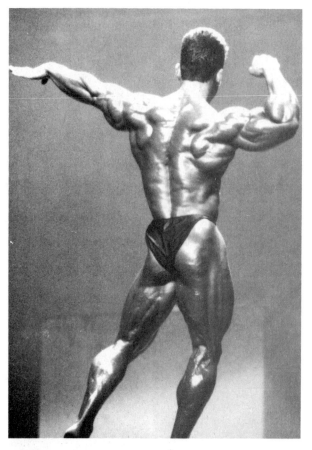
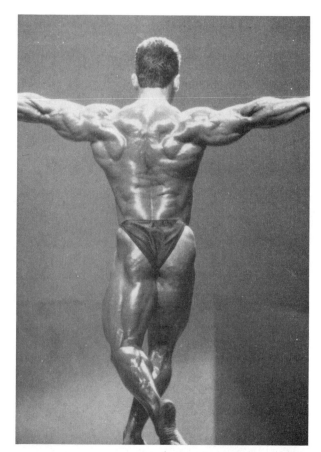
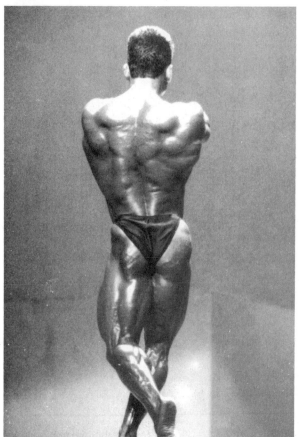
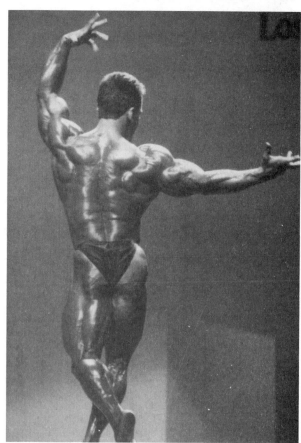

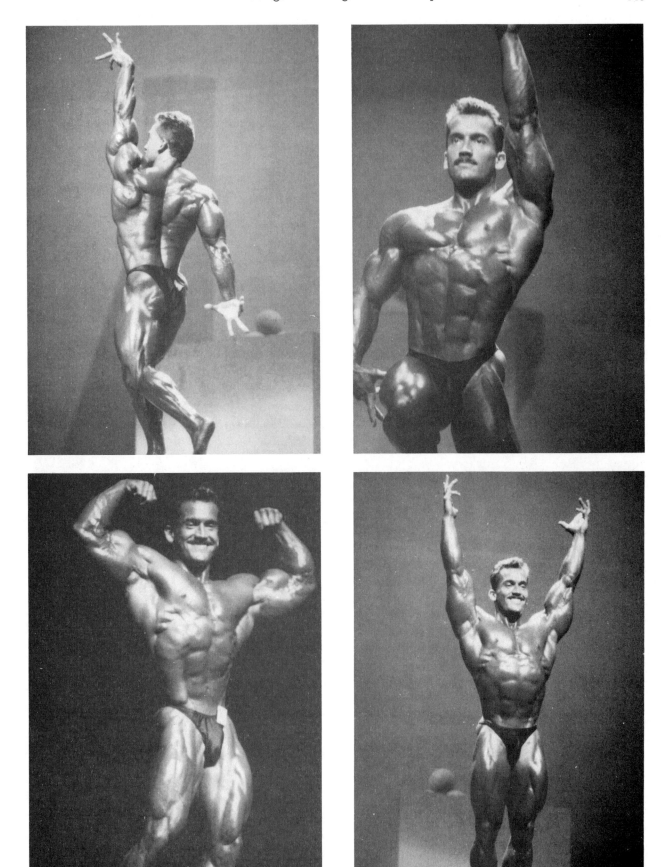

somehow from one round to the other. Just as one example, I do a side triceps pose in my free posing routine, but instead of standing when I do it—as is the case in Round One—I do it kneeling, a stance which totally changes the look of the pose.

"Your first individual poses will come from imitating shots you have seen depicted in various muscle magazines, but you are strongly encouraged to develop what may become your trademark shots, those poses that you alone do best.

"I have a lot of these signature poses in my own routine, but I'll tell you about only two. One of my most identifiable poses is my quadriceps isolation done with hands held in the small of my back. Another one, which invariably gets just as much audience response as the quad shot, is the one in which I smooth back my hair with one hand as it goes behind my head and the other arm is flexed. They go crazy for both of these poses, and everyone in any audience knows that they're uniquely Tom Platz poses.

"After careful observation, I've concluded that a good novice-level posing routine will consist of 10–12 shots. Still, you'll see plenty of young guys trying to pull off the 30-pose routine of a seasoned Olympian, but striking only 10 great shots and letting 20 bad poses overshadow the good ones. It's far better to do a smaller number of poses very well than many shots badly, then gradually increase the number of poses in your routine as your body matures.

"Concentrate on developing masterful individual poses, choose appropriate music, and choreograph a routine with artistic and effective transitions between poses. These transitions are very important because they indicate mastery of free-posing techniques.

"If you're having trouble coming up with good transitions between poses, I strongly suggest that you hire the services of a dance instructor, choreographer, or experienced bodybuilding poser for a few hours of intensive work. Such a man or woman can do wonders for your posing ability, and they can usually be located either by calling local dance studios or asking around at the gym where you are working out.

"Over months and years of posing practice, observing others onstage, and actually being onstage many times, you will learn little tricks of the trade that will endear you to both audience and judges. And when added up, these tricks will give you an indispensible quality: onstage charisma. Very little can defeat a bodybuilder in top shape who also has effective posing skills and a high degree of personal charisma."

THE POSEDOWN

Ah, the posedown. It's the *piece de resistance* of any bodybuilding competition, the time when the top five men can duke it out, man against man, for a few crucial points. I've often seen men jump up a place, or even two, in the final standings as a result of a hypereffective posedown. That's the main reason why a posedown is so energetic and animated.

According to *Chris Dickerson*, "There are two ways in which you can approach a posedown. My method is to remain aloof from the other contestants, no matter how hard they try to gain my attention. They come up and tempt me to duplicate all of their poses, but I just go through my preprogrammed posedown routine. By standing next to me and challenging me, they have admitted that I'm the man to beat. That's quite a compliment, and I'm sure the judges also notice it.

"The second method is to go ahead and respond to every challenge, and most bodybuilders can't resist the challenge of a heated posedown against a bodybuilder whom they feel they have to defeat in order to win the final competition. If you've ever seen a contest, you know that the audience responds readily to this approach, but I'm not sure that the judges do. They know what they're doing, and no amount of aggression in the posedowns can influence them to place you higher than you deserve. You might as well try my method. It's worked for me, and it will work for you, too."

I've only presented a bold outline of how you should pose at a bodybuilding competition. But it's difficult to advise you in detail how to go about posing, because it is such an individual activity. In the end, you'll make your best showing when you've spent many hours every week in front of the mirror gradually refining your poses. When you *know* you're good, you can go onstage and really shine!

CONTEST GROOMING

Personal appearance isn't supposed to count in your final competition score, but it always seems to. Whenever a competition is close, the man who is most healthy looking and well-groomed, who has the best skin tone and color, and who is wearing a posing suit which complements his native coloring always will place higher. And that's why I'm devoting a big section of this chapter to the vital topic of grooming.

SKIN COLOR AND TONE

Your skin is the biggest organ of your body. It's color and tone (these terms are often used interchangeably) play a great part in your general physical appearance. There are several things you can do to improve the appearance of your skin.

Taking a long-term approach to skin health should be a high priority for all competitive bodybuilders. The axiom "you are what you eat" applies more to the appearance of your skin than to the mass and density of your muscles. When you eat a lot of junk food, your skin shows it by appearing blotchy and pimply. Due to the fact that the skin is one of your body's eliminatory organs, toxins passing through the skin can cause eruptions that detract from your appearance.

Maintaining a well-balanced, junk-free diet will contribute greatly to skin health and appearance. It's particularly important to include lots of fresh vegetables in your diet. And you should consistently supplement your diet with a wide range of vitamin and mineral concentrates, particularly vitamin A supplements.

In order to keep your skin from appearing too loose once you reach peak shape—plus to limit the incidence of unsightly stretch marks—avoid bulking up by 30–50 pounds in the off-season. Bulking up really doesn't build significant muscle mass. It is most frequently the best available excuse a bodybuilder can find to eat like a pig for several months, then actually ending up looking like a pig. Your skin

will thank you if you maintain an off-season body weight no more than 8–10 pounds over competition level.

To make your skin soft and supple, I recommend rubbing vitamin E lotion into your skin each time you shower. Alternatively, you can use Nivea cream, but vitamin E lotion also helps to heal microscopic stretch marks before they become extensive enough to show up as ugly red scar lines in your skin. As you get older, those scars will turn white, but don't ask me which is worse.

It's essential (unless your skin is naturally dark) to have a deep tan for each competition. Not only do you look healthy, but dark skin displays the straitions and cuts in your muscles better than pale, sickly skin. This tanned appearance can be developed either naturally or chemically, or a combination of each type. A natural tan should be the preferred method. Many black bodybuilders lie out in the sun because of its skin dehydration properties. A natural tan gives you a thinner and darker looking skin, while chemicals only darken your skin.

Tom Platz has always been noted for his great natural tan, so I've asked him to tell you how he personally goes about tanning: "I have always relied solely on a natural tanning process, going out in the sun at least 3 or 4 months prior to a Mr. Olympia competition.

"You should allow at least 6–8 weeks in order to attain a deep, natural tan. Blitzing a tan and burning your skin in the process is counterproductive because a sunburn will draw water into your skin, making you appear much smoother than you actually are. It's much better to begin tanning early with short periods of exposure to the sun, then gradually work up exposure time as your skin darkens.

"I'd suggest starting with 10–15 minutes of sun exposure on both the front and back of your body. I personally prefer to lie out between the hours of 10:30 A.M. and 2:00 P.M., the hours of most direct sun exposure in Los Angeles. However, if your skin is rather fair, you should begin sun exposure before or after this peak-intensity time.

"Fair-skinned individuals should also consider using a sunscreen on their skin as they build up exposure time. Frequently reapplied, a

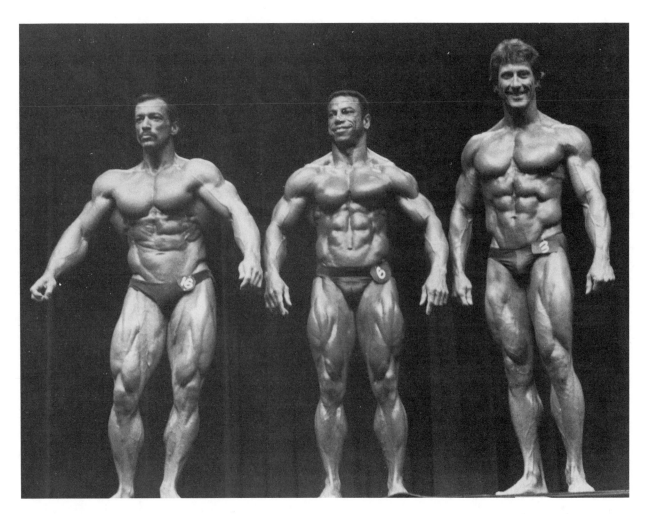

sunscreen filters out harmful, burning rays and permits the tanning rays to reach your skin. Sunscreens of varying strengths can be purchased at any pharmacy.

"I use a vegetable-oil coating on my skin when exposing myself to the sun. Commonly used oils, all available in bulk at health food stores, are almond, avocado, olive, and safflower. The oil keeps my skin soft and supple, as well as completely moisturized. And to further moisturize my skin when heavily into sunbathing, I rub Nivea cream on it both in the morning after my shower and at night before retiring.

"In addition to lying on your back and stomach, you should ultimately lie at various other angles to ensure an even tan over your entire body. And, you'll need to hold your hands above your head while lying on your back in order to tan your skin under your arms and along the sides of your torso.

"I prefer lying in the sun for both the depth of tan it affords, and also because regular sun-

bathing tends to dehydrate my skin, making it appear as though it's painted over my muscles. And the hotter the sun the last few days before a show, the better I like it. Therefore, it's not uncommon for me to pack my bags and jet off to Acapulco, Mexico for a few days just prior to competing in a Mr. Olympia show!"

During the winter, or at any other time when it is inconvenient to lie out in the sun, you can use a sun bed to darken your skin. Sun beds give you almost exclusively the tanning ultraviolet rays, but very few of the burning rays. You might still want to use a little sunscreen on your nose or other parts of your skin which tend to burn most easily.

Many bodybuilders can start out with a full 30 minutes in a sun bed, but very fair-skinned men should begin with about 15 minutes, then work it up to a half hour once or twice a day. You'll need to lie on your sides part of the time in order to achieve an even tan, particularly exposing the sides of your torso and legs, which are naturally shaded by the rest of your body.

If you live in the United States, you can obtain a prescription medication called Trisoralen, which augments skin pigmentation when you lie outdoors in the sun or inside in a sun bed. There are a couple of minor side effects your physician will tell you about, but as long as you guard against them you'll find Trisoralen a real help when tanning.

There is also a natural food substance called *canthaxin* which adds to skin pigmentation. You can find many ads for it in bodybuilding magazines. It's perfectly safe, and in conjunction with the sun, it's quite effective.

There are two types of chemical tanning agents: skin stains and make-ups. The most popular skin stain is Dyoderm, which lasts a day or two when applied at least 3–4 times on the skin. Dyoderm used to be available in most pharmacies, but was discontinued during the middle 1980s.

Several application methods are available for Dyoderm: spraying, rubbing on with a sponge, and rubbing on with a cotton ball. As long as you wear rubber gloves when putting on the goop and don't overlap strokes, you'll find 3–4 coats will give you a dark brown "tan" without running all over the place when you begin to sweat onstage.

There are several commercial "instant tans" on the market, and some bodybuilders use them. I personally believe they go on a few shades too yellow to look like a tan, but feel you should experiment with a couple of them in the off-season before making up your mind.

Makeups include tubes on "skin bronzer" and the powdered, dirt-like make-up used by many women as a cosmetic. The type in the tube is used on a man's face and washes right off. The problem with it is that it tends to run and streak.

The powder makeups can be purchased at women's cosmetics counters, and they go under names like Indian Earth and Beverly Hills Dirt. These *can* be rubbed on the skin with cotton balls, but they tend to streak a bit when you oil up. A better method is to mix the powder with some of your skin oil, then rub a couple coats of that goo on your skin.

Generally speaking, a deep natural tan is best. Next best is a combination of natural and chemical tans, the sun or solarium providing a good base for the skin stain. Chemical tans are a distant third when it comes to achieving a contest tan.

SHAVING DOWN

While a bodybuilder here and there might fail to remove all of his body hair for a competi-

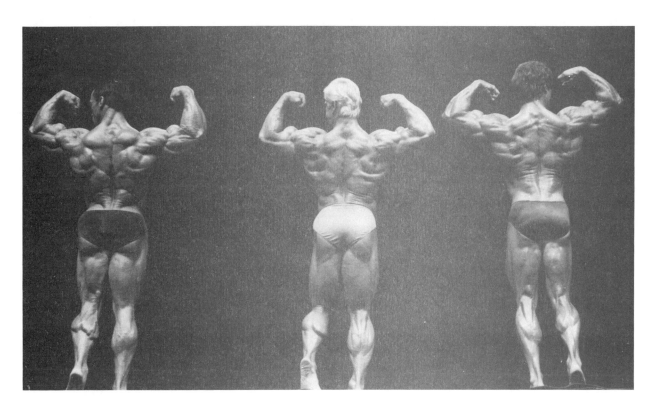

tion, virtually all iron athletes shave down prior to competing. Your hard-earned muscles should never be obscured by a thick pelt of body hair.

A few bodybuilders use chemical hair-removal cream, which is available without a prescription in most drug stores. But you should experiment with it on a small area of your body before using it wholesale. Allergic reactions are not uncommon, and there is an abrasive quality to these lotions that can leave your skin red or blotchy. That's why very few bodybuilders use any hair removal method besides shaving.

I'd suggest removing all body hair 2–3 months prior to competing, then keep it off with 1–2 shavings per week. This way, body hair won't get in the way when you are lying outdoors or in the sunbed getting a tan. Long-term body shaving also keeps you sufficiently in practice to keep you from nicking or abrading your skin a day or two prior to a show.

I took a survey and found that a majority of top bodybuilders like to shave down the first time while sitting in a tub of hot, soapy water, the way most women shave their legs. Simply use a safety razor over all of the hairy sections of your body, getting help to defur your back. After that first shaving, you can use an electric razor a couple of times each week to keep new hair from growing out of control.

If shaving down in a tub the first time doesn't appeal to you, an alternative method is dry shaving with a safety razor. This method is notorious for causing a few nicks and scrapes if you fail to do it very slowly and carefully. But shaving down a couple of months before competing allows plenty of time for your skin to heal.

HAIR STYLING

Cut and styling of both head and facial hair are important ingredients of a great personal appearance. When dieted down, virtually all competitive bodybuilders' faces are rather handsome. With your face leaned out, it's difficult not to be looking good.

You should always have your hair cut and styled prior to each competition, so you appear as clean-cut as possible. Be sure your hair is relatively short. Long hair can obscure your upper back muscularity. A hair style that makes your head appear large enough to detract from shoulder width is a mistake.

Unless you already have a hairstyle which complements your basic features, pay the $30 or so to have a professional stylist work with your hair to give you an appealing hairstyle. You can even have it styled the morning of a show. But whether freshly styled or restyled each day by yourself, use sufficient hairspray the day of a show to keep it looking fine while you are sweating through a warm-up and the long pre-judging rounds.

If you are balding, I strongly suggest that you consider getting hair transplants. This puts your own hair back where it belongs, and where it will never fall out again. Don't shortchange yourself in this matter. Be sure you get transplants from an experienced physician.

As long as a beard and/or mustache are neatly trimmed, I feel facial hair will never be a problem with the judges. More than 50% of all contemporary national and international champions have mustaches, and many of today's big winners sport beards as well.

POSING SUIT CHOICE

Experienced bodybuilders eventually discover their best posing suit cuts and colors, but first-time competitors *can* come up with an excellent suit choice before ever competing. All they need to do is follow the suit choice suggestions presented in this section. You'll get it okay alone, but if you have an experienced bodybuilder or knowledgeable gym owner handy, you should seek out his suggestions.

Suit color will be the least of your problems. By using the color chart on page 447, you can discover which colors harmonize with your basic hair color and skin tone. I strongly suggest you purchase two or three suits, perhaps in various colors. You'll invariably get oil on your suit at prejudging, so it's a great idea to have a fresh suit handy.

There are numerous suit cuts available. Some are cut high on the leg to display upper leg muscularity, or low to hide a lack of such development. Some others are cut low at the top to reveal lower abdominal muscularity, or high to hide a lack of such development. There are also several different cuts at the back of the suit.

Posing Trunks Color Chart

	Lightly Tanned	Darkly Tanned	Brown	Black
Red Hair	Medium Blue, Medium-to-Dark Green	Gold, Yellow		
Blond Hair	Red, Royal Blue, Black	Burgundy, Red, Medium Blue, Orange		
Brown Hair	Black, Navy Blue	Burgundy, Brown, Purple, Teal	Black, Yellow, Chocolate Brown	
Black Hair	Black, Navy Blue, Chocolate Brown	Yellow, Red, Gold, Orange, White	Lime Green, Kelly Green, Baby Blue	Bright Red, White, Red-Orange, Purple, Fusia

Source: The *Shape* magazine fashion editors.

You might hit on a perfectly cut and fitted set of posing briefs right off the bat, but you'll probably need to wear a variety of them to determine which fits best. Once you find a good cut, be sure to wear it when tanning, so you don't have untanned areas when you step onstage. (Alternatively, you can tan nude, a viable alternative if you use a sun bed.)

Some bodybuilders over the years have become closely identified with a particular suit color, so at the upper levels of the sport you might want to wear the same color from show to show. Frank Zane, for example, always wore burgundy, and it would be difficult to visualize him onstage in any other color.

YOUR COMPETITIVE WARBAG

Unless you use a checklist when packing for a show, you will invariably forget to take some vital piece of equipment with you. The following list was provided by *Ed Corney* (Mr. America, Mr. Universe), and all of the items in it can be carried in one medium-sized gym bag:

- Combination lock (if lockers are provided for valuables)
- 1-2 big, absorbent towels
- Shampoo and hair conditioner
- Comb
- Hair spray
- Tooth brush and tooth paste
- Eye wash
- Skin coloring (for touch ups) and applicator
- Hand mirror
- 2-3 posing suits
- 1-2 T-shirts
- 1-2 pairs of underwear shorts
- 2 cassette tapes of posing music (be sure to cue them both to the exact starting place for your music)
- Warm-up pants and jacket
- Oil (you'd be surprised at how many bodybuilders actually forget this little item!)
- High-energy snacks

With experience, you might wish to add one or two unique items to this list, items you personally need to take to every show. The key here is typing up a list based on the one above, then check off each piece as you put it into your gym bag. This way you can go to each show having to worry only about the competition, not about whether you brought your music cassette or oil.

PUBLICITY AND PHOTOGRAPHY

Far too many excellent bodybuilders seem to know so little about how to gain publicity for themselves in various bodybuilding magazines that they receive none. This is a shame, because there are a few easily followed procedures that will get you into virtually any bodybuilding magazine, provided you have a good, balanced, and aesthetic physique that is winning titles.

All of the English-language bodybuilding magazines worldwide are listed in the Bibliography in the back of this book. My own leading bodybuilding magazine, *Muscle & Fitness*, is pretty tough to get into, since it caters to the elite of the sport. You will probably have to have won a major national or international title to see your photos and an article about you in *Muscle & Fitness*.

My other muscle magazine, *Flex* (which is edited by Bill Reynolds, the coauthor of this book), is quite a bit easier to get into. *Flex* has several regular departments featuring new faces in the sport, and you can probably get into one of them—certainly your photo can be published, plus perhaps a short personality profile article—once you've won a local- or state-level competition.

The rest of the English-language bodybuilding journals are almost crying for quality

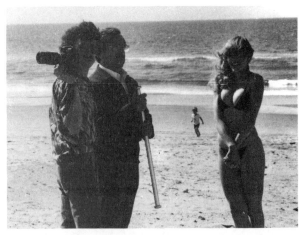

It's a dirty job, but someone's got to do it! The Master Blaster works with photog Craig Dietz to set up a beach bunny shot.

material, and any champion in the sport can see his or her photos published along with an article in any of these magazines. The key is having good quality photography and presenting yourself in fine written form.

The big casino is all of the scores of foreign-language magazines around the world. Most of them are independent, so they're always on the lookout for good quality black-and-white or color photos, plus articles, on promising bodybuilders on their way up in the sport. Every time you run across one of these foreign muscle magazines, make a note of the editor's name and the business address of the editorial office, so you can submit photos and article information to them once you have your publicity act together.

Let me give you an idea of how much national and international publicity you can generate for yourself. During the late 1970s, prior to winning his only big title, Mr. International, Andreas Cahling had won nothing bigger than the Mr. Venice Beach show, held each summer here in southern California. But he systematically had himself photographed by every available bodybuilding lensman every time he reached peak condition. By sending out a press release and different photos to each magazine on his extensive list, he made the cover of more than 20 magazines in the United States and abroad. Again, his biggest title was Mr. Venice Beach, and that's a smaller show than many readers who have never gotten publicity have won.

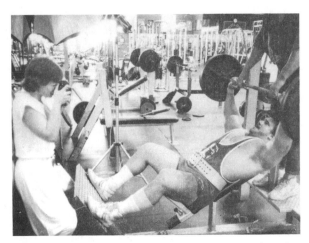

Paula Crane took many of the execise photos found in this book.

BODYBUILDING PHOTOGRAPHY

The first order of business when you set out to give yourself a burst of magazine publicity is to have high-quality photos taken of yourself. As long as a friend or family member has a 35 mm camera with a focusable lens, and the two of you follow the simple, sensible rules for good photography that I will outline in this section, you'll definitely get good-quality photos, good enough to be published in any bodybuilding magazine.

While you will see a lot of studio physique photos and gym training shots in the muscle mags, your best bet is to have your first physique photos taken outdoors with natural sunlight. These are relatively easy photos to take, and as long as you have mass, good proportions, and sharp cuts, you'll get superb photos.

Let's talk about camera, lens, and film selection first. As I said, a 35 mm camera with a focusable lens is essential, because you can never get a sharply focused shot using a cheap camera with a fixed-focus lens. Still, you won't have to spend hundreds of bucks on an expensive and elaborate Leica or Nikon camera, as nice as they might be for high-level physique photography. One that costs about $100 will do the trick nicely, and you undoubtedly know someone in your family or neighborhood who already owns such a camera or better.

The basic lens for most 35 mm cameras has a 50-millimeter focal length (the actual length of the lens). A 50-mm lens will work just fine for general outdoor physique photography. But if you happen to have access to a medium-range

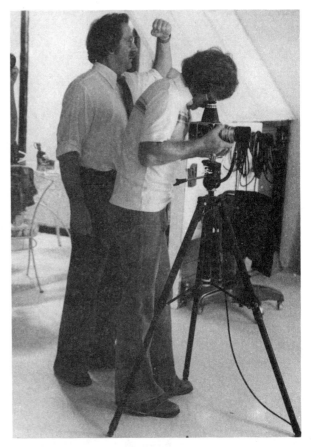

Joe Weider kibitzs behind the top flight Bob Gardner.

telephoto lens (something in the range of 85–135 mm), you can have your photographer friend blur out the background more easily on your pics, an advantage in physique photography work. Background can detract from the main subject of the photograph: you!

You will need color transparencies and good-quality black-and-white prints for magazine publication. The best 35 mm color transparency film is either Kodak Ektachrome 64 outdoor film (its a.s.a. rating is 64) or Kodak Kodachrome 64 outdoor film (again, it has an a.s.a. rating of 64). For black-and-white film, I suggest using Kodak Plus X (with an a.s.a. of 125).

After you have your photos taken, be certain that you send the color film to a Kodak lab for processing. The black-and-white film should be developed and printed on a proof sheet at a custom photo lab. The proof sheet allows you to preview all the photos from each roll of film and blow up only those which you want to submit to a magazine. Black-and-white prints should be the 8 × 10 standard size in width and height.

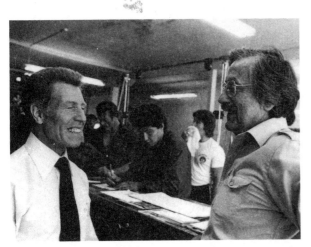

Jimmy Caruso is a legend among pro physique photographers.

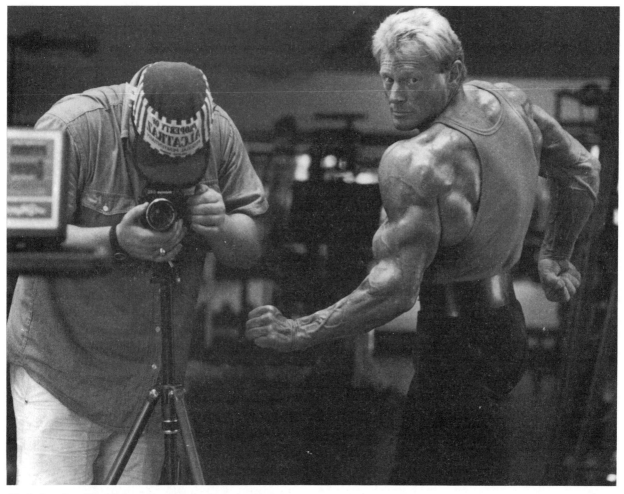

Chris Lund catches himself and the immortal Dave Draper in a mirror shot.

Next, you should think about your physical condition and personal appearance. Be sure you're in tight shape and have a good tan. Shave down like you would for a competition, be sure you have a fresh haircut, and wear solid-color posing trunks which fit you perfectly.

When you are completely prepared physically for a photo session, pick a location where you can be assured of having a monotonous background. Beaches with the water in the background are excellent, as is the top of a hill with only distant hills in the background. Be sure, however, that you don't pose in front of such "busy" backgrounds as bushes, shrubs, buildings, or the like.

All of your photos should be taken when the sun is at or below a 45-degree angle with the earth. Shooting during the middle of the day results in huge, distracting shadows all over your body. The best times to take physique photos outdoors is 8:00-9:00 in the morning and 3:30-4:30 in the afternoon. These times give you ideal sun angles.

Once you are at your photo location and your friend has the camera primed with film, he or she should use the camera's internal light meter to choose a perfect lens opening for $\frac{1}{500}$th of a second exposure interval *for each type of film used.* (A common mistake is forgetting to change the camera film speed (a.s.a.) setting when you switch from one film to another.)

Finally, every photo should be perfectly focused. Shoot all your black-and-white pics (two 36-exposure rolls of film will do the trick) with the indicated camera setting. But for the color shots, you should bracket your exposures, which means shoot one pic a half stop below the indicated exposure, one on the indicated exposure, and one a half stop above the indicated exposure. The middle exposure will usually be perfect, but to ensure getting a good shot you'll back that up with exposures on either side of the one the camera tells you to use.

After the session, get your film processed and sit down to prepare a package of photos and other information to send to magazines on your list. Just be sure that you don't send the same photos and information to several of the magazine editors, because they deserve a unique, exclusive view of you and your physique.

YOUR PUBLICITY PACKAGE

With the photos you send to each muscle magazine editor, you should also send a press release giving as much biographical information as possible. It's also a good idea to write out your

workout and dietary schedule and send them in with the photos. Be sure you include your home and work telephone numbers, just in case you didn't send in enough information, and the editor of the magazine needs more information to work up a story on you.

With a large manila envelope and a piece of cardboard the same size of the envelope to protect the photos, you can sit down to assemble your package. Address and stamp a return envelope in case your submission isn't appropriate for a particular magazine. Put in the self-addressed, stamped envelope, the cardboard, your black-and-white prints, and your color slides in plastic sheets that you have purchased for storage. Finally put in the biographical information and a short cover letter to the editor, ex-

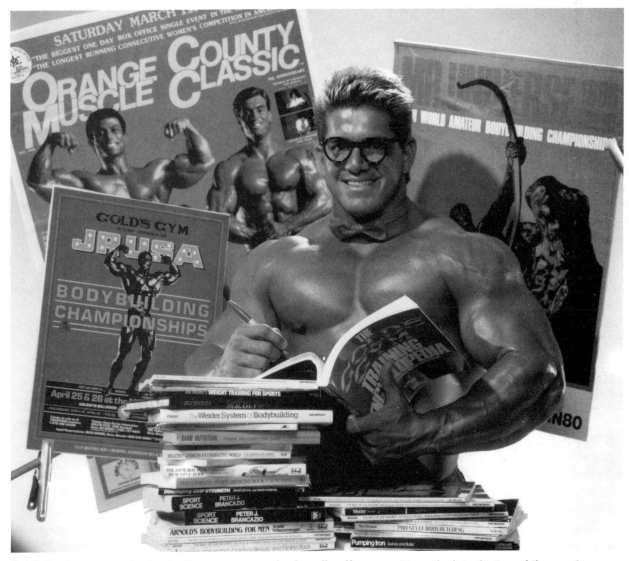

Publicity shot—those books, by the way, are required reading if you want to make it to the top of the sport.

plaining why you've sent your photos in and what titles you've won. Then send it off First Class mail, and keep your fingers crossed.

Occasionally, your photos may not make the grade, and you'll get them back as soon as the editor has decided not to use them. Feel free once you get them back to send the package out to another magazine.

KEEP TRYING

As soon as your physique is up to the standard of the bodybuilders you've seen depicted in various magazines, you're almost guaranteed of a photo and/or story publication. If you're really on the ball and lucky to boot, you might even end up on a cover, the goal of most serious bodybuilders.

Gradually, you'll meet up with the writers and photographers in the sport, and as your physique improves you'll gradually get more and more publicity. You deserve the best for all of your training efforts, so hang in there and keep submitting packages every time you're in good shape.

Ageless Albert Beckles (he was nearly 60 when this photo was taken) gets serious with a set of Cable Crossovers, an effective movement for the lower and outer pecs, carving deep striations across the muscle masses.

PART VI
BODYBUILDING
NUTRITION

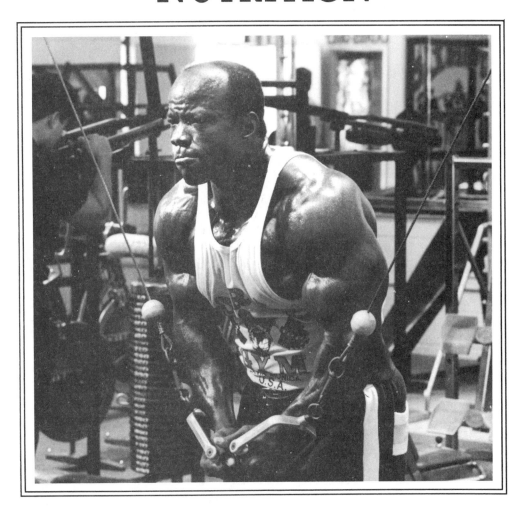

28
Nutrition and the
Competitive Bodybuilder

Like a skyrocket, *Gary Strydom* has streaked upward in bodybuilding. After winning U.S. and National Championships, he kicked off his professional career with an outstanding victory at Night of the Champions. Gary is typical of today's bodybuilders when he says, "All contemporary bodybuilders realize the importance of proper diet. Without it, all the training in the world won't build a contest-winning physique. I believe that diet and training are a 50–50 proposition off-season, with the importance of diet rising to 70%–75% of the battle as a competition approaches. I am truly what I eat, and so are you!

"Much has been learned about sports nutrition in the past few years. Five years ago, though, comparatively little nutritional information was available to me, so I had to formulate much of my nutritional philosophy through trial and error. I'd read about some new dietary practice, or hear about something from other bodybuilders in the gym, and would try it out. I could tell quickly if the variable worked for me. If it worked well, I kept it in the dietary rotation.

"Back in South Africa, my birthplace, my training partner, Ralph Piers, helped me a lot with my early dietary efforts. But since then I've relied on *Muscle & Fitness* and *Flex* magazines for nutrition information. Sure, I'd pick up a nugget of knowledge here and there, but I learned much more from reading than from experience in the gym.

"Whenever I have a new nutritional variable to try out, I rely on the Weider Instinctive Training Principle to determine how valuable it is to my unique system. Most bodybuilders think of this principle only in terms of training, but it's also extremely valuable when evaluating nutrition variables.

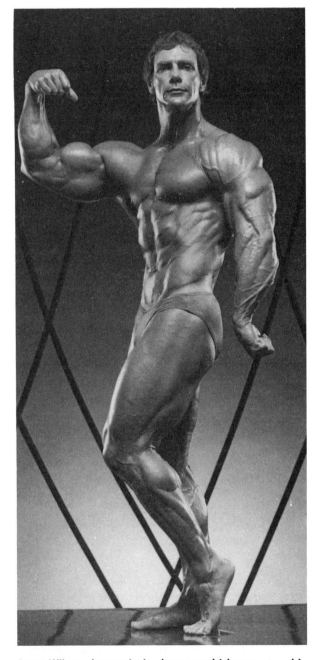

Scott Wilson demonstrates how good triceps can add to overall upper-arm impressiveness.

"It takes most bodybuilders six months to a year of monitoring their bodies' subtle biofeedback signals to master the Instinctive Training Principle, but all the effort is worthwhile. With good training instinct, you can rapidly evaluate any new training or nutritional variable. *That* saves a lot of time you might otherwise have wasted going down dead-end streets.

"I try to keep my nutritional philosophy as scientific as possible. My wife, Alyse, has a university degree in health and leisure, which involved a hell of a lot of nutrition study. Recently, she has been programming as many nutritional variables as possible into a computer to generate a profile of my ideal nutritional program.

"Some of the variables are data on the body's nutritional requirements to gain, lose, or maintain body fat and muscle tissue. Alyse inputs every change in my weight and aerobic workouts, changes in my mood, and which foods I actually prefer to eat. Each week she gets a readout of how many calories I should be eating each day and which foods (down to the ounce) I should actually eat at each meal.

"The computer comes very close in determining what I should eat each day. Its only real weakness is in its inability to take into account mood changes due to varying stresses from training. The computer also is unable to determine when I need to add a little fat in my diet, which normally occurs every 10-12 days."

While Gary Strydom has a very high metabolism and can therefore consume far more calories than many other bodybuilders, I feel his nutritional program presents a good example for other bodybuilders to follow. He continues: "I have leverage over most of my potential opponents because I have the ability to get ripped to shreds while maintaining relatively huge muscle mass. I have a good metabolism and the right nutritional knowledge.

"In the off-season I eat a few more calories than before a show (5,500-7,000 a day off-season versus 4,000-4,500 when peaking), but I still keep my consumption of fats under control. With a little extra body weight—no more than 15 pounds over contest level—in the off-season, I can train much heavier and make some significant improvements in my physique relatively quickly.

"I'd say that my off-season caloric intake is about 40% protein, 50% carbohydrates, and 10% (sometimes down to 5%) fat. This is very close to the ideal for hard-training athletes.

"Year-round I eat six times a day, consuming small meals at intervals of 2-3 hours. I never feel as though I'm stuffing myself, not even on 7,000 calories a day. I actually *need* every meal, because I'm training twice a day in the gym, plus doing aerobics every third day. My basal metabolic rate is very high, so with my activity level, I would lose weight on anything less than 5,500 calories. To gain muscular body weight I have to keep my intake up around 7,000 calories a day.

"In order to maintain the positive nitrogen balance necessary for muscle growth, a bodybuilder needs to take in plenty of high-quality, animal-source protein foods; however, I still eat very lean protein foods even in the off-season.

"Animal-source proteins are important because they have all the essential amino acids in sufficient quantities for muscle anabolism. Vegetarian protein foods usually lack one or more of the essential amino acids. So unless all the essential aminos are included in your dietary protein intake, your body won't be able to turn that protein into new muscle tissue.

"To be absolutely certain that I have a full range of essential amino acids in my system, I make heavy use of The Master Blaster's various protein and amino arid supplements. They supply any essential aminos that might be missing from my diet.

"If your budget doesn't allow you to buy the amounts of amino acid and protein supplements a serious bodybuilder needs, you can still make fairly certain that your body is getting them. You simply need to consume milk products—milk, cheese, cottage cheese, yogurt—and/or eggs with each meal. Milk and eggs are the natural foods that have the greatest supplies of each essential amino acid and consuming those two food groups will provide any essential amino acids that might be deficient.

"I'm very careful not to overload with protein and underload with carbs. With my low-fat diet and high-activity level, if I don't eat enough carbs, I can begin burning protein to meet my energy needs. Protein is a very poor source of energy, and it's required for muscle growth, so the natural solution is to keep my diet high in carbohydrates.

"In the off-season I eat complex carbs to provide a steady flow of energy, and consume simple carbs from fruit just before a workout for an energy burst. Eating too many complex carbs tends to smooth me out a bit, so I curtail them before a contest. I stick to the simplest carbs then, such as those found in baby food fruits.

"I take a *tremendous* amount of supplements during both off-season and precontest cycles, mainly amino acids, liver tablets, and multi-packs of vitamins and minerals. (I want to go on record saying most of these are Weider supplements.) I take a lot of mixed aminos before I train, plus individual arginine and ornithine in the evening before I go to bed.

"In addition to the multipacks, I take extra vitamin C, calcium, electrolyte replacement drinks, and a carboloading drink. I use protein powders to mix protein drinks only during the off-season. I always use milk-and-egg protein powder, because those foods are highest in biological protein quality. I always mix my protein drinks with juice, not milk, because I can't digest milk very well. Also, I like having both protein and carbohydrates in the same drink, because that helps spare the protein from being used for energy. You have to have carbs in your system in order to properly digest and assimilate protein. I use pineapple juice in my protein drinks, partly because the papaine in the juice is an enzyme which helps to digest the protein.

"My supplement intake goes up during a peaking cycle, especially the calcium, vitamin C and B-complex vitamins. I also take kelp close to a show to push my already high metabolism even higher in order to get *totally* ripped. And I take choline and liprotropics close to a show to assist in the cutting-up process.

"Through experimentation, I have found that I have to consume a lot of roughage. It's easier to consume protein and carbohydrates in liquid form throughout the day, but that doesn't provide the roughage I get from fruits and vegetables."

Strydom presented the following off-season day of nutrition and training:

- 0700—*Breakfast:* 5-6 eggs poached with only half of the yolks included, 2 slices of whole-grain dry toast, 2-3 pieces of fruit (perhaps a couple jars of baby food fruit), carbo drink, vitamin and mineral supplements
- 0830-1030—First workout of double-split
- 1100—*Lunch:* large tossed salad with tuna, sprouts, etc., whole-grain dry toast or slice of bread, glass or two of juice
- 1230—*Snack:* protein drink, vitamin and mineral supplements
- 1400-1530—Second workout of double-split
- 1700—*Snack:* tuna sandwich, 1-2 pieces of fruit, protein drink, vitamin and mineral supplements
- 1930—*Dinner:* steak (once every 4-5 days) or chicken or fish, baked potato (no butter or sour cream), steamed vegetables, fruit juice or iced tea, amino acid supplements
- 2200—*Snack:* bowl of whole-grain cereal with milk and plenty of fruit, arginine and ornithine.

"When peaking," Gary continues, "I eat pretty much the same foods as in the off-season. But instead of eating red meat twice a week, I may eat it only once. I cut my calories down to 4,000-4,200 per day. I really do get ripped up on a caloric intake this high. Many fellow bodybuilders envy my tremendous metabolism.

"Throughout the year I keep my body fat under control, no more than about 15 pounds above my projected contest weight. Then when peaking, I select the right foods and diet slowly and gradually, aiming at losing only one pound a week. If I'm 15 pounds away from my contest weight, I diet for 15 weeks.

"Concurrently, I increase my aerobic workouts from one every third day to one every other day. I also speed up my bodybuilding training, cutting my rest intervals between sets, sometimes by half. By eating less and exercising more, I lose about a pound a week and become muscular.

"Some weeks I'm not able to lose that pound. But as I get closer to the show, I may lose an extra 2-3 pounds during some of the weeks. I normally plan to be ready for a show 3-5 weeks out. Five weeks before the time I won the Nationals, I was low enough in body fat to compete. Then I allowed myself to eat my way to the show, gradually gaining a little body weight so my muscles looked full and my skin paper-thin. I gain a little muscle weight and lose a little fluid the last week, walking onstage ripped to shreds, massive, and very vascular.

"I sodium and carbo load during the last week. On sodium, I eat it for two days and then go off completely for 2-2½ days. With my muscles being 75% water, I don't want to lose much H_2O, especially since my body never seems to hold excess water. On carbs, I deplete for 3-4 days and then load for three full days.

"When I travel, I never leave home without food. For exhibitions, I leave late on Friday and then come back early on Sunday, so the food I take along helps me avoid eating the wrong foods. When I must eat out, I go into the kitchen and either prepare my food myself, or get someone to cook it exactly the way I want it. Then I'm back home early Sunday and back on my regular diet.

"I also take along a small bottle of distilled water to get me to the city I'm travelling to. I can always purchase distilled water in a grocery store once I'm at my destination. I keep the big bottle of water in my motel room.

"I've never had a problem with smoothing out after flying. I *have* had some problems with cramping, but eliminated that problem by being sure my electrolytes were perfectly balanced.

"I plan every show ahead of time and record everything so I can recreate a winning look over and over. I've seen far too many bodybuilders look great for one show and terrible for the next few because they don't analyze each peaking attempt to know *how* and *why* they reached a perfect degree of mass and muscularity.

"I write *everything* down. Instead of a hit-and-miss approach to peaking, I am able to consistently peak out perfectly because I keep very detailed records. You have to keep a record, and you have to trust your peaking formula once you have it down cold. Stick with whatever works for you and don't deviate by using other bodybuilders' suggestions. The person who knows your body best is *you*.

"If you feel like making small changes in your formula, that's okay. You can usually trust your instincts. If you do make a small mistake,

you'll have it written down in your training diary and can avoid making the same error for a subsequent competition.

"Listen to your body. It will tell you what you're doing right and/or wrong. Your body has many ways of showing the effects of nutritional variables.

"If you're not getting a good pump and you're going flat, maybe you aren't getting enough carbs, thereby giving you too little glycogen in your muscles to fuel your workout. If you're not sleeping at night, maybe you're overworking yourself and undereating. Or if you don't feel like eating all the food you need, perhaps you are overtraining.

"You *must* use the Weider Instinctive Training Principle in your nutritional program as well as in your training. Learn to recognize the biofeedback signals your body gives you. It's just as important to be instinctive in your diet as in your training."

Right on, Gary!

Each successful bodybuilder uses the Weider Instinctive Training Principle to gradually evolve a nutrition program—including food supplements—perfectly suited to his unique system. With an optimum nutritional schedule, you will make the fastest possible gains in muscle mass and quality.

Dietary instinct is easier to master than training instinct, because you can almost immediately notice the effects of nutritional variables on your body. In contrast, it may take months to notice the effects of some training variable on your physique.

Let me give you a couple of examples of how you can quickly tell how nutritional variables affect your body. Try eating a pint of Haagen Dasz ice cream (your choice of flavor) each night for two weeks. During the period you're eating the ice cream, keep an eye on your waistline. My guess is that you will see your waistline thickening almost from one day to the next because of the highly concentrated calories in this rich brand of ice cream. There isn't a pint of Haagen Dasz that comprises less than 1,000 calories, and that many extra calories each day will have a dramatic impact on your waistline.

A second example can be seen whenever you eat anything salty. Since sodium attracts more than 50 times its weight in water, you can notice a big jump in your body weight from one day to the next if you spend part of the previous evening chowing down on a salty pizza. I know bodybuilders who have mild allergies to milk and grains, who blow up 8–10 pounds after eating one medium pizza.

By monitoring the subtle, and not so subtle, biofeedback signals your body gives you each time you introduce a new variable into your nutritional equation, you will rapidly learn to tell almost from one day to the next whether a particular nutritional variable has a positive or negative effect on your physique.

FOOD SUPPLEMENTATION

In addition to macronutrients like protein, carbohydrates, fats, and water, you can use your dietary instincts to tell you which concentrated vitamins, minerals, proteins, and amino acids most enhance your bodybuilding efforts. With time, you will even be able to tell the relative effects of varying amounts of each micronutrient. When you master that delicate skill, you are on your way to becoming a superstar in the sport.

You'll need an approximate hierarchy of the value of various food supplements, because that will tell you which ones to run through first. Since you can only evaluate one food concentrate at a time, you should work from the most valuable down to the least valuable.

Here is a hierarchy of food supplements in approximate descending order of importance:
- Vitamin B-complex
- Vitamin C
- Powdered protein (preferably of milk and egg derivation)
- Calcium
- Potassium
- Magnesium
- Vitamin E
- Mixed free-form amino acids
- Iron
- Vitamin A
- Vitamin D
- Individual B-complex vitamins (start with B_{12} and B_{15})
- Inosine
- Carnitine
- Other individual minerals

- Desiccated liver tablets or powder
- Kelp tablets
- Arginine
- Ornithine
- Lysine and tryptophan

Be sure that all of the minerals you use to supplement your diet are protein chelated for more efficient metabolic utilization.

A FULL SUPPLEMENT PROGRAM

If you happen to have plenty of money to spend on food supplements, you might as well go for broke with a full program of food supplementation. I've known many bodybuilders over the years who have spent upwards of a grand per month for food supplements. Yes, they were almost living on concentrated food elements rather than everyday food. And many of these free-spending champs made absolutely fantastic progress on their out-of-sight programs of food supplementation.

When you can afford a Porsche, why drive a beat-up Honda? Instead of spending money on protein supplements, however, you should invest in free-form amino acids in capsule form. (You might try ingesting the powder itself, because that would get into your bloodstream more quickly, but bodybuilders who've tried this method say that the powder tastes somewhat like rotten eggs.)

The first kind of free-form amino acid formula would be one of mixed individual aminos. Some bodybuilders consume up to 75–100 of these capsules per day, which can mount up to a considerable investment each month.

In addition to mixed free-form aminos, you can invest in capsules of individual aminos that have an impact on muscle growth. Arginine and ornithine should be taken at bedtime to release human growth hormone, which enhances muscular development. You can also take tryptophan as a natural tranquilizer at bedtime; it will give you sound, restful sleep, no matter how jangled your nerves are each night. Lysine and Valine can also be taken individually during the day to foster muscle growth. And prior to each workout, both aerobics and weights, you can take capsules of branched-chain aminos.

Less affluent bodybuilders get by rather well

on one or two multipacks of vitamins, minerals, and trace elements per day. The affluent bodybuilders can take vitamins and minerals individually, gradually working out an intricate formula to be taken each day. You can take both B-Complex capsules and individual B vitamins. And you can take individual minerals, particularly the electrolyte minerals (calcium, potassium, and magnesium).

Some bodybuilders get heavily into desiccated liver supplements, taking as many as 50–60 tablets per day. That can add up to quite an investment. This is particularly true when you take liver capsules rather than compressed liver tablets.

The health food store owners will love you, because every time you come into their stores, you'll come with a handful of large denomination bills and a rucksack to carry off your bounty. But a lot of bodybuilders feel that such in-depth food supplement programs give them big gains.

BUDGET SUPPLEMENTATION

Most bodybuilders don't have the cash reserves that it would take to pay for the foregoing ultrasupplement program. If you could invest in only one food supplement, what should it be? I'd suggest investing in a high-potency B-Complex vitamin formula, because the B-Complex vitamins are vitally important in the cycle of muscle hypertrophy; without B-Complex vitamins, you won't make good gains in muscle mass or strength. And a bottle of 250 capsules cost less than $20.

As a second essential supplement, you might go to a drug store and purchase ascorbic acid (Vitamin C), which will keep your body detoxified. And that in turn will help you continue to make good gains in muscle mass.

For a budget protein supplement, I'd suggest going to a supermarket and purchasing a bag of non-fat milk powder. If you mix a heaping tablespoon of milk powder in regular milk, you essentially double the milk's protein content. And the protein in non-fat milk powder is of a very high biological quality, which can be readily digested and assimilated into muscle tissue.

With time and continued experimentation, you can expand your supplement program while still maintaining a tight budget. And you don't need to worry about making good gains in muscle mass, because with B-Complex, Vitamin C, and non-fat milk powder, you have all of the elements of a good food-supplementation program.

A health food store is a good place to shop around for supplements, although the prices in many stores are borderline out of sight. You definitely have to read labels when you are shopping in a health food store for vitamins, minerals, protein concentrates, and aminos. Check to see if each supplement is of high biological quality, then look to see what potencies are being sold by each distributer. Then you can compare prices for similar types of supplements of like potencies, purchasing only the one which is the best overall buy.

One of the best and most economical ways to purchase food supplements is to form a coalition with several of your bodybuilding friends, pool funds, and purchase the supplements at wholesale prices. In this manner, you can purchase large quantities, divide up the orders with your friends, and save a lot of money purchasing high-quality food supplements.

NOTES ON EATING OUT SAFELY

Since proper nutrition is so important in the bodybuilding process, you should learn how to eat out without blowing your diet. You will often be forced to eat away from home, perhaps at lunchtime or during a road trip lasting a day, week, or month.

The easiest way to blow your diet is to have any dish which is made up of two or more ingredients. For example, do you really know what food elements have been combined to make up that nice beef stroganoff? Probably not. There's bound to be one ingredient in that complicated entree that is on you no-no list. Eat it, and you've blown your diet.

The only sure way to maintain your diet is to consume only single-ingredient foods, such as charcoal-broiled chicken breasts with the skin removed before cooking and nothing on the meat. Even broiled lean ground beef is preferable to a dish with hidden fat and salt in it when you're dieting.

It's easiest to eat out at a broiler-type restaurant, such as the nationwide Sizzler chain. Most broilers will cook chicken, fish, or lean beef to your order, without adding any diet-threatening seasonings to the meat. All you need to do is discuss your meal with the waitress before ordering it.

Many restaurants douse their salad bars with sodium as a means of preserving the freshness of its ingredients; others don't because they are concerned with the cardiac health of their customers. You should ask the restaurant manager about this type of salad bar spray before ordering. Once you find a restaurant that doesn't add sodium to the salad bar, and *does* broil chicken to your liking, you should frequent it, and bring in some of your bodybuilding friends as a way of showing the manager your appreciation.

Dry-baked potatoes in a lot of restaurants can be a dietetic no-no, because the restaurants brush oil or butter on the skins before and/or during baking. Some of this oil or butter invariably soaks into the meat of the potato, thereby increasing its caloric value, and at least partially compromising your diet.

Rice pilaf in most restaurants is also contaminated with oil or butter. Restaurant cooks don't want rice sticking to their pans, so they add oil or butter to the water in which they boil their rice. And most cooks will also add salt to the mixture while it is boiling.

I also caution you to avoid drinking "diet" sodas unless you get one in an unopened, clearly labeled can. Waiters and waitresses tend to forget you want the cola without the sugar in it, bringing you the sugared variety instead. Some diet sodas also contain sodium. Even with the advent of low-sodium sodas, it is doubtful many restaurants carry them. To be on the safe side, drink either icewater or iced tea sweetened by you with aspartame.

If you are still in school or working at a day job, you might wish to pack your own lunch with foods that you *can* eat on your diet. These might include cold chicken, a small can of water-packed tuna, fruit, cold baked potatoes, and a green salad in a plastic dish. You can bring anything you want to drink in either the original can or a Thermos flask.

It's particularly important to pack and carry all of the food you'll need for the two or three days you'll be away from home for a competition. With carbo- and sodium-loading just prior to a competition, you have to be very careful of what you eat and drink for the final days prior to a show, as well as on the day of any competition. Bring your own food in individually wrapped packages, with the date and time each one should be consumed. And carry along your own distilled water. Don't forget your food supplements you'll require for the days you're away from home.

As an alternative, it is possible to rent hotel and motel rooms with refrigerators and cooking facilities. This way you can go to a local supermarket in the city where you will be competing, purchase your meal ingredients, and cook them yourself to be sure they don't contain no-no ingredients.

Michael Ashley (World Light-Heavyweight Champion) actually carries his own mini-microwave oven and electric frying pan, so he can cook all of his meals away from home. It's not unusual for the guys down the hall to stop by "just for a taste" when they begin to smell the delightful aroma of Mike's cooking.

The entire point of bodybuilding nutrition is to give you total control of how you will look onstage. You can stick 100% to your diet, and end up looking great onstage, probably winning the title for which you are competing. And, on the other hand, you can mess up your diet and end up smelling up the competition venue with the way you look. The choice is easy: stay in control of your diet!

29
Cycle Dieting

The Weider Cycle Training Principle advocates alternating off-season phases for performing heavy, low-rep training intended to enhance muscle mass and precontest phases for undertaking highly intense workouts required to reach a competitive peak. This way, muscle mass can be built up during an off-season cycle, and muscularity can be increased during a precontest phase.

The Weider Cycle Training Principle also applies to your year-round nutritional program. During the off-season you can consume plenty of calories—particularly from complex-carbohydrate and protein foods—to fuel heavy, high-intensity workouts. And during a peaking cycle, you must limit your caloric intake in order to slowly diet away body fat and reveal your muscular development very prominently.

It won't be difficult to master the theory behind cycle training and dieting. And once you have mastered the theory, you can greatly enhance your rate of muscle growth and degree of muscular definition onstage at each competition you enter.

Bodybuilders new to the sport are ultimately on an off-season mass-building program year-round, until they achieve the degree of muscle mass and balanced proportions needed to fare well in competition. For athletes currently competing, I recommend off-season cycles lasting at least 4–6 months, followed by a peaking cycle extending 6–12 weeks. Because there are so many individual nutrition variables to consider in a bodybuilder's personal dietary cycles, it's not as easy to recommend when you should begin peaking diets or off-season diets.

OFF-SEASON DIET

Your objective during an off-season cycle is to improve general muscle mass, and particularly to bring up any lagging body parts. It's easiest to build muscle mass when you follow a diet moderately high in calories (at least as high as your body weight maintenance level) and high in protein foods. There are also several food supplements you can add to your nutritional program which will also promote muscle mass.

I *must* caution you against using the old "bulk up and train down" plan which was so popular during the 1950s through early 1970s. Popularized by such superstars as *Bill Pearl* (four-time Mr. Universe), this system consisted of a period of heavy training and even heavier eating, which increased body weight up to 30–50 pounds over contest level. Then three months were devoted to a very strict low-carbohydrate diet which was intended to peel away all excess body fat and reveal a ripped-up physique with 6–8 pounds of additional muscle mass on it.

The problem with bulking up is that it really doesn't work. You might make a reasonable gain in muscle mass while bulking up, due to the use of heavier weights as a result of added tissue leverage when a bodybuilder is at a heavier weight. But what little extra muscle accrues when bulked up will very likely go by the wayside during the necessarily strict precontest diet.

Let *Lou Ferrigno* tell you about his experiment with bulking up: "When I was 18 I had worked my body weight up to 220 pounds in contest condition. Thinking it would help increase my lean body mass, I decided to spend an entire year bulking up and training down. I was aiming to add 10–15 pounds of muscle mass to my frame that year.

"So I ate everything that wasn't nailed down and trained like a demon on basic exercises with nearly back-breaking poundages. I ultimately got my body weight up to 305 pounds. Then I dieted down over a hellish three-month period. How much muscle did I gain that year? Only two pounds! Obviously bulking up and training down was not the answer to my problems with adding extra muscle mass.

"In reality, it's best to keep your body weight under control during the off-season and train hard and consistently when you're trying to add solid muscle to your physique. That way you will have plenty of energy for your workouts and won't have to diet off hard-earned muscle mass prior to a competition. That's the way all the superstars of bodybuilding go about adding muscle mass."

Enhancing Recovery Ability

To build muscle mass during the off-season you must be careful to recuperate fully between workouts. At its most basic level, your body cannot build extra muscle until it has recovered from the workouts before the present one. And there are food supplements that enhance recovery ability.

One miraculous food supplement has been used for many years by Soviet bloc athletes. However, it is new in the United States. It is called *inosine*, and news of the supplement reached the West when Dr. Fred Hatfield and Bill Reynolds returned from a sports training seminar in Moscow in the summer of 1984. Bill speaks Russian, and he and Fred were able to make friends with many of the best Soviet weightlifters. Those athletes told the intrepid pair about inosine, and Fred and Bill brought back samples. The substance can now be found in virtually every health food store in the Free World.

Inosine should be taken before and after every workout (whether aerobic or with weights) in strengths ranging between 1,500 and 3,000 milligrams per day. The inosine markedly increases training energy levels when used consistently.

Another recovery factor is Vitamin B_{15}, called pangamic acid by many nutritionists. For many years B_{15} was another secret of the great Eastern European athletes, who used it to improve oxygen transport to the working muscles. Like inosine, vitamin B_{15} can be purchased individually or in compounds with other food elements at most health food stores.

Desiccated liver tablets and powders, many feel, also increase training energy. There was a famous scientific study in which three groups of rats were fed different diets, then placed in drums of water to see how long they would swim before going under. One group was fed a normal rat diet; another, the rat diet supplemented by vitamins; and the third group, the normal lab-rat diet and all of the desiccated liver they wanted to consume.

Group two swam a bit longer than group one, but group three swam about three times as long as either of the other groups. Many bodybuilders and bodybuilding authorities believe that this experiment proves that liver enhances recovery ability and improves recovery between workouts. You'll have to experiment with liver tablets yourself to decide if they help.

Free-form amino acids (available most commonly in capsule form) is one of the best food supplements for promoting recuperative ability. Five or six capsules before and after each workout will go a long way toward enhancing recovery ability between sets.

Finally, you will recover much more quickly if you maintain a healthy, balanced diet as free of junk foods as possible. You had a good, basic diet menu listed in the last chapter, and later in this chapter, I'll provide suggestions for a weight-gain diet.

Anabolic Nutrition

Many bodybuilders take massive amounts of steroids in order to keep their muscles in an anabolic (muscle-increasing) state. To maintain an anabolic state without using steroids involves feeding enough protein and/or aminos to a bodybuilder to keep his system in a positive nitrogen balance.

When you break down muscle tissue, removing the water from it, the major constituent of muscle tissue is nitrogen. By placing stress on a skeletal muscle and feeding the body with plenty of protein to keep it in positive nitrogen balance, your muscles will constantly grow larger and stronger.

The best way to keep your nitrogen balance positive is to ingest plenty of free-form amino acid capsules every day. Free-form aminos rush right into the bloodstream, where they are available for assimilation into muscle tissue. Of course you could push amino acids into your circulatory system by eating regular food, but in comparison to free-form amino supplementation, eating normal protein foods is at best an inefficient process.

How many capsules of aminos should you take? Most top bodybuilders average about 20 capsules per day in the off-season and perhaps 30 close to a competition. I know of one top champ, though, who used to take more than 100 capsules of free-form amino acids per day prior to a competition.

Here is one good way to keep your system in positive nitrogen balance using free-form aminos. Every two hours or so, ingest 4–5 capsules of aminos and 250 milligrams of Vitamin C. Then train like a Trojan, and you'll increase muscle mass so fast that you won't believe you aren't taking anabolics.

SUGGESTED WEIGHT-GAIN DIET

Earlier in this book, Gary Strydom offered his weight-gain menu in which 5–6 smaller, protein-rich meals were consumed in one day. These meals must be high in milk and egg content, and also moderately high in complex carbohydrates. Following is such a daily weight-gain menu, in which you should eat every 2½–3 hours:

- *Meal One*—six-egg omelette with cheese, whole-grain toast, fruit, 1–2 glasses of milk, optional supplements
- *Meal Two*—broiled steak, 1–2 vegetables, baked potato, 1–2 glasses of milk
- *Meal Three*—tuna salad, 1–2 vegetables, 1–2 pieces of fruit, 1–2 glasses of milk, optional supplements
- *Meal Four (preworkout)*—protein drink (be sure it is made from milk-and-egg protein)
- *Meal Five*—roast chicken, 1–2 vegetables, rice, optional supplements, 1–2 glasses of milk
- *Meal Six*—boiled eggs, cold cuts, 1–2 glasses of milk

Overall, you should consume 300–500 calories above your maintenance level each day and at least one gram of high-quality protein per pound of body weight daily. With this much food, you will be able to meet your daily energy needs and have some calories/protein left over for building new muscle tissue. And this type of diet can be followed throughout an off-season cycle.

TRANSITION PERIODS

It would be a tremendous shock to your system to abruptly switch from a high-calorie off-season diet to one very low in calories. The same goes for moving from a low-cal diet to a normal, high-calorie off-season eating regimen. Therefore, you should program transitional phases lasting as much as 2–3 weeks between each major type of dietary cycle.

During a transitional period from off-season to precontest, you should gradually reduce your calories in stages of 200–300 calories each time you reduce food consumption. This way you won't shock your system so much that you end up binge eating because the tight precontest diet feels so restrictive.

It's also nonproductive to just pig out immediately after a competition. You should also have a transitional period between contest and off-season diets in which you gradually increase calories, allowing yourself some treat you've been craving from time to time.

PRECONTEST DIET

There are two main types of precontest diet—low-carbohydrate and low-calorie. The low-carb diet was almost universally followed by all bodybuilders during the 1950s and 1960s. It still has a few adherents, but nothing like the numbers who followed it during the golden days of the sport. One famous low-carbohydrate dieter was Frank Zane, three-times Mr. Olympia.

Starting about 1970, the low-fat/low-calorie precontest diet gradually won over bodybuilder after bodybuilder, until now the vast majority of all bodybuilders diet for a competition by gradually cutting back on caloric consumption by progressively limiting fat intake. A good example of a professional bodybuilder who diets on low calories would be four-time Mr. Olympia Lee Haney, who keeps his calories low all year (seldom more than 4,000 per day) to keep his body weight under control, then gradually reduces calories leading up to each Olympia.

Regardless of which precontest diet is followed, there are some food supplements that help you to get ripped up more quickly and to a greater extent. The first of these is lipotropic factors, which can be found naturally in such vegetables as safflower, or in capsules at a health food store.

While there is no conclusive scientific evidence to say it actually works that way, many top bodybuilders take kelp tablets prior to a competition. Kelp is rich in iodine, which could help to boost the output of your thyroid gland. Kelp is also rich in trace elements, but should be discontinued the last week prior to a competition because of its substantial sodium (water-retaining) content.

Choline and inositol, also available in concentrated form at health food stores, also help to metabolize body fat. One of the first great bodybuilders to discover this function of choline and inositol was Larry Scott, who won the first two Mr. Olympia titles in 1965 and 1966, and who reached his lifetime best condition at the age of 48.

LOW-CARBOHYDRATE DIETING

About 30 years ago, nutritionists discovered that eliminating carbohydrate foods from your diet will result in a rapid loss of body fat. You can actually consume a high number of calories in the form of fats, and still progressively reduce your body fat stores.

Low-carb diets do work, but they have some very undesirable side effects. One of the worst is a significant loss of muscle mass. It is not at all uncommon for a bodybuilder to lose 8–10 pounds of solid muscle tissue when limiting carbohydrates. Partly, this is due to the fact that you will have very low energy levels when low-carb dieting, which prevents you from getting in your normal heavy, high-intensity training sessions. The body also steals energy from muscles during anaerobic training.

Low-carbohydrate diets can also play hell with your mind, causing violent mood swings. It's not at all uncommon for a bodybuilder to become very depressed while on a low-carb diet

and binge eat as a result, wiping out all of his gains in contest muscularity.

In my experience, low-carb diets work best for ectomorphic (naturally thin and small-boned) bodybuilders. Many of them seem to thrive on the high-fat content of such a diet, because it seems to help them maintain a higher degree of muscle mass than is possible when low-calorie dieting. But this effect varies from one man to another, and you should experiment with both types of diet during the off-season to see which one works best for you.

If you plan to diet on limited carbohydrates, start out by consuming about 300 grams per day. (You can purchase an inexpensive carbohydrate gram counter at most drug stores.) Then each week, drop your carbohydrate consumption by 40–50 grams, until you are as low as about 30–40 grams per day. Some bodybuilders go to functional zero on carbs, but going so low on carbohydrate intake can turn virtually anyone into a moody maniac.

If you do choose to diet for a competition by limiting carbohydrates, it is essential that you progressively increase your intake of supplemental vitamins and minerals. When you are eating only meat, poultry, fish, eggs, and milk products, you are taking in very low amounts of many vitamins and minerals, which might cause a dietary deficiency which could retard your progress.

Following is a sample one-day menu for tight low-carb dieting, which you can experiment with in the off-season:

- *Breakfast*—fried or scrambled eggs, steak, half a cantaloupe, coffee, supplements
- *Lunch*—broiled chicken, green salad with safflower oil and vinegar dressing, iced tea, supplements
- *Dinner*—roast beef, green beans, iced tea, supplements
- *Snacks*—boiled eggs, hard cheese, cold cuts

As you experiment with a low-carbohydrate diet during an off-season cycle, you should take detailed written notes of what you are eating and photograph how your body is responding to the diet. Without these records, you really won't be able to tell over the long run whether you should use such a diet prior to a competition, and what to expect the next time you use it.

LOW-CALORIE DIETING

There is a considerable body of scientific research that proves you will lose body fat if you consume less calories than you expend in daily energy requirements for body metabolism and physical activity. To achieve a low caloric intake, you can limit intake of fats while keeping protein and carbohydrate intake up. And since you can consume large quantities of complex carbohydrate foods, you won't have the severe diminution of training energy, one of the undesirable side effects of a low-carb diet.

One gram of dietary fat yields about nine calories when it is metabolized (burned) to yield energy. One gram of body fat also yields the same number of calories when it is metabolized to meet your energy needs. In contrast, one gram of either protein or carbohydrate yields approximately four calories when metabolized. Therefore, fat contains about twice as many calories measure by measure than either protein or carbohydrate. So it just stands to reason that keeping protein and carbohydrate intake up while progressively reducing caloric-expensive fats in your diet, will place you into a negative-caloric balance. Result: you lose body fat.

While your body will gradually metabolize stored fat to meet its energy requirements, its preferred source of energy is carbohydrate foods. These natural sugars are turned into glycogen and other body sugars, and used to fuel your physical and mental activity.

There are simple and complex carbohydrates, and this designation refers to how difficult it is for your body to digest and metabolize the sugars in that food. Simple carbohydrate foods, such as those containing white sugar or white flour—rush through your bloodstream and immediately give you a blood-sugar spike. But this characteristic of simple carbohydrate foods has a negative affect in a bodybuilding diet, because your body releases insulin into your bloodstream to regulate your blood sugar down below normal, which results in a plunge in energy level.

In contrast, complex carbohydrate foods are digested slowly and released into the bloodstream slowly, where they supply a lower, yet steady, yield of training energy. These foods include potatoes, brown rice, seeds, nuts, vegetables, and some fruits. All of the top champions prefer to get their carbohydrates from these food groups.

You will need a calorie-counter book when low-calorie dieting. I usually recommend the calorie tables in *The Nutrition Almanac, Second Edition* (McGraw-Hill, NY, 1984), but there are also many calorie-counter booklets available. If you don't own a copy of *The Nutrition Almanac*, you can purchase it at most health food stores. This invaluable book lists many foods by their caloric, carbohydrate, sodium, and many other nutrient levels of most foods.

The best way to low-cal diet is to start your regimen 3–4 months out from a show, preferably after you have kept your body fat levels under control during your off-season cycle. This way you can diet slowly and less intensely over a long period, ultimately achieving intense contest muscularity without ever feeling like you had to deprive yourself of the foods you prefer to eat.

Determine your caloric maintenance level prior to starting your diet by writing down the amount of every food you consume during a week when your body weight remains stable. Total up your calories, divide by seven, and you have found a good working number of calories you must consume each day to maintain your body weight at a steady level.

When you start your diet, gradually reduce and then remove fatty foods and high-sugar junk foods from your diet. The foods with lots of fat in them include whole milk, beef, pork, egg yolks, poultry skin, avocados, corn, nuts, and seeds. By consulting your calorie table, you can determine which foods have significant fat content.

About 12 weeks out from a competition, you might be at about 3,500 calories per day, a typical maintenance level for an average-sized bodybuilder. Then each week you gradually reduce your daily diet by 100-200 calories, until you are down to perhaps 2,000 calories. Maintaining that level of caloric consumption and adding some aerobics will usually lean out virtually anyone. However, you might need to go lower than 2,000 calories if you get behind on your schedule.

Scott Wilson (Pro Portland Grand Prix

Champion) gives you a valuable bodybuilding dietary maxim: "Start your diet early and keep on schedule. Once you get behind on your diet, you can never get back on schedule without sacrificing valuable muscle size. Generally speaking, the more bland a diet is, the more valuable it is when seeking peak contest muscularity."

Following is a sample low-calorie diet which you can experiment with during the off-season to see if low-fat dieting is best for you:

- *Meal One*—egg whites, cooked whole-grain cereal, slice of watermelon, coffee, supplements
- *Meal Two*—water-packed tuna in a salad with minimum amount of Pritikin salad dressing, iced tea, supplements
- *Meal Three*—broiled fish, rice, green vegetable, iced tea, supplements
- *Meal Four*—broiled fish, dry-baked potato, green salad with Pritikin dressing, iced tea or coffee, supplements

BODY WATER BALANCE

Historically speaking, bodybuilders learned about 30 years ago that they could improve contest-day muscularity by dehydrating their bodies. At first this merely meant limiting water consumption for the last 2–3 days. But gradually, more and more bodybuilders resorted to harsh chemical diuretics.

Diuretics are dangerous because they leach electrolytes from your system, which can result in tachycardia (an irregular heart beat), which in turn can kill a bodybuilder. It took a couple of deaths, one being a former World Champion named Heinz Sallmayer, to convince bodybuilders that they should experiment with other means of changing the balance of water in their bodies.

Sodium control became an important way to temporarily reduce the body's water content. Sodium has a high affinity for water, as evidenced by the fact that it attracts and holds more than 50 times its weight in water. So by limiting sodium from the diet for 3–7 days prior to a competition, body water could be effectively eliminated.

SODIUM LOADING–DEPLETION

Some bodybuilders still had water retention problems, despite limiting sodium intake. *Samir Bannout* (Mr. Olympia in 1983) was one bodybuilder who suffered from water retention, despite controlling sodium. The reason for this problem was aldosterone secretion, which was the body's response to the stress situation prior to competition. Aldosterone retains sodium, which in turn retains water.

Aldosterone can be controlled with a prescription medication called Aldactone. But many bodybuilders prefer to limit aldosterone secretion naturally by sodium loading. Indeed, sodium loading–depletion is a favorite way of preventing the body from secreting aldosterone.

The sodium-loading cycle begins about 10 days prior to a competition. On the first day, you consume about 2–3 grams of sodium, and gradually work it up over a seven-day period to 8–10 grams of sodium per day. All of this sodium in your diet suppresses aldosterone secretion.

After seven days of sodium loading, you go completely off sodium for the final three days, even to the point of drinking distilled water to prevent you from getting any sodium from tap water. All of the sodium in your body will be flushed out in about 48 hours, leaving your body almost totally devoid of sodium content. Normally, the body will respond to this fact by again secreting aldosterone, but it takes some time for this to occur, more than three days. As a result of sodium loading–depletion, your body water content will be much lower-than-normal, and you will appear quite a bit more muscular than you would if you allowed aldosterone to spoil your hard-earned cuts.

CARB DEPLETION–LOADING

Carbohydrate depletion–loading is a means of pulling water out from under your skin and into your skeletal muscles, which allows your muscles to appear round and full, while your full-body muscularity improves. Carb loading takes advantage of the "supercompensation" carbohydrate factor discovered by Scandinavian exercise physiologists about 20 years ago.

The length of time you deplete and load, and the degrees to which you both deplete and load are highly individual, and you should experiment with various formulas in the off-season when a mistake isn't as disastrous as it would be when peaking. Over a period of time, you can discover the precise formula suited to your individual physique. But I can tell you generally the way it should be done.

Carbohydrate depletion–loading is a 5½-6 day cycle. It starts with 3 days of zero-carbdieting, while concurrently exhausting the body's supply of glycogen through long-lasting aerobic training and hard gym workouts. After 3 days of deprivation, you can load up on complex carbohydrates for the final 2½-3 days. The amount and type of complex carbohydrate foods vary, but rice and potatoes are commonly consumed, and 150-300 grams per day is about average among elite bodybuilders.

When your body has been starved of carbohydrates, it responds by supercompensating for this situation by storing amounts of sugar much higher than usual in the liver, muscles, and bloodstream. Each gram of carbohydrate attracts about four grams of water, which—when you limit water consumption to about two quarts per day—is pulled out of the tissues beneath the skin. This makes your muscles appear round and full, and gives you prominent vascularity.

It takes a strong mind to survive the combination of sodium loading–depletion and carbohydrate depletion–loading, because your physique will appear small and very smooth for the last few days before a competition. You will be sorely tempted to drop out of the competition. Many bodybuilders do bag competition at the last minute. But if you are able to stick it out, you will see a fantastic physique in the mirror the morning of your competition.

One other factor can have a bearing on how much excess water your body is retaining. When you have mild food allergies, they can also cause excess water retention. Most commonly, bodybuilders are allergic to milk and the gluten found in all grains except rice and millet. Simply by avoiding milk for the last few weeks and grains for the last couple of weeks, you will greatly improve your contest muscularity by reducing the possibility of water retention.

FINE TUNING YOUR DIET

It takes quite a bit of experience to peak perfectly for a competition. You have to have taken good photographic and written notes during other peaks, developing weekly checkpoints leading up to the competition and daily checkpoints over the last week. Then you can reduce food and increase aerobics if you are a little behind schedule, or increase food and decrease aerobics if you are a bit ahead of schedule. This ability to fine tune your diet is invaluable, and you can only obtain this ability primarily through experience. But be sure to always take notes about how you should appear at each of your checkpoints, and how your body reacts to various dietary and physical-activity factors.

PART VII
THE PSYCHOLOGY
OF BODYBUILDING

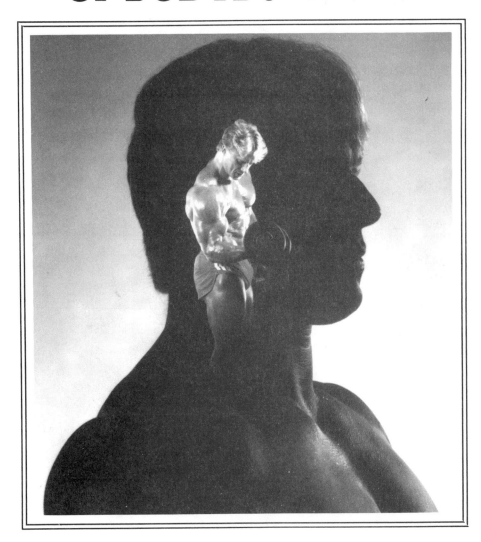

30
The Inner Game of Bodybuilding

Bodybuilders striving for ultimate development cannot afford anything but 100% effort, physical or mental. This means they cannot allow discouragement, a bad mood, superstitions, or anything else to keep them from making the most of their training. To be certain of success, this involves being sure you can train yourself mentally, just as you do physically.

POSITIVE THINKING

Since much of what we think and feel comes from habit, it can be dealt with using standard behavioral-modification techniques. Most temperament problems that keep bodybuilders from achieving their full potential are the result of negative thinking, cases of the mind getting in its own way. We all make mental mistakes that cloud our thinking, but I believe the following 10 mistakes are among the most significant obstacles for competitive bodybuilders seeking top titles.

The Either/Or Mistake—This is the error of expecting perfection. If you don't win the Mr. Universe title, you're a total failure. If everything isn't exactly right, it is all wrong. The truth of the matter is that everything is a matter of degree, and all measurements simply indicate how one thing relates to another, not to any absolute.

Solution—Learn to see things as matters of degree.

The Overgeneralization Mistake—This occurs when you jump to the conclusion that, because something didn't work out one time, that's the way things will always be. Somebody insults you, so you decide nobody likes you.

You don't win a competition, so you conclude you're a second-rate bodybuilder and that you'll never win. The truth is that not everything is part of a pattern. And even when things *do* indicate a general pattern, patterns can be altered and changed. The future is not inevitable.

Solution—Recognize that some events are isolated and unique, just as others are part of a general pattern.

The Negative Interpretation Mistake—We all see both good and bad around us practically all the time. When we're depressed, we tend to ignore the good and focus on the bad. If you do this for a while, you have to come to the conclusion that everything in your life is negative, and that simply is not true.

Solution—Practice seeing the positive as well as the negative in life situations.

The Negative-for-Positive Mistake—Some people just can't seem to accept compliments. They're the sort that have to twist any positive thing that happens to them so that it comes out negative.

Solution—Learn to accept and enjoy the positive aspects of life.

The Self-Fulfilling Prophecy—Because you believe something is going to happen, you actually help to bring it about. Suppose you're standing onstage in a contest and you find you're not called out for comparison often enough to suit you. So you assume that the judges don't think much of you, you get depressed, your energy sinks, and you don't present yourself to your best advantage. By doing this, you make sure that you won't score high. But actually, you did not know for certain what

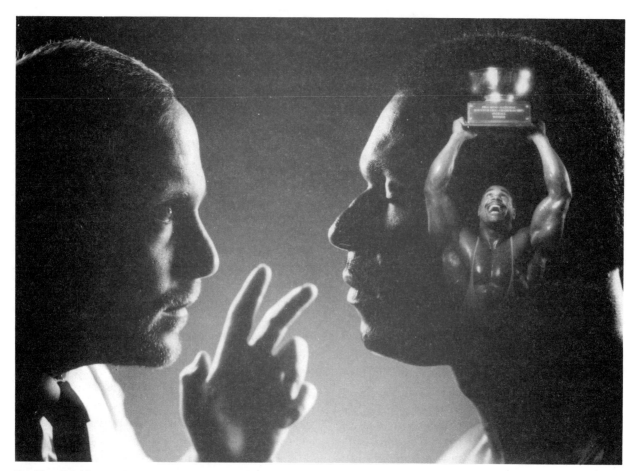

Positive thinking and the power of visualization are important in everything you undertake, including bodybuilding.

the judges thought of you, and it shouldn't have mattered. You were supposed to be up there doing your best, no matter what they thought. Besides, the first time Lee Haney won a Mr. Olympia competition, he was called out for only a couple of comparisons, because he was so obviously a winner.

Solution—Stick with conclusions that you can square with the facts, and don't go out of your way to create problems for yourself.

The Distortion Mistake—This involves making too much of your mistakes and not enough of your good points. If you insist on doing this, you're always going to make yourself feel inferior, no matter how well you really are doing. If you foul things up from time to time, you're no different than anyone else. But mistakes aren't the end of the world.

Solution—Learn to see your strengths and weaknesses in their true perspective; don't exaggerate or minimize.

The Feeling/Thinking Mistake—This is the error that happens when you assume that your feelings and emotions necessarily reflect reality. When you project your negative emotions onto the world around you, that world begins to seem negative, too. But in fact, what you do or don't like, do or don't want, prefer or disdain, frequently tell you nothing about reality. If you get into the "I feel overwhelmed, things are hopeless" habit of thinking every time the going gets tough, you will talk yourself into giving up.

Solution—Learn to distinguish between how things are and how you feel about them.

The Should Mistake—If you set your expectations too high, and convince yourself that there is some standard you have to live up to, some out-of-reach goal you have to attain, you are always going to see yourself as a failure. Perfection is simply not attainable . . . by anyone!

Solution—Learn to develop reasonable and attainable expectations.

The Inner Game of Bodybuilding

The Worst Possible Interpretation Mistake—

This is a form of overgeneralization and exaggeration in which you always end up assuming the worst. If you feel afraid, you assume that you're a coward; if you can't lift a certain weight, you assume that you're weak. In reality, we are all afraid sometimes, even the bravest of us, and weakness and strength are relative terms. You're stronger than some people, weaker than others. You're even stronger or weaker than yourself one day to the next.

Solution—Learn to recognize that you are not your mistakes. Don't label yourself automatically.

The Taking Blame Mistake—

Blame is the mother of guilt. If something goes wrong, it's not necessarily anyone's fault. If your workout partner doesn't do well in a contest, you shouldn't automatically assume that you didn't push him hard enough in the gym. Just remember, you may have a lot of influence on events around you, but you don't necessarily have to take the responsibility for them. After all, who put you in charge anyway? Let people take responsibility for themselves, and get on with your own life.

Solution—Don't assume responsibility where you don't have any control.

Putting all of these examples together, it should become pretty clear why some people make themselves suffer and become depressed when there's no real justification for it. It should also shed some light on the behavior of certain bodybuilders. When you read about Frank Zane meditating every day or working to develop nothing but a positive outlook on his career, you can see why. Zane was competing on a level where only a fraction of a percentage point may have separated him from a challenger. He needed to actualize every bit of potential that his mind and body possessed. That's the reason he stressed the mental aspect to such a degree, and that's what made him a three-time Mr. Olympia while competing against athletes who routinely outweighed him by up to 50 pounds!

Watching the film *Pumping Iron* on video, you can see how Arnold Schwarzenegger worked to create doubts in the mind of a young Lou Ferrigno prior to the Mr. Olympia competition in 1975. And you can see how Ken Waller tried to confuse Mike Katz prior to the Mr. Universe competition held with that Olympia. The film distorted these events to some degree, but the statement it made is true: the body cannot triumph if the mind is defeated.

Defeat more often comes from within rather than from outside ourselves. Some people learn to be very successful at failing. And those people do not become champions.

You don't develop a positive outlook just by willing it, however. You have to work at it, learn new habits by practicing them every day. But all this shouldn't convince us that negativism is all in our heads. It isn't. Sometimes negative information indicates what is really going on, tells us it shouldn't be ignored.

Pain is of this kind of information and it can be used positively. So is failure. When Arnold came to this country in 1968 to compete in the IFBB Mr. Universe competition, his defeat by Zane served to spur him to even greater efforts, and he was never defeated again. Taking responsibility for the failure, admitting he wasn't perfect, was the first step Arnold took toward making even greater progress.

Negative and positive feelings are a vital part of using the Weider Instinctive Training Principle in your workouts. By learning to pay attention to your feelings, and looking to see what realities they might represent, you can fine-tune your intuition so that it becomes a valuable asset in your progress.

Sometimes you may feel bad about something because you are doing the wrong thing. Maybe you're using the wrong kind of training routine, or you have allowed your dedication to training to unbalance the priorities by which you're leading your life.

The trick is not to overreact. Be aware of the positive and negative influences in your life, but don't let them sway you unduly. Life has ups and downs, but they have to be kept within limits. Otherwise, we just lose track of where we're going.

When you overreact, misinterpret, distort or jump to conclusions emotionally, you can't really listen to what your body and mind are telling you. The Instinctive Principle depends on your ability and willingness to pay careful attention, and not to make assumptions or create self-fulfilling prophecies.

Reality is a potent force. By working to regulate the swings of your individual temperament, you can get reality on your side so that it works for you, rather than against you.

INSPIRATION AND MOTIVATION

Past positive thinking, motivation is one of the most fundamental concepts in bodybuilding psychology. Without being highly motivated, you'll never become a champion. Highly motivated athletes are almost invariably highly successful athletes, particularly if they have good genetics for the sport.

Unfortunately, very few bodybuilders—even at the professional level—know how to become properly motivated to succeed in the competitive arena. If they give the concept any thought at all, most bodybuilders feel they're either born with high motivation, which will take them to victory in high-level competitions, or they'll never have enough motivation to become champs. This belief is definitely not true.

The father of motivation is inspiration. Three-time Mr. Olympia *Frank Zane* has commented at length on the subject of inspiration in bodybuilding:

"The dream is always there . . . you're center stage, the spotlight is yours, and the audience is in the palm of your hand as you explode with muscularity. Applause is deafening. You've won the Olympia!

"But it will always remain a dream without that singular quality that sets champions apart from the merely great: inspiration.

"Sure, you train with dedication, you train with skill, you use the latest most-effective techniques, and you pound the weights until you collapse, but if you lack inspiration, you'll always be an also-ran.

"To everyone, inspiration is a mystery, and most people will never know it, let alone be able to control it or summon it at will. But if you can, victory is yours! Of course, it's difficult, but with perseverance, you can 'train' yourself for inspiration just as you train yourself for bodybuilding perfection.

"Perhaps the best way to describe inspiration is 'being driven to be the best.' Naturally, this cannot be done if you are so egocentric as to ignore your environment, because your environment is the standard against which you judge yourself. I have always found it difficult to be inspired by myself alone; it takes other people, places, and events to evoke my competitive urge—precisely the reason why a great bodybuilding gym is so valuable. Compare yourself with the champs, then try to exceed them.

" 'Sure, you can talk, Frank,' you might say. 'You live in California and have access to the finest gyms in the world. But what about those of us who are stuck back in the boonies and have nothing but a cheap little barbell/dumbbell set?'

"Sorry friend, that's no excuse, because there was a day when I lived in Florida and was training for that year's Mr. Universe competition with nothing but a puny little home gym. But I found inspiration, nonetheless, and defeated Arnold Schwarzenegger for the title.

"Here's what I did: Constantly, I would visit back-date magazine shops and buy old copies of various bodybuilding magazines. In those days, they had their covers removed and cost only 5–10 cents, but I would study them, memorizing the photos and visualizing how I'd want to look.

"There's a saying that 'The conscious mind is smart, but the unconscious mind is smarter,' so if you continuously bombard your mind with images of the greatest bodybuilders, those images stay with you, and in your unconscious, you will always be striving to exceed their achievements.

"While visualization with photos is a great aid to inspiration, the ideal inspirational source is direct association with the champions themselves. In other words, if you have access to a gym in which those who are better than you train, your visualization image is right there in the flesh for you to observe. Alternatively, great bodybuilders give training seminars and guest-posing exhibitions all over the United States and the rest of the world.

"Many bodybuilders fall into the trap of becoming 'big fish in small ponds.' They actually believe themselves to be better than what they really are because there is no one around to give them critical feedback on their progress, or to apprise them of their weak points.

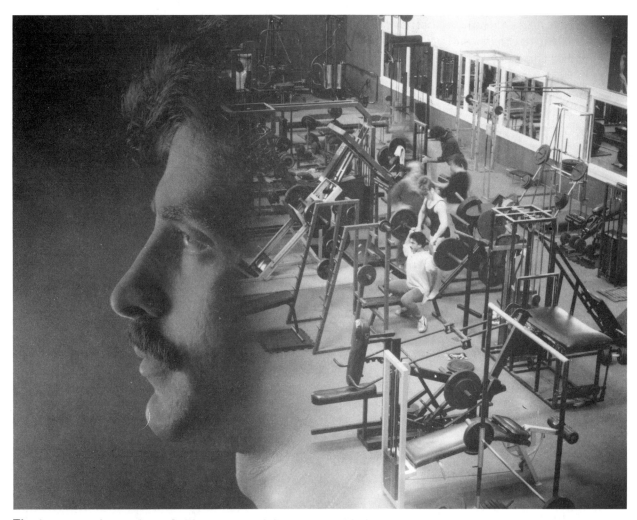

The top gyms, in southern California especially, can provide inspiration by allowing you to see the superstars of bodybuilding in action.

"I've seen this many times—guys out of shape, living on their reputations, not willing to admit to themselves that they are not as good as they used to be. If your training environment is good, this is not so likely to happen because you stay in the competitive mainstream and get the necessary objective criticism from your bodybuilding peers.

"There are several ways to use inspiration to train harder and improve. Aside from the inspiration you get from bodybuilding books and magazines, there is the motivation you get from seeing, and especially competing in, a physique contest. A top-calibre contest shows you that your dreams are possible after all. Some of my most outstanding inspirations came from seeing the champions in action: Scott winning Mr. Olympia in 1965, Arnold winning it in 1974—these were two of the best performances I've ever witnessed. And then there's inspira-

tion while actually competing: my wins in the Mr. Olympia in 1977, 1978, and particularly 1979 were gratifying.

"Remember that even losses in competition can inspire you to train harder. Some of my best training years followed my worst losses.

"The key to making gains is to get inspired enough to set a realistic goal and then constantly visualize it. Now close your eyes and imagine yourself in vivid detail reaching your goal, succeeding, winning—just as I described in the opening paragraph . . . except now the difference is that you are going to do something about it!

"Visualize your body as you'd like to see it look—this is where bodybuilding idols are helpful—then tell yourself that if another champion did it, then there's no reason why you can't too!

"In my early career, Steve Reeves inspired me

with his symmetry and proportions, Larry Scott with muscular roundness, and Arnold Schwarzenegger with his size, training intensity, and positive attitude. I trained to develop those characteristics using the examples my idols had set. In effect, all those who have gone before us can serve as our idols. We stand on the shoulders of giants in bodybuilding to become greater than our idols.

"It all starts with a goal. Make your goal provide you with a challenge, yet be realistic about it. Some set goals too low and don't think they can achieve greatness because they have low self-esteem. Others set goals too high because they haven't learned to realistically assess their potential. The ideal lies between these two extremes. Begin with small goals, then reward yourself on the achievement of each step. These accomplishments accumulate, and soon there seem to be no limits."

MENTAL CONCENTRATION

Frank Zane has won every possible bodybuilding title. He has become well-known for his Zen-oriented approach to the mental aspect of bodybuilding. His groundbreaking dissertation on workout concentration is here extracted from a two-part series of articles on the same subject, which appeared in *Muscle Builder & Power* magazine, the forerunner of *Muscle & Fitness*:

"Concentration is the key to bodybuilding success," claims Zane. "Concentration means you are better able to expand your awareness to fathom the meaning of unexplained phenomena. Whether you want to become a world-class bodybuilder, or merely want to look better than you do now, success depends on how well your brain devises and designs the training program that suits you best. Concentration allows you to transcend logic in your training, and you begin to see how the interaction of your senses carries you through a superlative training performance that creates bodybuilding excellence.

"Carrying it forward, according to Prabhavananda and Isherwood:

> . . . if the mind can be made to flow uninterruptedly toward the same object for 12 seconds, this may be called concentration. If the mind can continue in that concentra-

tion for 12 times 12 seconds—two minutes and 24 seconds—this may be called meditation. If the mind can continue in that meditation for 12 times two minutes and 24 seconds—28 minutes and 48 seconds—this will be the lower samadhi. (Samadhi may be defined as a deep state of meditation in which the mediator is oblivious to both internal and external stimuli, and the higher nervous system is in a state of ecstasy and bliss.)

"The difference between concentration and meditation is primarily one of time or duration. So in effect, meditation is an ongoing concentration. To make the mind flow uninterruptedly toward the same object for 12 seconds may seem easy, but in fact, it is not. It is even much more difficult to meditate perfectly. To do so would mean perfect concentration for two minutes and 24 seconds. This is almost impossible. The mind must always have something to do in order to occupy itself. When it runs out of interesting things, it fantasizes new diversions.

"This is the normal state of mind. To the mind, one-pointedness is boredom, and most minds are not willing to be bored. This point is, however, that power lies on the other side beyond boredom. In order to reach power the mind must be willing to experience boredom and go all the way through it.

"If you think you can concentrate to the point of actual meditation, try this simple experiment: Sit in a comfortable chair looking at your watch and see how long you can hold the thought 'I am sitting here looking at my watch' without getting distracted or actually forgetting what you are doing. Chances are it won't be very long before you find your mind somewhere else drifting off, forgetting the experiment, and looking for more interesting diversions.

"Some very interesting things can happen when a person becomes capable of total absorption of attention through the practice of concentration. For one thing, you notice the way a person experiences changes. I remember one of my first experiences of an altered sense of time which happened during my college years in the chemistry lab. I had been concentrating on one detail after another of the procedure of a com-

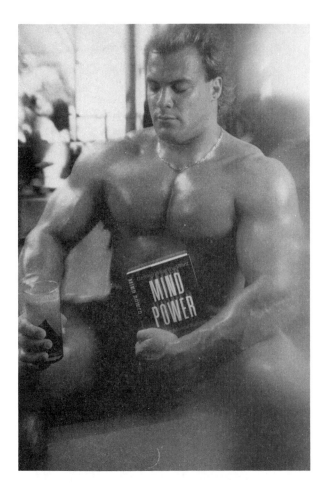

plicated experiment when I was suddenly told it was 6 P.M., and lab was closing.

"I had been in there eight hours, but it seemed like one hour! I was completely immersed in what I was doing and the result was that there was no such thing as time the way I normally experienced it.

"For the first time I realized that time is a mental construct—something people make up to keep track of events. I've since experienced this altered sense of time while training in the gym. When I'm totally involved in my training, my workout is always longer than it seems. It may seem like 45 minutes, but in fact two hours have passed!"

MEDITATION

"I'm sure everyone has had similar experiences at one time or another, and I urge you to cultivate the calm, clear, ecstatic experience that concentration through meditation can lead to. One good way to practice meditation is by paying attention to the mental repetition of a sound or mantra.

"The procedure is to sit comfortably in a quiet place and mentally repeat a standard mantra or a word of your own choosing which has a pleasant ringing sound. Some mantras commonly used are: OM. SO-HUM. AH-NAM. SHI-RIM. RAM-MAH. The mantra should ring through your mind and give you a feeling of serenity.

"For best results this should be done twice a day for 15-20 minutes each time. Before the workout is a good time for a bodybuilder because it helps clear the mind prior to the session. While at the gym, you may repeat the mantra silently to yourself between sets to help you maintain your inner calm. Also you'll be helping the frame of mind you achieve in sitting meditation carry over into your workout.

"The mantra sound becomes your mental point of reference. When distractions come up, you simply repeat your special sound. I have been doing this for many years and have been pleased with the results. Try it. It just may change your workout and your way of experiencing life."

PERCEPTIONS

Zane continued, "There are many analogies relative to the mind that tell us what it is like. The one I prefer is visualizing the mind as a computer with five inputs: seeing, hearing, smelling, tasting, and touching; and four outputs: thinking, feeling (or emotion), moving (in the sense of the mind initiating body movement), and opening (which I'll explain shortly).

"We perceive the world through our five senses. According to Prabhavananda and Isherwood:

> Ordinary sense perception is distorted and colored by the imagination of the perceiver. We decide in advance what it is we think we are going to see, and this preconception interferes with our vision.

"In other words, in ordinary (or untrained) sense perception we perceive our environment imperfectly, and as a result our thinking, feel-

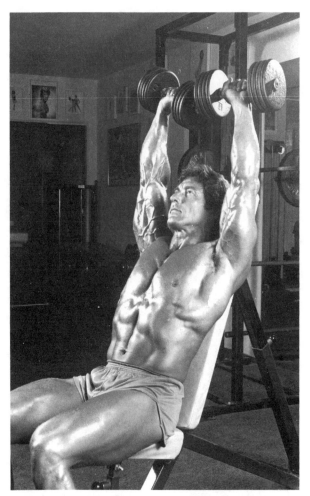

You can see the calm concentration on Frank Zane's face as he gets the most from his Arnold Presses.

ing, and body movements, do not have the force that these outputs could have.

"Sense perception can become clear and undistorted by practicing the fourth output, opening, which is our natural state. Young children are closer to this state than adults are, because they as yet have not become thoroughly into seeing things as they 'should and ought to be.' By age six, however, a child's conditioning is just about completed and eventually he accepts the same consensus reality of life as everyone else.

"The way to practice opening starts with concentration, or holding or fixing the mind on one object, center, or process. Concentration means one-pointedness, to hold one thing in mind to the exclusion of everything else. This is practically impossible for the untrained mind, which is constantly occupying itself with its own inner conversations. This 'mental chatter' goes on constantly. When we're awake, it shapes our actions. When we're asleep, it shapes our dreams.

"By practicing concentration we learn how to stop our mind's inner conversations; at first for very brief periods of time, and as we become more skilled in our practice, for longer periods.

"The idea is to quiet the mind by fixing your attention on one object. What does this have to do with the ideal workout? Simply this: if you had the ability to totally focus on each set of every exercise you did in your workout, your power and progress would become tremendous. The ideal workout means every set is perfectly performed and your concentration between each set is uninterrupted. Ordinary workouts become a thing of the past. and you become capable of super efforts.

"It's not easy. As a matter of fact, it's almost impossible. But there is that ever-so-narrow margin where anything can become possible, and this is only through discipline.

"The method for improving your concentration is simple and effective. The secret is disciplining yourself to practice and improve your concentration. You must sit and practice the method 20 minutes before each workout. Also remember to quiet the mind several times throughout the day.

"The tranquility you can develop with the method will carry over into your workout and your training will become more effective. All it takes is practice."

The method you can use to improve concentration is to sit down in a quiet place, close your eyes, and relax. Pick a single object and try to focus all of your concentration on that object for as long as possible. At first, your mind will almost immediately skip off to some other concept. Force it immediately back on your focal point. Keep forcing your attention back to the central point as soon as you discover that it has skipped away.

You might find it easier to focus all of your mental attention on the flame of a burning candle rather than on some manufactured object. Look at the flame, and think only of it. And every time your attention slips away, force it back on the candle.

Gradually, you will become more and more adept at keeping your entire conscious mental concentration on the flame, and nothing but the flame. You will remain focused for longer and longer periods of time on the object or thought you are using for your concentration practice.

As Zane mentioned, you can also concentrate on an aural concept, or mantra. Choose any soothing sound you wish, but it keep it simple. And keep bringing your mental attention back to center every time it has skipped away on you.

This no doubt sounds pretty simplified to you, but you have my assurance that it works. The better your concentration when practicing, the better it will be when you get into the gym. And perfect concentration on the working muscles is an essential ingredient in any bodybuilder's mental approach to championship competition.

31
Gaining the
Psychological Edge

Over the past few years, I have learned that hypnotism provides an exciting means of opening up a bodybuilder's mind and allowing him to reach his true physical potential. Champions such as Mike Christian and Andreas Cahling have proven the value of hypnotism in our sport. So I have asked *Peter C. Siegel, R.H.*, by far the best-known hypnotist working with bodybuilders, to explain some of his methods.

HYPNOTISM IN BODYBUILDING

"There is an inner voice in us all that, for the most part, is neither recognized nor utilized," Siegel states. "Hypnosis is the key to unlocking this power.

"What I intend to convey is a practical application of hypnosis for bodybuilding. It should be noted that all dimensions of life can be enhanced by hypnosis (i.e., social, emotional, financial, intellectual, etc.). But I will confine my energies mainly to a concise interpretation of hypnosis in the discipline of physique development.

"Before I get into specifics, I must clear up some widespread misconceptions about hypnotism. Many people still associate hypnosis with some mystic procedure involving the occult or some other magical activity. On the contrary, it is a discipline based on scientific fact, and there is nothing mystical about it. To date there is not one authenticated case of harm resulting from its application. Although the benefits and results of hypnosis are now widely documented, there still remains a resistance that originates from the fear of the unknown. That unknown is the energy or force that is hypnosis.

"That fear is now being replaced by acceptance and incorporation into their practice by doctors, psychiatrists, dentists, and other professionals who realize the undeniable value of hypnosis in dealing with stress-related—psychosomatic—illnesses and in bringing about positive changes in attitude. Simply stated, hypnosis is the positive use of your energy to improve yourself.

"Now that I have cleared the air I will get into specifics. Hypnosis involves reaching the subconscious portion of the mind so that a positive-directed suggestion can become part of one's behavior pattern. So that you will see how powerful and life-directing the subconscious mind is, a brief discussion of it is necessary.

"As a simple overview, your mind consists of three parts—the conscious, the unconscious, and the subconscious. The purpose of the conscious mind is to compare and evaluate each new idea introduced to it with previously accepted ideas. This level of consciousness is a sort of referee determining what is applicable and what is not. The conscious mind has the power to reason and be critical.

"The unconscious involves itself with the involuntary protection of the life of the organism—fight or flight.

"It is mainly the subconscious that I'll deal with, since it's the control center for all aspects of existence. You could compare it to a computer whose printout sheet is a direct result of the specific programming contained within.

"It must be mentioned here that the subconscious mind has no critical faculty, that is, it does not have the ability to reason. As a result of this lack, any idea or thought that reaches it becomes an accepted truth, consequently manifesting itself in your behavior pattern.

"The subconscious is a memory bank, storing all the information you have experienced from birth in an intricate web of memory pat-

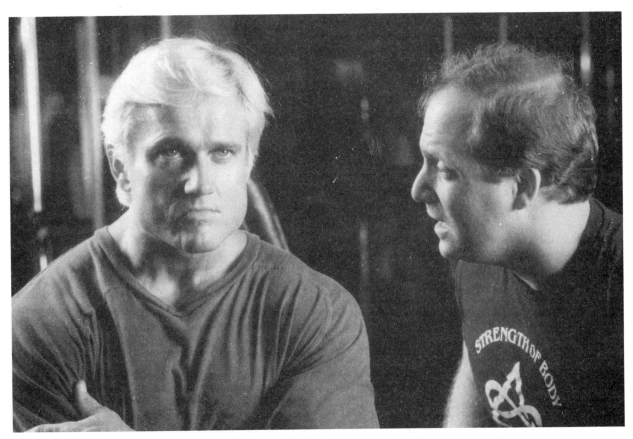

Peter Siegel works with Tom Platz on self-hypnosis techniques.

terns. It constantly feeds back information to the conscious mind. It is the seat of our imagination and emotions. To a great degree, emotions govern our desires, and our desires affect our behavior.

"The subconscious mind is the regulator of our energy and enables us to achieve our goals in life. If not controlled, this energy can be wasted on negative emotions. By the same token, however, the subconscious can be influenced to channel energy fully toward a positive life-improving goal.

"Earlier I mentioned that hypnosis can be a useful tool in all aspects of life. Here's why: You have the ability to direct your energies toward better health, success, or any other life-affirming concept by programming the subconscious mind to work for you rather than against you. The subconscious can be influenced to increase your strength, improve your ability to concentrate fully without any conflict resulting and, in general, to create a new self-image, combining the physical qualities you desire. The subconscious will do all these things—*if you want it to.*

EARLY INFLUENCES ON THE SUBCONSCIOUS

"Since your parents are your first teachers, they're the people who first influence your perception of the world, as well as the way you view yourself in relation to others. Unfortunately, parental perceptions of things are often incorrect. As a result, the child who hasn't developed the ability yet to distinguish between truth and untruth, accepts what they tell him. Thus, the parental perception reaches the subconscious mind, where it's accepted as truth. This acceptance eventually affects behavior patterns.

"One can see that after years of influence by unenlightened parents, or exposure to constant parental control, a person can develop a distorted emotional outlet as well as ultimately an unquestioning behavior problem. By 'unquestioning' I mean that many of the actions of a person are a direct result of early childhood conditioning by parents, and a set pattern is developed whereby the person will not question those actions. With the passage of years,

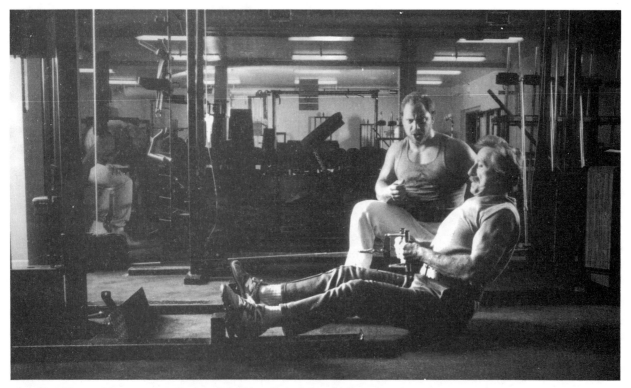

Even the Master Blaster subscribes to Pete Siegel's training advice when it comes to getting to the mental core of working out.

layer after layer of reinforcement of certain actions or ways of thinking build up, mainly by parental control in a person's mind, and a specific behavior pattern is formed.

"With respect to physique development, I raise these questions: What is your specific motivation to train? To what degree have you incorporated bodybuilding into your life? And, thirdly, are you getting sufficient gratification from the energy you have invested in all aspects of training?

"A set behavior problem is part of your life and bodybuilding is now a definite part of your lifestyle. To some degree it occupies a level of importance in your system of values.

"To tie in all the previous verbiage now with change effected through hypnosis is to simply state: The eventual good to be realized must become a burning desire. From birth on, your subconscious has made suggestions that affect your perceptions of the world. The degree of incorporation into one's life and vision of self through bodybuilding is a direct result of the way the subconscious has been programmed and, ultimately, how it perceives things. By reprogramming your subconscious mind, you may be able to realize a fuller existence. You

may influence your subconscious mind to bring you to greater heights of strength, motivation, and physique development.

"At this point I should state that some of the biggest names in bodybuilding today are clients of mine, and that all the information I give here concerning bodybuilding and hypnosis is a direct result of many hours of clinical work, experimentation, and research. I have seen champions become more intensely motivated, more confident, and more self-directed through the use of hypnosis. I have helped them to reach their inner minds and shown them how to utilize their own energies to rise to greater heights of self-awareness. In their imaginations, they grow to see themselves as they want to be, *coming to realize that what the mind can conceive, it can achieve.*

"These champions have developed a specific self-image in their imaginations and are taking the steps to become one with this image. The most significant outcome I have experienced to date is the ability to develop fully one's belief factor. Not only do these champions have a specific intent and image in mind, they also totally believe that they'll come to realize their expectations.

"To advance to the level of professional physique competition requires complete dedication and discipline. One must utilize all available avenues, 'all the tricks in the book,' to perfect a championship physique. Through positive reprogramming of your mind, you may come to realize a more intensified motivation and ultimately a greater direction of energy—physical, mental, emotional—toward your bodybuilding endeavors."

CHARTING YOUR DESIRES

"Some ground rules must first be established. First, *speak in terms of what you want, not what you want to avoid.* Example: If concentration is a problem for you, then, you must think like this: 'Whenever I'm involved in an activity that requires a focus of thought, I am able to see only the activity—or body part—I am engaged in. My mind automatically narrows down to one thing at a time.'

"Second, *see yourself as already having accomplished the goal.* Many bodybuilders, after looking at one of the professional champions at the gym, posing fully pumped, will utter something like, 'Man, what I wouldn't give to look like that.' Many can't envision themselves *ever* looking like that. In other words, their individual belief factor is grossly suppressed.

"Not everyone can become a champion. However, everyone has the capacity to reach a higher level of self-awareness (including physical size and proportion), greater emotional stability, and a full conceptual framework. You *must* create a self-image of the way you want to be. This must include physical proportions, and emotional characteristics as well.

"*If you want to be a success, you must visualize yourself as a success.* Here is a method I have successfully used with many champions to induce the state of hypnosis whereby the subconscious mind may be positively influenced. To effect change, the critical faculty must be bypassed and positive-improvement suggestions established. The process is twofold. First, I want you to write out a Personal Charter that includes four sections.

"The first section involves *physical image of self.* Include a precise description of yourself as you want to be. Remember, describe the size, shape, and proportion of each body part as

though you already possessed it. You beginners might be unable to picture what you want to look like in five years. You might do better at this point to see yourself 10–15 pounds more muscular with 1–2 inches of added muscle on each body part. The more advanced bodybuilders should see themselves as having the kind of physique they'd have to possess to win the next competition.

"A finished part of this section of the charter might look like this: *My bodyweight is 195 pounds. Thick, sinewy slabs of muscle cover my body from head to toe. I possess 19-inch arms, consisting of peaked, striated, vascular muscle. My thighs are 28 inches of rock-hard, striated muscle, packed with unbelievable power and strength. . . .*

The rest of the description is continued in this manner.

"You must create your own image, but remember, your mind will not accept excessive exaggerations—30-inch arms or 68-inch chest, for example. But you most definitely should see yourself as a champion. This in turn will create a more intense motivation and heighten your belief factor. The ideas and thoughts conveyed in this section are characterized by the key words 'ultimate champion.'

"Your second section should be concerned with *personality of image.* It's not enough to create a vision of self alone. You must also develop a specific personality and character as part of your new self-image. Include intangible factors such as self-confidence, concentration, leadership, self-discipline, and so forth. Your behavior is a direct result of the dominant thoughts held in your mind. Correct or incorrect, these dominant thoughts affect all aspects of perception. The mind will be attracted to those forces that coincide with the dominant thoughts: positive will attract positive, negative will attract negative.

"Some ground rules of the way to write this section will now be discussed. I want to repeat, your motivation must be extremely strong. Not to be confused with something you merely would like to have, the trait you desire must be a counterquality to replace a certain way of thinking you now maintain. Again, you must see yourself already in possession of this quality and use powerful descriptive words to heighten its effect.

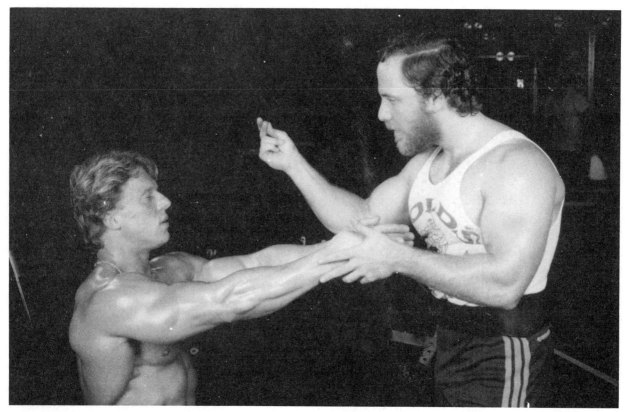

Hypnosis is a snap for Andreas Cahling.

"Initially, it might be difficult for you to see yourself in this new vein. But remember, as much as you believe, to that degree will you be successful.

"As your belief factor increases, you will continually lessen the limitations you have put upon yourself for so long. Gradually you will see yourself in a different and positive light. Keep all words positive and keep in mind that you desire to *achieve* something and not *avoid* something.

"Repeat and emphasize strongly the new positive quality you now want to adopt. Then symbolize it by giving it a key word that will reinforce the total picture you want to create. Finally, include in this section the concept that each day you're moving the new quality further along to total incorporation in your behavior pattern. A finished copy of this section might look like the following:

"Because I want to feel inner strength and rise to greater heights—physical, mental and emotional—I have growing confidence in myself. Each day I am more confident and more self-secure. I find it constantly easier to talk to people—both individually and in groups—

and know that what I have to say is important. People like me because of my new strength and warm, confident personality. I am calm and composed at all times and meet any challenge rationally and in good spirits. I view disagreements as a learning experience and benefit from them as an alternative viewpoint. I am poised, self-motivated, and directed, and do all that is necessary for my well-being and happiness. From this point forward, with each passing day, I grow stronger and more self-assured.

"All the ideas and concepts in this section are symbolized by the words 'inner strength.' I focused on self-confidence and composure in this section. However, you must pick the personality factors that are most important to you. You might deal with courage, concentration, relaxation, perseverance, success, or any other important character trait you desire to be part of your new image. Remember to write this section in positive terms and as already being part of you. Be specific and practical, and include only those traits you desire to attain. See yourself as successful right now!

"Your third section deals with *pre-workout declaration.* State explicitly what you intend to achieve during your next workout, including the frame of mind you'll maintain, as well as the feeling you want to realize and the intensity of effort you want to project. Again, word it positively and as you write it, picture yourself going through a grueling workout. Close your eyes for a moment, and let the image and the feeling fill your entire body. Then open your eyes and write down how you want to train from now on. An example follows:

"Because I have a strong desire to excel, win, and become a powerful being, I feel enthusiasm and excitement surge through my veins as I contemplate my next workout. With each workout I expect more and more from myself, and I find that as I intensify my effort, I benefit in terms of increased strength, stamina, and muscular size and shape.

"I will give 110% of myself with each and every workout, constantly destroying all past limitations of strength and endurance. Already, I feel adrenaline starting to flow, since I'll soon be using greater poundages, more intense sets, and will always be pushing myself to the ultimate. I will train each body part harder and faster, using more weight until each body part screams for mercy. Yet I will give it none. I will break through and ultimately conquer the pain barrier. From this point on, with each workout, I am more self-directed and self-motivated, and in the end, becoming physically supreme.

"All of the ideas and thoughts contained in this section are symbolized by the words 'intensity factor.' You may choose your own wording for this section, but you should now have a general understanding of what I am driving at. The idea here is to enter the gym with a definite purpose in mind and with a feeling of great desire.

"Your fourth section deals with *body talk*. This area deals with you communicating directly with your body before you go to sleep at night, telling it to relax, recover, and grow bigger. The finished part of this section might look like what follows:

"I am aware that I'm tapping the inner resources of my mind to create a stronger, more motivated me, and I'm realizing this internal power more fully every day. I will slumber deeply, and my body and mind will rest. I will recuperate fully and awaken refreshed and en-

thused, for I know that with each passing day I rise to greater heights of physique training performance.

"All ideas conveyed in this section can be represented by the words 'rebuild and rise above.' Once again you may word this section to suit your specific needs, but word it positively, specifically, and see it already happening in your imagination.

"It's most important that you compose your charter to reflect the attributes you wish to associate with yourself. Use strong, emotional wording. Read it to yourself upon awakening each morning, before your workouts, and before retiring for the night. The latter is especially important; no matter how late it is or how tired you are, read your charter. After each section, stop briefly and visualize and emotionalize the concepts and qualities as you want them. If you're not in a situation where you can read the charter out loud, then mouth the words as you read them. It's important that you read and feel every word three times each day.

"You may, after a period of time, find that you have advanced more than you had expected, then it's advisable to write a more-advanced charter. For the time being, develop each section exactly as outlined and keep the charter where it's easily accessible.

"Some words of advice before I continue are in order. One, keep your charter on a strictly personal basis. Discussion with friends, training partners, even family members, will undoubtedly raise some sort of negative criticism or other hindrance. Remember, the slightest bit of doubt will cause you to slip and see things as you did in the past. Your new attitude at this point is essential and quite fragile; any negatives will severely deter you from accomplishment, so keep your charter to yourself.

"Two, your initial charter may, in the beginning, sound incredible. Remember your mind is used to working on doubt and possible negative flows, and now you're introducing something positive and powerful into the spectrum. You'll gradually begin to accept and incorporate each section into your framework; but, remember, you must fully believe and have complete faith. With these ingredients, you can ultimately attain success."

The foregoing process is essential before entering hypnosis therapy. And after several hands-on sessions of hypnosis, you can begin to use this charter while performing self-hypnosis. But even if you don't go through hypnosis—the only excuse for not doing so is the unavailability of a good hypnotist—you can use this charter to improve your mental attitude toward your bodybuilding efforts.

Mental Visualization

"Visualization is the technique by which you can positively program your mind to help you reach your bodybuilding goals," says *Tom Platz*. "It involves a practical application of what psychologists call *self-actualization*. Through visualization you can actually program your subconscious mind in any manner you desire, much as a computer is programmed to perform a certain function.

"Think about someone you've known who wanted to become a physician, lawyer, piano virtuoso. Those who have successfully reached their goals are the ones whose desire to succeed was so strong that they actually lived the occupation of their choice in their daydreams. The subconscious mind can be programmed to pave the route to a desired goal. With a naturally strong desire provided by the subconscious mind, it becomes easy to sit down and practice a Brahms concerto time after time.

"In normal self-actualization one needn't do anything more than creatively daydream about becoming a certain type of person or holding a particular job. In visualization, we consciously program the mind to help us make bodybuilding decisions an easy task. When this is properly done, it's no longer an ordeal to diet intensely or train hard when energy has been depleted by such a strict diet. The entire bodybuilding process becomes a joyful, soaring experience, I can assure you of this because my own bodybuilding preparations for a professional competition are the best part of my life."

Psychologists have discovered several fundamental rules for proper visualization. First, it works best when you are relaxed and totally free from extraneous interruptions and distractions. It's also advantageous to visualize in the dark at first, since it facilitates the mental imagery necessary to properly program your subconscious mind.

At first you might require about 30 minutes to get totally into the visualization process, since it will be new to you and it takes some practice to learn how to do it correctly. Later, you probably won't need to spend more than about 15 minutes each session.

Platz agrees with these requisites to proper visualization: "When starting, I think you can best practice visualization while lying in bed preparing to sleep. Then you should be relaxed and have a minimum potential for disruption of your thought process. And it's a good idea to practice visualization in the dark, at bedtime."

You'll have to be perfectly relaxed to get the most out of your visualization practice, so you may actually drift off to sleep before you finish your mental routine. No problem. It's good to fall asleep toward the end of your visualization session, however, because it more vividly implants the mental image you have conjured up in your subconscious mind. But don't worry if you don't fall asleep immediately, because the main requisites to effective visualization are being fully relaxed and comfortable and free of extraneous distractions.

I always suggest lying on your back in bed with one pillow under your head and neck, another under your knees. Your legs should be held comfortably a few inches apart, and your arms should be naturally down at your sides. When you're fully relaxed, your head, torso, and limbs will assume a natural position, and you won't have to think about their positioning.

The next step is called *fractional relaxation*. It consists of systematically relaxing each part of your body in sequence, starting from your feet and ankles and then working upward. Take a minute or two to mentally will any existing tension out of your feet and ankles. When they are relaxed, work on your calves, and so on up your body to your neck and head.

When you are optimally relaxed, you probably will feel as though your body is actually floating in space. It's the same feeling you'll get the first time you are hypnotized, a process I recommend. Eventually, you'll be floating in space and won't be able to feel your arms and legs, or guess their positioning on the bed.

Platz continues his explanation of an initial visualization session, taking you from the point when you have achieved full relaxation: "As you lie in bed, imagine yourself as you would like to become one day. Gradually make this image more and more sharp, until it is almost as if you are projecting a film against the inside of your eyelids. Vividly visualize every ridge of muscle, every cut between muscle groups, every striation over each muscle belly, and every prominent vein winding over your musculature. And imagine in detail what it would like to be *inside* that new body, to walk onstage at a major competition, and to hear the audience shout its approval of your efforts."

When you first start to work on visualization, you'll find it difficult to keep your mind focused totally on the image you're developing. Your mind will tend to skip off to some other thought. This is a perfectly natural occurrence. And it's the reason why you should practice visualization when you are as free as possible from distractions—less external distractions will make it easier to focus all of your attention on your intended image.

As when perfecting your workout concentration, you must learn to focus your mind back on your mental image every time it skips off to wondering where to go on your next date, or what it's going to take to get your latest homework assignment done on time. The more consistently you keep refocusing your mind back on the task at hand, the longer you will ultimately be able to maintain your focus on your internal mental image each time before your attention again skips off. For proper visualization, your mind *must* stay focused on the image you have developed for at least 10 minutes.

An imperfect ability to focus only on this mental image is the reason why it will take you longer at first to get through your visualization practice. As you improve your ability to concentrate, it will take you less and less time to get through your ritual. After a couple of months, you'll be able to accomplish your task in only 15 minutes—5 to relax your body, and 10 minutes for the actual visualization procedure. And within a couple more months, you will probably find that your internal mental concentration has become so good you can do your visualization at odd times during the day, even when you don't have the security of a dark, comfortable bedroom.

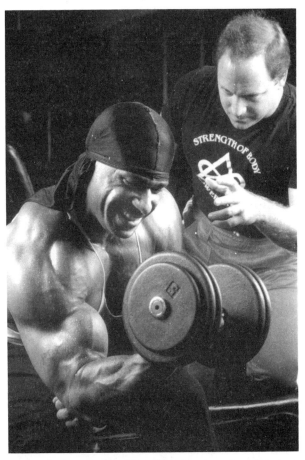

Peter Siegel coaches Mike Christian to wring the most from his muscles and his mind.

Once you have developed a good mental image of what you will soon look like, lie back and *enjoy* it. It's a very comfortable feeling. You deserve to take pleasure in it. And the more you like it—the comfortable, exciting feeling of being a truly great bodybuilder—the faster and more deeply you will be programming your subconscious mind to assist you in actually looking like the image you've conjured up, and it'll only take a few months to reach the physique you have visualized.

Platz comments, "The feeling of what it would be like *inside* a great physique is crucial to optimum visualization practice and results. Normally you would visualize yourself with only one of your five senses. And this is as far as virtually all bodybuilders and other athletes take visualization. But psychologists have determined that you can get a great deal more out of visualization practice if you also involve some of the other four senses—touch, hearing, taste, and smell—in your visualized image. They talk about a 'three out of five' rule, in which an athlete endeavors to involve at least three of his or her five senses in the visualization practice.

"In my own experience, visualization is more than twice as effective when I can visualize with at least three of my five senses. If you can involve all five senses—a relatively easy process once you know how to do it—I'm confident that you will triple the results of your visualization practice. As bodybuilders, we should consistently involve as many of our five senses as possible in our visualized images."

Once you can concentrate your mind totally on your "sighted" image for at least five minutes, you should be able to start working on incorporating some of your other four senses in this visual image. How?

Platz explains how: "Let's walk through an example of how you can involve sight, touch, hearing, taste, and smell in a single visualized image. Lie back in a comfortable position and fully relax your mind and body. Then begin to conjure up the image of your fantastic new physique. That involves the sense of sight, or at least the imagined sense of sight.

"Next imagine yourself inside that body, sensing your muscles straining to burst through your superthin skin. This is the imagined sense of touch. Savor it by walking about the room in your imagination, feeling your leg muscles powerfully contract and relax with each step. I do this image quite often myself. In my visualized image, I can feel myself walking onstage for a competition, and I can even look down at my feet and see them leading me toward the posing platform.

"The sense of hearing is relatively easy to add to your visualized image. I continue to imagine walking onstage for my Mr. Olympia competition by hearing the huge roar that comes up from the audience when they first see me step from behind the curtains, as well as when I am powerfully and confidently going through my posing routine. Alternatively, you can visualize yourself during a heavy workout, feel your muscles straining against the weights, and hear the deep-throated rattle of several 45-pound plates on the ends of the Olympic bar you're using.

"You can involve your sense of smell in a number of ways. Imagine the scent of the oil you've rubbed into your skin to highlight your body's amazing muscularity. You could simply add all of this into your image of the new you posing at a major competition. Other common olfactory experiences include the smell of honest sweat on your body as you blast away during a workout, and the aroma of the food you're eating while on a precontest diet.

"You're fifth sense, that of taste, most easily comes into play in imagining yourself eating one of your final precontest meals. That dry piece of fish or skinned chicken breast may not taste like much, but you can visualize how great your physique appears and feels as you are eating it. You can believe this: it'll feel absolutely great! This type of five-sense visualization will dramatically assist you in attaining your desired image."

Tom Platz concludes his discussion of mental visualization by revealing his personal visual images: "I visualize two things each day: how I will look at the next Mr. Olympia contest and how my entire superproductive workout will go. But I'm always realistic about my visualizations. If you are four feet tall, you aren't going to play professional basketball, are you? Take into consideration the strengths and weaknesses of your physique, as well as what you can realistically expect at contest time from your optimum training and dietary preparations. Set your target high, but not so high that you can't hit it.

"Each morning before I go to the gym, I picture every set and every rep of my workout, feeling the super pump I'll get from it. I do this every day, either just before breakfast or while drinking my cup of coffee. I used to also visualize my poundages for each set, but I don't anymore. Now my emphasis is more on how the working muscles *feel* than on the actual weight being used.

"While I recommend that you practice visualization before falling asleep, I've become so adept at this practice that I can do it throughout the day. When my posing music comes on the radio, for example, it automatically sets me to visualizing how I would pose to it.

"There are a lot of other tricks I use to put myself in the correct frame of mind to win a competition. Before my Mr. Universe win, for example, I had a sign that said, 'TOM PLATZ—MR. UNIVERSE hung over my posing mirror so

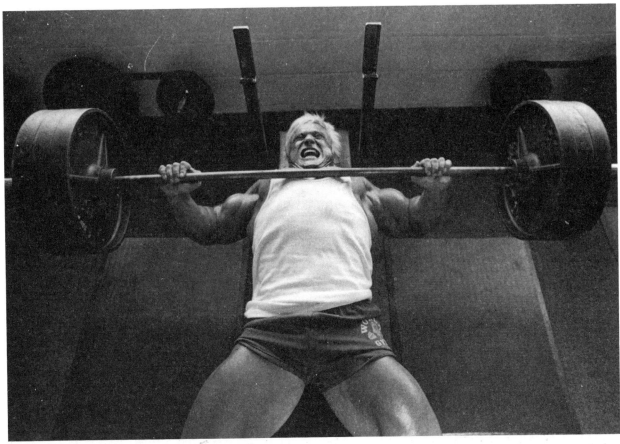

This is no visualization, just Tom blasting away at his chest.

I'd see it constantly. In my training and nutrition log I'd sometimes write out an autograph, 'Tom Platz—Mr. Universe.' Now I write 'Tom Platz—Mr. Olympia' in my diary, although I've yet to win it."

Regardless of how adept you might become at visualization, it won't do you any good to practice the technique if you don't do it on a daily basis. Regularity is vitally important, and it's probably the main way most bodybuilders go wrong—they forget to practice visualization every night, and after missing a couple of sessions here and there they stop using the technique altogether. Visualization is one of the most powerful mental tools in your arsenal, but you have to *use* it.

I know there's bound to be a couple of readers who will automatically think that this discussion of visualization is just so much hokum, something that would be a waste of time. But it *is* worth the time expenditure, because it *does* work wonders in helping ease the way toward a world-class physique.

The Psychological Edge

"You must consistently see yourself as a winner to establish a positive self-image," reveals *Tom Platz*. "I feel that you have to be truly willing to give your all as a bodybuilder in order to open the path to success. But you must be able to rationalize it if you don't get everything you've set as your goal in the sport, and still see yourself as a winner for achieving what you have.

"You must also realize that there's a risk involved in any venture, and especially in bodybuilding. Still, I always expect my training to work, because you have to expect and create success. Too much of anything—training, social life, or whatever—is counterproductive. And even though a risk is involved in your bodybuilding, it isn't a suicide mission, It's a calculated risk that you have to take in an effort to win. You might lose, but hopefully you will win every competition you enter."

Many times Mr. Universe, *Boyer Coe*, continues, "The spark that motivates the bodybuilder is set off in the mind. The desire—even the zeal—has to start there. You have to visualize what you want to be, and what in turn will generate your enthusiasm for training. Going to the gym day in and day out, and week in and week out, is not really a pleasant thing to do. It would be more fun, of course, to go out with your girl or take in a movie, or even stay home and watch television. But if your mind is made up to achieve all that you can with your body, you forget about what's outside the gym and concentrate on perfecting yourself. Without that motivating factor, that visual image of what you can become, you will fall by the wayside when something else beckons—and another once-bright dream turns to ashes.

"You won't, of course, achieve your dream overnight, or even in a couple of years. It will take persistence, determination, even courage sometimes, to stay on the road to that dream. The road requires hard work and an undying faith that you will reach out and touch that dream one day. But if you give it that—and, admittedly, that is a lot to ask of anyone—I'm convinced that you will succeed."

Coe goes on, "Along the way to reaching your goals in bodybuilding, there are little things you can learn to help keep your spirits up and your mind working in a positive direction. For example, I have always liked music a lot, so I use it as an asset to my training. Unlike some gyms I know, in which guys are afraid to talk very loud and in which no radios or stereos fill the air with a beat, I always have to have music when I train. Music, to me, is emotion. It can make a person very happy or very sad, and it can really get you motivated.

"I remember when I was a teenager that I couldn't do my bench presses unless there was a fast song on the radio. I would wait until one came on and got me going, before I would even try them. Now that may seem a little extreme, but it worked. I didn't think I could do my best until a fast number came on, therefore I couldn't. Music provided me with the emotional force I needed.

"Even today, music can get me back into the right frame of mind and ignite my training. Sometimes late at night after a busy day's work,

I just don't think I can put anything into my training. But my workout partner will come in and turn on the music, and in a little while I've shed that lackadaisical attitude and am moving to the beat and feeling good again. You really can't accomplish much in your training, or in anything else, for that matter, if you are feeling low and are just barely dragging. You have to be positive and go at it with a full head of steam.

"Another aid that will help you keep a positive mental attitude is the avoidance of distractions. That is why I like to come into the gym early in the morning when the only people there are me and my training partner. I realize that this might not be the best time to train, since the body is cold and not warmed up, but I make allowance for this by spending some time getting myself ready to handle the heavy weights that I like to use. I avoid the distraction of a lot of people around me and the temptation to spend time socializing with them.

"So many people—and I was guilty of this when I was younger—waste valuable time in the gym just horsing around and killing a good workout with too much talk. Instead, they should be visualizing their muscles contracting, extending, and growing. Frank Zane has had a lot to say about seeing yourself in your own mind and eliminating all the negative thoughts around you which distract you from your goals. He has learned how to control his mind, and look what this ability has done for him: three Mr. Olympia titles! He has learned, probably as well as anybody, how to put 100% of himself into his workouts.

"Before he could do this, however, he had to have that spark of imagination that led him to visualize what he wanted. Once that image comes to the bodybuilder, he has to hold it in his mind and strive to make that image a reality. That reality may be far down the road, but once you are on the right track, the journey will take you directly toward the dream. One day you will get there, if you believe that you will. Accept criticism for what it is—constructive criticism is a great help to the bodybuilder—but maintain that dream. That's what bodybuilding is all about."

The Last Word

One of the worst things you can do is make bodybuilding your entire life. I see many men in the gym who do nothing but eat, sleep, and do bodybuilding. And many of these men are athletes who have very little physical potential. But everything is bodybuilding, bodybuilding, bodybuilding. The best champions in the sport are men who have well-rounded lifestyles. They have good relationships, good jobs, good family ties, and good hobbies outside of the sport.

"My own life is very full," says *Tom Platz*. "I am a bodybuilder only in the morning when I am training; the rest of the day I am a human being. I work on my business affairs, I work on my social life, and I work at furthering my education. In short, I stop to smell the roses, and I'm far better off for it. If I hadn't done this, I would be a less-complete person, and I am very sure that I would never have reached my correct level of physical and mental development."

This is our last set together. I hope you have learned from reading this book, and that you will refer to it often in the future. The best-informed bodybuilders eventually rise to the top of the competitive hierarchy. You know as much as anyone in the sport at this point. Keep that mental edge on your side, and you'll undoubtedly become a great champion!

Glossary

Aerobic Exercise. Prolonged, moderate-intensity work that uses up oxygen at or below the level at which your cardiorespiratory (heart–lung) system can replenish oxygen in the working muscles. *Aerobic* literally means *with oxygen*, and it is the only type of exercise which burns body fat to meet its energy needs. Bodybuilders engage in aerobic workouts to develop additional cardiorespiratory fitness, as well as to burn off excess body fat to achieve peak contest muscularity. Common aerobic activities include running, cycling, swimming, dancing, and walking. Depending on how vigorously you play them, most racquet sports can also be aerobic exercise.

AMDR. An abbreviation for the Adult Minimum Daily Requirement of certain nutrients as established by the United States Food and Drug Administration (FDA).

Anabolic Drugs. Also called anabolic steroids, these are artificial male hormones that aid in nitrogen retention and thereby add to a male bodybuilder's muscle mass and strength. These drugs are not without hazardous side effects, however, and they are legally available only through a physician's prescription. Steroids are available in most gyms via the black market, but it is very dangerous to use such unknown substances to increase muscle mass.

Anaerobic Exercise. Exercise of much higher intensity than aerobic work, which uses up oxygen more quickly than the body can replenish it in the working muscles. Anaerobic exercise eventually builds up a significant oxygen debt that forces an athlete to terminate the exercise session rather quickly. Anaerobic exercise (the kind of exercise to which bodybuilding training belongs) burns up glycogen (muscle sugar) to supply its energy needs. Fast sprinting is a typical anaerobic form of exercise.

Androgenic Drugs. Androgenics are drugs that simulate the effects of the male hormone testosterone in the human body. Androgens do build a degree of strength and muscle mass, but they also stimulate secondary sex characteristics such as increased body hair, a deepened voice, and high levels of aggression. Indeed, many bodybuilders and powerlifters take androgens to stimulate aggressiveness in the gym, resulting in more productive workouts.

Balance. A term referring to an even relationship of body proportions in a man's physique. Perfectly balanced physical proportions are a much-sought-after trait among competitive bodybuilders.

Bar. The steel shaft that forms the basic part of a barbell or dumbbell. These bars are normally about one inch thick, and they are often encased in a revolving metal sleeve.

Barbell. Normally measuring between four and six feet in length, a barbell is the most basic piece of weight-training and bodybuilding equipment. Indeed, you can train every major skeletal muscle group in your body using only a barbell. There are two major types of exercise barbells in common use, adjustable sets (in which you can easily add or subtract plates by removing a detachable outside collar held in place on each side by a set screw) and fixed barbells (in which the plates are either welded or bolted permanently in place). Fixed weights are arranged in a variety of poundages on long racks in commercial bodybuilding gyms, the approximate poundage for each one painted or etched on the bar. Fixed weights relieve you of the problem of changing plates on your barbell for each new exercise. While fixed barbells and dumbbells are normally found in large commercial gyms, adjustable barbell and dumbbell sets are more frequently used at home.

Basic Exercise. A bodybuilding exercise which stresses the largest muscle groups of your body (e.g., the thighs, back, and/or chest), often in combination with smaller muscles. You will be able to use very heavy weights in basic exercises in order to build great muscle mass and physical power. Typical basic movements include squats, bench presses, and deadlifts. (You should also see the listing for *Isolation Exercise*.)

Benches. A wide variety of exercise benches is available for use in doing barbell and dumbbell exercises either lying or seated on a bench. The most common type of bench, a flat exercise bench, can be used for chest, shoulder, and arm movements. Incline and decline benches (which are angled at about 30–45 degrees) also allow movements for the chest, shoulders, and arms.

Biomechanics. The scientific study of body positions, or form, in sport. In bodybuilding, biomechanics studies body form when exercising with weights. When you have good biomechanics in a bodybuilding exercise, you will be safely placing maximum beneficial stress on your working muscles.

BMR. Your basal metabolic rate, or the speed at which your resting body burns calories to provide for its basic survival needs. You can elevate your BMR and more easily achieve lean body mass through consistent exercise, and particularly through aerobic workouts.

Bodybuilding. A type of weight training applied in conjunction with sound nutritional practices to alter the shape or form of one's body. In the context of this book, bodybuilding is a competitive sport nationally and internationally in both amateur and professional categories for men, women, and mixed pairs. However, a majority of individuals use bodybuilding methods merely to lose excess body fat or build up a too thin part of the body.

Burn. A beneficial burning sensation in a muscle that you are training. This burn is caused by a rapid buildup of fatigue toxins in the muscle and is a good indication that you are optimally working a muscle group. The best bodybuilders consistently forge past the pain barrier erected by muscle burn and consequently build very massive, highly defined muscles.

Burns. A training technique used to push a set past the normal failure point, and thereby to stimulate it to greater hypertrophy. Burns consist of short, quick, bouncy reps 4–6 inches in range of motion. Most bodybuilders do 8–12 burns at the end of a set that has already been taken to failure. They generate terrific burn in the muscles, hence the name of this technique.

CAFB. The Canadian Amateur Federation of Bodybuilders, the sports federation responsible in Canada for administering amateur bodybuilding for men, women, and mixed pairs. The CAFB is one of the more than 120 national bodybuilding federations affiliated internationally with the IFBB.

Cardiorespiratory Fitness. Physical fitness of the heart, circulatory system and lungs that is indicative of good aerobic fitness.

Cheating. A method of pushing a muscle to keep working far past the point at which it would normally fail to continue contracting due to excessive fatigue buildup. In cheating you will use a self-administered body swing, jerk, or otherwise poor exercise form once you have reached the failure point to take some of the pressure off the muscles and allow them to continue a set for two or three repetitions past failure.

Chinning Bar. A bar attached high on the wall or gym ceiling, on which you can do chins, hanging leg raises, and other movements for your upper body. A chinning bar is analogous to the high bar male gymnasts use in national and international competitions.

Circuit Training. A special form of bodybuilding through which you can simultaneously increase aerobic conditioning, muscle mass, and strength. In circuit training, you will plan a series of 10–20 exercises in a circuit around the gym. The exercises chosen should stress all parts of the body. These movements are performed with an absolute minimum of rest between exercises. Then at the end of a circuit, a rest interval of 2–5 minutes is taken before going through the circuit again. Three–five circuits would constitute a circuit training program.

Clean. The movement of raising a barbell or two dumbbells from the floor to your shoulders in one smooth motion to prepare for an overhead lift. To properly execute a clean movement, you must use the coordinated strength of your legs, back, shoulders, and arms.

Collar. The clamp that is used to hold plates securely in place on a barbell or dumbbell bar. The cylindrical metal clamps are held in place on the bar by means of a set screw threaded through the collar and tightened securely against the bar. Inside collars keep plates from sliding inward and injuring your hands, while outside collars keep plates from sliding off the barbell in the middle of an exercise.

Couples' Competition. A relatively new form of bodybuilding competition in which man–woman teams compete against others with particularly appealing posing routines featuring *adagio* and other dance movements and lifts. More frequently called "Mixed Pairs Competition,"

this event is rapidly gaining international popularity with the bodybuilding community and general public, and is held in both amateur and professional World Championships.

Cut Up (or Cut). A term used to denote a bodybuilder who has an extremely high degree of muscular definition due to a low degree of body fat.

Definition. The absence of fat over clearly delineated muscular movement. Definition is often referred to as "muscularity," and a highly defined bodybuilder has so little body fat that very fine grooves of muscularity called "striations" will be clearly visible over each major muscle group.

Density. Muscle hardness, which is also related to muscular definition. A bodybuilder can be well-defined and still have excess fat within each major muscle complex. But when he has muscle density, even this intramuscular fat has been eliminated. A combination of muscle mass and muscle density is highly prized among all competitive bodybuilders.

Dipping Bars. Parallel bars set high enough above the floor to allow you to do dips between them, leg raises for your abdominals, and a variety of other exercises. Some gyms have dipping bars which are angled inward at one end; these can be used when changing your grip width on dips.

Diuretics. Sometimes called "water pills," these are drugs and herbal preparations that remove excess water from a bodybuilder's system just prior to a show, thereby revealing greater muscular detail. Harsh chemical diuretics can be quite harmful to your health, particularly if they are used on a chronic basis. Two of the side effects of excessive chemical diuretic use are muscle cramps and heart arrhythmias (irregular heart beats).

Dumbbell. For all intents and purposes, a dumbbell is a short-handled barbell (usually 10–12 inches in length) intended primarily for use with one in each hand. Dumbbells are especially valuable when training the arms and shoulders, but can be used to build up almost any muscles.

Exercise. Each individual movement (e.g., a seated pulley row, barbell curl, or seated calf raise) that you perform in your bodybuilding workouts.

EZ-Curl Bar. A special type of barbell used in many arm exercises, but particularly for standing EZ-bar curls wherein it removes strain from your wrists. An EX-curl bar is also occasionally called a "cambered curling bar." Albert Beckles, one of the sport's most successful professionals, whimsically calls this piece of equipment a "wiggly bar" because of its shape.

Failure. That point in an exercise at which you have so fully fatigued your working muscles that they can no longer complete an additional repetition of a movement with strict biomechanics. You should always take your post-warm-up sets at least to the point of momentary muscular failure, and frequently past that point.

Flexibility. A suppleness of joints, muscle masses, and connective tissues which lets you move your limbs over an exaggerated range of motion, a valuable quality in bodybuilding training, since it promotes optimum physical development. Flexibility can only be attained through systematic stretching training, which should form a cornerstone of your overall bodybuilding philosophy.

Forced Reps. Forced reps are a frequently used method of extending a set past the point of failure to induce greater gains in muscle mass and quality. With forced reps, a training partner pulls upward on the bar just enough for you to grind out two or three reps past the failure threshold.

Form. This is simply another word to indicate the biomechanics used during the performance of any bodybuilding or weight-training movement. Perfect form involves moving only the muscles specified in an exercise description, while moving the weight over the fullest possible range.

Free Weights. Barbells, dumbbells, and related equipment. Serious bodybuilders use a combination of free weights and such exercise machines as those manufactured by Nautilus and Universal Gyms, but they primarily use free weights in their workouts.

Giant Sets. Series of 4-6 exercises done with little or no rest between movements and a rest interval of 3-4 minutes between giant sets. You can perform giant sets for either two antagonistic muscle groups or a single body part.

Hypertrophy. The scientific term denoting an increase in muscle mass and an improvement in relative muscular strength. Hypertrophy is induced by placing an "overload" on the working muscles with various training techniques during a bodybuilding workout.

IFBB. The International Federation of Bodybuilders, the gigantic sports federation founded in 1946 by Joe and Ben Weider. With more than 120 member nations, the IFBB proves that bodybuilding is one of the most popular of all sports on the international level. Through its member national federations, the IFBB oversees competitions in each nation, and it directly administers amateur and professional competition for men, women, and mixed pairs internationally.

Intensity. The relative degree of effort that you put into each set of every exercise in a bodybuilding workout. The more intensity you place on a working muscle, the more quickly it will increase in hypertrophy. The most basic methods of increasing intensity are to use heavier weights in good form in each exercise, do more reps with a set weight, or perform a consistent number of sets and reps with a particular weight in a movement, but progressively reducing the length of rest intervals between sets.

Isolation Exercise. In contrast to a basic exercise, an isolation movement stresses a single muscle group (or sometimes just part of a single muscle) in relative isolation from the remainder of the body. Isolation exercises are good for shaping and defining various muscle groups. For your thighs, squats would be a typical basic movement, while leg extensions would be the equivalent isolation exercise.

Judging Rounds. In the universally accepted and applied IFBB system of judging, bodybuilders are evaluated in three distinctly different rounds of judging, plus a final posedown round for only the top five competitors after the first three rounds have been adjudicated. In Round One, the competitors are viewed in groups and individually in seven well-defined compulsory poses; in Round Two, they are viewed semi-relaxed from the front, both sides, and back; and in Round Three, they perform their own uniquely personal free-posing routines to their own choice of music. Overall, this use of three rounds of judging and a posedown round results in a very fair choice of the final winners of a bodybuilding championship.

Juice. A slang term for anabolic steroids, e.g., being "on the juice."

Layoff. Most intelligent bodybuilders take a one- or two-week layoff from bodybuilding training from time to time, during which they totally avoid the gym. A layoff after a period of intense precompetition preparation is particularly beneficial as a means of allowing the body to completely rest, recuperate, and heal any minor training injuries that might have cropped up during the peaking cycle.

Lifting Belt. This is a leather belt 4-6 inches wide at the back that is fastened tightly around your waist when you do squats, heavy back work, and overhead pressing movements. A lifting belt adds stability to your midsection, preventing lower back and abdominal injuries.

Mass. The relative size of each muscle group, or of the entire physique. As long as you also have a high degree of muscularity and good balance of physical proportions, muscle mass is a highly prized quality among competitive bodybuilders.

Mixed Pairs Competition. Couples' competition, a relatively new form of bodybuilding competition in which man–woman teams compete against others with particularly appealing posing routines featuring *adagio* and other dance movements.

Muscularity. An alternative term for "definition" or "cuts."

Nautilus. A brand of exercise machine in common use in large gyms.

NPC. The National Physique Committee, Inc., which administers men's and women's amateur bodybuilding competitions in the United States. The NPC National Champions in each weight division are annually sent abroad to compete in the IFBB World Championships.

Nutrition. The applied science of eating to foster greater health, fitness, and muscular gains. Through correct application of nutritional practices, you can selectively add muscle mass to your physique, or totally strip away all body fat, revealing the hard-earned muscles lying beneath your skin.

Olympian. A term reserved for use when referring only to a bodybuilder who has competed in the Mr. Olympia or Ms. Olympia competitions.

Olympic Barbell. A special type of barbell used in weightlifting and powerlifting competitions, but also used by bodybuilders in heavy basic exercises such as squats, bench presses, barbell bent rows, standing barbell curls, standing barbell presses, and deadlifts. An Olympic barbell sans collars weighs 45 pounds, and each collar weighs five pounds.

Olympic Lifting. The type of weightlifting competition contested at the Olympic Games every four years, as well as at national and international competitions each year. Two lifts (the snatch and the clean and jerk) are contested in a wide variety of weight classes.

Overload. The amount of weight that you force a muscle to use that is over and above its normal strength ability. Applying an overload to a muscle forces it to increase in hypertrophy.

Peak. The absolute zenith of competitive condition achieved by a bodybuilder. To peak out optimally for a bodybuilding show, you must intelligently combine bodybuilding training, aerobic workouts, diet, mental conditioning, tanning, and a large number of other preparatory factors.

PHA. The abbreviation for "peripheral heart action," a system of circuit training in which short 4–6-exercise circuits are performed in order to stimulate cardiorespiratory conditioning and further physical development.

Plates. The flat discs placed on the ends of barbell and dumbbell bars to increase the weight of the apparati. Although some plates are made from vinyl-covered concrete, the best and most durable plates are manufactured from metal.

Pose. Each individual stance that a bodybuilder does onstage in order to highlight his muscular development.

Poundage. The amount of weight that you use in an exercise, whether that weight is on a barbell, dumbbell, or exercise machine.

Power Lifting. A second form of competitive weightlifting (not contested in the Olympics, however) featuring three lifts: the squat, bench press, and deadlift. Power lifting is contested both nationally and internationally in a wide variety of weight classes for both men and women.

Progression. The act of gradually adding to the amount of resistance that you use in each exercise. Without consistent progression in your workouts, you won't overload your muscles sufficiently to promote optimum increases in hypertrophy.

Pump. The tight, blood-congested feeling in a muscle after it has been intensely trained. Muscle pump is caused by a rapid influx of blood into the muscles to remove fatigue toxins and replace supplies of fuel and oxygen. A good muscle pump indicates that you have optimally worked a muscle group.

Quality Training. A type of workout used just prior to a competition in which the lengths of rest intervals between sets are progressively reduced to increase overall training intensity and help further define the physique.

Repetition (or Rep). Each individual count of an exercise that is performed. Series of repetitions called "sets" are performed on each exercise in your training program.

Resistance. The actual amount of weight that you are using in any exercise.

Rest Interval. The brief pause lasting 30–90 seconds between sets that allows your body to partially recuperate prior to initiating the succeeding set.

Ripped. The same as *cut up*.

Routine. Also called a training schedule or program, a routine is the total list of exercises, sets, and reps (and sometimes weights) used in one training session.

Set. A grouping of repetitions (usually in the range of 6–15) that is followed by a rest interval and usually another set. Three to five sets are usually performed of each exercise.

Sleeve. The hollow metal tube fit over the bar on most exercise barbell and dumbbell sets. This sleeve makes it easier for the bar to rotate in your hands as you do an exercise.

Spotters. Training partners who stand by to act as safety helpers when you perform such heavy exercises as squats and bench presses. If you get stuck under the weight or begin to lose control of it, spotters can rescue you and prevent needless injuries.

Steroids. Prescription drugs which mimic male hormones, but without most of the androgenic side effects of actual testosterone. Many bodybuilders use these dangerous drugs to help increase muscle mass and strength.

Sticking Point. A stalling out of bodybuilding progress.

Stretching. A type of exercise program in which you assume exaggerated postures that stretch muscles, joints, and connective tissues, hold these positions for several seconds, relax and then repeat the postures. Regular stretching exercise promotes body flexibility.

Stretch Marks. Tiny tears in a bodybuilder's skin caused by poor diet and too rapid increases in bodyweight. If you notice stretch marks forming on your own body (usually around your pectoral–deltoid tie-ins), rub vitamin E cream over them two or three times per day, and try cutting back on your body weight by reducing body fat levels.

Striations. The tiny grooves of muscle across major muscle groups in a highly defined bodybuilder.

Supersets. Series of two exercises performed with no rest between sets and a normal rest interval between supersets. Supersets increase training intensity by reducing the average length of rest interval between sets.

Supplements. Concentrated vitamins, minerals, and proteins used by bodybuilders to improve the overall quality of their diets. Many bodybuilders believe that food supplements help to promote quality muscle growth.

Symmetry. The shape or general outline of a person's body, as when seen in silhouette. If you have good symmetry, you will have relatively wide shoulders, flaring lats, a small waist–hip structure, and generally small joints.

Testosterone. The male hormone primarily responsible for the maintenance of muscle mass and strength induced by heavy training. Testosterone is secondarily responsible for developing such secondary male sex characteristics as a deep voice, body hair, and male pattern baldness.

Trisets. Series of three exercises performed with no rest between movements and a normal rest interval between trisets. Trisets increase training intensity by reducing the average length of rest interval between sets.

Vascularity. A prominence of veins and arteries over the muscles and beneath the skin of a well-defined bodybuilder.

Warm-up. The 10–15-minute session of light calisthenics, aerobic exercise, and stretching taken prior to handling heavy bodybuilding training movements. A good warm-up helps to prevent injuries and actually allows you to get more out of your training than if you went into a workout totally cold.

Weight. The same as *Poundage* or *Resistance*.

Weight Class. In order for bodybuilders to compete against men of similar size, the IFBB has instituted weight classes for all amateur competition. The normal men's weight classes are 70 kilograms (kg), 154 pounds (lbs); 80 kg, 176 lbs; 90 kg, 198 lbs; and over 90 kg. In a minority of competitions, particularly in the Far East, one additional class 65 kg, or 143 lbs is also contested.

Weightlifting. The competitive form of weight training in which each athlete attempts to lift as much as he can in well-defined exercises. Olympic lifting and power lifting are the two types of weightlifting competition.

Weight Training. An umbrella term used to categorize all acts of using resistance training. Weight training can be used to improve the body, rehabilitate injuries, improve sports conditioning, or as a competitive activity in terms of bodybuilding and weightlifting.

Workout. A bodybuilding or weight-training session.

Index